INTERNAL MEDICINE
Essentials
for
Students

A Companion to
MKSAP® for Students 5

Patrick C. Alguire, MD, FACP

SENIOR VICE PRESIDENT
MEDICAL EDUCATION
AMERICAN COLLEGE OF PHYSICIANS
EDITOR-IN-CHIEF

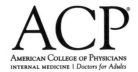

AMERICAN COLLEGE OF PHYSICIANS
INTERNAL MEDICINE | *Doctors for Adults*

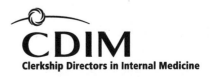

CDIM
Clerkship Directors in Internal Medicine

Editorial Production: Helen Kitzmiller
Design: Michael E. Ripca
Composition: ACP Graphic Services

Printed in the United States of America by RR Donnelley

ISBN: 978-1-934465-43-1

The authors and publisher have exerted every effort to ensure that the drug selection and dosages set forth in this book are in accordance with current recommendations and practice at the time of publication. In view of ongoing research, occasional changes in government regulations, and the constant flow of information relating to drug therapy and drug reactions, however, the reader is urged to check the package insert for each drug for any change in indications and dosage and for added warnings and precautions. This care is particularly important when the recommended agent is a new or infrequently used drug.

11 12 13 14 15 16 / 10 9 8 7 6 5 4 3 2 1

Section Editors

Thomas M. DeFer, MD, FACP
Clerkship Director
Division of Medical Education
Department of Internal Medicine
Washington University School of Medicine
St Louis, Missouri

Mark J. Fagan, MD, FACP
Clerkship Director
Department of Medicine
Alpert Medical School of Brown University
Providence, Rhode Island

Sara B. Fazio, MD, FACP
Associate Professor, Harvard Medical School
Director, Core I Medicine Clerkship
Division of General Internal Medicine
Beth Israel Deaconess Medical Center
Boston, Massachusetts

Robert L. Trowbridge, MD, FACP
Assistant Professor of Medicine
Tufts University School of Medicine
Director of Undergraduate Medical Education
Department of Medicine
Maine Medical Center
Portland, Maine

T. Robert Vu, MD, FACP
Associate Professor of Clinical Medicine
Director, Internal Medicine Clerkship
Indiana University School of Medicine
Indianapolis, Indiana

Contributors

Arlina Ahluwalia, MD, FACP
Associate Professor of Medicine
Medicine Clerkship Site Director, Palo Alto VAHCS
Stanford University School of Medicine
Palo Alto, California

Erik K. Alexander, MD, FACP
Director, Medical Student Education
Brigham and Women's Hospital
Associate Professor of Medicine
Harvard Medical School
Boston, Massachusetts

Irene Alexandraki, MD, MPH, FACP
Assistant Professor, Department of Medicine
Medicine Clerkship Director
University of Florida College of Medicine
Jacksonville, Florida

Eyad Al-Hihi, MD, MBA, FACP
Associate Professor of Medicine
Section Chief, Division of General Internal Medicine
Clerkship Director, Medicine Continuing Care Clinic
University of Missouri-Kansas City School of Medicine
Medical Director, Medicine Primary Care Clinics
Truman Medical Center-Hospital Hill
Kansas City, Missouri

Mark Allee, MD, FACP
Associate Professor of Medicine
Clerkship Director
Department of Internal Medicine
University of Oklahoma College of Medicine
Oklahoma City, Oklahoma

Alpesh N. Amin, MD, MBA, FACP
Professor of Medicine
Medicine Clerkship Director
University of California, Irvine
Orange, California

Joel Appel, DO
Director, Ambulatory and Subinternship Programs
Wayne State University School of Medicine
Detroit, Michigan

Jonathan S. Appelbaum, MD, FACP
Associate Professor, Clinical Sciences Department
Director, Internal Medicine Education
Florida State University College of Medicine
Tallahassee, Florida

Mary Jane Barchman, MD, FACP, FASN
Professor of Medicine
Internal Medicine Clerkship Director
Section of Nephrology and Hypertension
Brody School of Medicine at East Carolina University
Greenville, North Carolina

Gonzalo Bearman, MD, MPH
Associate Professor of Medicine
Associate Hospital Epidemiologist
Medicine Clerkship Director
Virginia Commonwealth University
Richmond, Virginia

Seth Mark Berney, MD, FACP
Professor of Medicine
Chief, Section of Rheumatology
Director, Center of Excellence for Arthritis and
  Rheumatology
Louisiana State University Health Sciences Center
  School of Medicine in Shreveport
Shreveport, Louisiana

Jennifer Bierman, MD, FACP
Primary Care Clerkship Director
Northwestern University Feinberg School of Medicine
Chicago, Illinois

Cynthia A. Burns, MD, FACP
Assistant Professor
Internal Medicine Clerkship Director
Department of Internal Medicine
Section on Endocrinology & Metabolism
Wake Forest University School of Medicine
Winston Salem, North Carolina

Danelle Cayea, MD, MS
Assistant Professor of Medicine
Medicine Clerkship Director
Johns Hopkins University School of Medicine
Baltimore, Maryland

Joseph Charles, MD, FACP, FHM
Assistant Professor of Medicine
Division Education Coordinator
Mayo Clinic Hospital
Phoenix, Arizona

Amanda Cooper, MD
Assistant Professor of Medicine
University of Pittsburgh Medical Center
University of Pittsburgh School of Medicine
Pittsburgh, Pennsylvania

Mark D. Corriere, MD, FACP
Associate Clerkship Director, Department of Medicine
Uniformed Services University of the Health Sciences
Bethesda, Maryland

Thomas M. DeFer, MD, FACP
Clerkship Director
Division of Medical Education
Department of Internal Medicine
Washington University School of Medicine
Saint Louis, Missouri

Gretchen Diemer, MD, FACP
Assistant Professor of Internal Medicine
Clerkship Director Internal Medicine
Director of Undergraduate Medical Education
Associate Program Director Internal Medicine
Thomas Jefferson University
Philadelphia, Pennsylvania

Reed E. Drews, MD, FACP
Associate Professor
Harvard Medical School
Program Director, Hematology-Oncology Fellowship
Beth Israel Deaconess Medical Center
Boston, Massachusetts

Anne Eacker, MD, FACP
Associate Professor, Department of Medicine
Medical Director, General Internal Medicine Center
University of Washington
Seattle, Washington

Richard S. Eisenstaedt, MD, FACP
Chair, Department of Medicine
Abington Memorial Hospital
Clinical Professor of Medicine
Temple University School of Medicine
Philadelphia, Pennsylvania

D. Michael Elnicki, MD, FACP
Professor and Chief, Section of General Internal
  Medicine
UPMC Shadyside
Ambulatory Clerkship Director
University of Pittsburgh
Pittsburgh, Pennsylvania

Mark J. Fagan, MD, FACP
Clerkship Director
Department of Medicine
Alpert Medical School of Brown University
Providence, Rhode Island

Sara B. Fazio, MD, FACP
Associate Professor, Harvard Medical School
Director, Core I Medicine Clerkship
Division of General Internal Medicine
Beth Israel Deaconess Medical Center
Boston, Massachusetts

J. Michael Finley, DO, FACP, FACOI
Associate Professor of Medicine
Chief, Division of Rheumatology
Associate Dean for Graduate Medical Education
Western University College of Osteopathic Medicine
Pomona, California

Jane P. Gagliardi, MD, MHS
Assistant Professor of Psychiatry & Behavioral Sciences
Assistant Professor of Medicine
Director of UME, Department of Medicine
Medicine Clerkship and Subinternship Director
Duke University School of Medicine
Durham, North Carolina

Peter Gliatto, MD, FACP
Associate Dean for Undergraduate Medical Education
  and Student Affairs
Mount Sinai School of Medicine
New York, New York

Eric H. Green, MD, MSc, FACP
Clinical Associate Professor of Medicine
Drexel University College of Medicine
Associate Program Director
Mercy Catholic Medical Center
Darby, Pennsylvania

Heather Harrell, MD, FACP
Associate Professor, Department of Medicine
Medicine Clerkship Director
Director of Fourth Year Programs
University of Florida College of Medicine
Gainesville, Florida

Warren Y. Hershman, MD, MPH
Director of Student Education
Boston University School of Medicine
Department of Medicine
Boston, Massachusetts

Susan T. Hingle, MD, FACP
Associate Professor of Medicine
Internal Medicine Clerkship Director
Internal Medicine Residency Associate Program
  Director
Southern Illinois University School of Medicine
Springfield, Illinois

Bryan Ho, MD
Assistant Professor, Department of Neurology
Neurology Clerkship Director
Tufts University School of Medicine
Boston, Massachusetts

Mark D. Holden, MD, FACP
Vice-Chair for Undergraduate Education
Department of Internal Medicine
University of Texas Medical Branch
Galveston, Texas

Eric Hsieh, MD
Director, Internal Medicine Clerkship
Sr. Associate Director, Internal Medicine Residency
Department of Medicine
Keck School of Medicine
University of Southern California
Los Angeles, California

Robert Jablonover, MD
Assistant Professor in Internal Medicine
Clerkship Director in Internal Medicine
George Washington University School of Medicine
Washington, District of Columbia

Asra R. Khan, MD, FACP
Assistant Professor of Clinical Medicine
Associate Program Director, Medicine
Medicine Clerkship Director
University of Illinois College of Medicine
Chicago, Illinois

Saba Khan, MD
Fellow, Section of Rheumatology
Louisiana State University Health Sciences Center
School of Medicine in Shreveport
Shreveport, Louisiana

Sarang Kim, MD, FACP
Assistant Professor of Medicine
Division of General Internal Medicine
University of Medicine and Dentistry of New Jersey,
  Robert Wood Johnson Medical School
New Brunswick, New Jersey

Karen E. Kirkham, MD
Associate Professor of Medicine
Vice-Chair for Undergraduate Medical Education
Department of Internal Medicine
Wright State Boonshoft School of Medicine
Dayton, Ohio

Christopher A. Klipstein, MD
Associate Professor of Medicine
Director, Internal Medicine Clerkship
University of North Carolina School of Medicine
Chapel Hill, North Carolina

Valerie J. Lang, MD, FACP
Director, Inpatient Medicine Clerkship
Hospital Medicine Division
University of Rochester School of Medicine
  and Dentistry
Rochester, New York

Rosa Lee, MD
Clinical Assistant Professor, Department of Medicine
Albert Einstein College of Medicine
Site Leader, Medicine Clerkship
Montefiore Medical Center
Bronx, New York

Bruce Leff, MD, FACP
Professor of Medicine
Co-Director, Basic Medicine Clerkship
Johns Hopkins University School of Medicine
Baltimore, Maryland

Kyle Lokitz, MD
Fellow, Section of Rheumatology
Louisiana State University Health Sciences Center
School of Medicine in Shreveport
Shreveport, Louisiana

Fred A. Lopez, MD, FACP
Richard Vial Professor and Vice Chair
Department of Medicine
Louisiana State University Health Sciences Center
New Orleans, Louisiana

Kevin M. McKown, MD, FACP
Associate Professor and Head, Division of
  Rheumatology
Co-Director M3 and M4 Student Programs
Department of Medicine
School of Medicine and Public Health
University of Wisconsin
Madison, Wisconsin

Chad S. Miller, MD, FACP
Director, Student Programs
Associate Program Director, Residency
Department of Internal Medicine
Tulane University Health Sciences Center
New Orleans, Louisiana

Katherine Nickerson, MD
Professor of Clinical Medicine
Vice Chair, Department of Medicine
Clerkship Director, Internal Medicine
College of Physicians & Surgeons
Columbia University
New York, New York

L. James Nixon, MD
Vice Chair for Education, Department of Medicine
Medicine Clerkship Director
University of Minnesota Medical School
Minneapolis, Minnesota

Isaac O. Opole, MD, PhD, FACP
Assistant Dean for Student Affairs
Internal Medicine Clerkship Director
Kansas University Medical Center
Kansas City, Kansas

Carlos Palacio, MD, MPH, FACP
Associate Professor of Medicine, Department of
  Medicine
Clerkship Director
University of Florida College of Medicine-Jacksonville
Jacksonville, Florida

Alyssa C. Perroy, MD
Assistant Clerkship Director, Department of Medicine
Uniformed Services University of the Health Sciences
Bethesda, Maryland

Suma Pokala, MD, FACP
Associate Professor, Department of Medicine
Texas A&M Health Sciences Center
Central Texas Veterans Health Care System
Temple, Texas

Nora L. Porter, MD, MPH, FACP
Co-director, Internal Medicine Clerkship
Saint Louis University School of Medicine
Saint Louis, Missouri

Shalini Reddy, MD
Associate Dean
Student Programs and Professional Development
The University of Chicago Pritzker School of Medicine
Chicago, Illinois

Joseph Rencic, MD, FACP
Associate Professor of Medicine
Medicine Site Clerkship Director
Medicine Associate Program Director
Tufts University School of Medicine
Boston, Massachusetts

Klara J. Rosenquist, MD
Clinical/Research Fellow
Division of Endocrinology, Diabetes and
  Hypertension
Brigham & Women's Hospital
Harvard Medical School
Boston, Massachusetts

Kathleen F. Ryan, MD, FACP
Associate Professor of Medicine
Department of Medicine
Drexel University College of Medicine
Philadelphia, Pennsylvania

Mysti D.W. Schott, MD, FACP
Associate Professor of Medicine
Course Director, Advanced Clinical Evaluation Skills
Department of Medicine, Division of General
  Medicine and Office of Educational Programs
University of Texas Health Science Center San
  Antonio
San Antonio, Texas

Amy Wiegner Shaheen, MD
Ambulatory Medicine Clerkship Director
University of North Carolina School of Medicine
Chapel Hill, North Carolina

Monica Ann Shaw, MD, FACP
Associate Professor and Chief
Division of General Internal Medicine, Palliative
  Medicine and Medical Education
Medicine Clerkship Director
University of Louisville
Louisville, Kentucky

Patricia Short, MD, FACP
Assistant Professor of Medicine
Associate Clerkship Director
Uniformed Services University of the Health Sciences
Madigan Army Medical Center
Tacoma, Washington

Karen Szauter, MD, FACP
Professor, Department of Internal Medicine and
  Office of Educational Development
Co-Director, Internal Medicine Clerkship
University of Texas Medical Branch
Galveston, Texas

Harold M. Szerlip, MD, FACP, FCCP, FASN
Professor and Vice-Chair, Department of Medicine
Chief, Medical Service, UPH Hospital
University of Arizona College of Medicine
Tucson, Arizona

Gary Tabas, MD, FACP
Associate Professor of Medicine
University of Pittsburgh School of Medicine
Pittsburgh, Pennsylvania

David C. Tompkins, MD
Vice Chairman, Department of Medicine
Head, Division of Infectious Diseases
Lutheran Medical Center
Brooklyn, New York

Dario M. Torre, MD, MPH, PhD, FACP
Associate Professor of Medicine
Associate Program Director Internal Medicine
  University of Pittsburgh-Shadyside
University of Pittsburgh School of Medicine
Pittsburgh, Pennsylvania

Robert L. Trowbridge, MD, FACP
Assistant Professor of Medicine
Tufts University School of Medicine
Director of Undergraduate Medical Education
Department of Medicine
Maine Medical Center
Portland, Maine

John Varras, MD
Associate Professor
Interim Chair
Clerkship Director
Department of Internal Medicine
University of Nevada School of Medicine
Las Vegas, Nevada

H. Douglas Walden, MD, MPH, FACP
Professor of Medicine
Co-Director, Internal Medicine Clerkship
Saint Louis University School of Medicine
Saint Louis, Missouri

John A. Walker, MD, FACP
Professor and Vice-Chair for Education
Department of Medicine
Medicine Clerkship Director
University of Medicine and Dentistry of New Jersey
Robert Wood Johnson Medical School
New Brunswick, New Jersey

Joseph T. Wayne, MD, MPH, FACP
Internal Medicine Clerkship Director
Department of Internal Medicine
Albany Medical College
Albany, New York

John Jason White, MD, FASN
Associate Professor of Medicine
Section of Nephrology, Hypertension and
  Transplantation
Georgia Health Sciences University
Augusta, Georgia

Jenny Wright, MD
Acting Instructor, Department of Medicine
Associate Director, Medicine Core Clerkship
University of Washington School of Medicine
Seattle, Washington

Contents

IV General Internal Medicine

V Hematology

VI Infectious Disease Medicine

VII Nephrology

VIII Neurology

IX Oncology

X Pulmonary Medicine

XI Rheumatology

Foreword

Internal Medicine Essentials for Students is a collaborative project of the American College of Physicians (ACP) and the Clerkship Directors in Internal Medicine (CDIM), the organization of individuals responsible for teaching internal medicine to medical students. The purpose of Internal Medicine Essentials is to provide medical students with an authoritative educational resource that can be used to augment learning during the third-year internal medicine clerkship. Much of the content is based upon two evidence-based resources of the ACP: the Medical Knowledge Self-Assessment Program (MKSAP) and the Physician Information and Education Resource (PIER); in most instances, content was taken directly from these authoritative sources and edited to meet the learning needs of students on the medicine clerkship. Other sources include recently published practice guidelines and review articles. IM Essentials is updated every 3 years with the best available evidence and is designed to be read cover-to-cover during the clerkship.

Like preceding editions, Internal Medicine Essentials contains multiple color plates, electrocardiograms, radiographs, tables, and algorithms designed to enhance learning (and pass tests!). The Book Enhancement section cited at the end of each chapter has been enhanced to contain hundreds of web-based links to additional content. Importantly, the Book Enhancement section identifies specific chapter-related self-assessment questions published in the companion book, MKSAP for Students 5.

MKSAP for Students 5 consists of a collection of patient-centered self-assessment questions and answers. The questions begin with a clinical vignette, just as in the medicine clerkship examination and the USMLE Step 2 licensing examination. The questions are organized into 11 sections that match the 11 sections found in Internal Medicine Essentials. The authors and editors of Internal Medicine Essentials have made every effort to ensure that relevant content is included in the textbook to answer every question in MKSAP for Students 5. Each of the more than 450 questions has been specifically edited by a group of clerkship directors to meet the learning needs of students participating in the medicine clerkship. Each question comes with an answer critique that supplies the correct answer, an explanation of why that answer is correct and the incorrect options are not, and a short bibliography. We recommend that students first read the appropriate chapter in Internal Medicine Essentials, and then assess their understanding by answering the designated questions in MKSAP for Students 5.

The content of Internal Medicine Essentials is based upon The Core Medicine Clerkship Curriculum Guide (available at www.im.org/CDIM), a nationally recognized curriculum for the required third-year internal medicine clerkship, created and published by the CDIM and the Society for General Internal Medicine. A collaboration of 77 authors, all of whom are either internal medicine clerkship directors or clerkship faculty, representing 45 different medical schools, Internal Medicine Essentials is unique in that it is created by faculty who helped design the internal medicine curriculum and who are actively involved in teaching and advising students on the internal medicine clerkship.

*   *   *   *   *

Founded in 1915, the American College of Physicians is the nation's largest medical specialty society. Its mission is to enhance the quality and effectiveness of health care by fostering excellence and professionalism in the practice of medicine. Its 130,000 members include allied health professionals, medical students, medical residents, and practicing physicians. Physician members practice general internal medicine and related subspecialties, including cardiology, gastroenterology, nephrology, endocrinology, hematology, rheumatology, neurology, pulmonary disease, oncology, infectious diseases, allergy and immunology, and geriatrics.

The Clerkship Directors in Internal Medicine is the national organization of individuals responsible for teaching internal medicine to medical students. Founded in 1989, CDIM promotes excellence in the education of medical students in internal medicine. CDIM serves internal medicine faculty and staff by providing a forum to share ideas, generate solutions to common problems, and create opportunities for career development; participating in the development and dissemination of innovations for curriculum, evaluation, and faculty development; encouraging research and collaborative initiatives among medical educators; and advocating for issues concerning undergraduate medical education.

*   *   *   *   *

Internal Medicine Essentials for Students would have been impossible without the valuable and entirely voluntary contributions of many people, some of whom are named in the Acknowledgments section. Others, not specifically named, were representatives of a wide spectrum of constituencies and organizations such as the Clerkship Directors in Internal Medicine and various committees within the American College of Physicians, including the Education and Publication Committee and the Council of Student Members.

Patrick C. Alguire, MD, FACP
Editor-in-Chief,
Internal Medicine Essentials for Students
Senior Vice President for Medical Education
American College of Physicians

Acknowledgments

The American College of Physicians and the Clerkship Directors in Internal Medicine gratefully acknowledge the special contributions to *Internal Medicine Essentials for Students, A Companion to MKSAP for Students 5*; Sheila Costa, Interim Director of Operations, Alliance for Academic Internal Medicine; Rosemarie Houton, Administrative Representative, American College of Physicians; Lisa Rockey, Education and Career Development Coordinator, American College of Physicians; and Scott Hurd, Senior Systems Analyst/Developer, American College of Physicians. We also thank the many others, too numerous to mention, who have contributed to this project. Without the dedicated efforts of them all, publication of this volume would not have been possible.

Chapter 1

Approach to Chest Pain

Dario M. Torre, MD

Chest pain is one of the most common complaints in internal medicine. The differential diagnosis of chest pain includes cardiac, pulmonary, gastrointestinal, musculoskeletal, and psychiatric causes (Table 1). In the outpatient setting, the most common cause is musculoskeletal chest pain, although up to 12% of patients may have chest pain secondary to myocardial ischemia. A prudent approach to patients with acute chest pain focuses the initial evaluation on six potentially lethal conditions (the "serious six"): acute coronary syndrome, pericarditis/pericardial tamponade, pulmonary embolism, pneumothorax, aortic dissection, and esophageal rupture.

Cardiac Causes

Acute coronary syndrome (ACS) is an important cause of acute chest pain. ACS refers to a spectrum of diseases, including unstable angina, non–ST-elevation myocardial infarction (NSTEMI), and ST-elevation myocardial infarction (STEMI), which are classified on the basis of electrocardiographic (ECG) changes and presence of cardiac biomarkers (see Chapter 3). Acute cardiac ischemia classically presents as substernal pressure, tightness, or heaviness, with radiation to the jaw, shoulders, back, or arms. The pain may be accompanied by dyspnea, diaphoresis, and nausea. Patients with diabetes mellitus, women, and the elderly may present with atypical symptoms, such as dyspnea without chest pain. The most powerful clinical features that increase the probability of myocardial infarction (MI) include chest pain that simultaneously radiates to both arms (positive likelihood ratio = 9.7), an S_3 (positive likelihood ratio = 3.2), and hypotension (positive likelihood ratio = 3.1). Features that make an ischemic cause less likely include a normal electrocardiogram (ECG) (negative likelihood ratio = 0.1-0.3), chest pain that is positional (negative likelihood ratio = 0.3), chest pain reproduced by palpation (negative likelihood ratio = 0.2-0.4), or chest pain that is sharp or stabbing (negative likelihood ratio = 0.3). Patients suspected of having ACS are hospitalized and evaluated with serial ECGs and cardiac biomarkers, chest radiography, and, at times, echocardiography. Echocardiography is most helpful in the evaluation of acute chest pain that is present at the time of the examination; detection of regional wall motion abnormalities suggests focal myocardial ischemia (Table 2). Low-risk patients without evidence of MI are evaluated with exercise or pharmacologic stress testing.

Coronary artery vasospasm (Prinzmetal angina) classically presents as rest pain, similar to ACS, and may be associated with ST-segment elevation on a resting ECG. Cocaine use can cause chest pain and ST-segment changes due to ischemia or secondary to vasospasm, without evidence of direct myocardial injury.

Pericarditis is characterized by sudden onset of sharp, stabbing, substernal chest pain with radiation along the trapezius ridge.

Table 1. Differential Diagnosis of Chest Pain

Disorder	Clinical Features/Notes
Acute coronary syndrome (see Chapter 3)	Chest pain, nausea, dyspnea. Associated with specific ECG and echocardiographic changes. Cardiac enzymes help establish diagnosis of MI.
Aortic dissection	Substernal chest pain with radiation to the back or mid-scapular region; often described as "tearing" or "ripping" pain. Chest radiograph may show a widened mediastinal silhouette, pleural effusion, or both.
Aortic stenosis (see Chapter 8)	Chest pain with exertion, heart failure, syncope. Typical systolic murmur at the base of the heart radiating to the neck.
Esophagitis (see Chapter 20)	Burning-type chest discomfort; usually precipitated by meals and not related to exertion; often worse lying down and improved with sitting.
Musculoskeletal pain	Typically more reproducible chest pain. Includes muscle strain, costochondritis, and fracture. Should be a diagnosis of exclusion.
Panic attack	May be indistinguishable from angina. Often diagnosed after a negative evaluation for ischemic heart disease. Often associated with palpitations, sweating, and anxiety.
Pericarditis	Substernal chest discomfort that can be sharp, dull, or pressure-like in nature, often relieved with sitting forward; usually pleuritic. ECG changes may include ST-segment elevation (usually diffuse) or more specifically (but less commonly) PR-segment depression.
Pneumothorax (see Chapter 81)	Sudden onset of pleuritic chest pain and dyspnea. Chest radiograph or CT scan confirms the diagnosis.
Pulmonary embolism (see Chapter 87)	Commonly presents as dyspnea; pleuritic chest pain is present in 45%-75% of patients. Look for risk factors (immobilization, recent surgery, stroke, cancer, previous VTE).

ECG = electrocardiographic; MI = myocardial infarction; VTE = venous thromboembolism.

Table 2. Laboratory and Other Tests for Chest Pain

Test	Notes
Electrocardiography	CAD: >50% of patients have normal resting ECGs. The presence of pathologic Q waves or ST-T–wave abnormalities consistent with ischemia increases the likelihood of CAD. Many but not all patients will have some abnormality on an ECG obtained during an episode of chest pain.
	Pericarditis: ST-segment elevations and other abnormalities are present in approximately 90% of patients.
	PE: Abnormalities are present in 70% of patients, most commonly, nonspecific ST-segment and T-wave changes. P pulmonale, right axis deviation, right bundle branch block, and right ventricular hypertrophy occur less frequently.
Arterial blood gas analysis	Distributions of arterial Po_2 and alveolar-arterial oxygen gradient are similar in patients with and without PE.
Chest radiography	Used to diagnose pneumothorax and pneumonia; widened mediastinum suggests aortic dissection.
Cardiac enzyme studies	CK, CK-MB, and cTnI are obtained as indicated by clinical history, with elevations signifying active myocardial ischemia or injury. cTnI may be elevated in PE.
Echocardiography	Improves diagnostic accuracy in patients with chest discomfort when diagnosis is uncertain. May help differentiate ACS from aortic dissection. Transthoracic or transesophageal echocardiography may rarely identify central pulmonary artery emboli or intracardiac thrombi. Echocardiography can detect very small pericardial effusions that may help with the diagnosis of pericarditis.
Exercise ECG	For patients considered at low risk for ACS (i.e., atypical chest pain, normal cardiac markers, normal ECG), can be used as an early, rapid diagnostic tool for CAD.
D-Dimer (ELISA)	Helpful to exclude PE in patients with low pretest probability or nondiagnostic lung scan.
Contrast-enhanced spiral CT	Often preferred test for PE. An advantage of CT is the diagnosis of other pulmonary parenchymal, pleural, or cardiovascular processes causing or contributing to symptoms (dissection, aneurysms, malignancy).

ACS = acute coronary syndrome; CAD = coronary artery disease; CK = creatine kinase; CK-MB = MB isoenzyme of creatine kinase; cTnI = cardiac troponin I; ECG = electrocardiogram; ELISA = enzyme-linked immunosorbent assay; PE = pulmonary embolism.

Often, the pain is worse with inspiration and lying flat and is alleviated with sitting and leaning forward. A pericardial friction rub is present in 85% to 100% of cases at some time during the course of pericarditis. The classic rub consists of three components: occuring during atrial systole, ventricular systole, and ventricular diastole. A confirmatory ECG will show diffuse ST-segment elevation and PR-segment depression, findings that are specific but not sensitive (Figure 1). An echocardiogram may be helpful if there is suspicion of significant pericardial effusion or pericardial tamponade. Acute pericarditis secondary to infection (viral or bacterial) may be preceded or accompanied by symptoms of an upper respiratory tract infection and fever. Acute pericarditis may also occur within 1 or 2 days of an acute MI. Post–myocardial infarction syndrome, or Dressler syndrome, develops several weeks to months after an MI and accounts for fewer cases of pericarditis. In patients with acute pericarditis, hospitalization is prompted by an associated MI, pyogenic infection, or tamponade. Outpatient management is appropriate if other potentially serious causes of chest pain are excluded, hemodynamic status is normal, and a moderate or large pericardial effusion is excluded by echocardiography. In the absence of a specific cause for acute pericarditis, anti-inflammatory therapy is the mainstay of treatment.

Patients with dissection of the thoracic aorta typically present with abrupt onset of severe, sharp, or "tearing" chest pain often radiating to the abdomen, or with back pain. Aortic dissection can be associated with syncope due to decreased cardiac output; stroke, and MI caused by carotid or coronary artery occlusion/dissection; cardiac tamponade, and sudden death due to rupture of the aorta. Hypertension is present in 50% of patients and is not helpful diagnostically. A pulse differential (diminished pulse compared with the contralateral side) on palpation of the carotid, radial, or femoral arteries is one of the most useful findings but is uncommon (sensitivity of 30%; positive likelihood ratio = 5.7). An early diastolic murmur due to acute aortic insufficiency may be heard, particularly if the dissection involves the ascending aorta, but the presence or absence of a diastolic murmur is not useful in ruling in or ruling out dissection. Focal deficits on neurologic examination can be present in a few patients but are highly suggestive in the proper clinical context (positive likelihood ratio = 6.6 to 33.0).

In patients with dissection of the thoracic aorta, a wide mediastinum on a chest radiograph is the most common initial finding (sensitivity of 85%); the absence of this finding helps rule out dissection (negative likelihood ratio = 0.3). When aortic dissection is suspected, imaging the aorta is indicated. CT or MRI of the chest, transesophageal echocardiography, and aortic root angiography all have a high sensitivity and specificity for detection of a dissection flap; the specific diagnostic modality chosen depends on the rapidity with which the examination can be performed and the stability of the patient. Dissections involving the ascending aorta and aortic arch are surgical emergencies. Dissections distal to the subclavian artery usually are treated medically to reduce the blood pressure (intravenous β-blockers followed by sodium nitroprusside, fenoldopam, or enalaprilat).

Aortic stenosis is a cause of exertional chest pain and may also be accompanied by dyspnea, palpitations, and exertional syncope due to a diminished cardiac output. Physical examination reveals a systolic, crescendo-decrescendo murmur best heard at the second right intercostal space, with radiation to the right carotid artery. A transthoracic echocardiogram is the diagnostic test of choice for suspected aortic stenosis.

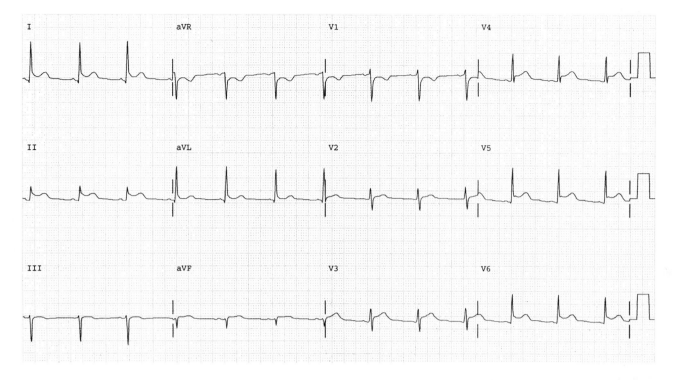

Figure 1. Electrocardiogram showing sinus rhythm with diffuse ST-segment elevation consistent with acute pericarditis. Note also the PR-segment depression in leads I, II, and V_4-V_6.

Syndrome X is a cause of angina-like chest pain in young women. It is characterized by anginal symptoms, ST-segment depression on exercise testing, and normal coronary arteries on angiography. The cause of the pain is unknown, but there is a strong correlation with psychiatric disorders.

Pulmonary Causes

Pulmonary embolism may present as acute pleuritic chest pain (45% to 75% of cases), dyspnea, and, less often, cough and hemoptysis. The presence of risk factors for pulmonary embolism (e.g., recent surgery, immobilization, previous venous thromboembolism, malignancy) may suggest the diagnosis. Physical examination findings are nonspecific but may include tachycardia, tachypnea, and wheezing. A right-sided S_3 and a right ventricular heave may be present if there is acute right heart failure secondary to pulmonary hypertension.

Pleuritic chest pain also can be a manifestation of pneumonia and is associated with fever, chills, cough, purulent sputum, and dyspnea. The physical examination may show wheezing or crackles and signs of consolidation, such as dullness to percussion, egophony, and bronchophony.

Pneumothorax should be considered in any patient with sudden onset of pleuritic chest pain and dyspnea. The physical examination may reveal decreased breath sounds on the affected side; if a tension pneumothorax is present, hypotension and tracheal deviation to the opposite side of the pneumothorax may be noted. Chest radiography shows a lack of lung markings on the affected side. In addition, in tension pneumothorax, there is a shift of the mediastinum away from the side of the pneumothorax, whereas hydropneumothorax is identified by the presence of concomitant pleural fluid.

Pulmonary causes of chest pain are initially evaluated with a chest radiograph. In patients with dyspnea, pulse oximetry or arterial blood gas analysis is indicated. If there is moderate to high suspicion for pulmonary embolism, a spiral CT scan of the chest or a ventilation-perfusion lung scan with or without duplex Doppler examination of lower extremities is an appropriate initial approach. A negative D-dimer test result helps exclude the diagnosis of pulmonary embolism and is most helpful when the clinical suspicion is low.

Gastrointestinal Causes

Gastroesophageal reflux disease (GERD) can mimic ischemic chest pain. Important distinctions include pain lasting minutes to hours and pain resolving spontaneously or with antacids. Chest discomfort associated with GERD often is positional, is worse when lying down and after meals, or awakens the patient from sleep. Other symptoms may include heartburn, regurgitation, chronic cough, sore throat, and hoarseness. On physical examination, patients may exhibit wheezing, halitosis, dental erosions, and pharyngeal erythema. In unclear cases, it is most appropriate to exclude cardiac causes of chest pain before evaluating gastrointestinal causes. For patients with a high probability of GERD, empiric treatment with a proton pump inhibitor for 4 to 6 weeks is an appropriate initial diagnostic and therapeutic approach.

Patients with spontaneous esophageal rupture typically have severe retching and vomiting followed by excruciating retrosternal chest and upper abdominal pain. These symptoms are followed by the rapid development of odynophagia, tachypnea, dyspnea, cyanosis, fever, and shock. Many cases are related to excessive alcohol ingestion.

Acute cholecystitis presents as right upper quadrant pain that may radiate to the right shoulder and is associated with nausea, vomiting, and fever. On physical examination, deep palpation during inspiration can elicit pain in the right upper quadrant and cause inspiratory arrest (Murphy sign).

Patients with acute pancreatitis usually have sudden onset of epigastric or, occasionally, lower anterior chest pain. The pain often radiates to the back and is accompanied by nausea, vomiting, fever, and tachycardia. The physical examination shows epigastric tenderness, abdominal distention, hypoactive bowel sounds, and occasional guarding.

Musculoskeletal Causes

Musculoskeletal causes of chest pain are more common in women than in men. Frequent causes include costochondritis, arthritis, and fibromyalgia. Musculoskeletal chest pain has an insidious onset and may last for hours to weeks. It is most recognizable when sharp and localized to a specific area of the chest; however, it also can be poorly localized. The pain may be worsened by turning, deep breathing, or arm movement. Chest pain may or may not be reproducible by chest palpation; pain reproduced by palpation does not exclude ischemic heart disease. The cardiovascular examination often is normal. The presence of tender points in the upper chest increases the likelihood of fibromyalgia. For musculoskeletal chest pain, the history and physical examination are keys to the diagnosis; selected radiographic studies and laboratory tests may be indicated depending on the clinical circumstances.

Psychiatric Causes

Chest pain can be a manifestation of severe anxiety and panic attacks. Patients may complain of sweating, trembling, or shaking; sensations of choking, shortness of breath, or smothering; nausea or abdominal distress; or feeling dizzy, unsteady, or lightheaded. On physical examination, tachycardia and tachypnea may be present, but the cardiovascular and pulmonary examinations are otherwise unremarkable. Generalized anxiety and panic attacks may be treated with cognitive behavioral therapy and selective serotonin reuptake inhibitors or venlafaxine. Panic disorder stands alone among the anxiety spectrum disorders as a condition for which there is evidence that the combination of cognitive behavioral therapy and pharmacotherapy is superior to either treatment modality alone. Psychosomatic chest pain is a clinical diagnosis; other causes of chest pain usually are excluded by a careful history and physical examination.

Book Enhancement

Go to www.acponline.org/essentials/cardiovascular-section.html. In *MKSAP for Students 5*, assess your knowledge with items 2, 4, 6, 8, and 11 in the **Cardiovascular Medicine** section.

Bibliography

Lee TH, Goldman L. Evaluation of the patient with acute chest pain. N Engl J Med. 2000;342:1187-1195. [PMID: 10770985]

Chapter 2

Chronic Stable Angina

John Varras, MD

Angina is a sensation of chest discomfort secondary to myocardial ischemia, which occurs with exertion and is relieved by rest. Chronic stable angina often occurs with a predictable amount of exertion and is relieved by a predictable amount of rest or nitroglycerin, but can vary based on several factors. Conditions that provoke angina do so by increasing myocardial oxygen demand, decreasing myocardial oxygen supply, or both. Myocardial oxygen demand is determined by heart rate, systolic blood pressure (afterload), myocardial contractility, and left ventricular wall stress, which is proportional to left ventricular end-diastolic volume (preload) and myocardial mass. Myocardial oxygen supply is dependent on coronary blood flow and perfusion pressure. The subendocardium, which is at greatest risk for ischemia, receives most of its blood supply during diastole; tachycardia, which shortens diastole, may cause ischemia. Some patients may not present with classic chest pain but may have other symptoms referred to as *anginal equivalents*. These symptoms can include dyspnea, weakness, syncope, and mental status changes. Dyspnea is the most frequent anginal equivalent and is difficult to differentiate from heart failure or pulmonary disease. The pathogenesis is an elevated left ventricular filling pressure induced by ischemia, which leads to vascular congestion. The most common cause of angina is coronary artery disease (CAD); inflammation plays an important role in the development of CAD. Angina also may be present in the absence of coronary artery obstruction; these patients may have coronary vasospasm, aortic stenosis, hypertrophic cardiomyopathy, or systemic arterial hypertension.

Prevention

Cardiovascular risk factors should be identified and modified. Risk reduction efforts are particularly important in patients at high risk for CAD. Smoking cessation should be encouraged in all patients who smoke. All adults aged ≥20 years should be assessed for dyslipidemia, and blood pressure should be checked at each office visit to identify and treat hypertension. In patients with diabetes mellitus, risk factors for CAD should be treated aggressively; strict blood pressure and lipid control appears to provide additional benefits to patients with diabetes above those seen in the general population. The Framingham risk score allows estimation of the 10-year risk of CAD using a patient's age, gender, and other risk factors (www.acponline.org/acp_press/essentials/calculator.htm).

Primary prevention with aspirin (75-325 mg/day) should be considered in asymptomatic patients with a moderate (10%-20%) 10-year absolute risk of a first CAD event, barring any contraindication or risk factors for bleeding. All patients should be encour-

aged to engage in regular physical activity, such as brisk walking for ≥30 minutes 5 to 7 times per week. Dietary advice to all patients should include limiting refined sugars, cholesterol, and fat, particularly saturated fats, and eating a diet rich in fruits, vegetables, and fiber and low in sodium. Consideration also should be given to daily intake of 250 to 500 mg of omega-3 fatty acids. Use of antioxidant vitamins or hormone replacement therapy in postmenopausal women is not recommended for CAD risk reduction. Although elevated homocysteine levels are associated with coronary events, reducing homocysteine levels has not been shown to improve outcomes. Cohort studies of healthy persons have shown that the concentration of C-reactive protein measured by high-sensitivity assay (hs-CRP) modestly correlates with future risk of CAD independent of conventional risk factors. The American Heart Association and Centers for Disease Control and Prevention do not recommend routine measurement of hs-CRP, but measurement may be useful in patients with a moderate (10%-20%) 10-year risk of a first CAD event. Measurement of hs-CRP has been found to reclassify up to 30% of moderate-risk patients to either low-risk or high-risk status.

Screening

Asymptomatic persons without cardiovascular risk factors should not undergo routine screening for CAD. Although exercise testing may identify persons with CAD, two factors limit the utility of routine stress testing in asymptomatic adults: false-positive results are common, and abnormalities of exercise testing do not accurately predict major cardiac events. CT-based coronary artery calcium scoring is an evolving technology. It may be reasonable to use calcium scoring in select patients with an estimated 10% to 20% 10-year risk of coronary events, based on the possibility that such patients might be reclassified to a higher risk status and offered more aggressive risk management interventions. It is unclear if calcium scoring adds to traditional risk-prediction tools.

Diagnosis

The pretest probability for CAD can be estimated (Table 1) based on the type of chest pain, patient age and gender, and presence of cardiac risk factors (i.e., smoking history, hyperlipidemia, diabetes, hypertension, physical inactivity, and family history). *Typical angina* consists of three components: (1) substernal chest pain or discomfort of a usual duration and quality, (2) provocation by exertion or stress and (3) relief by rest or nitroglycerin. *Atypical angina* has two of the three components, and noncardiac chest pain has

Table 1. Clinical Assessment of Pretest Probability of Coronary Artery Disease

	Pretest Probability					
	Noncardiac Chest Pain[a]		Atypical Chest Pain[b]		Typical Chest Pain[c]	
Age (y)	Men	Women	Men	Women	Men	Women
30-39	4	2	34	12	76	26
40-49	13	3	51	22	87	55
50-59	20	7	65	31	93	73
60-69	27	14	72	51	94	86

[a]Noncardiac chest pain has one or none of the components for typical chest pain.
[b]Atypical chest pain has two of the three components for typical chest pain.
[c]Typical chest pain has three components: (1) substernal chest pain or discomfort, (2) provocation by exertion or emotional stress, and (3) relief by rest and/or nitroglycerin.

Data from Diamond GA, Forrester JS. Analysis of probability as an aid in the clinical diagnosis of coronary-artery disease. N Engl J Med. 1979;300:1350-1358. [PMID: 440357]

one or none of the components. Physical examination findings suggesting peripheral vascular or cerebrovascular disease increase the likelihood of CAD. Patients should be assessed for conditions that increase myocardial oxygen demand (e.g., aortic stenosis, hypertrophic cardiomyopathy, uncontrolled hypertension, tachyarrhythmias, hyperthyroidism), conditions that diminish tissue oxygenation (e.g., anemia, hypoxemia), and conditions that cause hyperviscosity (e.g., polycythemia), all of which may precipitate angina in the setting of nonsignificant CAD. A complete blood count, thyroid-stimulating hormone level, or drug screen (e.g., cocaine) should be obtained as indicated by the clinical situation.

A resting electrocardiogram (ECG) is obtained in all patients without an obvious noncardiac cause of chest pain. Chest radiography is useful in all patients with signs or symptoms of heart failure, valvular heart disease, pericardial disease, aortic dissection, or aneurysm. Standard echocardiography is obtained in patients with possible valvular disease, signs or symptoms of heart failure, or a history of myocardial infarction (MI). In patients with stable angina, reduced left ventricular function is associated with a worse prognosis.

Various noninvasive stress tests can be performed in patients with angina. The choice of test is based on the patient's pretest

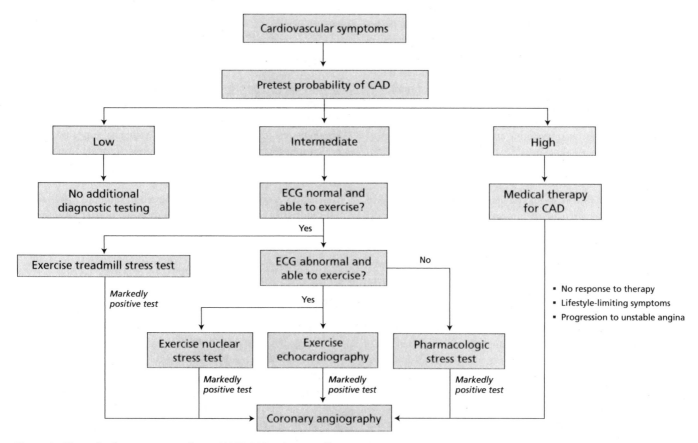

Figure 1 Diagnosis of coronary artery disease (CAD). ECG = electrocardiogram.

Table 2. Choice of Diagnostic Stress Test

Test	Notes
Exercise electrocardiography without imaging	Obtain in patients who have a moderate probability of CAD and are able to exercise, including patients with <1-mm ST-segment depression or complete right bundle branch block on resting ECG. Left ventricular hypertrophy with repolarization abnormality on resting ECG reduces the specificity of exercise treadmill testing.
Exercise electrocardiography with myocardial perfusion imaging or exercise echocardiography	Obtain in patients who have a moderate probability of CAD, are able to exercise, and have preexcitation (Wolff-Parkinson-White syndrome) or >1-mm ST-segment depression on resting ECG. Also appropriate in patients with a moderate probability of CAD and a history of previous revascularization (PTCA or CABG). Stress imaging is recommended to further stratify patients.
Pharmacologic stress myocardial perfusion imaging or dobutamine echocardiography	Obtain in patients with a moderate probability of CAD and an electronically paced ventricular rhythm or left bundle branch block. Also appropriate in patients with a moderate probability of CAD who are unable to exercise.

CABG = coronary artery bypass grafting; CAD = coronary artery disease; ECG = electrocardiogram; PTCA = percutaneous transluminal coronary angiography.

probability of CAD, ability to exercise, and baseline ECG (Table 2). Patients with a low probability of CAD do not require stress testing, and patients with a high probability of CAD should be started immediately on medical management, with consideration of coronary angiography if there is no response to therapy or severe disease is suspected. Noninvasive tests provide the most diagnostic information about patients with a moderate probability of CAD (Figure 1).

Patients who are able to exercise and do not have baseline resting ECG abnormalities are evaluated with exercise electrocardiography, which has a sensitivity of 65% to 70% and a specificity of 70% for diagnosing CAD; the sensitivity increases to 85% in patients with a normal baseline ECG. Myocardial perfusion imaging or stress echocardiography is preferred in settings in which exercise electrocardiography alone is difficult to interpret (e.g., abnormal baseline ECG); myocardial perfusion imaging and stress echocardiography have similar sensitivity (80%-85%) and specificity (77%-88%). Exercise stress testing is preferred whenever possible, because it provides additional prognostic information relating to the level of exercise attained. Pharmacologic stress tests are used in patients who cannot exercise. In general, patients with normal results on exercise electrocardiography, myocardial perfusion imaging, or stress echocardiography have a good prognosis. Patients with indeterminate results or suspicious clinical histories may require additional testing based on the clinical scenario. Those with markedly abnormal stress tests indicative of multivessel disease should be considered for cardiac catheterization and possible revascularization.

CT angiography can provide information about the coronary anatomy but does not assess ischemia. Although noninvasive, CT angiography requires intravenous contrast, exposes the patient to radiation, and is prone to discovering incidental findings (lung nodules). Initial trials show good sensitivity (85%-96%) and specificity (74%-90%). Current guidelines suggest CT angiography as an option in moderate-risk patients, but the overall role of this test is still evolving.

Coronary angiography should be considered in patients at high risk for CAD, patients with diagnostic difficulties or inconclusive results on noninvasive testing, patients with chronic angina that is increasing in severity, patients with markedly abnormal stress tests (suspicious for two- or three-vessel disease), and

patients with an episode of sudden cardiac death or ventricular tachycardia. Coronary angiography is the gold standard test for diagnosing CAD and is useful for assessing options for revascularization. Risks associated with angiography include use of contrast, cholesterol emboli, and bleeding.

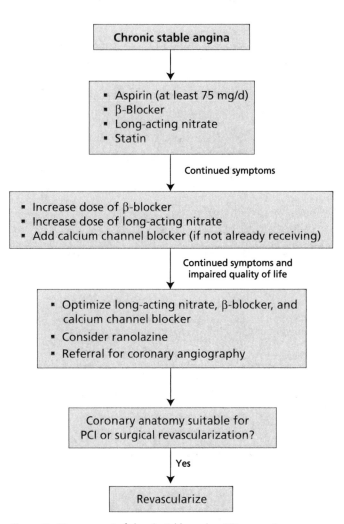

Figure 2. Management of chronic stable angina. PCI = percutaneous coronary intervention.

In the evaluation of patients with chest pain, always consider potentially life-threatening causes of chest pain, such as myocardial ischemia, pericardial tamponade, aortic dissection, pulmonary embolism, and pneumothorax (see Chapter 1). Although chest pain may have a benign cause, the initial diagnostic efforts should exclude a life-threatening cause.

Therapy

Risk factor modification is vital to the treatment of patients with chronic stable angina. Patients who smoke should be advised to stop smoking. All patients should be encouraged to engage in at least 30 to 60 minutes of moderate physical activity 5 to 7 days a week and to maintain a normal body weight. In addition, all patients should be encouraged to eat a heart-healthy diet low in saturated fat and cholesterol and rich in plant stanols/sterols; the diet should also include 1000 mg/day of omega-3 fatty acids.

Medical therapy is the key to treating chronic stable angina. A recent trial showed that medical management was as effective as early intervention (revascularization). Drug therapy for chronic stable angina is directed at reducing the incidence of MI and death and relieving symptoms. Drug therapy can be divided in to antianginal medications (β-blockers, calcium channel blockers, nitrates) and vascular protective medications (antiplatelet agents, statins, ACE inhibitors) (Figure 2).

β-Blockers are first-line therapy in most patients with chronic stable angina; these medications reduce angina severity and frequency by reducing heart rate and myocardial contractility. β-Blockers have been shown to reduce mortality after MI and are used to treat heart failure. Absolute contraindications include severe reactive airway disease, severe bradycardia, and decompensated heart failure. β-Blockers often are well tolerated by patients with mild to moderate COPD, asthma, and diabetes.

Calcium channel blockers are indicated for patients who cannot tolerate β-blockers or whose symptoms are inadequately controlled with β-blockers. Calcium channel blockers produce vasodilation, increase coronary blood flow, and reduce myocardial contractility. Non-dihydropyridine agents (verapamil, diltiazem) have a greater effect on myocardial contractility and conduction and should be avoided in patients with heart failure or bradycardia. Dihydropyridine agents exert a relatively greater effect on vasodilatation and can be used together with β-blockers and in patients with heart failure. Short-acting calcium channel blockers are contraindicated because of their association with increased risk of MI and, possibly, mortality.

Long-acting nitrates can be used in combination with or instead of β-blockers or calcium channel blockers (if these agents are not tolerated). Nitrates alleviate symptoms of angina by causing dilation of epicardial coronary vessels and increasing capacitance of the venous system, resulting in diminished cardiac preload and myocardial oxygen demand. Patients are taken off nitrates at night to mitigate nitrate tolerance. Nitrates must be avoided in patients taking phosphodiesterase-5 inhibitors (sildenafil, vardenafil, tadalafil).

Ranolazine is available for patients with inadequate response to standard antianginal therapy. Ranolazine is a selective inhibitor of a late sodium channel. The medication reduces angina by about one episode per week and does not affect heart rate or blood pres-

Table 3. Drug Treatment of Chronic Stable Angina

Agent	Notes
β-Blockers	First-line agents. Reduce heart rate, myocardial contractility, and arterial pressure, resulting in decreased myocardial oxygen demand. Used in patients with a history of MI and in heart failure.
Dihydropyridine calcium channel	Second-line agents. Reduce blood pressure; do not affect heart rate and can be used with β-blockers. Avoid blockers (amlodipine, nifedipine) and short-acting nifedipine.
Non-dihydropyridine calcium channel blockers (verapamil, diltiazem)	Second-line agents. Reduce blood pressure; negative chronotropy and inotropy reduce myocardial oxygen demand. Avoid in patients with heart failure; use with caution in patients taking β-blockers (bradycardia).
ACE inhibitors	Reduce blood pressure and afterload by a reduction. Reduce ventricular remodeling and fibrosis after infarction. Improve long-term survival in patients with LVEF ≤40% and, possibly, in patients with high cardiovascular risk (e.g., diabetes mellitus, PVD). Improve short-term survival in subsets of patients with acute MI. Side effects include cough, hyperkalemia, kidney failure, and angioedema.
Long-acting nitrates	Second-line agents. Can be used with β-blockers and calcium channel blockers. Tachyphylaxis occurs with continued use; requires nitrate-free period (8-12 h/d). Side effects include headache. Avoid in patients taking PDE-5 inhibitors.
Short-acting nitrates	Dilate coronary arteries and reduce preload. Indicated for all patients with chronic stable angina for use on an as-needed basis.
Ranolazine	Indicated for patients not responding to standard therapy; used in combination with a nitrate, β-blocker, or calcium channel blocker. Avoid using with verapamil or diltiazem (prolongs QT interval).
Aspirin	Indicated for all patients with stable angina, barring contraindications; reduces major cardiovascular events by 33%.
Thienopyridine derivatives (clopidogrel, ticlopidine, prasugrel)	Aspirin alternatives, but significantly more expensive. Improve outcomes in patients with recent ACS or stent placement. In patients with stable CAD, thienopyridine derivatives do not clearly improve outcomes and are associated with an increased risk of bleeding.
Statins	In patients with mild to moderate elevations in total and LDL cholesterol and a history of MI, statins are associated with a 24% risk reduction for fatal and nonfatal MI.

ACS = acute coronary syndrome; CAD = coronary artery disease; LDL = low-density lipoprotein; LVEF = left ventricular ejection fraction; MI = myocardial infarction; PDE-5 = phosphodiesterase-5; PVD = peripheral vascular disease.

sure. Ranolazine interacts with diltiazem and verapamil, resulting in a prolonged QT interval.

Aspirin is prescribed unless there is a history of significant gastrointestinal bleeding or aspirin allergy. Aspirin reduces platelet aggregation and acute coronary events and decreases the risk of MI and death. It should be used in all patients with CAD, especially those who have had an MI.

Thienopyridine derivatives (clopidogrel, ticlopidine, prasugrel) should be used in patients who have contraindications to aspirin or who have other indications (recent stent placement, acute coronary syndrome). The data do not provide convincing support for the use of these agents in the setting of chronic stable angina, where the risk of bleeding may outweigh the benefits.

Statins should be used to reduce low-density lipoprotein (LDL) cholesterol to <100 mg/dL (2.6 mmol/L); LDL cholesterol reduction is associated with improved survival and reduced risk of major coronary events. An optional LDL goal of <70 mg/dL (1.8 mmol/L) is recommended for patients at high risk for CAD. High-risk patients include those with recent acute coronary syndrome, diabetes, or multiple poorly controlled risk factors. Consider the use of niacin or fibrates for patients with elevated triglycerides or low levels of high-density lipoprotein cholesterol.

Treatment with an ACE inhibitor reduces mortality most dramatically in patients with heart failure and reduced left ventricular function (ejection fraction <40%). Treatment also reduces mortality and cardiovascular events in high-risk patients with vascular disease, diabetes, and other risk factors as well as patients with stable CAD and preserved left ventricular function who are at higher risk. Table 3 summarizes drug treatment options for chronic stable angina.

Percutaneous coronary intervention (PCI; angioplasty and stent placement) has not been shown to reduce mortality or cardiovascular events in patients with stable CAD, but it has been shown to reduce angina and to improve quality of life. PCI is most appropriately used in patients who do not respond to medical therapy.

Coronary artery bypass grafting (CABG) is used to treat patients with extensive CAD. It has been shown to improve mortality in patients with left main coronary artery stenosis, three-vessel disease, and, possibly, two-vessel disease (if it includes the left anterior descending coronary artery). In patients with diabetes, CABG is associated with improved clinical outcomes (death, MI, stroke, revascularization) as compared with PCI.

Follow-Up

Regular follow-up visits should address angina symptoms, medication use, and modifiable risk factors; patients should be seen every 4 to 12 months, depending on their stability. Routine resting ECGs are not recommended if there have been no changes in symptoms, examination findings, or medications. A repeat stress test is indicated if there is a change in symptoms but should not be performed routinely.

Book Enhancement

Go to www.acponline.org/essentials/cardiovascular-section.html. In *MKSAP for Students 5*, assess your knowledge with items 10, 12, 14, 16, and 18 in the **Cardiovascular Medicine** section.

Acknowledgment

We would like to thank Dr. Anna C. Maio, who contributed to an earlier version of this chapter.

Bibliography

Snow V, Barry P, Fihn SD, et al; American College of Physicians; American College of Cardiology Chronic Stable Angina Panel. Primary care management of chronic stable angina and asymptomatic suspected or known coronary artery disease: a clinical practice guideline from the American College of Physicians [published erratum appears in Ann Intern Med. 2005;142:79]. Ann Intern Med. 2004;141:562-567. [PMID: 15466774]

Chapter 3

Acute Coronary Syndrome

Patrick C. Alguire, MD

The term *acute coronary syndrome* (ACS) refers to any component of the clinical syndromes caused by acute myocardial ischemia. ACS encompasses unstable angina, non–ST-elevation myocardial infarction (NSTEMI), and ST-elevation myocardial infarction (STEMI). STEMI has a clinical presentation consistent with acute myocardial infarction (MI) and electrocardiographic (ECG) evidence of ST-segment elevation. Unstable angina and NSTEMI are closely related and differ only in the severity of ischemia. NSTEMI is associated with elevated biomarkers of myocardial injury, whereas unstable angina is not; the principles of risk stratification and therapy are identical for both. It is important to distinguish between STEMI, unstable angina, and NSTEMI. Patients with STEMI benefit from immediate reperfusion therapy typically consisting of thrombolytic therapy or coronary angiography, angioplasty, and stenting (percutaneous coronary intervention [PCI]). Patients with NSTEMI or unstable angina require immediate medical therapy followed by risk stratification to determine the risk for death or nonfatal MI, which determines the need for PCI versus a more conservative approach with medical therapy alone.

The pathophysiology of ACS is characterized by atherosclerotic plaque rupture, formation of a platelet and fibrin thrombus, and local release of vasoactive substances. Unstable angina and NSTEMI are most commonly caused by a nonocclusive thrombus. The most common cause of STEMI is an occlusive thrombus. Rare causes of ACS include spontaneous vasospasm of an epicardial coronary artery (variant or Prinzmetal angina), coronary artery spasm due to cocaine use, and non–coronary artery conditions (e.g., hypoxemia, anemia, tachycardia, thyrotoxicosis).

Prevention and Screening

The principles of primary prevention and screening for ACS are discussed in Chapter 2, Chronic Stable Angina.

Diagnosis

The pain of ACS is usually retrosternal in location, may radiate to the shoulders or arms, and may be associated with nausea and vomiting (more common with an inferior MI), diaphoresis, or shortness of breath. A strong clinical predictor of ACS is character of the chest discomfort. Typical angina, characterized by substernal discomfort, exertional onset, and prompt relief with nitroglycerin or rest, is associated with a 94% probability of coronary artery disease in certain patients. The most common reason for failure to diagnose ACS is that the patient has either "noncardiac" or "atypical" symptoms of dyspnea, fatigue, nausea, abdominal discomfort, or syncope; thus, any of these symptoms, with or without chest discomfort, should always prompt consideration of ACS.

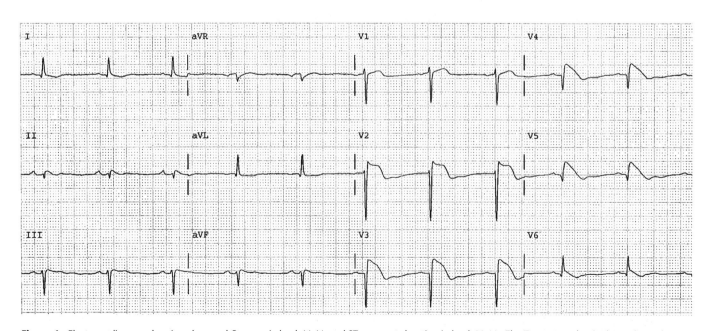

Figure 1. Electrocardiogram showing abnormal Q waves in leads V_3-V_5 and ST-segment elevation in leads V_2-V_5. The T waves are beginning to invert in leads V_3-V_6. This pattern is most consistent with a recent anterolateral myocardial infarction.

Table 1. Electrocardiographic (ECG) Localization of Acute Myocardial Infarction

Anatomic Location	ST-Segment Change	Indicative ECG Leads
Inferior	Elevation	II, III, aVF
Anteroseptal	Elevation	V_1-V_3
Lateral and apical	Elevation	V_4-V_6; possible elevations in I and aVL
Posterior wall[a]	Depression	Tall R waves in V_1-V_3
Right ventricle[a]	Elevation	V_4R; tall R waves in V_1-V_3

[a]Often associated with inferior and/or lateral ST-elevation infarctions.

Up to 25% of patients with ACS—particularly women, elderly persons, and patients with diabetes—present with atypical symptoms. Chest pain that is pleuritic, sharp, stabbing, or positional significantly decreases the likelihood of ACS.

The physical examination should focus on conditions that can mimic ACS (e.g., aortic dissection, pericarditis) and conditions that influence prognosis and treatment decisions (e.g., heart failure). Physical examination signs most predictive of ACS include hypotension (positive likelihood ratio = 3.1), S_3 (positive likelihood ratio = 3.2), and bibasilar crackles (positive likelihood ratio = 2.1). A new murmur may suggest valvular incompetence caused by papillary muscle dysfunction or rupture. Heart failure may be present if ischemia results in left ventricular diastolic or systolic dysfunction or valvular incompetence and is a high-risk feature for death. Normal findings do not exclude ACS.

The initial electrocardiogram (ECG) may be nondiagnostic in half of patients; therefore, serial ECGs are recommended (e.g., every 20 minutes for 2 hours). The diagnostic yield of the ECG is improved if a tracing can be recorded during an episode of chest discomfort. STEMI is characterized by ST-segment elevations >1 mm in two or more contiguous leads (Figure 1), new left bundle branch block, or evidence of true posterior infarction on electrocardiography (Table 1). NSTEMI is defined by elevated cardiac biomarkers and absence of ST-segment elevation. NSTEMI often is associated with ST-segment depression, but a persistently normal ECG decreases the probability of ACS.

With prolonged ischemia, cardiac myocytes lose membrane integrity and leak proteins (creatine kinase, myoglobin, cardiac troponin) into the serum; by serially measuring cardiac marker proteins at 0, 6 and 12 hours, evidence of myocardial damage within the previous 24 hours can be detected. In patients with acute ST-segment elevations, do not delay reperfusion therapy pending return of biomarker studies.

In patients with a nondiagnostic ECG and pending biomarkers, an echocardiogram may detect regional wall motion abnormalities suggesting ACS. In patients with ongoing chest pain, the sensitivity of echocardiography for regional wall motion abnormalities may approach 90%. A normal echocardiogram excludes extensive myocardial damage but does not rule out small infarctions. Echocardiography can identify nonischemic conditions that cause chest pain (e.g., myocarditis, aortic stenosis, aortic dissection, pulmonary embolism; see Chapter 1, Approach to Chest Pain), mechanical complications of acute infarction (e.g., papillary muscle dysfunction, rupture), and ventricular septal defect.

Coronary angiography provides detailed information about the coronary anatomy and facilitates invasive management of occluded coronary arteries. It is most often considered in the evaluation of patients with STEMI, new left bundle branch block, or true posterior infarction in whom immediate angioplasty is an option; in patients with unstable angina or NSTEMI and high-risk features (discussed later); and in patients with repeated episodes of ACS despite optimal therapy.

Right ventricular infarction should be considered in the setting of an inferior wall infarction complicated by hypotension. Right ventricular ischemia impairs the systolic function of the right ventricle, causing limited filling to the left ventricle, which results in the clinical triad of hypotension, clear lung fields, and jugular venous distention. Treatment of right ventricular infarction includes early revascularization to restore blood flow to the ischemic right ventricle, aggressive volume loading to increase filling to the left ventricle and cardiac output, and inotropic support with dopamine or dobutamine if hypotension persists after volume loading.

Mechanical complications occur between days 2 and 7. These complications include ventricular septal defect, papillary muscle rupture leading to acute mitral valve regurgitation, and left ventricular free wall rupture leading to cardiac tamponade. Ventricular septal defect and papillary muscle rupture usually lead to a new, loud systolic murmur and acute pulmonary edema or hypotension. Diagnosis is critical because the 24-hour survival rate is approximately 25% with medical therapy alone but increases to 50% with emergency surgical intervention. Pericardial tamponade from free wall rupture usually leads to sudden hypotension, pulseless electrical activity on electrocardiography, and death.

Therapy

Effective analgesia early in the course of ACS is an important therapeutic intervention. Morphine sulfate reduces sympathetic tone through a centrally mediated anxiolytic affect. Morphine also reduces myocardial oxygen demand by reducing preload and by a vagally mediated reduction in pulse rate.

Unless there are compelling contraindications, all patients presenting with presumed ACS should be treated with antiplatelet therapy, β-blockers, nitrates, and heparin. Thienopyridines (e.g., clopidogrel, prasugrel) block the adenosine diphosphate $P2Y_{12}$ receptor on platelets, preventing aggregation. A thienopyridine should be added to background aspirin therapy (162-325 mg/day) in all patients, unless there is an increased risk of bleeding. For patients requiring surgical revascularization, thienopyridines must be stopped 5 days prior to surgery to avoid excessive bleeding. Patients should chew the aspirin tablet in order to quickly achieve therapeutic blood levels.

β-Blockers should be given to all patients except those with decompensated heart failure, systolic blood pressure <90 mm Hg, pulse rate <50/min, or second-degree atrioventricular block. Oral β-blockers typically are used for patients with unstable angina or NSTEMI. Calcium channel blockers, with the exception of nifedipine, can be used in patients with contraindications to β-blockers and in those with continued angina despite optimal doses of β-blockers and nitrates. For STEMI patients, intravenous β-blockers are commonly given. β-Blockers should not be used in patients with STEMI precipitated by cocaine or those with variant angina because of the risk of potentiating coronary artery spasm.

Sublingual nitroglycerin should be given to all patients except those with an inferior STEMI and presumed right ventricular infarction who may experience treatment-related hypotension. Following sublingual nitroglycerin and in the absence of hypotension, intravenous nitroglycerin should be initiated for patients with continued chest pain. Nitrates may reduce infarct size, improve regional myocardial function, and provide a small relative reduction in mortality rate. Transdermal or oral nitrates should be used for patients with unstable angina or NSTEMI who have had recent episodes of chest pain but have no active symptoms at presentation.

Unstable angina and NSTEMI are treated with unfractionated heparin (UFH) or low-molecular-weight heparin (LMWH). Advantages of LMWH include twice daily subcutaneous administration and achievement of predictable levels of anticoagulation without the need for laboratory monitoring. LMWH should be avoided in patients with obesity or chronic kidney disease. Patients treated with stenting also require heparin therapy; UFH often is preferred to LMWH because of the ease with which the degree of anticoagulation can be assessed with the activated clotting time during PCI.

PCI is the preferred reperfusion therapy in specific subsets of patients with ACS (i.e., STEMI, new left bundle branch block, or true posterior infarction). In these patients, PCI is associated with a lower 30-day mortality rate compared with thrombolytic therapy. The incorporation of drug-eluting stents has further increased the clinical advantage of PCI over thrombolytic therapy. A drug-eluting stent is a metallic stent with a polymer covering containing an antirestenotic drug that is released over a period of 14 to 30 days. Antiplatelet therapy with a thienopyridine should be given upon hospital presentation, because most patients will subsequently receive a coronary stent during PCI, and there appears to be a benefit of pretreatment. Glycoprotein IIb/IIIa inhibitors (discussed later) also are beneficial in patients undergoing PCI, and early administration improves coronary patency.

Transfer of patients to a facility with PCI capabilities may be beneficial but is contingent on the ability to initiate PCI within 90 minutes of initial medical contact, which rarely is achievable. PCI also is indicated in patients with a contraindication to thrombolytic therapy and in patients with cardiogenic shock. PCI is most effective if completed within 12 hours of the onset of chest pain; the earlier the intervention, the better the outcome.

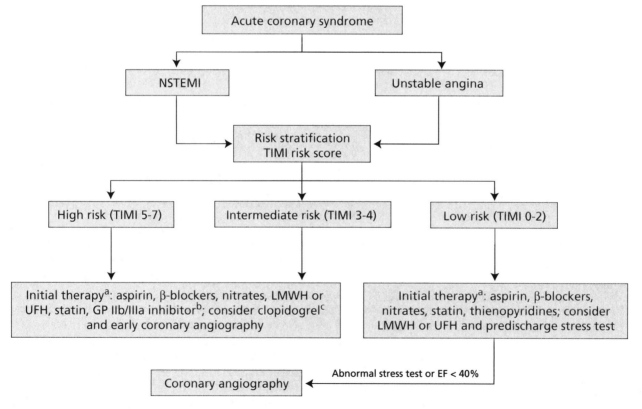

Figure 2. Initial management of unstable angina/non–ST-elevation myocardial infarction (NSTEMI). EF = ejection fraction; GP = glycoprotein; LMWH = low-molecular-weight heparin; TIMI = Thrombolysis in Myocardial Infarction; UFH = unfractionated heparin. [a] For patients with continued symptoms despite initial medical therapy, consider GP IIb/IIIa inhibitor and emergent coronary angiography. [b] Indications for GP IIb/IIIa inhibitor include ongoing chest pain, dynamic electrocardiographic changes, elevated troponin on presentation, heart failure, and diabetes mellitus. [c] A thienopryidinel can be given prior to coronary angiography. If coronary artery bypass grafting is required, the thienopryidinel should be stopped and surgery delayed for at least 5 days.

In the United States, approximately 70% of patients with STEMI present to hospitals without onsite PCI capabilities; therefore, thrombolytic therapy is the predominant method of reperfusion. By lysing the clot that is limiting blood flow to the myocardium, thrombolytics restore perfusion to the ischemic area, reduce infarct size, and improve survival. Thrombolytics should be administered within 12 hours after the onset of chest pain; the earlier the administration, the better the outcome. Patients receiving thrombolytic therapy with fibrin-specific agents (e.g., reteplase, tenecteplase) require concomitant heparin therapy; LMWH appears to be superior to UFH. Absolute contraindications to thrombolytic therapy include any prior intracerebral hemorrhage, known cerebrovascular lesions (e.g., arteriovenous malformation), ischemic stroke within 3 months, suspected aortic dissection, active bleeding or bleeding diathesis, and significant closed head or facial trauma within 3 months.

The 14-day risk for death or nonfatal MI in patients presenting with unstable angina or NSTEMI can be estimated using the Thrombolysis in Myocardial Infarction (TIMI) risk score (www.mdcalc.com/timi-risk-score-for-uanstemi). The TIMI risk score identifies patients who will derive the greatest benefit from aggressive medical therapy with glycoprotein IIb/IIIa inhibitors and early PCI (Figure 2). Glycoprotein IIb/IIIa inhibitors (tirofiban, eptifibatide, abciximab) act by occupying platelet receptors that would otherwise bind with fibrinogen, thus preventing platelet aggregation. Patients with a TIMI risk score ≥3 benefit most from the use of these agents. The main adverse effect of glycoprotein IIb/IIIa inhibitors is increased bleeding events.

The role of coronary bypass surgery in the treatment of ACS is evolving. Bypass surgery is preferred in patients who have a large amount of myocardium at ischemic risk due to proximal left main disease or multivessel disease, especially if the left ventricular ejection fraction is reduced. Bypass surgery may be preferred in patients with diabetes mellitus because of better long-term vessel patency and improved clinical outcomes. However, there is increasing evidence that drug-eluting stents may produce outcomes comparable to bypass surgery.

An intra-aortic balloon pump is indicated for ACS with cardiogenic shock unresponsive to medical therapy, acute mitral regurgitation secondary to papillary muscle dysfunction, ventricular septal rupture, or refractory angina. The intra-aortic balloon pump reduces afterload during ventricular systole and increases coronary perfusion during diastole. Patients with refractory cardiogenic shock who are treated with an intra-aortic balloon pump have a lower in-hospital mortality rate than patients who are not treated with this device.

The final phase of hospital therapy for ACS includes initiation of ACE inhibitor therapy, statin therapy, and, in certain patients, eplerenone. ACE inhibitors can attenuate ventricular remodeling, resulting in a reduction in the development of heart failure and risk of death. ACE inhibitors may also reduce the risk of recurrent infarction and other vascular events. In patients who cannot tolerate an ACE inhibitor due to cough, an angiotensin-receptor blocker is a reasonable alternative. Early statin therapy appears to improve endothelial function and to reduce the risk of future coronary events. The concept of plaque stabilization and improvement in endothelial function with statin therapy suggests that there is an emerging benefit to statins in ACS beyond reducing low-density lipoprotein (LDL) cholesterol. Eplerenone is a selective aldosterone blocker that limits collagen formation and ventricular remodeling and also has a favorable effect on the neurohormonal profile. Eplerenone reduces mortality when started 3 to 14 days after ACS presentation in patients with a left ventricular ejection fraction ≤40% and clinical heart failure or diabetes. Aldosterone antagonists should be used with great caution or not at all in patients with kidney disease (creatinine >2.5 mg/dL [88.4 μmol/L]) or preexisting hyperkalemia (potassium >5.0 meq/L [5 mmol/L]).

Follow-Up

Early cardiac catheterization during hospitalization for ACS should be considered for patients with recurrent ischemic symptoms, serious complications, or other intermediate- to high-risk features (e.g., heart failure, left ventricular dysfunction, ventricular arrhythmias). These complications and high-risk features are associated with more severe coronary artery disease and subsequent cardiac events. Cardiac catheterization also is routinely indicated for stable high-risk patients following successful thrombolytic therapy.

Post-MI exercise testing in patients without high-risk features is performed as a prognostic assessment. By doing stress testing early post-MI, the clinician can assess functional capacity, evaluate efficacy of the patient's current medical regimen, and assess the risk of future cardiac events. The finding of nonsustained ventricular tachycardia >48 hours after MI usually prompts electrophysiologic testing or placement of an implantable cardioverter-defibrillator (ICD). Patients with an ejection fraction <35% also are at high risk for sudden death and have improved survival when treated with an ICD.

Secondary prevention measures are an essential component of outpatient management following ACS and include management of hypertension and diabetes, lipid lowering, smoking cessation, and an exercise program. Aspirin, β-blockers, and ACE inhibitors should be continued indefinitely. Statins should be used to achieve an optional LDL cholesterol goal of <70 mg/dL (1.8 mmol/L) and should be continued indefinitely. A thienopyridine should be continued for at least 1 year for patients who receive medical or thrombolytic therapy. Patients with coronary stents should receive aspirin and a thienopyridine for at least 1 month for a bare metal stent and for at least 1 year following placement of a drug-eluting stent.

Studies indicate that approximately 20% of patients experience depression after acute MI and that the presence of depression is associated with increased risk for recurrent hospitalization and death. Post-MI, patients should be screened for depression.

Book Enhancement

Go to www.acponline.org/essentials/cardiovascular-section.html. In *MKSAP for Students 5*, assess your knowledge with items 1, 3, 5, 20, 22, 24, and 25 in the **Cardiovascular Medicine** section.

Bibliography

Kumar A, Cannon CP. Acute coronary syndromes: diagnosis and management, part I. Mayo Clin Proc. 2009;84:917-938. [PMID: 19797781]

Kumar A, Cannon CP. Acute coronary syndromes: diagnosis and management, part II. Mayo Clin Proc. 2009;84:1021-1036. [PMID: 19880693]

Chapter 4

Conduction Blocks and Bradyarrhythmias

Robert Trowbridge, MD

Cardiac conduction defects and bradyarrhythmias most commonly are the result of idiopathic degeneration of the conduction system, myocardial disease (coronary artery disease, amyloidosis, Lyme disease, hypertension), or medication effects (calcium channel blockers, β-blockers, digoxin, cholinesterase inhibitors). Any level of the conduction system may be affected, including the sinoatrial (SA) node, the atrioventricular (AV) node, and the ventricular system (bundle of His, right and left bundle branches). Depending on the level and severity of the conduction defect, clinical manifestations range from electrocardiographic (ECG) abnormalities without clinical effects (e.g., right bundle branch block, first-degree AV block) to symptomatic bradycardia manifesting as lightheadedness, syncope, and sudden death.

Bradyarrhythmias

Evaluation of bradyarrhythmia centers on identifying underlying cardiac and systemic disease as well as assessing potential medication effects. Accordingly, therapy includes removal of offending agents, treatment of underlying disorders, and consideration of permanent pacemaker placement. In general, pacemaker placement is not appropriate unless symptoms are present or there is a high likelihood of progression to symptomatic disease (Table 1).

SA node disease (sick sinus syndrome) is common in the elderly as a result of idiopathic degeneration of the cardiac conducting system. The spectrum of SA node disease includes sinus bradycardia, sinus arrest, carotid sinus hypersensitivity, and the bradycardia-tachycardia (brady-tachy) syndrome. Sinus bradycardia often is asymptomatic but, if severe, may manifest as lightheadedness, weakness, or syncope. Most cases do not require intervention. Sinus arrest appears as prolonged sinus pauses on electrocardiography and may also cause syncope. Carotid sinus hypersensitivity is a common cause of syncope in the elderly and results from increased vagal tone following manipulation of the neck (e.g., turning the head, wearing a tight collar). Brady-tachy syndrome is a subtype of SA node disease in which bradycardia or pauses occur following episodes of supraventricular tachyarrhythmias, most commonly atrial fibrillation. SA node disease may require pacemaker implantation if symptomatic. Brady-tachy syndrome requires concomitant therapy for the tachycardia as well as pacemaker placement.

Atrioventricular Block

AV block is classified as first-degree, second-degree, or third-degree. First-degree AV block may occur at several levels in the

---

Table 1. American College of Cardiology/American Heart Association Recommendations for Permanent Pacing in Acquired Atrioventricular (AV) Block in Adults

Conditions for which there is evidence or agreement that pacemaker implantation is beneficial, useful, and effective:

Third-degree and advanced second-degree AV block associated with any one of the following conditions:

Bradycardia with symptoms (including heart failure) or ventricular arrhythmias presumed to be due to AV block

Arrhythmias and other medical conditions that require drug therapy that results in symptomatic bradycardia

Asystole ≥3.0 sec or any escape rate <40/min, or with an escape rhythm that is below the AV node in awake, symptom-free patients in sinus rhythm

Atrial fibrillation and bradycardia with one or more pauses ≥5 sec in awake, symptom-free patients

Following catheter ablation of the AV junction

Postoperative AV block that is not expected to resolve after cardiac surgery

Neuromuscular diseases with AV block

AV block during exercise in the absence of myocardial ischemia

Second-degree AV block (regardless of type or site of block) with associated symptomatic bradycardia

Asymptomatic persistent third-degree AV block with average awake ventricular rates ≥40/min if cardiomegaly or left ventricular dysfunction is present or if the site of block is below the AV node

Type II second-degree AV block with a wide QRS complex, including isolated right bundle branch block

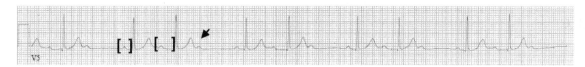

Figure 1. Electrocardiogram showing Mobitz type I second-degree atrioventricular block (Wenckebach block). Note prolongation of PR intervals (*brackets*) followed by nonconducted P waves (*arrow*).

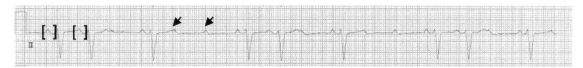

Figure 2. Electrocardiogram showing Mobitz type II second-degree atrioventricular block. Note absence of PR prolongation (*brackets*) and successive nonconducted P waves (*arrows*).

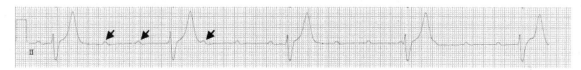

Figure 3. Electrocardiogram showing complete heart block. Note stable R-R intervals and lack of relation of P waves (*arrows*) to the QRS complex.

conduction system and is defined as prolongation of the PR interval to >200 msec. First-degree AV block is asymptomatic but weakly associated with an increased risk of syncope and death. It does not require intervention.

There are two types of second-degree AV block, both recognized electrocardiographically by the presence of a P wave that is not followed by a ventricular complex. Mobitz type I block (Wenckebach block) manifests as a progressive prolongation of the PR interval until there is a dropped ventricular beat (Figure 1). Mobitz type I block usually is secondary to a block at the level of the AV node and only rarely causes symptoms or progresses to higher-grade AV block. Mobitz type II block manifests as dropped ventricular beats without antecedent PR prolongation (Figure 2). In contrast to the defect in Mobitz type I, the conduction defect in Mobitz type II block usually is infranodal (e.g., within the ventricular conduction system). Mobitz type II block often is accompanied by an intraventricular conduction delay (which manifests as a widened QRS complex) or a left bundle branch block and typically progresses to third-degree AV block. Mobitz type I block usually does not require therapy, but Mobitz type II block is an indication for permanent pacemaker placement.

Third-degree AV block (complete heart block) occurs when there is no conduction of the atrial beats to the ventricles, resulting in the two chambers beating asynchronously. The atrial and ventricular rates are independent, and the QRS complex may be wide or narrow, depending on the origin of the ventricular escape rhythm (Figure 3). The conduction defect in third-degree AV block may be at the level of the AV node but more typically is within the infranodal system. It is often associated with significant bradycardia (pulse rates near 30/min) and, if untreated, may result in lightheadedness, syncope, and death. Third-degree AV block is an indication for permanent pacemaker placement.

Bundle Branch and Fascicular Blocks

Conduction defects at the level of the individual components of the ventricular conduction system may also be electrocardiographically apparent without causing bradycardia. Left bundle branch block (LBBB) manifests electrocardiographically as a wide QRS complex (>120 msec), loss of Q waves in leads V_5 and V_6, and wide R waves in the lateral leads (I, V_5, and V_6) (Figure 4). LBBB is common in the elderly and, as with other manifestations of conduction disease, may reflect degeneration of the conduction system or myocardial disease. LBBB usually is asymptomatic but when new may be the ECG representation of an acute anterior wall myocardial infarction in patients with an acute coronary syndrome; specific criteria (Sgarbossa criteria) can be used to help determine the likelihood of acute myocardial infarction in patients with LBBB. Left anterior hemiblock (LAHB) and left posterior hemiblock (LPHB) occur when the conduction block is limited to one of the two fascicles of the left bundle branch. LAFB is recognized by a positive QRS in lead I and a negative QRS in aVF. LPHB is recognized by a negative QRS in lead I and a positive QRS in aVF. The QRS duration is normal in both LAFB and LPFB. Isolated LAFB or LPFB is asymptomatic but may indicate underlying myocardial disease.

Right bundle branch block (RBBB) is diagnosed by a widened QRS complex (>120 msec), an rsR' pattern (small initial upward

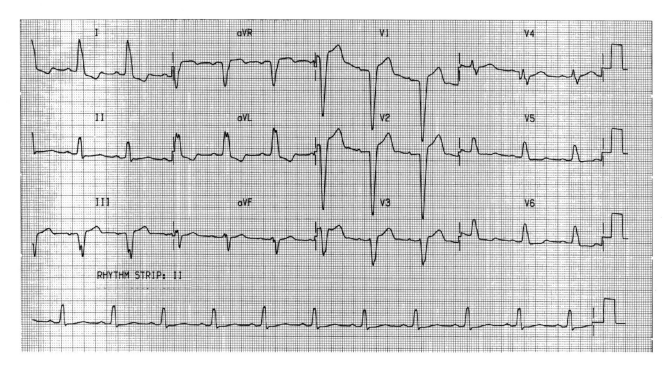

Figure 4. Electrocardiogram showing left bundle branch block pattern, including a wide QRS complex (>120 msec), absent Q waves in leads V_5 and V_6, and wide R waves in leads I, V_5, and V_6.

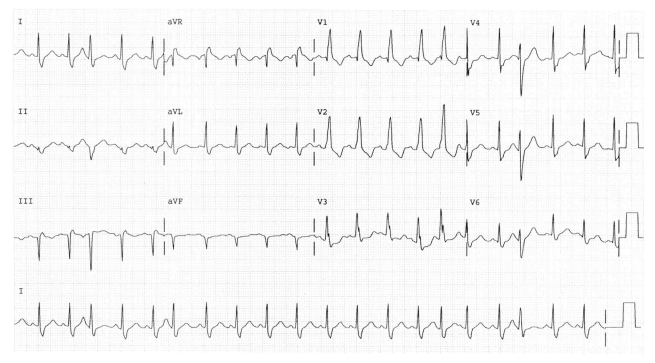

Figure 5. Electrocardiogram showing right bundle branch block pattern, including a wide QRS complex (>120 msec), rsR' pattern in lead V_1, and a wide negative S wave in leads I, V_5, and V_6.

deflection followed by a small downward deflection then a large upward deflection) in lead V_1, and a wide negative S wave in leads I, V_5, and V_6 (Figure 5). RBBB is asymptomatic and may be the result of degenerative disease. It can also be a marker of right heart strain secondary to primary arterial hypertension, chronic obstructive or restrictive pulmonary diseases, congenital heart disease, or pulmonary embolism. No specific therapy is indicated for RBBB.

Bifascicular block refers to the combination of RBBB with either LAFB or LAHB. Trifascicular block refers to the combination of RBBB, bifascicular block, and first-degree AV block. By definition, LBBB cannot be present with either bi- or trifascicular block. Bifascicular block and trifascicular block both can progress to third-degree AV block.

Book Enhancement

Go to www.acponline.org/acp_press/essentials/cardiovascular-section.html. In *MKSAP for Students 5*, assess your knowledge with items 7, 9, 23, 26, and 27 in the **Cardiovascular Medicine** section.

Bibliography

Da Costa D, Brady WJ, Edhouse J. Bradycardias and atrioventricular conduction block. BMJ. 2002;324:535-538. [PMID: 11872557]

Chapter 5

Supraventricular Arrhythmias

Chad S. Miller, MD

Enhanced automaticity and reentry are the mechanisms responsible for most episodes of supraventricular tachyarrhythmia (SVT). Enhanced automaticity is the accelerated generation of an action potential, which occurs normally in the sinoatrial (SA) node but also can occur abnormally in diseased myocardial tissue. Enhanced automaticity is responsible for atrial tachycardia, a subtype of SVT. Reentry is responsible for most other forms of SVT and is characterized by an electrical circuit that continuously reexcites the myocardium. Reentry is dependent on the presence of two interconnected conduction pathways. The first pathway initially is refractory to new impulse conduction because of a recent depolarization, whereas an alternative pathway is able to conduct the impulse. The conduction down the alternative pathway is slow enough to allow the first pathway to recover from its refractory period from the prior conducted impulse and become susceptible to depolarization by the impulse conducted by the alternative pathway. The reentrant circuit is completed when the conduction along the first pathway restimulates the alternative pathway to form a repeating electrical loop (Figure 1). Reentrant SVTs are classified by their conduction within or around the atrioventricular (AV) node. AV nodal reentrant tachycardia (AVNRT) describes a reentrant circuit within the AV node, whereas AV reentrant tachycardia (AVRT) describes a circuit that may involve the AV node but is not entirely contained within the node itself. Most SVTs (atrial tachycardia, AVNRT, and AVRT) are characterized by a rapid heart rate and a QRS complex <120 msec; the narrow QRS complex proves that electrical activation of the ventricles begins above or within the AV node (including the bundle of His). Less commonly, some forms of AVRT are associated with a wide QRS complex. SVTs can be further categorized as regular or irregular (Figure 2).

Diagnosis

Symptoms of SVT include palpitations, syncope, chest pain, dyspnea, and fatigue. The cardinal rule for diagnosing any arrhythmia is to document the heart rhythm at the time of symptoms with electrocardiography or another recording device. If a suspected arrhythmia cannot be documented on a resting electrocardiogram (ECG) or cardiac monitor during the initial evaluation, it can be evaluated with an event monitor that is activated by the patient at the time of symptoms. For symptoms that are very brief or prevent the patient from activating the event monitor (e.g., syncope), a continuous loop recorder activated by the patient after the event will save cardiac rhythm data from the previous 30 seconds to 2 minutes. If symptoms are very infrequent, an implantable recorder can be used. This small device is placed subcutaneously, similar to a

pacemaker, but there are no leads in the heart chambers. Cardiac rhythm data can be retrieved noninvasively; 24-hour ambulatory (Holter) monitors can record a full 24 or 48 hours of cardiac rhythm data, but this technique rarely provides useful diagnostic information unless the patient's symptoms are very frequent.

Sinus Tachycardia

Sinus tachycardia is the result of increased automaticity at the SA node. The most common causes are normal physiologic responses to exercise and increased sympathetic activity. Because sinus tachycardia originates from the SA node and is propagated normally through the AV node to the ventricles, it generally is not included in the SVT category. Heart rate is between 100/min and 150/min. The onset and conclusion of sinus tachycardia are gradual in con-

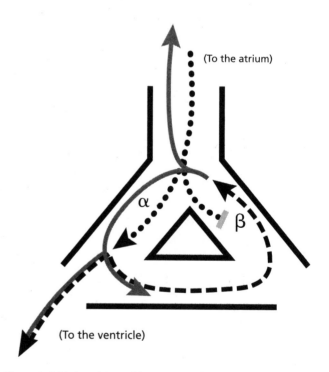

Figure 1. Initiation of AV nodal reentrant tachycardia (AVNRT). The α pathway has a short refractory period, and the β pathway has a long refractory period. The *dotted line* represents antegrade conduction down the α pathway; conduction does not occur down the β pathway because it is refractory. The *dashed line* represents impulse conduction into the ventricle and retrograde up the β pathway, which is no longer refractory. The *grey line* represents completion of the circuit, with activation of the atria and ventricles.

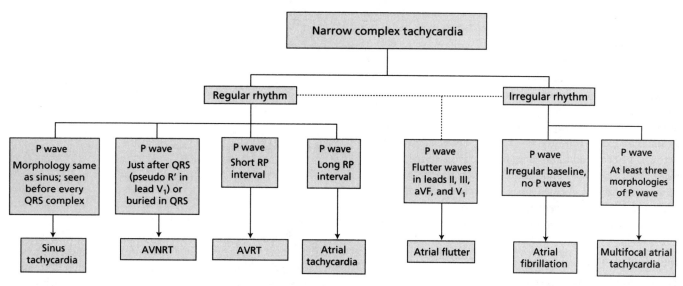

Figure 2. Classification of narrow complex tachycardias. AVNRT = atrioventricular nodal reentrant tachycardia; AVRT = atrioventricular reentrant tachycardia.

trast to SVTs, which begin and end suddenly. The P wave has normal morphology but may be difficult to identify with very rapid rates; slowing the heart rate with carotid sinus massage may allow identification of the normal P wave morphology and help establish the diagnosis. Once the diagnosis of sinus tachycardia is established, treatment is guided by the underlying cause. Fever, exercise, anxiety, pain, anemia, thyrotoxicosis, hypoxemia, cocaine use, and alcohol withdrawal are common causes of sinus tachycardia.

Regular Supraventricular Tachyarrhythmia

Atrial tachycardia usually results from increased automaticity of a group of atrial cells separate from the SA node. Heart rate is between 150/min and 200/min. The P wave morphology is abnormal, often upright, biphasic, or inverted in the inferior leads. The PR interval often is short, because the origin of the depolarizing impulse typically is located close to the ventricles. Atrial tachycardia commonly occurs in patients with coronary artery disease or cor pulmonale. Other causes include pulmonary embolization, thyrotoxicosis, digitalis toxicity, and acute noncardiac illness. Atrial tachycardia occasionally is seen in patients without structural heart disease.

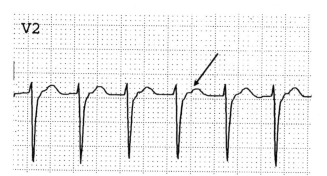

Figure 3. Atrioventricular nodal reentrant tachycardia is a narrow complex tachycardia with P waves buried in the T wave, most easily seen in lead V_2.

AVNRT accounts for approximately 60% of all SVTs that present as a regular rhythm. AVNRT is diagnosed by its characteristic findings on an ECG; the P wave is seen either just after the QRS complex, which accounts for a short RP interval, or is concealed within the QRS complex (no visible P wave) (Figure 3). Heart rate typically is between 120/min and 220/min. AVNRT often occurs in the absence of structural heart disease and typically is benign.

AVRT is associated with an accessory pathway between the atria and ventricle that is not contained within the AV node itself. This is also called the Wolff-Parkinson-White (WPW) syndrome. During the tachycardia, the reentrant impulses may travel antegrade (from atria to ventricles) down the AV node and then retrograde (from ventricles to atria) via the accessory pathway (orthodromic AVRT), or they may travel anterograde down the accessory pathway and back up to the atria via the AV node (antidromic

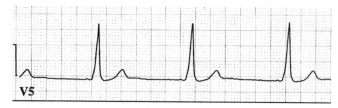

Figure 4. Preexcitation pattern typical of the Wolff-Parkinson-White syndrome showing a delta wave (upsloping of initial QRS wave), short PR interval, and wide QRS.

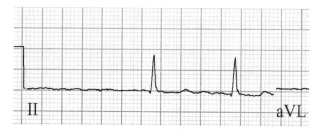

Figure 5. Atrial fibrillation showing atrial fibrillatory waves, best seen in lead II, and an irregular ventricular response.

AVRT). Antegrade-conducting AVRT accessory pathways can be identified on routine electrocardiography by two characteristics: a short PR interval, and the presence of a delta wave (a sloping upstroke initiating the QRS complex, which may be wide due to sequential rather than parallel depolarization of the ventricles) (Figure 4). A WPW accessory pathway that conducts impulses retrograde cannot be identified on routine electrocardiography. In a given patient, the defining features of WPW may not be present at all times and can even vary beat to beat. Heart rate typically is between 140/min and 250/min. Because the accessory pathway may be capable of rapid antegrade conduction, patients who develop atrial fibrillation can experience a very rapid ventricular response that can degenerate into ventricular fibrillation. The risk of sudden cardiac death in these patients is 0.15% to 0.39% over 3 to 10 years.

Irregular Supraventricular Tachyarrhythmia

Atrial fibrillation is associated with loss of sinus node function, leading to uncoordinated atrial activity. The ECG is characterized by absent P waves and irregularity of the ventricular response (Figure 5). Atrial fibrillation is classified as paroxysmal (lasting <7 days), persistent (lasting >7 days), or permanent (lasting >1 year or associated with failed cardioversion). Most cases of atrial fibrillation are associated with structural heart disease, such as valvular disease (especially mitral valve disease), dilated cardiomyopathy, hypertension, and coronary artery disease. Heart failure, pulmonary hypertension, and increasing age also are strongly associated with atrial fibrillation. Noncardiac causes include substance abuse (alcohol, caffeine, cocaine, amphetamines) inhaled β-agonists, hypoxemia, COPD, pulmonary embolization, obstructive sleep apnea, and hyperthyroidism. Lone atrial fibrillation is a form of paroxysmal atrial fibrillation occurring within an otherwise normal heart in the absence of precipitating or predisposing factors.

In patients with long-standing, uncontrolled ventricular rates >130/min, a tachycardia-related cardiomyopathy can develop. Systemic embolization is another major adverse event, of which stroke is the most common manifestation. Ineffectual atrial contraction results in stasis of blood, especially in the atrial appendages, allowing for the formation of thrombi, which may embolize to other organs. The annual risk of stroke in patients with atrial fibrillation is between 1% and 18%. The risk is particularly high in patients with valvular atrial fibrillation and prior stroke or transient ischemic attack (TIA). The CHADS$_2$ risk score is used to predict the likelihood of stroke in patients with nonvalvular atrial fibrillation. The CHADS$_2$ acronym is derived from the individual stroke risk factors (i.e., congestive heart failure, hypertension, age >75 years, diabetes mellitus, and prior stroke or TIA). Patients are assigned 2 points for a previous stroke or TIA and 1 point for each of the other risk factors. The higher the CHADS$_2$ score, the greater the risk of stroke.

Atrial flutter is characterized by regular atrial contractions (flutter waves) on electrocardiography (Figure 6). The atrial rate is between 240/min and 300/min and usually is associated with a 2:1 or 3:1 AV block, resulting in a ventricular rate of approximately 100-150/min. Sustained atrial flutter is uncommon, and flutter

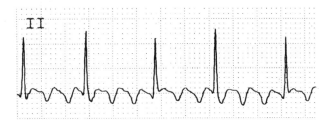

Figure 6. Electrocardiogram showing an irregular rate and a saw-tooth pattern in lead II characteristic of atrial flutter.

typically converts to atrial fibrillation over time. The cause of atrial flutter is the same as for atrial fibrillation.

Multifocal atrial tachycardia (MAT) is diagnosed by the presence of three or more morphologically distinct P waves and a heart rate between 100/min and 140/min. MAT is due to multiple areas of increased automaticity or triggered activity within the atria. MAT occurs most often in patients with severe COPD.

Therapy

With the exception of sinus tachycardia, electrical cardioversion is indicated for any hemodynamically unstable rhythm. In patients with sinus tachycardia, addressing the underlying cause is the key therapeutic principle.

Atrial tachycardia often terminates without intervention once the underlying cause is treated. First-line drug therapies for stable atrial tachycardia are β-blockers and non-dihydropyridine calcium channel blockers (verapamil, diltiazem). Adenosine and electrical cardioversion are relatively ineffective. If atrial tachycardia fails to respond to first-line therapy, cardiology consultation to guide antiarrhythmic therapy is recommended. Typical antiarrhythmic agents include amiodarone, flecainide, and sotalol. These drugs have significant side effects and can be proarrhythmic. For recurrent atrial tachycardia, long-term therapy with β-blockers and non-dihydropyridine calcium channel blockers is the treatment of choice. For refractory cases, radiofrequency catheter ablation of the abnormal impulse generation site is an option.

AVNRT may be terminated by maneuvers to increase vagal tone, such as Valsalva or unilateral carotid massage (after careful carotid artery auscultation for bruits). Intravenous adenosine, a non-dihydropyridine calcium channel blocker, and β-blockers often are successful in terminating AVNRT not responding to vagal maneuvers. Intravenous adenosine has a very rapid onset and is extremely short-acting, with a half-life of 10 seconds, making it an excellent first therapeutic choice. Adenosine is contraindicated in patients with severe bronchospastic disease. β-Blockers and non-dihydropyridine calcium-channel blockers also can be used chronically to prevent frequent recurrence of AVNRT. In refractory cases, catheter radiofrequency ablation is between 95% and 99% successful in preventing recurrence of AVNRT. Because of the success of this procedure, antiarrhythmic drugs are seldom used.

Narrow-complex AVRT is treated in the same manner as AVNRT. AV nodal blocking drugs are contraindicated when AVRT is associated with a wide QRS complex secondary to antegrade conduction over the accessory pathway, because the medications are associated with accelerated conduction down the bypass tract and may result in rapid ventricular rates and possible induction of ventricular arrhythmias. Procainamide is the drug of choice for wide-complex AVRT, because it will increase refractoriness in the accessory pathway. Catheter radiofrequency ablation has similar success rates as in AVNRT and can prevent sudden death associated with AVRT.

Treatment of atrial fibrillation is guided by three basic principles: rate control, restoration/maintenance of sinus rhythm, and stroke prevention. Atrial fibrillation with a rapid ventricular rate is treated acutely with intravenous non-dihydropyridine calcium channel blockers and β-blockers. The goal of rate control is to reduce the ventricular rate to <80/min at rest and <100/min during exercise. Digitalis is not recommended as a single agent for rate control due to its slower onset, increased toxicity, and lack of efficacy for controlling the ventricular rate during exercise, but digitalis can be a useful adjunctive therapy, especially in patients with relative hypotension or systolic heart failure. Other options to control ventricular rate include full or partial catheter radiofrequency ablation of the AV node, which may require concomitant pacemaker placement.

Conversion to normal sinus rhythm should be considered in all patients with atrial fibrillation. In most patients, however, a rate control and anticoagulation strategy is likely as efficacious as a rhythm control approach. In patients aged >65 years, heart rate control is preferred to antiarrhythmic therapy, because it results in fewer hospitalizations and serious drug reactions. In younger patients, restoration of sinus rhythm may be associated with improved quality of life. Synchronized direct-current cardioversion and pharmacologic therapy (dofetilide, flecainide, ibutilide) both are effective for converting atrial fibrillation to sinus rhythm. For atrial fibrillation of <48 hours' duration, cardioversion can proceed safely without anticoagulation. For atrial fibrillation of >48 hours' duration or of unknown duration, cardioversion is performed after anticoagulation with warfarin for 3 weeks (target INR of 2.0-3.0). If cardioversion is desired more quickly, a transesophageal echocardiogram can be performed to evaluate for the presence of left atrial thrombus. In the absence of thrombus, the patient is anticoagulated with heparin, cardioverted, and maintained on warfarin for at least 4 weeks. The antiarrhythmic agents amiodarone, flecainide, ibutilide, propafenone, and sotalol are used to maintain patients in sinus rhythm following cardioversion. Amiodarone is the antiarrhythmic drug of choice in patients with underlying heart disease because of its relatively low proarrhythmic potential compared to other agents. Even with antiarrhythmic drugs, the long-term (>1 year) recurrence rate of symptomatic atrial fibrillation is 20% to 50%.

Stroke prevention must be considered in all patients with atrial fibrillation. All patients with atrial fibrillation due to valvular heart disease and patients with previous TIA or stroke require lifelong anticoagulation with warfarin to prevent stroke. Warfarin (target INR of 2.0-3.0) reduces the risk of stroke by an average of 64% in nonvalvular atrial fibrillation. For patients at intermediate risk for stroke (CHADS$_2$ score of 1 or 2), need for warfarin therapy should be assessed individually, taking into account the risk of major hemorrhage and patient preference. Most of these patients will benefit from warfarin therapy, although aspirin may be a rea-

sonable choice in those with a CHADS$_2$ score of 1. In patients in whom full anticoagulation is contraindicated, aspirin decreases stroke risk by 22%. In patients with a CHADS$_2$ score of 0, the risk of stroke is low, and anticoagulation is not required. Chronic anticoagulation also is considered if there is high risk for recurrence of atrial fibrillation following successful cardioversion, evidence of intracardiac thrombus, or other risk factors for thromboembolism.

An emerging strategy is to use pulmonary vein catheter radiofrequency ablation to prevent recurrent atrial fibrillation. Foci for atrial fibrillation are commonly located around the ostia of the pulmonary veins and can be isolated with catheter radiofrequency ablation. Up to 80% of patients with paroxysmal atrial fibrillation will remain arrhythmia-free after pulmonary vein catheter radiofrequency ablation. Alternatively, the "maze" surgical procedure consists of multiple atrial incisions to reduce effective atrial size and prevent formation of atrial fibrillation wavelets; it is 70% to 95% effective. The maze procedure requires open cardiac surgery and is considered only in patients undergoing heart surgery for other reasons.

Follow-Up

A 12-lead ECG should be obtained to check QRS complexes and QT intervals for evidence of drug toxicity in patients on antiarrhythmic drugs. Antiarrhythmic drug levels should be monitored when feasible in all patients who are taking medications for supraventricular tachycardia, and patients should be routinely screened for side effects of antiarrhythmic therapy. Periodic thyroid function tests, liver chemistry tests, and pulmonary function tests (including diffusing capacity for carbon dioxide) should be obtained in patients treated with amiodarone, and periodic complete blood counts should be obtained for patients treated with procainamide. Amiodarone has several serious side effects, including pulmonary fibrosis, hyperthyroidism, hypothyroidism, and hepatitis. Procainamide can cause agranulocytosis.

In patients with atrial fibrillation, assess rate control by asking about easy fatigability and exertional dyspnea, and measure heart rate after walking. If the heart rate is >100/min, increase the AV nodal blockade. Maintain the INR at 2.0 to 3.0 in patients with nonvalvular atrial fibrillation or at 2.5 to 3.5 in patients with valvular atrial fibrillation.

Book Enhancement

Go to www.acponline.org/essentials/cardiovascular-section.html. In *MKSAP for Students 5*, assess your knowledge with items 13, 15, 17, 28-30 in the **Cardiovascular Medicine** section.

Acknowledgment

We would like to thank Dr. Charin L. Hanlon, who contributed to an earlier version of this chapter.

Bibliography

Delacrétaz E. Clinical practice. Supraventricular tachycardia. N Engl J Med. 2006;354:1039-1051. [PMID: 16525141]

Chapter 6

Ventricular Arrhythmias

Suma Pokala, MD

Ventricular arrhythmias are the most important causes of sudden cardiac death, particularly in patients with structural heart disease and a low ventricular ejection fraction. In general, the ventricular arrhythmias associated with structural heart disease are more malignant than those associated with a structurally normal heart. Ventricular arrhythmias can be categorized into premature ventricular contractions, ventricular tachycardia, and ventricular fibrillation.

Premature ventricular contractions (PVCs) are extraventricular beats that occur individually or as couplets. Although PVCs appear to be more frequent in patients with heart disease, they have minimal prognostic significance if left ventricular function is preserved. Ventricular tachycardia (VT) is a potentially life-threatening arrhythmia due to rapid, depolarizing impulses originating from the His-Purkinje system, the ventricular myocardium, or both. VT is subdivided into sustained VT and nonsustained VT. VT is sustained when it persists >30 seconds or requires termination due to hemodynamic collapse. Nonsustained VT has ≥3 beats but is <30 seconds in duration. VT also is categorized by the morphology of the QRS complexes. VT is monomorphic if QRS complexes in the

same leads do not vary in contour (Figure 1); VT is polymorphic if the QRS complexes in the same leads do vary in contour (Figure 2). Proper use of these terms and the patient context in which VT occurs are essential for accurate diagnosis and therapy. Ventricular fibrillation (VF) reflects a lack of organized ventricular activity and, unless terminated, results in sudden death.

The pathophysiology of VT most commonly relates to abnormalities of impulse conduction, usually by a reentrant pathway. Reentry occurs when an impulse fails to extinguish after normal activation of myocardial tissue and continues to propagate after the refractory period. Once the reentrant pathway is initiated, repetitive circulation of the impulse over the loop can produce VT. VT also may arise through abnormal impulse formation, such as enhanced automaticity or triggered activity. Enhancement of normal automaticity in latent pacemaker fibers or the development of abnormal automaticity due to partial resting membrane depolarization can serve as a nidus for VT. Triggered activity does not occur spontaneously; it requires a change in cardiac electrical frequency as a trigger, such as early depolarization (i.e., PVCs). VT often accompanies structural heart disease, most commonly

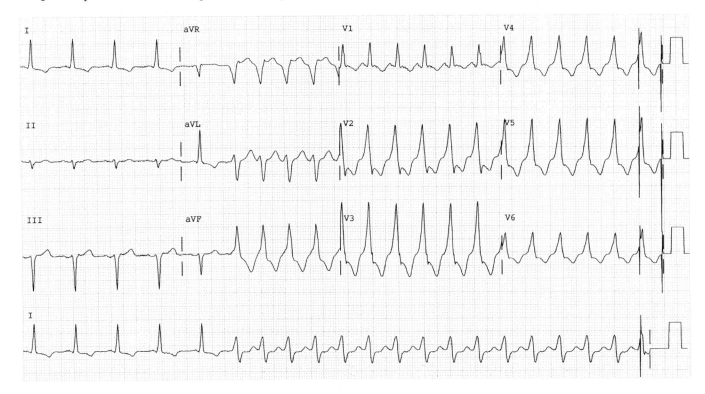

Figure 1. Approximately one quarter of the way into this electrocardiogram, monomorphic ventricular tachycardia begins; it is associated with an abrupt change in the QRS axis.

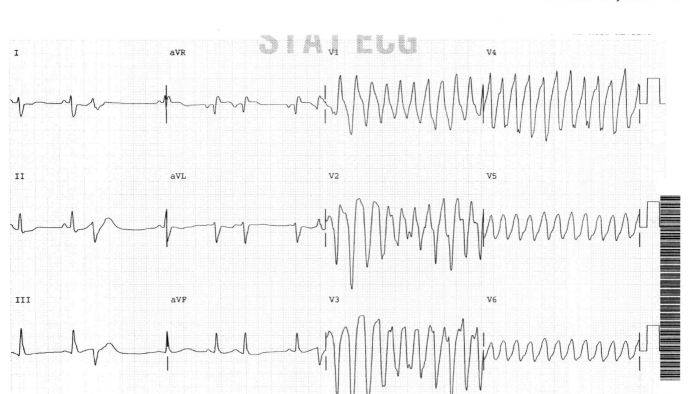

Figure 2. Electrocardiogram showing degeneration of sinus rhythm into polymorphic ventricular tachycardia.

ischemic heart disease, and is associated with electrolyte disorders (e.g., hypokalemia, hypomagnesemia), drug toxicity, valvular heart disease, nonischemic cardiomyopathy, and long QT syndrome.

Prevention

Because VT and VF often occur in the setting of ischemic heart disease, identification and reduction of risk factors for coronary artery disease are indicated.

Screening

Routine screening for VT in asymptomatic persons is not recommended. However, a screening electrocardiogram (ECG) is reasonable in asymptomatic persons with a family history of sudden cardiac death, as these individuals may have long QT syndrome, arrhythmogenic right ventricular dysplasia, or Brugada syndrome (an ion channel disorder associated with incomplete right bundle branch block).

Diagnosis

Symptoms are dependent on several factors, including the ventricular rate, the duration of tachycardia, and the presence of underlying heart disease. Patients with PVCs usually are asymptomatic but may complain of palpitations or a sensation that the heart has stopped, owing to the post-PVC compensatory pause. Patients with nonsustained VT usually are asymptomatic but may

experience palpitations, dizziness, or syncope. Patients with sustained VT usually present with syncope or near syncope and can also present with sudden cardiac death. Patients with VF often present with sudden cardiac death.

Ventricular tachyarrhythmias are characterized by wide-complex QRS morphology (QRS >120 msec) and ventricular rate >100/min. In VT, the ventricular rate typically ranges from 140/min to 250/min; in VF, the rate typically is >300/min. In torsades de pointes, a special subset of polymorphic VT, the ventricular rate ranges from 200/min to 300/min. Torsades de pointes is associated with long QT syndrome, which may be congenital or acquired. Long QT syndrome is characterized by prolonged ventricular repolarization and a predisposition to the development of polymorphic VT and sudden cardiac death. Patients can be diagnosed after presenting with syncope, or a prolonged QT interval (>500 msec, corrected for heart rate) can be an incidental finding on an ECG. Risk factors for acquired long QT syndrome include female sex, hypokalemia, hypomagnesemia, structural heart disease, and a history of previous long QT or drug-induced arrhythmias. An extensive list of agents that can cause torsades de pointes can be found at www.torsades.org.

Supraventricular tachycardia with a wide QRS complex can mimic VT and usually is due to coexisting bundle branch block or preexcitation syndrome (Wolff-Parkinson-White syndrome). Differentiating VT from supraventricular tachycardia with aberrant conduction is important, because the treatment differs markedly. VT is more common than supraventricular tachycardia with aberrancy, particularly in patients with structural heart disease. A key point is that any wide QRS tachycardia should be con-

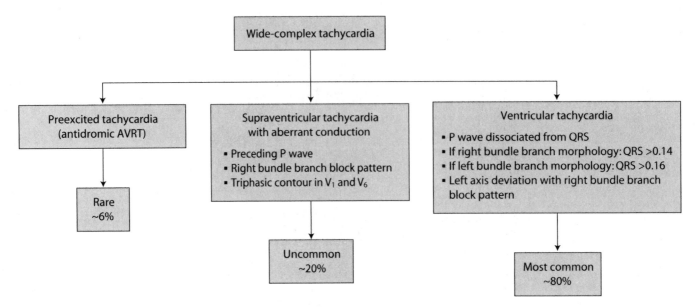

Figure 3. Differentiating ventricular tachycardia from supraventricular tachycardia with aberrancy. AVRT = atrioventricular reentrant tachycardia.

sidered to be VT until proven otherwise (Figure 3). The most important differentiating point is a history of ischemic heart disease. In the presence of known structural heart disease, particularly a prior myocardial infarction (MI), the diagnosis of VT is almost certain. Another clue is more profound hemodynamic deterioration in VT; however, a normal blood pressure does not rule out VT. Additionally, supraventricular tachycardia and VT may be distinguished at times by looking for evidence of atrioventricular dissociation on physical examination, which is present in VT. The presence of cannon *a* waves (large *a* waves) in the jugular venous pulsations and varying intensity of S_1 support atrioventricular dissociation and the diagnosis of VT. At times, physical examination and electrocardiography are insufficient to identify the cause of a wide-complex tachycardia; electrophysiologic testing provides definitive diagnosis and is indicated in these patients. In the absence of immediate expert consultation, it is always preferable to assume the patient has VT and to treat accordingly with immediate cardioversion.

The key points in the evaluation of VT include (1) reviewing the history for evidence of ischemic heart disease; (2) examining prior ECGs for evidence of long QT syndrome and baseline electrocardiographic abnormalities (prior MI, Wolff-Parkinson-White syndrome); and (3) searching for reversible causes, including electrolyte abnormalities, heart failure, and drug toxicity.

Therapy

Among persons with no evidence of heart disease, frequent PVCs are of uncertain significance. Among persons with a depressed ejection fraction, frequent PVCs are associated with increased mortality, but suppression of PVCs with antiarrhythmic drugs does not improve mortality. If symptoms can be clearly correlated with PVCs, treatment may be appropriate, although many patients respond well to reassurance. If symptoms are intolerable, first-line therapy almost always is a β-blocker or a non-dihy-

dropyridine calcium channel blocker. Class IC and class III antiarrhythmic agents also can be useful but have a high incidence of side effects; class IC drugs are proarrhythmic in patients with coronary artery disease. Radiofrequency ablation may be appropriate for patients with severe symptoms that are refractory to drug therapy.

In general, medical therapy does not improve survival in patients with VT. Pharmacologic therapy for nonsustained VT usually is avoided unless the patient has a history of structural heart disease or long QT syndrome or (rarely) intolerable symptoms. Therapy for symptomatic nonsustained VT is similar to treatment for PVCs; β-blockers are the mainstay, although non-dihydropyridine calcium channel blockers also may be used in patients with structurally normal hearts. The most frequently used class III antiarrhythmic agents are amiodarone and sotalol; class IC agents (e.g., flecainide, propafenone) are limited to use in patients without coronary artery disease. Patients in whom drug therapy for nonsustained VT fails or is not tolerated can be referred for radiofrequency ablation.

Suppression of nonsustained VT by medical therapy has not shown a mortality benefit in patients with a high risk of sudden death, including those with coronary artery disease or depressed left ventricular function. Nonsustained VT within 48 hrs of an acute coronary syndrome or reperfusion therapy does not confer additional mortality risk so need not be treated. However, nonsustained VT occurring in the year following MI is associated with increased mortality. In these patients, management includes treatment of reversible ischemia.

The prognosis for a patient with monomorphic sustained VT is dependent on the presence or absence of structural heart disease. In contrast, polymorphic VT most often is related to an underlying genetic defect predisposing to often-fatal cardiac arrhythmias. Sustained, symptomatic VT in ischemic or nonischemic cardiomyopathy is an adverse prognostic indicator with a high risk of recurrence.

Large clinical trials have demonstrated that implantable cardioverter-defibrillator (ICD) therapy improves survival rates in select patients with VT. An ICD is an internal defibrillator that senses dangerous cardiac arrhythmias and automatically converts the rhythm to sinus rhythm by either administering a high-energy shock or delivering a short series of paced beats. Accepted indications for an ICD include (1) ischemic or nonischemic cardiomyopathy and an ejection fraction <35%, (2) a prior episode of resuscitated VT/VF or hemodynamically unstable VT, (3) sustained VT in a patient with structural heart disease, and (4) a prior MI and an ejection fraction <35%.

Immediate cardioversion is the treatment of choice for hemodynamically unstable patients (regardless of the rhythm disorder) and often is the safest choice even in hemodynamically stable patients, particularly those with wide-complex tachycardia. Survival in cardiac arrest is proportional to intervention time for cardioversion or defibrillation. Epinephrine or vasopressin is recommended for hemodynamic support, and amiodarone has largely replaced other antiarrhythmic agents for resistant VT, although lidocaine can be useful in coronary ischemia. After termination of the arrhythmia, the ECG can provide clues regarding the presence of a prior MI, left ventricular hypertrophy, or long QT syndrome; an ECG also provides evaluation for structural heart disease and assessment of left ventricular function. Exercise testing can screen for significant coronary artery disease and provoke exercise-associated tachycardias. In newly diagnosed cardiomyopathy, cardiac catheterization often is necessary to evaluate for coronary artery disease as the cause of myocardial dysfunction.

The treatment of torsades de pointes is complex and will require consultation with a specialist. Recommendations that have strong supporting evidence include withdrawal of any offending drugs, correction of electrolyte abnormalities, and initiation of β-blocker therapy for patients with congenital prolonged QT syndrome. Patients who continue to have recurrent arrhythmias despite β-blocker therapy should be considered for ICD placement.

Follow-Up

Appropriate treatment for heart failure, including β-blockers, ACE inhibitors, and spironolactone, has been shown to reduce the incidence of sudden death in selected patients with systolic dysfunction.

Book Enhancement

Go to www.acponline.org/essentials/cardiovascular-section.html. In *MKSAP for Students 5*, assess your knowledge with items 19, 31-34 in the **Cardiovascular Medicine** section.

Acknowledgment

We would like to thank Drs. Steven J. Durning and Mark C. Haigney, who contributed to an earlier version of this chapter.

Bibliography

Thavendiranathan P, Bagai A, Khoo C, Dorian P, Choudhry NK. Does this patient with palpitations have a cardiac arrhythmia? JAMA. 2009; 302:2135-2143. [PMID: 19920238]

Chapter 7

Heart Failure

Alpesh N. Amin, MD

Heart failure is a complex clinical syndrome resulting from a structural or functional abnormality that impairs the ability of the ventricles to fill with or eject blood. New-onset heart failure often results from acute pump dysfunction caused by myocardial ischemia or infarction. In chronic heart failure, the left ventricle dilates and/or hypertrophies, causing the chamber to become more spherical in a process called *ventricular remodeling*. The geometric changes that affect the left ventricle increase wall stress, depress myocardial performance, and activate various neurohormonal compensatory responses that result in salt and water retention despite the presence of excess intravascular volume. In addition to causing peripheral vasoconstriction, elevated levels of circulating neurohormones (e.g., epinephrine, aldosterone, angiotensin II) may exert direct toxic effects on cardiac cells by promoting further hypertrophy, stimulating myocardial fibrosis and triggering programmed cell death (apoptosis).

The important causes of heart failure are best understood by reviewing the population attributable risk (PAR) calculations, which take into account the relative risk of the condition and its prevalence in the population. Using this methodology, the first National Health and Nutrition Examination Survey (NHANES I) calculated PARs for conditions causing heart failure as follows: coronary heart disease, 62%; cigarette smoking, 17%; hypertension, 10%; overweight, 8%; diabetes, 3%; and valvular heart disease, 2%.

Prevention

Based on the PARs for heart failure, important preventive measures include controlling risk factors for coronary artery disease, such as dyslipidemia, hypertension, and cigarette smoking. Aggressive blood pressure and lipid control appears to provide benefits to patients with diabetes above those seen in the general population. ACE inhibitors and angiotensin receptor blockers (ARBs) can prevent the development of heart failure and also provide kidney protection in patients with diabetes.

Advise patients to avoid exposure to cardiotoxic substances, such as alcohol, tobacco, and illicit drugs, particularly cocaine. Alcohol is a direct myocardial toxin and can cause heart failure. In some patients, abstinence from alcohol can reverse left ventricular dysfunction. Cocaine has both direct and indirect effects on the myocardium that increase the risk of heart failure and sudden cardiac death.

Prolonged tachycardia may be associated with the development of a reversible form of left ventricular dysfunction. Control of rapid ventricular responses in patients with atrial fibrillation and other supraventricular tachycardias can prevent the development of tachycardia-induced cardiomyopathy.

Screening

Look for familial patterns of unexplained heart failure, sudden cardiac death, and progressive heart failure in young family members. Dilated cardiomyopathies may be familial in a significant percentage of cases. A personal or family history of hemochromatosis, hypertrophic cardiomyopathy, or amyloidosis may warrant echocardiographic or genetic screening of asymptomatic family members.

Diagnosis

Among patients presenting to the emergency department with dyspnea, several signs and symptoms influence the likelihood of heart failure. Features that increase the likelihood of heart failure include the presence of paroxysmal nocturnal dyspnea (>2-fold likelihood) and the presence of an S_3 (11 times greater likelihood). The likelihood of heart failure is decreased 50% by the absence of dyspnea on exertion and by the absence of crackles on pulmonary auscultation. Elevated jugular venous pressure and an S_3 are independently associated with adverse outcomes, including progression of heart failure.

Symptoms are used to assess functional capacity. Functional capacity most commonly is expressed in terms of the New York Heart Association (NYHA) classification, which describes the effort needed to elicit symptoms (Table 1). Such classification schemes are used to determine prognosis and to guide therapy.

Laboratory Evaluation

A resting 12-lead electrocardiogram (ECG) should be obtained in any patient with new-onset heart failure or an exacerbation of preexisting heart failure to identify the cardiac rhythm and determine the presence of ischemia, prior infarction, left ventricular hypertrophy, and/or conduction system abnormalities. In addition, the ECG may be used in decision making regarding cardiac resynchronization therapy.

Initial laboratory evaluation should include serum electrolytes, kidney and liver function testing, a complete blood count, and, if indicated, assessment of thyroid function along with tests to screen for specific cardiomyopathies (e.g., hemochromatosis). Measurement of serum B-type natriuretic peptide (BNP), a sensitive marker of ventricular pressure and volume overload, should be considered in the evaluation when diagnostic uncertainty exists. BNP levels may help in differentiating heart failure from noncardiac causes of dyspnea in the acute care setting. Higher BNP levels suggest heart failure and may provide additional prognostic information, where-

Table 1. Clinical Stages of Chronic Heart Failure

ACC/AHA Stage	NYHA Functional Class	Estimated 1-Year Mortality
A (at risk; no structural disease or symptoms)	—	Mortality associated with any existing comorbidities
B (structural disease but no symptoms)	I (asymptomatic)	5%-10%
C (structural disease with prior or current symptoms)	II (symptomatic; slight limitation of physical activity)	15%-30%
	IIIª (symptomatic; marked limitation of physical activity)	15%-30%
D (refractory disease)	IIIª (symptomatic; marked limitation of physical activity)	15%-30%
	IV (inability to perform any physical activity without symptoms)	50%-60%

ACC/AHA = American College of Cardiology/American Heart Association; NYHA = New York Heart Association.
ªNYHA class III overlaps with ACC/AHA stages C and D.
Adapted with permission from Givertz MM, Colucci WS, Braunwald E. Clinical aspects of heart failure; pulmonary edema, high-output failure. In: Zipes DP, Libby P, Bonow RO, Braunwald E, eds. Heart Disease: A Textbook of Cardiovascular Medicine. 7th ed. Philadelphia, PA: WB Saunders; 2005:552. Copyright 2005, Elsevier.

as low serum BNP levels help to exclude a diagnosis of heart failure in patients with symptoms of acute dyspnea. In one recent review, a serum BNP level <100 pg/mL was the most useful test for ruling out heart failure in an emergency department setting, with a negative likelihood ratio of 0.11. In a second study, BNP level >100 pg/mL was 90% sensitive and 73% specific in the diagnosis of heart failure in the emergency department and had improved accuracy compared with clinical judgment alone. Caution should be used in interpreting BNP levels outside the acute setting. Patients with chronic heart failure may have BNP levels <100 pg/mL. In addition, other conditions that cause increased wall stress, such as acute myocardial infarction (MI) and pulmonary embolism, can raise BNP levels. Factors other than ventricular wall stress that increase BNP levels include chronic kidney disease, older age, and female sex; BNP is reduced by obesity.

Common radiographic findings in heart failure include cardiomegaly, pulmonary vascular congestion, and pleural effusions (often bilateral). Although a chest radiograph may be helpful in determining the cause of dyspnea, serial chest radiographs are not sensitive to small changes in pulmonary vascular congestion and are not recommended.

Echocardiography can help identify specific causes of heart failure, including hypertensive heart disease, ischemic disease, hypertrophic or infiltrative cardiomyopathy, and primary valvular heart disease. Coronary artery disease, which is the underlying cause of systolic heart failure in about two thirds of patients, may show echocardiographic evidence of regional wall motion abnormalities and/or post-MI ventricular remodeling. Echocardiography is necessary for distinguishing systolic heart failure from heart failure with preserved systolic function. Heart failure with preserved systolic function is diagnosed when signs and symptoms of systolic heart failure are present, but an echocardiogram reveals a normal left ventricular ejection fraction and the absence of significant valvular or pericardial abnormalities. Heart failure with preserved systolic function is common, especially in elderly patients, and in conditions causing significant left ventricular hypertrophy (e.g., hypertension, aortic stenosis, hypertrophic cardiomyopathy).

Ischemia is a significant cause of ventricular dysfunction, either as a primary cause or an exacerbating factor. In appropriate patients, revascularization can result in improved ventricular function, reduced symptoms, and increased survival. Evaluation for the presence of ischemia is necessary in almost all cases of new-onset or worsening heart failure, unless the clinical evidence strongly suggests a cause other than ischemia. The American College of Cardiology/American Heart Association guidelines recommend coronary angiography for patients with new-onset heart failure who have angina or significant ischemia and are potential candidates for revascularization. In general, the weight of evidence and expert opinion also favor performing coronary angiography for patients who have chest pain and unknown coronary anatomy. For patients with known coronary disease who present with heart failure, noninvasive imaging to assess for myocardial ischemia and viability also is reasonable.

Cardiomyopathies

Specific cardiomyopathies may require specific testing or treatment beyond that generally recommended for systolic heart failure. A diagnosis of dilated cardiomyopathy requires evidence of dilatation and impaired contraction of the left ventricle or both ventricles. Dilated cardiomyopathy has many causes, with the most common being idiopathic (50%), myocarditis (9%), ischemic (7%), peripartum (4%), and toxic (3%). Idiopathic cardiomyopathy is diagnosed if there is no evidence of coronary artery obstruction, myocarditis, or a primary or secondary form of heart muscle disease. Acute myocarditis is immunologically mediated damage to the myocardium; cardiac troponin levels typically are elevated, indicating some degree of myocardial necrosis, and ventricular dysfunction may be global or regional. Peripartum cardiomyopathy occurs during the last trimester of pregnancy or up to 6 months postpartum in the absence of an identifiable cause. Peripartum cardiomyopathy is a major cause of pregnancy-related death in North America; maternal death is related to heart failure, thromboembolic events, and arrhythmias. Left ventricular function improves within 6 months after delivery in approximately 50% of women with peripartum cardiomyopathy.

Restrictive cardiomyopathy is a disease of ventricular myocardium that typically results in delayed diastolic relaxation, decreased compliance, and elevated filling pressures with nondilated ventricles. Amyloidosis is the most common diagnosis when a cause can be identified; other common causes include sarcoidosis and hemochromatosis. Prominent symptoms of restrictive cardiomyopathy include fatigue, weakness, anorexia, and edema. Physical examination may reveal peripheral edema, jugular venous distention, hepatojugular reflux, and Kussmaul sign (an increase in jugular venous distention during inspiration). The apical impulse may be forceful, a loud S_3 usually is present, and regurgitant murmurs are common.

Amyloidosis is suggested by neuropathy, marked proteinuria, and hepatomegaly disproportionate to other signs of right-sided heart failure. Characteristic echocardiographic features of amyloidosis include increased ventricular wall thickness, thickened atrioventricular valves, a thickened atrial septum, and pericardial effusion. The combination of low voltage on ECG and thick ventricular walls on echocardiogram suggests amyloidosis (or another infiltrative process). Bilateral hilar lymphadenopathy with or without pulmonary reticular opacities and skin, joint, or eye lesions are common presenting signs of sarcoidosis. In patients with sarcoidosis, cardiac involvement is suggested by the presence of arrhythmias, conduction blocks, or heart failure. Cardiac symptoms are the initial presentation of hemochromatosis in up to 15% of patients. In patients with hemochromatosis and restrictive cardiomyopathy by echocardiography, a presumptive diagnosis of myocardial hemochromatosis is appropriate.

Therapy

Limiting dietary sodium to 2 g daily and fluid to 2 liters per day results in fewer hospitalizations for decompensated heart failure. Because exercise may improve both physical and psychological well-being, it is important to encourage patients to participate in a long-term aerobic exercise program that is tailored to their functional capacity. Exercise conditioning also improves metabolic and hemodynamic indices in patients with heart failure.

All forms of sleep-disordered breathing are common in patients with cardiovascular disease, especially heart failure and hypertension. Effective treatment of sleep-disordered breathing is associated with significant improvement in blood pressure control, exercise capacity, and quality of life, as well as decreased rates of disease progression and rehospitalization for heart failure.

Drug Therapy

Table 2 outlines medical therapy for chronic heart failure by functional status. ACE inhibitors are indicated for treatment of all NYHA functional classes of systolic heart failure, including asymptomatic (NYHA class I) disease. ACE inhibitors delay the onset of clinical heart failure in patients with asymptomatic left ventricular dysfunction, and they reduce morbidity and mortality. Overall, ACE inhibitor therapy reduces mortality by about 20%, risk for MI by about 20%, and risk for hospitalization for heart failure by 30% to 40%. ARBs also reduce mortality and morbidity in patients with systolic heart failure. The primary reason to use an ARB instead of an ACE inhibitor is to avoid the side effect of cough. Combined treatment with an ACE inhibitor and an ARB generally is not recommended, as additional benefit of using these two medications together is not well established; furthermore, concurrent therapy is significantly associated with increased risk of worsening kidney function, hyperkalemia, and hypotension.

Table 2. Medical Therapy for Systolic Heart Failure by Functional Status

Initial Therapy

All NYHA classes (I–IV)

ACE inhibitor (if ACE inhibitor is not tolerated because of cough, an ARB can be used; if ACE inhibitor is contraindicated because of hyperkalemia or renal insufficiency, combined hydralazine and isosorbide dinitrate can be used)

β-Blocker

Additional Therapy

NYHA class I or II (asymptomatic or mild symptoms)

Diuretic as needed to maintain euvolemia

NYHA class III or IV (moderate to severe symptoms)

Spironolactone (if gynecomastia occurs, eplerenone can be used)

Combined hydralazine and isosorbide dinitrate (for black patients)

Digoxin

Diuretic as needed to maintain euvolemia

ARB = angiotensin receptor blocker; NYHA = New York Heart Association.

As with ACE inhibitors, β-blockers are indicated for treatment of systolic heart failure of any NYHA functional class, including asymptomatic (NYHA class I) and severe (NYHA class IV) disease. Treatment with a β-blocker is consistently associated with a 30% reduction in total mortality. Both sudden death and death due to pump failure are reduced. In the United States, carvedilol and extended-release metoprolol (metoprolol succinate) are approved for the treatment of heart failure. In general, β-blockers should not be initiated when a patient is acutely decompensated (hypotensive or volume overloaded), as initiation of therapy is associated with a transient decline in cardiac output. β-Blockers can be initiated and tolerated once euvolemia or near-euvolemia has been established. The risk of exacerbating bronchospastic pulmonary disease with β-blockers is low, except in patients with the most refractory pulmonary disease. If reactive airway disease is a concern, more cardioselective (β₁-receptor–selective) agents such as metoprolol should be used.

Diuretics are used for the management of volume overload and typically are needed acutely to achieve euvolemia before starting β-blocker therapy and on a long-term basis to prevent recurrent volume overload. Spironolactone is the only diuretic that has been shown to improve survival in heart failure (for NYHA class III or IV); however, the diuretic effect is weak at the doses typically used for heart failure treatment. Spironolactone further blocks the actions of aldosterone, which is not completely suppressed by chronic ACE inhibitor therapy; aldosterone has adverse effects of sodium retention, potassium wasting, and myocardial fibrosis. In general, loop diuretics (e.g., furosemide, bumetanide, torsemide) are used for volume management in heart failure because of their superior natriuretic effects compared with other classes of diuretics.

In patients in sinus rhythm, digoxin is used primarily for symptom control. Treatment with digoxin has not been shown to affect mortality but has been shown to reduce hospitalizations.

One study demonstrated that black patients with severe heart failure (NYHA class III or IV) had a significant (approximately 40%) reduction in mortality with the addition of hydralazine and isosorbide dinitrate to standard heart failure therapy (i.e., ACE inhibitor or ARB, β-blocker, spironolactone, digoxin, and diuretics).

First-generation calcium channel blockers (e.g., nifedipine) have been shown to increase the risk of heart failure decompensation and hospitalization; however, second-generation dihydropyridine calcium channel blockers do not appear to increase the risk of decompensation or to adversely affect mortality. These agents can be used in patients with heart failure for the management of hypertension or angina not adequately controlled with other agents (e.g., ACE inhibitors, β-blockers). Amlodipine and felodipine are the only calcium channel blockers with demonstrated neutral effects on mortality in patients with heart failure.

Management of peripartum cardiomyopathy includes early delivery and standard medical therapy with β-blockers, digoxin, and diuretics prior to delivery. Because of teratogenicity, ACE inhibitors and ARBs are withheld until after delivery.

The management of patients with heart failure and preserved left ventricular function is based largely on theoretical concepts and extrapolation from trials in patients with low ejection fractions. There is general agreement that the approach to such patients includes control of heart rate and blood pressure, maintenance of normal sinus rhythm, and identification and management of myocardial ischemia.

Device Therapy and Cardiac Transplantation

Patients with NYHA class III or IV heart failure, an ejection fraction ≤35%, and a prolonged QRS duration (>120 msec) on electrocardiography should be referred for biventricular pacing. Cardiac resynchronization therapy in these patients improves functional capacity, quality of life, and mortality. Cardiac resynchronization therapy is not indicated for patients with heart failure and preserved left ventricular function.

In patients with significant left ventricular systolic dysfunction (ejection fraction ≤35%), NYHA class II or III heart failure while on optimal medical therapy, and life expectancy >1 year, implantation of a cardioverter-defibrillator is associated with a reduction in mortality regardless of whether the underlying cardiomyopathy is secondary to an ischemic or nonischemic cause (Table 3).

Cardiac transplantation improves survival, functional status, and quality of life in patients with NYHA class III or IV heart failure. Relative contraindications to cardiac transplantation include age >65 years, end-organ damage from diabetes or vascular disease, malignancy, previous stroke, lack of psychosocial support, or active psychiatric illness.

Follow-Up

The Seattle Heart Failure Model (www.SeattleHeartFailureModel.org) is a multivariate model that can help estimate 1-, 2-, and 5-year survival. Once the diagnosis and underlying cause of heart failure are established, factors responsible for any symptomatic exacerbations need to be identified and corrected. Common rea-

Table 3. Indications for Device Therapy in Heart Failure

Implantable Cardioverter-Defibrillator

NYHA class II or III while on optimal medical therapy[a] *and*

Life expectancy >1 year *and*

Either of the following:

> Ischemic or nonischemic cardiomyopathy with ejection fraction ≤35% (primary prevention)

> History of hemodynamically significant ventricular arrhythmia or cardiac arrest (secondary prevention)

Cardiac Resynchronization Therapy

All of the following:

> NYHA class III or IV

> Ejection fraction ≤35%

> Ventricular dyssynchrony (QRS >120 msec)

NYHA = New York Heart Association.
[a] NYHA class I and ejection fraction ≤30% also is an accepted indication.
Recommendations from Epstein AE, Dimarco JP, Ellenbogen KA, et al; American College of Cardiology; American Heart Association Task Force on Practice Guidelines; American Association for Thoracic Surgery; Society of Thoracic Surgeons. ACC/AHA/HRS 2008 Guidelines for device-based therapy of cardiac rhythm abnormalities [published erratum appears in Heart Rhythm. 2009;6:e2]. Heart Rhythm. 2008;5:e1-62. [PMID: 18534360]

sons for an increase in symptoms or a decline in functional status include myocardial ischemia or infarction, cardiac arrhythmias (i.e., atrial fibrillation), severe hypertension, worsening kidney function, and nonadherence with medications or dietary recommendations. In general, any condition that causes tachycardia (e.g., fever, infection, anemia, thyrotoxicosis) has the potential to worsen heat failure symptoms by shortening diastole and impairing left ventricular filling. It is important to be aware that concomitant use of noncardiac medications (e.g., NSAIDs, thiazolidinediones) may cause significant fluid retention and worsen heart failure.

Serial measurements of a patient's weight will determine clinical stability or the need to adjust diuretic doses. Electrolyte disturbances in heart failure are common due to the effect of medications as well as the pathophysiology of heart failure. Echocardiographic reassessment of ejection fraction is most useful when there is a notable change in clinical status rather than at regular or arbitrary intervals.

Book Enhancement

Go to www.acponline.org/essentials/cardiovascular-section.html. In *MKSAP for Students 5*, assess your knowledge with items 35-41 in the **Cardiovascular Medicine** section.

Acknowledgment

We would like to thank Dr. James L. Sebastian, who contributed to an earlier version of this chapter.

Bibliography

Goldberg LR. Heart failure. Ann Intern Med. 2010;152:ITC61-15; quiz ITC616. [PMID: 20513825]

Chapter 8

Valvular Heart Disease

H. Douglas Walden, MD

Prevention

Antibiotic treatment of group A streptococcal infections and long-term prophylactic antibiotic therapy for patients with a history of rheumatic carditis may decrease the likelihood of rheumatic valvular heart disease (see Chapter 58).

Screening

Routine screening for valvular heart disease is not recommended, although a high degree of suspicion is appropriate whenever a patient presents with chest pain, heart failure, arrhythmias, congenital abnormalities (e.g., Marfan syndrome), or a history of rheumatic fever.

Approach to Cardiac Murmurs

Cardiac murmurs result from increased blood flow across a normal orifice (e.g., anemia, thyrotoxicosis, pregnancy, atrial septal defect), turbulent flow through a narrowed orifice (e.g., aortic stenosis, mitral stenosis), or regurgitant flow through an incompetent valve (e.g., aortic regurgitation, mitral regurgitation). Timing in the cardiac cycle, chest wall location, radiation, intensity (Table 1), configuration, duration, and pitch all assist in the differential diagnosis (Table 2). Not all systolic murmurs are pathologic. Short, soft systolic murmurs (grade <3) that are asymptomatic often do not require further investigation. The presence of any diastolic or continuous murmur, cardiac symptoms (e.g., chest pain, dyspnea, syncope), or abnormalities on examination (e.g., clicks, abnormal S_2, abnormal pulses) requires evaluation by echocardiography.

Various interventions may alter the intensity of murmurs. The murmur of hypertrophic cardiomyopathy may increase with standing or Valsalva maneuver (decreased venous return decreases left ventricular chamber size and increases the degree of obstruction). The click and murmur of mitral valve prolapse may move earlier in systole and increase in intensity with standing or Valsalva maneuver (mitral prolapse increases with decreased ventricular volume and chamber size).

Aortic outflow murmurs increase in the intensity in the beat following a premature ventricular contraction (increased left ventricular volume). Murmurs of mitral regurgitation, ventricular septal defect, and aortic regurgitation increase with handgrip (increased cardiac output and peripheral resistance). Right-sided heart murmurs may increase during inspiration (increased venous return).

Characteristics of the S_2 may assist in determining the severity of a valvular lesion. A fixed split of S_2 (present during inspiration and expiration) results from a delay in right ventricular emptying (atrial septal defect). A paradoxical split of S_2 (present during expi-

ration) indicates a delay in left ventricular emptying (severe aortic stenosis). Presence of a physiologic split (present during inspiration) is helpful for excluding severe aortic stenosis.

Aortic Stenosis

In adults, aortic stenosis occurs as a result of rheumatic heart disease (patients aged 30-40 years), degeneration of a congenital bicuspid valve (patients aged 50-60 years), or senile degeneration of a normal trileaflet valve (patients aged ≥70 years). A prolonged asymptomatic period of many years is marked by progressive left ventricular hypertrophy and is followed by a shorter symptomatic period (1-3 years) characterized by angina, syncope, and heart failure. Surgical valve replacement is the definitive therapy.

Diagnosis

Exercise intolerance is an early symptom; symptoms of more advanced disease include dyspnea, angina, or exertional syncope. Physical examination reveals a crescendo-decrescendo systolic murmur loudest at the second right intercostal space, with radiation to the carotid arteries. The murmur becomes longer and peaks later in systole with more advanced disease. It may soften in the presence of left ventricular dysfunction; the intensity of the murmur does not correlate with severity of disease. The S_2 may be diminished in intensity, because the valve loses mobility in patients with calcific disease. In younger patients with mild to moderate aortic stenosis due to a bicuspid valve, S_2 may be accentuated and associated with an aortic ejection click heard best at the right upper sternal border just prior to the murmur. An S_4 gallop may accompany left ventricular hypertrophy. Pulsus parvus et tardus (dampened and delayed carotid pulsations) may be present, but carotid upstrokes can be brisk in elderly patients with noncompliant vessels.

Grade	Description
1	Murmur heard with the stethoscope, but not at first
2	Faint murmur heard with the stethoscope on the chest wall
3	Murmur heard with the stethoscope on the chest wall; louder than grade 2 but without a thrill
4	Murmur associated with a thrill
5	Murmur heard with just the rim of the stethoscope held against the chest
6	Murmur heard with the stethoscope held close to but not touching the chest wall

Table 1. Grading the Intensity of Cardiac Murmurs

Table 2. Cardiac Murmurs and Associated Findings

Cause of Murmur	Characteristic	Location	Radiation	Associated Findings
Systolic Murmurs				
Innocent flow murmur	Soft, midsystolic	Base	None	Normal splitting of S_2
Aortic stenosis	Crescendo-decrescendo, midsystolic	Base	Carotids	Single S_2, pulsus parvus, S_4
Hypertrophic obstructive cardiomyopathy	Crescendo, mid- or late systolic	Lower left sternal border	Carotids	Bifid carotid impulse; murmur decreases with passive leg elevation or handgrip, increases with Valsalva
Mitral regurgitation	Holo- or late systolic	Apex	Axilla or back	Murmur increases with isometric exercise; best heard with patient in left lateral decubitus position
Mitral valve prolapse with mitral regurgitation	Late systolic	Apex	Axilla	With Valsalva, murmur and midsystolic click move closer to S_1, and murmur increases in intensity
Tricuspid regurgitation	Holosystolic	Lower left sternal border	Lower right sternal border	Prominent *v* waves in neck; murmur increases with inspiration
Diastolic Murmurs				
Aortic regurgitation	Decrescendo	Second right or third to fourth left intercostal space	None	Widened pulse pressure, bounding carotid pulses; murmur best heard with patient in upright position, leaning forward, at end-expiration
Pulmonic regurgitation	Mid-diastolic	Upper left sternal border	None	Loud S_2 if pulmonary hypertension is present
Mitral stenosis	Low-pitched rumble	Apex	None	Murmur best heard with patient in left lateral decubitus position; opening snap

Chest radiographs often are normal but may demonstrate a boot-shaped silhouette of left ventricular hypertrophy. Electrocardiograms (ECGs) may demonstrate changes consistent with left atrial or left ventricular enlargement. Echocardiograms often demonstrate thickened and calcified aortic valve leaflets with restricted motion. Doppler studies can estimate the transvalvular pressure gradient and aortic valve area. CT can be helpful in evaluating the aortic root to exclude aortic aneurysm, which is particularly common in patients with a bicuspid aortic valve. A coronary angiogram is obtained in patients aged >35 years prior to aortic valve surgery and most patients aged <35 years with left ventricular systolic dysfunction or risk factors for premature coronary disease.

Therapy

Aortic valve replacement is indicated in patients with symptomatic severe disease (valve area <1.0 cm^2) but not for most asymptomatic patients. Left ventricular failure is associated with an increased mortality rate but is not a contraindication to surgery. Ventricular function often improves after valve replacement. Balloon aortic valvuloplasty does not improve survival and is associated with a high rate of restenosis but can be considered as a temporizing measure in select patients.

Atrial fibrillation often is poorly tolerated due to loss of the atrial contractile kick and inadequate diastolic filling with faster heart rates. Cardioversion or atrioventricular nodal blocking agents (e.g., diltiazem, metoprolol) are used to manage atrial fibrillation. Careful use of ACE inhibitors, digoxin, and diuretics may result in symptomatic improvement in heart failure, but these medications are of limited value if surgical therapy is not possible.

Follow-Up

Asymptomatic patients with mild disease typically remain stable for years. The degree of aortic valve calcification, the presence of coronary disease, and more severe valvular disease predict worse outcomes without surgery. A history and physical examination and transthoracic echocardiography are performed at least annually, with more frequent clinical evaluations in patients with more advanced disease. Transthoracic echocardiography is repeated periodically, depending upon the severity of the valvular stenosis.

Aortic Insufficiency

Acute, severe aortic insufficiency is caused by infective endocarditis, aortic dissection, or trauma; it often presents as cardiogenic shock and usually requires emergent valve replacement. Chronic aortic insufficiency may result from rheumatic heart disease, previous endocarditis, a bicuspid aortic valve, aortic root disease, or tertiary syphilis. Acute disease and chronic disease differ in clinical presentation.

Diagnosis

The diagnosis of acute aortic insufficiency is suggested in patients with rapid onset of dyspnea, exercise intolerance, or chest pain (aortic dissection). Physical findings include tachycardia, hypotension, a soft S_1 (due to premature closure of the mitral valve), an S_3 gallop, an accentuated pulmonic valve closure sound (P_2), and pulmonary crackles. Heart size may be normal, and pulse pressure may not be widened. The typical murmur of aortic insufficiency may not be prominent in acute disease, as aortic and left ventricular diastolic pressures equilibrate quickly, resulting in a short and soft (sometimes inaudible) diastolic murmur.

Symptoms of chronic disease include dyspnea on exertion, orthopnea, paroxysmal nocturnal dyspnea, angina, and palpitations. Some patients remain asymptomatic for long periods as the left ventricle insidiously dilates. Physical findings include cardiomegaly, tachycardia, a widened pulse pressure, a thrill at the base of the heart, a soft S_1 and sometimes absent aortic valve closure sound (A_2), and an S_3 gallop. The characteristic high-pitched diastolic murmur begins immediately after S_2 and is heard at the second right or third left intercostal space; it is heard best with the patient seated and leaning forward at end-expiration. Manifestations of the widened pulse pressure may include Traube sign (pistol shot sounds over the peripheral arteries), Musset sign (head bobs with each heartbeat), Duroziez murmur (systolic and diastolic murmur heard over the femoral artery), and Quincke pulse (systolic plethora and diastolic blanching in the nail bed with nail compression).

Chest radiographs may reveal cardiomegaly, valve calcification, enlargement of the aortic root, or pulmonary congestion. ECG findings can include left axis deviation and left ventricular hypertrophy. A serologic test (i.e., VDRL, rapid plasma reagin) is needed to exclude tertiary syphilis. Doppler echocardiography with color flow can confirm the presence and severity of disease and assess cause.

Therapy

Immediate aortic valve replacement is indicated in acute disease, because a normal left ventricle cannot accommodate the large regurgitant volume. Aortic valve replacement also is the treatment of choice for patients with severe chronic disease. Left ventricular systolic function is the most important determinant of survival. Valve replacement is indicated for all patients with more than mild symptoms, patients with progressive left ventricular dilatation, and patients with a left ventricular ejection fraction <50%.

In acute disease, sodium nitroprusside or intravenous nitroglycerin leads to augmentation of forward cardiac output, reduction of regurgitant flow, and an improved ejection fraction as a bridge to valve replacement. Intravenous diuretics and inotropic agents (dobutamine) also may support blood pressure and improve cardiac contractility. In chronic aortic insufficiency, the role of vasodilators is unclear. Nifedipine, hydralazine, or an ACE inhibitor may be helpful as a short-term measure in symptomatic patients or for patients with left ventricular dysfunction who are unable to undergo surgical valve replacement. Prognosis for asymptomatic patients with a preserved ejection fraction is excellent without drug therapy; there is no clear benefit of vasodilators in this group.

Follow-Up

A history and physical examination and echocardiography are performed every 2 to 3 years in asymptomatic patients with normal left ventricular size and function. Evaluation every 6 to 12 months is needed in asymptomatic patients with severe aortic insufficiency and in patients with dilated left ventricles. Echocardiography also should be obtained in patients with new or changing symptoms, worsening exercise tolerance, or clinical findings suggestive of progressive disease. Transthoracic echocardiography is repeated periodically, depending upon the severity of the valvular stenosis.

Mitral Stenosis

Nearly all mitral stenosis in adults is due to rheumatic heart disease. Rare causes include malignant carcinoid syndrome, systemic lupus erythematosus, rheumatoid arthritis, and amyloidosis. Thickening and calcification of the valve impair flow from the left atrium to the left ventricle, leading to pulmonary hypertension and right-sided heart failure. Symptoms develop after years of valvular dysfunction. Surgical valve repair is the definitive treatment of severe disease.

Diagnosis

Symptoms of mitral stenosis include dyspnea, fatigue, edema, orthopnea, paroxysmal nocturnal dyspnea, cough, hemoptysis, hoarseness, chest pain, palpitations, and symptoms suggestive of systemic embolism. Exertional symptoms often develop when the valve area is <1.5 cm^2, whereas resting symptoms can be present when the valve area is <1.0 cm^2. Symptoms may develop with larger valve areas during exercise, pregnancy, or infection or with atrial fibrillation. Physical findings include a prominent a wave in the jugular pulse (decreased right ventricular compliance with pulmonary hypertension), a palpable thrill at the apex, a right ventricular heave, and signs of right-sided heart failure (e.g., jugular venous distention, hepatomegaly, ascites, edema). Cardiac auscultation reveals an accentuated P_2 (evidence of elevated pulmonary artery pressure), an opening snap (a high-pitched apical sound best heard with the diaphragm), and a low-pitched, rumbling diastolic murmur best heard at the apex using the bell, with the patient in the left lateral decubitus position. Presystolic accentuation of the murmur may be present in both sinus rhythm and atrial fibrillation. As the severity of the stenosis worsens, the opening snap moves closer to S_2 as a result of increased left atrial pressure, and the murmur increases in duration.

A chest radiograph may reveal chamber enlargement and interstitial edema. ECG findings often include rhythm abnormalities (i.e., atrial fibrillation in 30% of symptomatic patients), right axis deviation, and left atrial and right ventricular enlargement. Transthoracic Doppler echocardiography can assess mitral valve morphology, involvement of other valves, chamber size and function, and presence of a left atrial thrombus and can exclude other conditions that mimic mitral stenosis. The valve area, the pressure gradient across the valve, and concomitant mitral regurgitation can be determined using Doppler techniques.

Therapy

Mitral valvotomy or valve replacement is the treatment of choice in symptomatic patients. Percutaneous balloon valvotomy is suitable in symptomatic patients with moderate to severe disease and pliable noncalcified leaflets with minimal mitral regurgitation. Valve replacement is recommended for patients with moderate or severe disease (marked limitation of physical activity or inability to perform any physical activity) who are not candidates for valvotomy or valve repair, or for patients with severe pulmonary hypertension. Mortality associated with mitral valve replacement depends on functional status, age, left ventricular function, and the presence of coronary artery disease but may be as high as 10% to 20% in older patients with comorbidities.

β-Blockers or calcium channel blockers with negative chronotropic properties increase diastolic filling time and are used for patients with symptoms associated with tachycardia. Diuretics are useful if pulmonary vascular congestion is present. Atrial fibrillation usually is treated with anticoagulants and atrioventricular nodal blocking agents to control heart rate, but antiarrhythmic agents or cardioversion may be considered for worsening symptoms. Warfarin therapy (goal INR of 2.0-3.0) is recommended for patients with a history of prior embolic events and for patients with atrial fibrillation, sinus rhythm and an enlarged left atrium, or left atrial thrombi.

Follow-Up

Asymptomatic and mildly symptomatic patients are evaluated annually with a history and physical examination, electrocardiography, and chest radiography. Patients who have undergone percutaneous or surgical mitral valvuloplasty are evaluated with postprocedure echocardiography and an annual evaluation thereafter. An echocardiogram is obtained if symptoms recur or if a change is noted on physical examination.

Mitral Regurgitation

Acute mitral regurgitation may result from chordae tendineae rupture, papillary muscle rupture or dysfunction in patients with acute coronary syndrome, myxomatous degeneration, infective endocarditis, trauma, or acute myocardial ischemia. Mitral valve prolapse currently is the most common cause of chronic disease, followed by ischemic mitral valve disease and damage from infective endocarditis. Mitral annular calcification is a common cause of mitral regurgitation in older patients, whereas rheumatic heart disease is now a relatively uncommon cause.

Diagnosis

Acute, severe mitral regurgitation causes abrupt onset of dyspnea, pulmonary edema, or cardiogenic shock. Physical findings may include hypotension, an apical holosystolic murmur radiating to the axilla (the murmur may be short or absent), an S_3 or S_4 gallop, pulmonary crackles, and signs of right-sided heart failure (e.g., jugular venous distention, hepatomegaly, edema).

Chronic mitral regurgitation results in exercise intolerance, dyspnea, or fatigue. Physical findings include brisk carotid upstrokes, a laterally displaced apical impulse, decreased intensity

of S_1, increased intensity of P_2, a widely split S_2 during inspiration, and an S_3 gallop. The holosystolic murmur is best heard with the diaphragm at the apex, with the patient in the left lateral decubitus position; the murmur may radiate to the left axilla and left scapular region. In advanced cases, chest radiographs may reveal cardiomegaly and pulmonary vascular congestion. An ECG may demonstrate an abnormal rhythm (i.e., atrial fibrillation) and findings consistent with left atrial enlargement and left ventricular hypertrophy. Doppler echocardiography allows for assessment of left atrial and left ventricular volumes, ejection fraction, and other valvular disease. The left ventricular ejection fraction may be normal or falsely elevated due to systolic ejection of a portion of left ventricular volume into the low-pressure left atrium.

Therapy

Repair or replacement of the mitral valve is indicated in symptomatic patients with acute disease. Vasodilators (sodium nitroprusside, nitroglycerin) and diuretics reduce pulmonary congestion and improve forward cardiac output. An inotropic agent (dobutamine) may be used if hypotension develops. Intra-aortic balloon counterpulsation can improve coronary perfusion and reduce afterload in hemodynamically unstable patients as a bridge to valve replacement.

In chronic disease, survival is dependent on left ventricular function, and surgery is most effective prior to development of heart failure, atrial fibrillation, and pulmonary hypertension. Patients who display echocardiographic features of left ventricular dilatation and/or depressed function are candidates for surgical intervention. Valve repair has advantages over replacement, including the avoidance of anticoagulants and future mechanical valve failure. In chronic mitral regurgitation with depressed left ventricular function, diuretics, β-blockers, and ACE inhibitors (or angiotensin receptor blockers) are indicated. Anticoagulants and atrioventricular nodal blocking agents are used in patients with atrial fibrillation.

Follow-Up

Annual history, physical examination, and echocardiography are appropriate for mild disease. More frequent monitoring is indicated for advanced disease. Patients with evidence of progressive left ventricular dysfunction require surgical intervention.

Mitral Valve Prolapse

Mitral valve prolapse results from myxomatous degeneration and is the most common congenital valvular abnormality, with a prevalence of up to 4% to 5%. Many patients are asymptomatic, others require symptomatic treatment, and occasional patients may progress to severe mitral regurgitation requiring valve replacement or repair.

Diagnosis

Patients may experience chest pain, palpitations, dizziness, syncope, dyspnea, fatigue, or symptoms of embolic phenomena. Many symptoms cannot be attributed directly to valvular dysfunction. Auscultation may reveal a high-pitched, midsystolic click sometimes followed by a late systolic murmur that is loudest at the apex. The click and murmur are accentuated and move earlier into systole as left ventricular volume decreases (standing or Valsalva maneuver).

Chest radiographs may reveal chamber enlargement, thoracic aneurysm formation, and skeletal abnormalities (e.g., pectus excavatum or carinatum, abnormalities of the thoracic spine). An ECG may reveal a prolonged QT interval and arrhythmias. Echocardiography is used to assess severity of mitral regurgitation, mitral leaflet morphology, and left ventricular size and function. Severe regurgitation, thick and redundant leaflets, flail leaflets, and left atrial and left ventricular enlargement are associated with adverse outcomes.

Therapy

Dietary and lifestyle modifications (i.e., restriction of alcohol and caffeine intake, smoking cessation) are the initial treatment of palpitations, chest pain, anxiety, and fatigue. If symptoms persist, β-blockers are used. Anticoagulation with warfarin is indicated if structural cardiac disease and atrial fibrillation are present. Surgical intervention (mitral valve repair or replacement) is indicated for severe mitral regurgitation.

Follow-Up

Serial echocardiograms are useful for patients with thickened, redundant mitral leaflets, chest pain, syncope, or left ventricular dysfunction/mitral regurgitation. Development of significant mitral regurgitation may ultimately lead to the need for mitral valve surgery.

Tricuspid Valve Disease

Tricuspid valve regurgitation is almost always an acquired process, not a primary valvular disease. Pulmonary hypertension due to chronic lung disease or left-sided heart failure causes right ventricular enlargement, with stretching of the tricuspid annulus. Other causes may include carcinoid heart disease, irradiation, and drug exposure (e.g., fenfluramine, dexfenfluramine, pergolide, ergotamine, methysergide).

Diagnosis

Most patients are asymptomatic, with mild to moderate tricuspid regurgitation. Dyspnea, ascites, and edema can appear with severe regurgitation. Examination reveals a systolic murmur, which is loudest at the lower left sternal border and may increase with inspiration. An ECG may reveal right axis deviation and changes consistent with right atrial enlargement and right ventricular enlargement. Echocardiography can confirm the diagnosis.

Treatment

Diuretics may be helpful for management of ascites and edema. Valve replacement or repair usually is not required but may be needed in refractory cases.

Pregnancy

The increased plasma volume and increased heart rate present during pregnancy may lead to cardiac decompensation in patients with impaired left ventricular function or moderate to severe valvular heart disease. Regurgitant lesions may be tolerated, but stenotic lesions often pose clinical problems due to inadequate diastolic filling with faster heart rates. Mitral stenosis, in particular, may first come to attention during pregnancy. For women with prosthetic heart valves, issues pertaining to anticoagulation during pregnancy require careful attention and discussion among the patient, obstetrician, and cardiologist.

Prosthetic Heart Valves

Decisions regarding the timing of surgical intervention for valvular disease can be difficult and are best made in consultation with a cardiologist and cardiac surgeon. Preservation of left ventricular function is important to optimal cardiac function after surgery, particularly in mitral valve disease.

The choice of a bioprosthetic valve or a mechanical prosthetic valve is an individualized decision based primarily on patient age and suitability or desirability of warfarin anticoagulation. Mechanical valves are more durable than bioprostheses, but they require long-term warfarin anticoagulation to a goal INR of 2.5 to 3.5 (with the addition of aspirin, assuming no contraindication to its use). Bioprostheses are reasonable choices for older patients but also may be used in younger patients who understand the potential future need for a second valve procedure. The development and future use of less invasive techniques of valve replacement (e.g., percutaneous catheter-based aortic valve replacement) may make selection of bioprostheses even more reasonable as an initial choice. Patients with bioprostheses in the aortic or mitral position and without known risk factors for embolic events (e.g., atrial fibrillation, left ventricular dysfunction, previous thromboembolism, hypercoagulable state) may be treated with aspirin without the addition of warfarin. All patients with prosthetic heart valves should receive antibiotic prophylaxis for prevention of infective endocarditis.

Patients with prosthetic valves should be monitored clinically for evidence of valvular dysfunction. Findings suggestive of prosthetic aortic valvular dysfunction can include loss of a sharp valve click and development of the diastolic murmur of aortic regurgitation. A systolic ejection murmur secondary to turbulent flow is common after aortic valve replacement and is not evidence of valvular dysfunction. Evidence suggesting prosthetic mitral valvular dysfunction includes loss of a sharp valve click and development of the blowing murmur of mitral regurgitation. Routine serial echocardiography is not needed in asymptomatic patients. Echocardiography is indicated when clinical symptoms or clinical examination suggests the presence of prosthetic valvular dysfunction.

Book Enhancement

Go to www.acponline.org/essentials/cardiovascular-section.html. In *MKSAP for Students 5*, assess your knowledge with items 21, 42-49 in the **Cardiovascular Medicine** section.

Bibliography

Etchells E, Bell C, Robb K. Does this patient have an abnormal systolic murmur? JAMA. 1997;277:564-571. [PMID: 9032164]

Chapter 9

Diabetes Mellitus

Erik K. Alexander, MD

Diabetes mellitus is a heterogeneous disorder with a common clinical phenotype of inappropriate glucose metabolism. Nearly 20 million people in the United States have been diagnosed with diabetes, the vast majority of whom have type 2 diabetes. This number is increasing and largely parallels the epidemic of obesity. Diabetes remains a major contributor to heart disease, blindness, kidney failure, and other complications, making it a major focus for public health initiatives.

Two processes are central to the development of all forms of diabetes mellitus: β-cell failure to produce insulin in a sufficient and reliable manner and/or insulin resistance of peripheral tissues (i.e., muscle and liver). Type 1 diabetes is primarily a disease of complete β-cell failure and lack of circulating insulin; insulin sensitivity usually remains quite normal. This is evident by the fact that insulin doses required to treat patients with type 1 diabetes are similar to a healthy individual's daily endogenous insulin production (30-60 U/day). Type 1 diabetes can occur any time throughout life but most often presents in childhood or early adulthood. Because of the acute onset of symptoms, most cases are detected soon after disease onset.

Type 2 diabetes often is asymptomatic and not diagnosed for several years because of the lack of initial symptoms. Type 2 diabetes is almost always associated with significant insulin resistance. In insulin-treated patients, a total of 100-200 U/day of insulin often is required, confirming the resistance of peripheral tissues to the effects of insulin. Although initial resistance results in augmented insulin secretion from β-cells, this is unsustainable over the long term; this fact is crucial toward understanding the natural history of type 2 diabetes. Over 5 to 10 years, most patients with type 2 diabetes require increased medication (or increased insulin) to maintain glycemic control.

Diabetes can also be rarely attributable to other concurrent illness, other endocrine disorders, genetic syndromes, or medication use (Table 1).

Table 1. Classification of Diabetes Mellitus

Type 1 Diabetes

Autoimmune β-cell destruction, usually leading to absolute insulin deficiency

Type 2 Diabetes

Defect ranging from predominant insulin resistance with relative insulin deficiency to profound insulin deficiency and resistance

Gestational Diabetes Mellitus

Similar pathogenesis to that of type 2 diabetes

Other Specific Types

Genetic defects in β-cell function

Genetic defects in insulin action

Diseases of the exocrine pancreas (pancreatitis, pancreatic cancer, cystic fibrosis, hemochromatosis, pancreatectomy)

Endocrinopathies (Cushing syndrome, acromegaly, glucagonoma, pheochromocytoma)

Drug- or chemical-induced diabetes (corticosteroids, niacin, diazoxide)

Infections associated with β-cell destruction (cytomegalovirus infection, congenital rubella)

Other genetic syndromes associated with diabetes (Down, Turner, Klinefelter, Prader-Willi, Laurence-Moon-Biedl syndromes; myotonic dystrophy; Huntington chorea)

Adapted with permission from American Diabetes Association. Diagnosis and classification of diabetes mellitus. Diabetes Care. 2010;33 Suppl 1:S65. [PMID: 20042775]

prediabetes, a lifestyle modification program reduced the incidence of diabetes from 29% to 14% over a 3-year period. A separate cohort of patients received metformin therapy. This intervention reduced the incidence of diabetes from 29% to 22%. Thus, while beneficial, the medication intervention was less powerful than lifestyle changes. Several other investigations have confirmed these findings.

Prevention

There are no data to suggest any available lifestyle or pharmacologic intervention can delay the onset of type 1 diabetes. However, several randomized trials confirm that lifestyle interventions and certain medications can reduce the incidence of type 2 diabetes. Dietary and exercise programs that lead to mild to moderate weight loss (5%-7% reduction) in overweight or obese patients are associated with most impressive clinical outcomes. Perhaps the most commonly cited investigation is the Diabetes Prevention Program. In this randomized, controlled trial of 3234 adults with

Screening

There is no recommendation to screen individuals for type 1 diabetes. Screening the general population for type 2 diabetes also is not recommended. The U.S. Preventive Services Task Force (USPSTF) has concluded that the current evidence is insufficient to assess the benefit versus harm of routine screening for type 2 diabetes in asymptomatic adults with blood pressure ≤135/80 mm Hg. The USPSTF recommends screening for type 2 diabetes in asymptomatic adults with sustained blood pressure (treated or untreated) >135/80 mm Hg, because in patients with diabetes, lowering the blood pressure to <130/80 mm Hg reduces cardiovascular events and cardiovascular mortality. This case-finding approach to screening is recommended because diabetic status alters the management goals for such patients.

Diagnosis

Medical history, physical examination, and appropriate laboratory testing are required for the diagnosis of diabetes. Target any patient with symptoms consistent with the disease (e.g., unexplained weight loss, frequent infections, polyuria, impotence) or relevant physical findings (e.g., acanthosis nigricans, peripheral neuropathy, recurrent vaginal yeast infections, proliferative retinopathy).

A random plasma glucose value ≥200 mg/dL (11.1 mmol/L) is predictive of diabetes, although it should be confirmed on repeat analysis in a fasting state. Fasting plasma glucose ≥126 mg/dL (7.0 mmol/L) is highly specific for the diagnosis. A hemoglobin A_{1c} (HbA_{1c}) value ≥6.5% also is considered diagnostic of diabetes mellitus (Table 2). A level between 6.0% and 6.4% may identify patients most likely to benefit from strategies aimed at preventing diabetes. Once diabetes is diagnosed, HbA_{1c} measurement, fasting lipid profile, serum electrolyte panel, urinalysis (including testing for microalbuminuria), and electrocardiography are performed to screen for complications and establish baseline values.

Therapy

Improved control of blood glucose levels lowers the incidence of microvascular complications (retinopathy, nephropathy) in patients with type 1 and type 2 diabetes. There is conflicting evidence about whether improving glucose levels also benefits macrovascular complications (myocardial infarction, stroke, peripheral arterial disease). The most reliable assessment of overall glycemic status is a periodic measurement of the HbA_{1c} value. This test allows practitioners to determine the average degree of glycemia over the previous 2 to 3 months. Ideally, the HbA_{1c} value should be <7.0% (normal range, 4.0%-6.0%).

Several large studies have evaluated the benefit of more strict glucose control (HbA_{1c} <6%-6.5%) on cardiovascular outcomes and mortality. These studies did not demonstrate a decreased incidence of myocardial infarction, stroke, or death, but there was an increased incidence of hypoglycemia and, in some studies, an increased mortality rate. At present, while a modest further reduction in microvascular complications can be demonstrated with very low HbA_{1c} targets (<6.5%), the lack of other demonstrated benefit and possible harm currently prohibit widespread adoption. Most importantly, glycemic targets must be individualized, taking into account a patient's risk for hypoglycemia, comorbid conditions that could limit life expectancy, and interpretation of other factors that may limit the safety of attempting more aggressive glucose control.

Patient education and self-management are critical in the management of diabetes. Patient education should be individualized for a patient's specific needs and include information about the disease process, its complications, its relationship to metabolic control, and the key role of diet and exercise in diabetes management. Glucose-monitoring techniques, the proper administration of oral agents and insulin, the treatment of hypoglycemia, and the situations in which medical care should be sought must also be carefully reviewed. Diabetes self-management training is optimally provided outside of routine physician office visits by an interdisciplinary team composed of, at minimum, a diabetes educator and a nutritionist who work in conjunction with the patient's primary care physician.

Home glucose monitoring allows patients and providers to assess glucose control longitudinally. Home monitoring should be considered for all patients with diabetes, particularly those on insulin therapy. Home monitoring allows real-time assessment of glucose concentrations. This in turn allows patients and physicians to carefully assess treatment strategies. Symptoms can also be monitored to see if they are related to hypoglycemia. Although fasting glucose concentrations usually are most helpful, postprandial measurements also are informative, especially in patients with an elevated HbA_{1c} despite normal fasting glucose levels.

Type 2 Diabetes

Type 2 diabetes is conventionally treated first with diet, weight loss (for overweight or obese patients), and exercise. Such lifestyle modifications reduce insulin resistance and blood glucose levels and also improve cardiovascular risk factors. However, these steps usually are insufficient to attain glucose targets.

Drug therapy is initiated in type 2 diabetes if diet and exercise do not adequately control hyperglycemia. Noninsulin medications available to treat type 2 diabetes are summarized in Table 3. Available insulin preparations are described in Table 4.

Metformin often is a first-line agent in patients with creatinine levels <1.6 mg/dL [141.4 µmol/L] in men, <1.5 mg/dL [132.6 µmol/L] in women and without known liver disease or alcohol abuse. Metformin must be stopped prior to receiving radiocontrast agents. Patients should be counseled about the risk of loose stools, bloating, gas, or other gastrointestinal side effects.

Sulfonylureas also are first-line agents or can be given in combination with metformin. Sulfonylureas are well tolerated and have few contraindications, although they can cause hypoglycemia and should be used with caution in the elderly, especially in the presence of chronic kidney disease.

Table 2. Screening and Diagnostic Tests for Diabetes Mellitus

Test	Threshold Value
Fasting plasma glucose[a]	≥126 mg/dL (7.0 mmol/L)
	100-125 mg/dL (5.6-6.9 mmol/L) = impaired fasting glucose
Random plasma glucose	≥200 mg/dL (11.1 mmol/L) plus hyperglycemia symptoms
Hemoglobin A_{1c}[a]	≥6.5%
Oral glucose tolerance test (2-h)[a]	≥200 mg/dL dL (11.1 mmol/L)
	140-199 mg/dL (7.8-11.0 mmol/L) = impaired glucose tolerance

[a]In the absence of unequivocal hyperglycemia, these tests should be confirmed by repeat testing.

Table 3. Commonly Used Noninsulin Antihyperglycemic Agents for Type 2 Diabetes

Drug Class (examples)	Mechanism of Action	Benefits	Risks/Concerns
Sulfonylureas (glyburide, glipizide, glimepiride)	Bind to sulfonylurea receptor on β-cells, stimulating insulin release; long duration of action	Improved microvascular outcomes; low cost	Hypoglycemia; weight gain
Glinides (repaglinide, nateglinide)	Bind to sulfonylurea receptor on β-cells, stimulating insulin release; short duration of action	Target postprandial glucose	Hypoglycemia; weight gain; no long-term studies; expensive
Biguanides (metformin)	Decrease hepatic glucose production	No hypoglycemia; weight loss or weight neutral; improved macrovascular outcomes; low cost	Diarrhea, abdominal discomfort; many contraindications; lowers vitamin B_{12} levels; avoid in chronic kidney disease
Thiazolidinediones (pioglitazone, rosiglitazone)	Activate the nuclear receptor PPARγ, increasing peripheral insulin sensitivity; may also reduce hepatic glucose production	No hypoglycemia	Edema and heart failure risk; weight gain; possible increased myocardial infarction risk with rosiglitazone; expensive
Incretin modulators (exenatide)	Activate GLP-1 receptors, increasing glucose-dependent insulin secretion, decreasing glucagon secretion, delaying gastric emptying, and enhancing satiety	No hypoglycemia; weight loss	Nausea, vomiting; possible pancreatitis (rare); requires injection; expensive
DPP-4 inhibitors (sitagliptin, saxagliptin)	Inhibit degradation of endogenous GLP-1 and GIP, thereby enhancing the effect of these incretins on insulin and glucagon secretion	No hypoglycemia; weight neutral; once-daily dosing	Possible urticaria/angioedema (rare); no long-term studies; expensive

DPP-4 = dipeptidyl peptidase-4; GIP = gastric inhibitory peptide; GLP-1 = glucagon-like peptide-1; PPARγ = peroxisome proliferator–activated receptor-gamma.

Table 4. Pharmacokinetic Properties of Insulin Products

Human Insulins and Insulin Analogues	Onset	Peak	Duration
Rapid-acting (lispro, aspart, glulisine)	10-15 min	1-2 h	3-5 h
Short-acting (regular)	0.5-1 h	2-4 h	4-8 h
Intermediate-acting (NPH)	1-3 h	4-10 h	10-18 h
Long-acting			
Glargine	2-3 h	none	24+ h
Detemir	1 h	none	12-24 h

NPH = neutral protamine Hagedorn.

Many patients fail to achieve optimal glucose control with metformin and/or sulfonylureas. In such patients, available therapeutic strategies include:

- Initiating an incretin-based therapy while continuing oral medications. Currently available incretin therapies include a glucagon-like peptide-1 (GLP-1) receptor agonist (exenitide) and dipeptidyl peptidase-4 (DPP-4) inhibitors (sitagliptin, saxagliptin). Exenatide is a twice-daily injectable medication that can result in HbA_{1c} reductions of approximately 0.5% to 1.5%; the drug also promotes modest weight loss. Up to 40% of patients using exenatide experience mild nausea, at times precluding continuation of the drug. DPP-4 inhibitors are oral agents that also can result in HbA_{1c} reductions of approximately 0.5% to 1.5%, although without a change in body weight. These drugs are administered once or twice daily and are often associated with mild-to-moderate nausea.

- Initiating insulin therapy while continuing oral medications. Because type 2 diabetes is associated with loss of β-cell function, insulin therapy is a rational option. Initially, a single dose of intermediate or long-acting insulin can be given in the evening. Glycemic control throughout the day is improved if morning fasting glucose concentrations are <100 mg/dL (5.6 mmol/L).

- Initiating a third oral medication. Thiazolidinediones (pioglitazone, rosiglitazone) can result in further reductions in HbA_{1c} of approximately 0.5% to 1.0%. However, recent meta-analyses have suggested that rosiglitazone is associated with increased cardiovascular adverse events compared with placebo. As a result, the FDA has significantly restricted the use of rosiglitazone and warns of the need to continually monitor patients who use the drug. Current evidence of the risks and benefits of using rosiglitazone (and possibly pioglitazone) suggest that these drugs are not optimal for treating type 2 diabetes. They may have a role in unique circumstances, although risks and benefits must be carefully weighed and discussed with the patient in advance. Thiazolidinediones require routine monitoring of liver chemistry tests during the first year of use, and fluid retention is a common side effect. These agents are contraindicated in patients with heart failure or liver dysfunction.

Most experts initiate insulin therapy if the desired level of glycemic control is not achieved with these strategies. The most popular method is to begin with a single, typically nighttime injection of basal (long-acting) insulin, because this simple approach minimizes the risk of hypoglycemia. Basal insulin, although effective in many patients, does not address postprandial glucose excursions. To address postprandial glucose excursions, short- or rapid-acting insulin is added before breakfast and dinner. Another method is twice-daily use of a premixed product that contains both intermediate- and short- or rapid-acting insulins in fixed ratios. Oral agents usually are continued when basal insulin is initiated, although insulin secretagogues (sulfonyluyreas, glinides) can be stopped once prandial insulin is added to the treatment regimen. Regardless, patients should be counseled that consistency in their routine (both time of insulin administration and eating patterns) is paramount to success. Many patients with type 2 diabetes will require a total daily insulin dose equal to 1 U/kg body weight, although highly insulin-resistant patients may require a higher daily dose. Insulin therapy is also considered the standard of care for treating diabetes mellitus during pregnancy, although some recent studies suggest certain oral agents may prove to be safe.

Type 1 Diabetes

Insulin is the primary therapeutic intervention for patients with type 1 diabetes and is required to avoid ketoacidosis. Without insulin, patients will become hyperglycemic (and ultimately ketotic) within 24 to 48 hours. Insulin therapy most frequently consists of multiple daily subcutaneous injections of long- and short- or rapid-acting insulins. A common regimen is a combination of evening basal insulin and short- or rapid-acting insulin before each meal (bolus). An alternative regimen is to administer intermediate-acting insulin twice daily and rapid-acting insulin at breakfast and dinner.

A further option for basal-bolus insulin delivery is the use of an insulin pump. With this therapy, a continuous infusion of short-acting insulin is delivered through a subcutaneous needle implanted under the skin every 72 hours. Patients are able to deliver standard basal rates of insulin throughout the day and bolus insulin at mealtimes. This strategy allows for greater flexibility and precision.

Achieving the therapeutic goal of HbA_{1c} <7% commonly results in mild hypoglycemia. Patients need to be educated about how to avoid hypoglycemia and how to recognize and treat hypoglycemia if it occurs. Frequent daily monitoring of capillary blood glucose is required.

Prevention of Chronic Complications

Microvascular complications of diabetes involve the kidneys (diabetic nephropathy), the retinae (diabetic retinopathy), and the peripheral nerves (diabetic neuropathy). To screen for nephropathy, test all patients with diabetes for urine albumin excretion with a spot urine albumin-creatinine ratio. The presence of microalbuminuria (approximately 30-300 mg/g) should prompt initiation of an angiotensin-converting enzyme inhibitor (ACE) or angiotensin receptor blocker (ARB) for its renoprotective effects.

The highly vascular retina is often affected in patients with long-standing diabetes mellitus and diabetic retinopathy is responsible for most cases of legal blindness in adults in the United States. Hard exudates, microaneurysms, and minor hemorrhages (background diabetic retinopathy) are among the early changes. Although diabetic background retinopathy is not typically associated with any decline in visual acuity, it is associated with an increased risk for the development of significant abnormalities that can lead to visual loss including retinal infarcts and growth of abnormally fragile blood vessels (neovascularization) that predispose to retinal and vitreous hemorrhage. Macular edema may also occur. Laser photocoagulation can preserve sight in these individuals. In addition, blood pressure reduction and glycemic control slows the progression of eye disease.

To prevent foot ulcers, institute foot-care strategies for all patients with diabetes, particularly those with documented diabetic neuropathy. A foot ulcer, defined as any transdermal interruption of skin integrity, is predictive of amputation. Educate patients about inspecting feet daily, wearing appropriate shoes, avoiding high-impact exercise, not going barefoot, and testing water temperature before bathing. Emphasize increased surveillance by the patient and health care team for decreased foot sensation, callus formation, deformities, and structural changes. Prescribe orthotic footwear for patients with foot deformities and to cushion high-pressure areas. Testing sensation with a 5.07/10-g monofilament has been shown to predict ulcer and amputation risk (Plate 1) and to have superior predictive value compared with other sensory test modalities (128-Hz tuning fork, pinprick, cotton wisps) or the presence or absence of neuropathic symptoms. Refer patients with foot ulcers to a multidisciplinary foot clinic, if available; multidisciplinary clinics that specialize in diabetic foot care can reduce amputation rates.

To reduce the risk of macrovascular complications, blood pressure and cholesterol levels are aggressively managed. The American Diabetes Association (ADA) recommends a blood pressure target <130/80 mmHg. The USPSTF and American College of Physicians have adopted a blood pressure target <135/80 mm Hg. Lipid control is usually achieved with the assistance of statin therapy. A low-density lipoprotein (LDL) cholesterol concentration <100 mg/dL (2.6 mmol/L) is desired; an optional goal <70 mm/dL [1.8 mmol/L] should be considered in patients at highest risk for coronary artery disease.

The ADA and American Heart Association recommend aspirin for secondary prevention in patients with a history of myocardial infarction, vascular bypass, stroke or transient ischemic attack, peripheral arterial disease, claudication, or angina. Aspirin is also recommended for primary prevention in patients with diabetes and a 10-year risk of cardiovascular disease >10% (based on the Framingham risk score), which would include most men aged >50 years and women aged >60 years who have at least one additional cardiovascular risk factor.

Hospital Management

Current recommendations for the treatment of hyperglycemia during hospitalization are to use insulin infusions to reduce blood glucose levels to 140 to 180 mg/dL (7.8 to 10.0 mmol/L) in critically ill patients. In noncritically ill patients, insulin generally replaces oral medications. Insulin therapy is adjusted to achieve premeal blood glucose concentrations <140 mg/dL (7.8 mmol/L) and a random glucose target <180 mg/dL (10.0 mmol/L). Current guidelines also emphasize the need to reconsider the widespread use of regular insulin sliding scales as the sole antihyperglycemic therapy in hospitalized patients with diabetes. Instead, more proactive, physiologic insulin regimens, such as a basal-bolus approach, are advised.

Follow-Up

Monitor glycemic control with HbA_{1c} measurements every 3 to 6 months. Obtain an annual fasting lipid profile, including LDL cholesterol, triglyceride, high-density lipoprotein cholesterol, and total cholesterol levels, and adjust treatment to meet goals. Screen annually for diabetic nephropathy with a spot urine test for microalbuminuria. Perform a foot examination at each visit. Obtain an annual dilated funduscopic examination from a specialist, unless otherwise dictated by the specialist. Reinforce the key issues of diabetes self-management, hypoglycemia prevention and treatment, appropriate use of medications, blood glucose monitoring, and lifestyle measures.

Book Enhancement

Go to www.acponline.org/essentials/endocrinology-section.html. In *MKSAP for Students 5*, assess your knowledge with items 1-7 in the **Endocrinology and Metabolism** section.

Bibliography

American Diabetes Association. Standards of medical care in diabetes—2010. Diabetes Care. 2010;33 Suppl 1:S11-61 [published erratum appears in Diabetes Care. 2010;33:692]. [PMID: 20042772]

Chapter 10

Diabetic Ketoacidosis and Hyperglycemic Hyperosmolar Syndrome

Klara J. Rosenquist, MD
Erik K. Alexander, MD

The most life-threatening acute complication of type 1 diabetes mellitus is diabetic ketoacidosis (DKA), occurring in 10% to 20% of patients at the initial presentation of their illness. DKA develops when significant insulin deficiency is coupled with excess circulating levels of counter-regulatory hormones, including glucagon. Insufficient insulin prevents glucose uptake by muscle and liver cells, resulting in profound hyperglycemia and excessive hepatic glucose production. The hyperglycemia is responsible for osmotic diuresis and hypovolemia. The excess glucose is metabolized via the fatty acid degradation pathway to free fatty acids that are converted to β-hydroxybutyrate and acetoacetate by the liver, resulting in ketoacidosis, ketonuria, and electrolyte abnormalities.

Hyperglycemic hyperosmolar syndrome (HHS) is associated with type 2 diabetes. Although HHS shares similar pathophysiology to DKA, residual circulating insulin precludes the onset of ketosis; therefore, acidosis does not occur (Table 1).

Prevention

Once type 1 diabetes has been diagnosed, patient education is paramount in preventing DKA. Patients should be instructed on how to manage their diabetes during illness. When ill, patients with type 1 diabetes must increase the frequency of home blood glucose monitoring, measure urinary or fingerstick ketones regularly, continue insulin (even if not eating), and maintain fluid and carbohydrate intake. Insulin deficiency of even 6 to 12 hours can lead to significant ketosis. Patients should be advised to seek emergent medical care if nausea or vomiting limits oral hydration or if ketone testing is positive.

Diagnosis

Diabetic Ketoacidosis

Symptoms of DKA include polyuria, polydipsia, blurred vision, nausea, vomiting, and abdominal pain. If DKA is severe, patients may have altered mental status or be unresponsive. Symptoms usually occur following infection, trauma, cardiovascular events, and changes in medications such as corticosteroids and thiazide diuretics. However, the most common precipitating event for DKA is insulin nonadherence.

Physical examination will reveal signs of hypovolemia, including tachycardia, hypotension, dry mucous membranes, and poor skin turgor. Kussmaul respiration (deep and frequent breathing) is a sign of metabolic acidosis, and a fruity breath odor is often noted due to acetone elimination by the lungs. The diagnosis is based on a triad of hyperglycemia (blood glucose >250 mg/dL [13.9 mmol/L]), increased anion gap metabolic acidosis (arterial pH <7.30, serum bicarbonate <15 meq/L [15 mmol/L]), and positive serum or urine ketones. Blood urea nitrogen and serum creatinine levels usually are elevated secondary to hypovolemia.

The serum sodium level will often be low due to the hyperglycemia-induced osmotic shifts of fluid into the vascular system. Serum potassium may be elevated due to extracellular potassium shifts caused by acidosis, but total body potassium stores often are depleted because of urinary losses.

Hyperglycemic Hyperosmolar Syndrome

HHS is almost exclusively seen in patients with type 2 diabetes. Signs and symptoms often include altered mental status and evi-

Table 1. Comparison of Diabetic Ketoacidosis and Hyperglycemic Hyperosmolar Syndrome

	Diabetic Ketoacidosis	Hyperglycemic Hyperosmolar Syndrome
Diabetes mellitus classification	Type 1	Type 2
Serum glucose	250 mg/dL- 600 mg/dL (13.9- 33.3 mmol/L)	>600 mg/dL (33.3 mmol/L); often >1,000 mg/dL (55.5 mmol/L)
Serum and urine ketones	Positive	Negative
Anion gap	Elevated	Normal
Serum pH	<7.2	>7.3
Serum osmolality	Variable	>320 mosm/kg (320 mmol/kg)
Serum bicarbonate	<18 meq/L (18 mmol/L)	>18 meq/L (18 mmol/L)

dence of hypovolemia. Common precipitating conditions include infection, trauma, and in some cases myocardial infarction.

Diagnostic criteria for HHS include: plasma glucose >600 mg/dL (33.3 mmol/L); arterial pH >7.30; serum bicarbonate >15 meg/L (15 mmol/L); serum osmolality >320 mosm/kg (320 mmol/kg), and absent urine or serum ketones. The anion gap is usually normal but can be increased in the setting of hypovolemia-induced prerenal azotemia.

Therapy

Diabetic Ketoacidosis

Diabetic ketoacidosis is a life-threatening condition. Patients require hospitalization, often in the intensive care unit. The goals of treatment are the resolution of ketosis (anion gap normalization), volume repletion, and restoration of electrolyte abnormalities. An intravenous (IV) infusion of 0.9% saline is started immediately, along with IV regular insulin. From 2 to 6 L of IV fluid may be required to achieve a euvolemic status. An initial IV bolus of regular insulin (0.15 U/kg) is administered, followed by a constant IV infusion of approximately 0.1 U/kg/h. Blood glucose is monitored hourly, targeting a reduction in serum glucose of 50-100 mg/dL (2.8-5.6 mmol/L) per hour. When serum glucose reaches 250 mg/dL (13.9 mmol/L), the IV solution is changed to 0.45% saline with 5% or 10% dextrose to avoid hypoglycemia. The insulin infusion is continued until the anion gap has normalized and ketones are no longer present. Premature discontinuation of insulin may lead to rebound acidosis. Once ketones are cleared and the anion gap is normalized, patients are begun on subcutaneous insulin with a 2- to 6-hour period of overlapping subcutaneous and IV insulin before the IV insulin is discontinued.

Insulin will cause substantial shifts of potassium and phosphorus from the extracellular to the intracellular space. Therefore, it is important to measure serum potassium every 1 to 2 hours and to replace potassium intravenously. Phosphate repletion typically is not required. Bicarbonate therapy is reserved for severe acidosis (pH <6.9).

The most dangerous complication of DKA treatment is the development of cerebral edema signaled by symptoms of headache and altered mental status. It is most common during the treatment of children and can be fatal. The exact cause is unknown but may be due in part to aggressive hydration with hypotonic fluids.

Hyperglycemic Hyperosmolar Syndrome

Patients with HHS often are hemodynamically unstable and require care in the intensive unit care. The mainstay of treatment is correction of hypovolemia with 0.9% saline, infusing at least 1 L before the initiation of insulin. Half of the fluid deficit should be replaced during the first 24 hours, with the remainder replaced during the following 2 to 3 days (see Chapter 64, Acid-Base Disorders). IV insulin is initiated with a bolus of 0.1 U/kg and continued at a rate of 0.1 U/kg. The goal is to decrease serum glucose by 50-100 mg/dL (2.8-5.6 mmol/L) per hour until glucose is <200 mg/dL (11.1 mmol/L) and the patient is eating, at which point the patient is changed to subcutaneous insulin.

Potassium is monitored closely, as patients may become hypokalemic. IV or oral potassium is provided to maintain serum potassium concentrations between 4.0 and 5.0 meq/L (4-5 mmol/L). Bicarbonate therapy typically is not required. Serum osmolarity is monitored, with a goal of decreasing it by <3 mosm/kg (3 mmol/kg) per hour.

Book Enhancement

Go to www.acponline.org/essentials/endocrinology-section.html. In *MKSAP for Students 5*, assess your knowledge with items 8-10 in the **Endocrinology and Metabolism** section.

Bibliography

Wilson JF. In the clinic. Diabetic ketoacidosis. Ann Intern Med. 2010; 152(1):ITC1-15 [PMID: 20048266]

Chapter 11

Dyslipidemia

D. Michael Elnicki, MD
Gary Tabas, MD

Lipoproteins are protein-bound lipids in the blood. Low-density lipoprotein (LDL) comprises 60% to 70% of total serum cholesterol, is the major atherogenic component, and is the main target for lipid-lowering therapy. High-density lipoprotein (HDL) accounts for 20% to 30% of total serum cholesterol. HDL level is inversely related to coronary heart disease (CHD) risk, but HDL generally is not a target of primary preventive therapy; there is no established goal for HDL. Very-low-density lipoproteins (VLDL) are triglyceride-rich precursors of LDL that are produced by the liver and contain highly atherogenic remnant particles. Intermediate-density lipoproteins (IDL) also are atherogenic and included in the LDL measurement. Chylomicrons are formed in the intestine, are rich in triglyceride, and when partially degraded are atherogenic.

Other lipoproteins are likely involved in the formation of an atheroma. Lp(a) lipoprotein is associated with increased risk for CHD, but treatment with statins does not lower Lp(a) lipoprotein levels or risk. Small LDL particles and HDL subfractions are related to CHD but are not superior to LDL or HDL in predicting risk. Measurement of these other lipoproteins is not routinely indicated.

Prevention

All patients should be advised about lifestyle measures that will reduce lipid levels. These include a healthy diet, regular exercise, weight control, avoidance of tobacco, and moderation of alcohol intake. A healthy diet is one that does not exceed caloric needs, contains less than 25% to 35% of calories from all fat sources (less than 7% from saturated fat), and includes less than 200 mg (5.2 mmol/L) of cholesterol per day. Increasing dietary intake of vegetables, fruits, and high-fiber foods will help lower lipid levels. In particular, LDL cholesterol will be lowered by eating foods with high levels of plant stanols (2 g/day) and increased amounts of soluble fiber (10-25 g/day). Aerobic exercise has beneficial effects on lipid profiles and should be done most days for at least 30 minutes per session. However, any amount of exercise is of benefit, and more is better. Body weight should be brought as close as possible to the ideal BMI. All forms of tobacco should be avoided, and alcohol intake should be moderated to ≤2 drinks per day for men and ≤1 drink per day for women.

Screening

Initiate screening for lipid disorders in men aged 20 to 35 years and in women aged 20 to 40 years using fasting lipid profiles. Repeat screening every 5 years in average-risk patients with normal lipids at initial screening and more frequently in patients with other CHD risk factors or whose diet, weight, or both have changed significantly. Screening for lipid disorders should be continued into advanced age unless patients have a short life expectancy (<1-2 years). Lipid disorders are more common in the elderly and, due to the higher burden of disease, carry as high a CHD-attributable risk as in middle-aged patients, even if the relative risk change is not as great. Lowering lipids also lowers the risk of stroke, an important problem in the elderly.

If a fasting lipid profile is not feasible, total and HDL cholesterol levels can be used for initial screening. If either of these is abnormal, a fasting lipid profile should be obtained. A fasting lipid profile consists of total and HDL cholesterol and triglyceride measurements and calculated LDL cholesterol. LDL cholesterol is calculated using the Friedewald formula:

$$LDL = [total\ cholesterol] - [HDL] - [triglycerides/5]$$
$$(all\ units\ are\ mg/dL)$$

Triglyceride levels >400 mg/dL (4.5 mmol/L) invalidate the Friedewald formula. In this case, LDL cholesterol can be directly measured.

Diagnosis

Perform a thorough history to identify other cardiovascular risk factors, such as cigarette smoking, hypertension, or a family history of premature heart disease. A variety of drugs can cause dyslipidemia, including estrogens, corticosteroids, thiazide diuretics, β-blockers, and androgenic steroids. History can identify CHD risk equivalents such as diabetes mellitus, peripheral vascular disease (aortic aneurysm, claudication), stroke, or a 10-year risk of CHD >20%. Physical examination also can identify CHD risks or CHD equivalents. The examination should include measurement of blood pressure and BMI. Patients with existing cardiovascular disease may have abnormal cardiac examinations, diminished pulses, bruits, or other signs of peripheral vascular disease.

Patients with very high lipids often have cutaneous xanthomas. Eruptive xanthomas are small yellow papules on the trunk or extremities; they are seen when triglycerides are elevated, particularly in familial hypertriglyceridemia.

Tendinous xanthomas are nodules deposited within the extensor tendons; they are seen with high LDL levels, particularly in familial hypercholesterolemia. Tuberous xanthomas are soft yellow papules or nodules that can form lobular masses on extensor surfaces; they are seen with elevations of LDL or triglycerides. Plane

Table 1. Laboratory Tests for Evaluation of Dyslipidemia

Test	Notes
Fasting lipid profile with calculated LDL-C	Obtain two measurements at least 1 wk apart to confirm diagnosis. Results unreliable >24 hr after myocardial infarction, major surgery, or trauma and for 6-8 wk after event onset.
Direct LDL-C measurement	Obtain if triglycerides >400 mg/dL (4.5 mmol/L), which makes Friedewald equation unreliable for calculating LDL-C.
Thyroid-stimulating hormone	Identify hypothyroidism as secondary cause.
Fasting blood glucose (FBG)	Identify uncontrolled diabetes as secondary cause with FBG >126 mg/dL (7.0 mmol/L) on two fasting samples.
Direct bilirubin	Identify obstructive jaundice as a secondary cause if bilirubin >50% above normal.
Alkaline phosphatase, AST/ALT	Identify liver disease as contraindication to some lipid-lowering drugs.
Urine protein	Begin with urine dipstick for overt proteinuria to identify nephrotic syndrome as secondary cause.

ALT = alanine aminotransferase; AST = aspartate aminotransferase; LDL-C = low-density lipoprotein cholesterol.

xanthomas are yellow plaques found in skin folds in the neck, face, upper trunk, and arms; they are seen with elevations of LDL or triglycerides. Xanthelasma are flat yellow papules or plaques around the eyelids seen in familial hypercholesterolemia.

Secondary causes of dyslipidemia—important because they often are treatable (Table 1)—include hypothyroidism, obstructive liver disease, nephrotic syndrome, alcoholism, uncontrolled diabetes, smoking, and kidney failure.

Before making the diagnosis of hyperlipidemia, obtain at least two measures of LDL cholesterol at least 1 week apart. LDL levels are the primary targets of therapy. LDL cholesterol risk categories are shown in Table 2. Further stratification of risk in patients who are above the LDL cholesterol goal of 130 mg/dL (3.4 mmol/L) can be calculated using the Framingham risk equation (www.acponline.org/essentials/endocrinology-section.html), which predicts 10-year risk of CHD. Triglyceride levels are secondary targets for therapy. Levels are classified as normal (<150 mg/dL [1.7 mmol/L]), borderline (150-199 mg/dL [1.7-2.2 mmol/L]), high (200-499 mg/dL [2.3-5.7 mmol/L]), and very high (>500 mg/ dL [5.7 mmol/L]). Very high triglyceride levels can cause pancreatitis and are treated regardless of cardiovascular risk. Low HDL cholesterol (<40 mg/dL [1.0 mmol/L] in men)

is a CHD risk factor and is treated in patients with CHD, as secondary prevention.

Cardiovascular risk factors often occur in clusters. One example of particular importance is the metabolic syndrome, the diagnostic criteria for which are shown in Table 3. The National Cholesterol Education Program Adult Treatment Panel III (ATP III) recommendations state that the metabolic syndrome should be considered a secondary target for risk reduction therapy after LDL cholesterol is evaluated and managed as a primary target. Any person at high or moderately high risk who has lifestyle-related risk factors such as the metabolic syndrome is a candidate for therapeutic lifestyle changes to modify these risk factors regardless of LDL cholesterol level. However, it is not clear whether the metabolic syndrome in itself confers an independent risk beyond that associated with the specific individual risk factors that comprise this syndrome.

Therapy

In patients with moderate-to-low risk for CHD, dietary interventions to reduce LDL cholesterol are appropriate. Switching to a diet low in saturated fat can result in a 5% to 15% reduction in

Table 2. Adult Treatment Panel III Recommendations for LDL Cholesterol Level Management

Risk Category	LDL Cholesterol Goal	Initiate TLC	Consider Drug Therapy
High risk: CHD[a] or CHD risk equivalents[a] (10-y risk >20%)	<100 mg/dL (2.6 mmol/L) (optional goal: <70 mg/dL [1.8 mmol/L])	≥100 mg/dL (2.6 mmol/L)	≥100 mg/dL (3.4 mmol/L)
Moderately high risk: ≥2 risk factors[b] (10-y risk 10%-20%)	<130 mg/dL (3.4 mmol/L)	≥130 mg/dL (3.4 mmol/L)	≥130 mg/dL (3.4 mmol/L)
Moderate risk: ≥2 risk factors (10-y risk <10%)	<130 mg/dL (3.4 mmol/L)	≥130 mg/dL (3.4 mmol/L)	≥160 mg/dL (4.1 mmol/L)
Lower risk: 0 to 1 risk factor	<160 mg/dL (4.1 mmol/L)	≥160 mg/dL (4.1 mmol/L)	≥190 mg/dL (4.9 mmol/L); (160 to 189 mg/dL [4.1 to 4.9 mmol/L]: drug optional)

CHD = coronary heart disease; HDL = high-density lipoprotein; LDL = low-density lipoprotein; TLC = therapeutic lifestyle changes.
[a]CHD includes history of myocardial infarction, unstable angina, stable angina, coronary artery procedure, or evidence of clinically significant myocardial ischemia; CHD risk equivalents include clinical manifestations of noncoronary atherosclerosis (peripheral vascular disease, abdominal aortic aneurysm, carotid disease, stroke), diabetes, and ≥2 risk factors with 10-y risk for CHD >20%.
[b]Risk factors include cigarette smoking, hypertension (blood pressure ≥140/90 mm Hg or on medication), low HDL cholesterol (<40 mg/dL [1.0 mmol/L]), family history of premature CHD (CHD in first-degree male relative <55 y or first-degree female relative <65 y), and age (men, ≥45 y; women, ≥55 y).
Data adapted from the National Heart Lung and Blood Institute. National Cholesterol Education Program. Third Report of the Expert Panel on Detection, Evaluation, and Treatment of High Blood Cholesterol in Adults (Adult Treatment Panel III): Executive Summary. www.nhlbi.nih.gov/guidelines/cholesterol/atp_iii.htm. Published May 2001. Accessed January 2011.

Table 3. Criteria for Diagnosis of Metabolic Syndrome

Any Three of the Following Risk Factors	Defining Level
Abdominal obesity (waist circumference)	Men, >40 in (102 cm)
	Women, >35 in (88 cm)
Triglycerides[a]	≥150 mg/dL (1.7 mmol/L)
HDL cholesterol	Men, <40 mg/dL (1.0 mmol/L)
	Women, <50 mg/dL (1.3 mmol/L)
Blood pressure	≥130/85 mm Hg
Fasting glucose	≥110 mg/dL (6.1 mmol/L)

[a]Triglycerides ≥150 mg/dL (1.7 mmol/L) as a single factor correlates highly with presence of metabolic syndrome.

Data adapted from the National Heart Lung and Blood Institute. National Cholesterol Education Program. Third Report of the Expert Panel on Detection, Evaluation, and Treatment of High Blood Cholesterol in Adults (Adult Treatment Panel III): Executive Summary. www.nhlbi.nih.gov/guidelines/cholesterol/atp_iii.htm. Published May 2001.

Table 4. Drug Therapy for Dyslipidemia

Class/Agent	Notes
Bile acid sequestrants (colestipol hydrochloride, colesevelam hydrochloride)	Interrupt bile acid reabsorption and lower LDL-C by 10%-15%. Often used as second-line agents with statins to synergistically induce LDL receptors. Do not use in patients with triglycerides >300 mg/dL (3.4 mmol/L) or in those with gastrointestinal motility disorders. Can interfere with absorption of other drugs given at the same time. **Clinical Outcomes:** Clinical trials show that bile acid sequestrants reduce CHD incidence and mortality.
Statins (atorvastatin, lovastatin, pravastatin, simvastatin)	Partially inhibit HMG-CoA reductase, inducing LDL receptor formation. Lower LDL-C by 20%-60%, raise HDL-C by 5%-10%, and lower triglycerides by 15%-25%. Drugs of choice for elevated LDL-C. Use in combination with bile acid sequestrants to synergistically lower LDL-C. Use in combination with niacin and fibrates in patients with combined hyperlipidemia. Side effects include increased aminotransferase levels and myalgia/myositis. Use cautiously in patients on fibrates due to increased risk of myalgia/myositis. Pravastatin is least likely to cause myalgia. **Clinical Outcomes:** Primary prevention trials show that statins reduce risk for major coronary events and coronary death. In patients with CHD (secondary prevention), clinical trials demonstrate that statins reduce total mortality, coronary mortality, major coronary events, and stroke.
Fibrates (gemfibrozil, fenofibrate)	Reduce VLDL synthesis and induce lipoprotein lipase. Lower triglycerides by 50%, raise HDL-C by 15%, and lower LDL-C. Use cautiously in combination with statins due to increased risk of myalgia/myositis. Use with caution in patients with renal insufficiency or gallbladder disease. **Clinical Outcomes:** Fibrates reduce the risk for coronary events but not cardiovascular mortality or all-cause mortality.
Niacin	Reduces hepatic production of β-containing lipoproteins and increases HDL production. Lowers LDL-C and triglycerides by 10%-30%. Most effective drug to raise HDL-C (25%-35%). Drug of choice for combined hyperlipidemia and in patients with low HDL-C. Use in combination with statins or bile acid sequestrants in combined hyperlipidemia. Can cause nausea, glucose intolerance, gout, and elevated uric acid levels. Extended-release preparations limit flushing and aminotransferase abnormalities. To minimize flushing, aspirin can be taken 1 h before dose. Over-the-counter, long-acting niacin preparations are not recommended because they increase the incidence of hepatotoxicity. **Clinical Outcomes:** Niacin treatment reduces cardiovascular events and the progression of atherosclerosis.
Intestinal cholesterol absorption blockers (ezetimibe)	Selectively inhibit intestinal absorption of cholesterol. Lower LDL-C by 18% and triglycerides by 8%. When used in combination with statins, yield an additional LDL-C reduction of 12% (total reduction, 26% to 60%), an increase in HDL-C of 3%, and a triglyceride reduction of 8%. Do not use in combination with bile acid sequestrants or fibrates. Contraindicated in patients with liver disease or elevated aminotransferase levels. **Clinical Outcomes:** The effect of intestinal cholesterol absorption blockers on cardiovascular mortality or morbidity is unknown.

CHD = coronary heart disease; HDL-C = high-density lipoprotein cholesterol; HMG-CoA = 3-hydroxy-3-methylglutaryl-coenzyme A; LDL-C = low-density lipoprotein cholesterol; VLDL-C = very-low-density lipoprotein cholesterol.

LDL cholesterol, and incorporating high-fiber foods can result in a 5% further reduction. Diets rich in fruits, vegetables, nuts, whole grains, and monounsaturated oils (olive oil, canola oil) and low in animal fat reduce cardiovascular risk even without changing lipid levels. Diets rich in omega-3 fatty acids, from fish intake or supplements, improve lipid profiles and reduce risk of CHD by 20% to 30%.

Overweight patients should be encouraged to lose weight by reducing caloric intake, particularly calories from fats and simple carbohydrates. Regular physical activity is encouraged, and both weight loss and exercise are particularly encouraged for patients with a BMI >25. Regular aerobic exercise facilitates weight loss and improves lipid profiles. The beneficial effects are related to the amount of exercise, rather than exercise intensity or overall fitness. Patients should begin structured exercise programs lasting at least 30 minutes on most days. Smoking cessation improves lipid ratios and reduces CHD risk and should be an integral part of lifestyle therapy.

In low-risk patients, 6 months of diet and exercise are appropriate before starting drugs. Drug therapy is started earlier in patients with higher overall CHD risk and in those whose LDL cholesterol is greater than 30 mg/dL (0.8 mmol/L) above their goal, because lowering LDL cholesterol pharmacologically has been shown to reduce CHD and stroke in primary and secondary prevention studies.

Drug therapy is initiated in high-risk patients who are not responsive to lifestyle interventions, at least to the point of reaching ATP III target LDL cholesterol levels (Table 2). Drug classes available for lipid lowering include HMG-CoA reductase inhibitors (statins), fibrates, niacin, bile acid sequestrants, and intestinal cholesterol absorption blockers (Table 4). Statins, the most effective drugs for lowering LDL cholesterol, can cause hepatotoxicity and myopathy, particularly when used in combination with other lipid-lowering drugs. Patients should routinely be asked about symptoms such as nausea, abdominal pain, or myalgias. Because statins can cause aminotransferase elevations and fatal acute hepatic failure has occurred rarely in patients taking statins, there is controversy regarding the frequency of monitoring aminotransferase levels. Many clinicians measure serum aminotransferase levels at the start of therapy, after 12 weeks, after dosage increases, and if clinically indicated by new symptoms; other recommendations call for less or more frequent testing. If a statin-induced myopathy is suspected, confirm the diagnosis by measuring serum creatine phosphokinase.

Follow-Up

Patients are seen at regular intervals even after lipids are normalized. Patients who are on drug therapy need to be seen at 4- to 6-month intervals. A fasting lipid profile should be obtained at least yearly, with monitoring for drug toxicity.

Book Enhancement

Go to www.acponline.org/essentials/endocrinology-section.html. In *MKSAP for Students 5*, assess your knowledge with items 11-15 in the **Endocrinology and Metabolism** section.

Bibliography
Kopin L, Lowenstein C. In the clinic. Dyslipidemia. Ann Intern Med. 2010;153(3): ITC2-1-ITC2-14. [PMID: 20679557]

Chapter 12

Thyroid Disease

Erik K. Alexander, MD

The thyroid gland releases two forms of thyroid hormone: thyroxine (T_4) and triiodothyronine (T_3). All T_4 in the body is made within the thyroid gland, whereas 80% of T_3 is derived from the peripheral conversion of T_4. Conversion of T_4 to T_3 is down-regulated during the course of nonthyroid illness and is decreased by various medications, including propranolol, corticosteroids, propylthiouracil, and amiodarone. The synthesis and release of thyroid hormone are controlled by pituitary-derived thyroid-stimulating hormone (TSH) under the influence of thyrotropin-releasing hormone from the hypothalamus. TSH also stimulates basic thyrocyte functions, such as iodine uptake and organification. Both T_3 and T_4 are predominantly bound to circulating carrier proteins (thyroxine-binding globulin [TBG], transthyretin, albumin); binding serves to prevent excessive tissue uptake and maintain a readily accessible reserve of thyroid hormone. Several medications (e.g., estrogens, corticosteroids) affect levels of TBG without generally affecting the levels of free (unbound) thyroid hormone.

Screening

Screening for hyperthyroidism is not recommended for the general population, although screening for hypothyroidism is considered for certain higher-risk populations. It is reasonable to screen women aged >50 years using a sensitive TSH test, given the increased prevalence of hypothyroidism in this population. It is also appropriate to measure TSH in the following high-risk individuals, even in the absence of symptoms:

* Patients with a first-degree relative with Hashimoto disease or Graves disease
* Patients with other autoimmune diseases such as type 1 diabetes mellitus
* Patients with a history of any prior thyroid dysfunction
* Patients living in an iodine-deficient region of the world
* Women who are anticipating a pregnancy or currently pregnant

Young women on thyroid replacement for hypothyroidism should be counseled to contact their physician as soon as pregnancy is suspected or confirmed so that the levothyroxine dose can be adjusted to maintain a euthyroid state. The daily thyroid hormone requirement increases by approximately 40% beginning very early in gestation, making it essential to increase the dose of levothyroxine. Failure to do so results in maternal (and possibly fetal) hypothyroidism. For this reason, prepregnancy or pregnancy screening for hypothyroidism is important in women of child-bearing age.

Diagnosis

Effective examination of the thyroid is critical for accurate diagnosis of nodules or a simple goiter (an enlarged thyroid gland without nodules). Examination of the thyroid includes anterior and lateral inspection and palpation. To enhance visualization, have the patient tilt the head back slightly, which stretches the tissues overlying the thyroid. On the lateral view, there should be a smooth, straight contour from the cricoid cartilage to the suprasternal notch; disruption of this smooth contour suggests thyroid enlargement. Observe movement of the thyroid when the patient swallows a sip of water. Next, standing behind the patient, attempt to locate the thyroid isthmus by palpating between the cricoid cartilage and suprasternal notch; examination from in front of the patient is also acceptable. Move the sternocleidomastoid muscle aside with one hand, and use the opposite hand to palpate the thyroid. Attempt to feel for thyroid fullness beneath the sternocleidomastoid muscle. Palpate the thyroid again while the patient is swallowing a sip of water.

Numerous tests are available to assess thyroid function and anatomy. Serum TSH is the most sensitive test of thyroid function. Although total thyroid hormone (T_4 and T_3) levels exhibit wide interindividual variation, serum TSH is tightly regulated and effectively signals normal or abnormal thyroid function with great precision. Free T_4 represents the prohormone available for conversion to active T_3, and its measurement is imperative for accurate assessment of thyroid status. In most cases, serum T_3 (or free T_3) testing is not helpful. When serum TSH is abnormal, free T_4 should be measured to assess the degree of hyper- or hypothyroidism. A free T_4 test also should be done to detect secondary hypothyroidism in patients with hypothyroidism and TSH levels that are low or inappropriately normal. Because total T_4 levels are greatly affected by any variation in binding proteins, they may not accurately reflect free T_4 levels. Thyroid peroxidase (TPO) antibody is an excellent marker of autoimmune thyroid disease. A positive titer is associated with Hashimoto thyroiditis. Thyroglobulin is a glycoprotein integral in follicular storage of thyroid hormone and can normally be detected in serum. Thyroglobulin levels can be elevated in both hyperthyroidism and destructive thyroiditis. Levels are suppressed by intake of exogenous thyroid hormone, making thyroglobulin measurement useful to detect thyrotoxicosis caused by surreptitious use of thyroid hormone. The radioactive iodine uptake (RAIU) test measures thyroid gland iodine uptake over a timed period, usually 24 hours. Patients with hyperthyroidism typically have an elevated RAIU, which is inappropriate in the context of a suppressed TSH level. In patients with thyroiditis or exposure to exogenous thyroid hormone, the RAIU will be low (<5%). A thyroid scan shows the location(s) of radioactive iodine uptake within the thyroid gland (diffusely in Graves disease or focally within autonomous nodules). Radionuclide studies should not be performed during pregnancy or in women who are breast feeding. Thyroid ultrasonography is most useful in the evaluation of thyroid nodules.

Thyrotoxicosis

The term *thyrotoxicosis* encompasses all forms of thyroid hormone excess, whether endogenous or exogenous. Most thyrotoxicosis is caused by excess thyroid hormone production (hyperthyroidism) or by increased thyroid hormone release from a damaged thyroid (thyroiditis). The most common cause of hyperthyroidism is Graves disease. Rarely, a toxic ("hot") adenoma, toxic multinodular goiter, factitious hyperthyroidism due to thyroid hormone consumption, or a struma ovarii may be the cause. Certain drugs such as amiodarone or lithium also can cause thyrotoxicosis, usually by inducing thyroiditis.

Consider the diagnosis of hyperthyroidism in patients with signs or symptoms of thyrotoxicosis (Table 1) or in those with diseases known to be caused or aggravated by thyrotoxicosis (e.g., atrial fibrillation, osteoporosis, weight loss, anxiety). In hyperthyroidism, serum TSH is low or undetectable and free T_4 is elevated. If TSH is suppressed and free T_4 is normal, measure the serum T_3 concentration. T_3 thyrotoxicosis (suppressed TSH, normal T_4, elevated T_3) is occasionally seen in patients with toxic multinodular goiter and autonomously functioning thyroid nodules.

Look for "apathetic thyrotoxicosis" in elderly patients, a condition characterized by a lower frequency of goiter (found in 25%-50% of patients), fewer hyperadrenergic symptoms, and cardiac findings including heart failure and atrial fibrillation. Patients with a low or undetectable TSH and a normal free T_4 have subclinical hyperthyroidism. This distinction is important, because subclinical hyperthyroidism can be followed with periodic thyroid function tests in otherwise healthy patients aged <60 years. RAIU is the optimal test to differentiate between hyperthyroidism and thyroiditis. An elevated RAIU is consistent with hyperthyroidism, whereas a suppressed RAIU (usually <5%) is consistent with thyroiditis (Figure 1).

Thyroid storm is a life-threatening condition characterized by exaggerated clinical signs and symptoms of thyrotoxicosis accompanied by systemic decompensation. Thyroid storm is usually caused by rapid release of thyroid hormone (e.g., following a large iodine load, withdrawal of antithyroid drugs, or treatment with radioactive iodine) in the setting of other conditions such as surgery, infection, or trauma. Early recognition, prompt hospitalization, and endocrinology consultation are key to a successful outcome. Thyroid storm is a clinical diagnosis; there is no thyroid hormone concentration that is diagnostic.

The risks of hyperthyroidism are primarily related to cardiac function and arrhythmias, osteoporosis, and a hypermetabolic state. Graves ophthalmopathy (soft tissue inflammation, proptosis, extraocular muscle dysfunction, optic neuropathy) is present in 10% to 25% of affected patients, although up to 70% of patients may have subclinical enlargement of extraocular muscles without overt eye disease. Pretibial myxedema (infiltrative dermopathy characterized by nonpitting scaly thickening and induration of the

Table 1. Signs and Symptoms of Hyperthyroidism and Hypothyroidism

Hyperthyroidism (% frequency)	Hypothyroidism (% frequency)
Common symptoms	**Common symptoms**
Nervousness or emotional lability (99)	Sluggish affect or depression (91)
Increased sweating (91)	Fatigue (87)
Heat intolerance (89)	Cold intolerance (70)
Palpitations (89)	Constipation (70)
Fatigue (88)	Weight gain (56)
Weight loss (85)	Alopecia (44)
Hyperdefecation (33)	**Common signs**
Menstrual irregularity (22)	Dry, coarse skin and hair (75)
Common signs	Periorbital puffiness (75)
Tachycardia or atrial fibrillation (100)	Bradycardia (55)
Goiter (99)	Slow movements and speech (53)
Tremor (97)	Hoarseness (50)
Proptosis of the eyes or extraocular muscle palsy (40)	Diastolic hypertension (30)
Stare, lid lag, or signs of optic neuropathy (40)	Goiter (27)
Pretibial myxedema (NA)	Loss of the lateral portion of the eyebrow (NA)
	Delayed deep tendon reflexes (NA)

NA = not available.

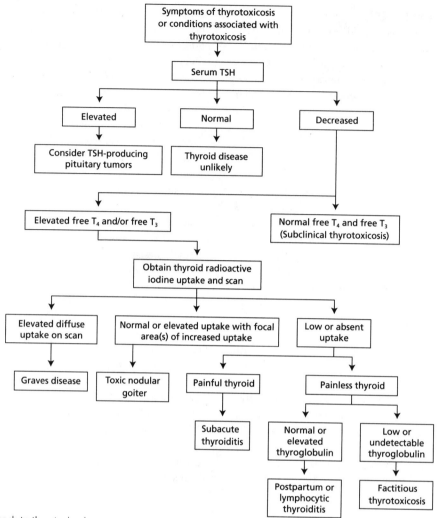

Figure 1. Diagnostic approach to thyrotoxicosis.

skin) is a rare complication of Graves disease. Once hyperthyroidism is treated effectively, the overall risks associated with hyperthyroidism can be substantially diminished.

Hypothyroidism

Hypothyroidism has a wide range of clinical signs and symptoms (Table 1). Serum TSH is elevated (>10 µU/mL [10 mU/L]) in primary hypothyroidism (thyroid gland failure), whereas TSH is low or normal in conjunction with a low free T_4 in rare cases of hypothyroidism due to pituitary or hypothalamic disease (secondary hypothyroidism). Patients with a mildly elevated TSH (5-10 µU/mL [5-10 mU/L]) and a normal free T_4 have subclinical hypothyroidism. This distinction is important, because patients with subclinical hypothyroidism may not require treatment if they are asymptomatic or are women not desiring pregnancy or currently pregnant.

The most common causes of hypothyroidism are chronic lymphocytic thyroiditis (Hashimoto disease), post-thyroidectomy, and radioiodine therapy (Table 2). Hashimoto disease is an autoimmune disease that may present at any time but increases in prevalence with age. Onset is usually insidious and associated with

a goiter. The presence of TPO antibody is highly correlated with Hashimoto disease. Hashimoto disease is the most common cause of chronic hypothyroidism, and confirmation of the diagnosis with measurement of TPO antibody is usually not necessary. Measurement of TPO antibody may be helpful in patients with subclinical hypothyroidism (elevated TSH level but normal free T_4). In these patients, increased TPO antibody titers confer an increased risk of hypothyroidism (approximately 4% per year), which escalates as TSH levels rise above the reference range. These patients warrant close monitoring for the development of hypothyroidism. Subacute or painful thyroiditis also can lead to hypothyroidism. Most patients demonstrate a triphasic thyroid hormone response: mild hyperthyroidism, followed by mild hypothyroidism, followed by a return to normal thyroid function. If the final phase of thyroid normalization is not attained, TSH will remain elevated and hypothyroidism will persist.

Myxedema coma is severe hypothyroidism. Similar to thyroid storm, there is no concentration of thyroid hormone that is diagnostic. Mental status changes and hypothermia are hallmark findings of myxedema coma, with hypothermia occurring in nearly 90% of patients. Additional common findings are hypoxemia and hypercapnia. The combination of mental status changes, hypother-

Table 2. Differential Diagnosis of Hypothyroidism

Cause	Notes
Hashimoto disease	TSH high; positive family history for hypothyroidism; TPO antibodies present; slowly progressive
Iodine deficiency	TSH high; iodine-deficient area; rare in United States
Postpartum thyroiditis	TSH triphasic (low, high, normal) over 2-4 mo but often ultimately elevated; recent pregnancy
Silent thyroiditis	TSH triphasic (low, high, normal) over 2-4 mo; self-limited in most cases
Subacute thyroiditis	TSH triphasic (low, high, normal) over 2-4 mo; ESR elevated; painful thyroid
Drug-induced hypothyroidism	TSH high; use of amiodarone, lithium, sunitinib, interferon, iodine, or thioamides in past 1-6 mo
Pituitary/hypothalamic mass	TSH low or normal; FT_4 low; headaches; most often a pituitary or sellar lesion noted on MRI/CT scan or evidence of prior pituitary surgery
Pituitary/hypothalamic radiation therapy	TSH low or normal; FT_4 low; history of cranial radiation therapy

ESR = erythrocyte sedimentation rate; FT_4 = free T_4; TPO = thyroid peroxidase; TSH = thyroid-stimulating hormone.

mia, hypoventilation, and hyponatremia in a patient whose clinical picture is consistent with hypothyroidism strongly suggests the diagnosis of myxedema coma.

Effects of Nonthyroid Illness on Thyroid Function

Patients with acute nonthyroid illness may have TSH suppression that is part of the "euthyroid sick syndrome" and not due to underlying thyrotoxicosis. Most commonly, T_3 levels decline sharply and T_4 levels remain relatively unchanged, although low T_4 levels have been reported in patients with prolonged severe illness. The TSH response is less consistent, with low, normal, or elevated levels reported. The thyroid hormone patterns associated with nonthyroid illness appear to be an adaptive response to mitigate catabolism associated with severe stress. Thyroid hormone therapy is not beneficial or indicated. Thyroid hormone levels typically normalize 4 to 8 weeks after recovery from the nonthyroid illness.

Thyroid Nodules

Thyroid nodules usually occur in euthyroid patients, and most are benign. Clinically, the focus is on detecting the few malignant thyroid nodules. Factors associated with increased cancer risk include young age (<30 years), male sex, a history of head or neck irradiation, a family history of thyroid cancer (especially medullary thyroid cancer), rapid nodule growth, larger nodules, and hoarseness. Evaluation of serum TSH is recommended to diagnose functional ("toxic" or "hot") nodules; these nodules are rarely malignant (<1% cancer risk). All euthyroid patients with possible nodular disease should undergo thyroid ultrasonography. Ultrasonography allows accurate detection and sizing of all nodules on the thyroid gland, and ultrasound characteristics can be used to further delineate cancer risk. According to several guidelines, biopsy of any nodule greater than 1 cm in diameter is reasonable (10%-15% cancer risk), and biopsy of smaller nodules should be considered in patients with thyroid cancer risk factors.

Therapy

Thyrotoxicosis

Early in the treatment of thyrotoxicosis, iodine avoidance (e.g., the contrast agent used in CT scans) and exercise restriction are recommended. If immediate control of severe thyrotoxicosis is required, inorganic iodine (saturated solution of potassium iodide [SSKI]) can be administered orally and is highly effective. However, this therapy is self-limited in duration (3 weeks) and precludes further use of radioiodine (^{131}I) for months thereafter.

Thyrotoxicosis due to thyroiditis is often self-limited and managed conservatively. β-Blockers can be used for sympathomimetic symptoms (tachycardia, tremor, anxiety). Nonsteroidal anti-inflammatory drugs and, rarely, corticosteroids are administered to reduce inflammation and discomfort.

Graves disease and autonomously functioning thyroid nodules can be treated with antithyroid drugs or radioiodine, although patient preference, patient age, comorbidities, severity of thyrotoxicosis, and the presence of Graves ophthalmopathy must be taken into account. The response of Graves ophthalmopathy to the treatment of hyperthyroidism is complex and requires consultation with an ophthalmologist and endocrinologist. Antithyroid drugs (propylthiouracil, methimazole) are preferred to radioiodine in the presence of severe Graves ophthalmopathy and thyroid storm. Between 20% and 40% of patients with Graves disease will achieve drug-free remission rates after 1 year of treatment with antithyroid drugs. Methimazole is generally recommended as first-line antithyroid therapy, as propylthiouracil has been associated with elevated aminotransferase levels and a higher rate of serious adverse effects on the liver than occur with methimazole. An exception is women who are in the first trimester of pregnancy, during which methimazole has been associated with possible teratogenicity. Propylthiouracil is also preferred in patients with an allergy to methimazole. With either drug, patients should be counseled about the risk of the rare but severe side effects of agranulocytosis, hepatitis, and vasculitis. Rarely, severe hepatic necrosis has been reported, predominantly with propylthiouracil.

Most patients select radioiodine as therapy for thyrotoxicosis caused by Graves disease, toxic multinodular goiter, or autonomously functioning thyroid nodules. Radioiodine is also indicated in patients failing to achieve remission after a course of antithyroid drugs. Thyroidectomy is a reasonable choice in thyrotoxic patients with concomitant suspicious (malignant) nodules and in patients who cannot tolerate or refuse radioiodine or antithyroid drugs.

Hypothyroidism

Levothyroxine is the preferred treatment of hypothyroidism. Levothyroxine is converted to T_3 primarily in peripheral tissues at an appropriate rate for overall metabolic needs. Treatment with a combination of T_4 and T_3 is not recommended. Although all patients with overt hypothyroidism (TSH >10 µU/mL [10 mU/L]) should be treated, there is limited evidence that treatment of subclinical hypothyroidism is beneficial in nonpregnant patients. At present, most patients can be safely monitored for disease progression with TSH measurements every 4 to 6 months. This recommendation excludes women seeking pregnancy or currently pregnant, who should be treated once TSH is outside the normal range because of greater maternal and fetal risk. For pregnant women, baseline levothyroxine dosing should be increased by approximately 30% as soon as pregnancy is confirmed. Thyroid function should be measured every 4 weeks through midpregnancy, as subsequent changes in levothyroxine dose may be required. In general, serum TSH should be maintained at <2.5 µU/mL [2.5 mU/L] throughout gestation.

Follow-Up

Following treatment for hyperthyroidism, TSH and free T_4 are monitored every 3 to 6 months for the first year and every 6 to 12 months thereafter. Therapeutic radioiodine is likely to cause permanent thyroid destruction requiring lifelong levothyroxine therapy.

Once initiated for the treatment of hypothyroidism, levothyroxine therapy is lifelong. Serum TSH should be monitored 6 to 8 weeks after initiating therapy, with adjustments in levothyroxine dose made to achieve a TSH value within the normal range. A full replacement dose of levothyroxine is approximately 1.7 µg/kg, although many patients require a lower dose due to partial thyroid function. Finally, an annual evaluation of serum TSH is recommended in patients receiving levothyroxine therapy; studies have demonstrated that up to 30% of such patients may be unintentionally under- or overtreated.

Book Enhancement

Go to www.acponline.org/essentials/endocrinology-section.html. In *MKSAP for Students 5*, assess your knowledge with items 16-21 in the **Endocrinology and Metabolism** section.

Bibliography

Brent GA. Clinical practice. Graves' disease. N Engl J Med. 2008;358:2594-2605. [PMID: 18550875]

McDermott MT. In the clinic. Hypothyroidism. Ann Intern Med. 2009; 151(11):ITC61. [PMID: 19949140]

Chapter 13

Adrenal Disease

Cynthia A. Burns, MD

This chapter reviews four types of adrenal disease: adrenal insufficiency, hyperadrenocorticism (Cushing syndrome), hyperaldosteronism, and pheochromocytoma. Adrenal nodules discovered incidentally on abdominal imaging also are reviewed.

Adrenal Insufficiency

Adrenal insufficiency may be due to disease of the adrenal glands (primary) or disorders of the pituitary gland (central). Autoimmune adrenalitis is the most common cause of primary adrenal insufficiency in the United States; exogenous corticosteroid use is the most common cause of central adrenal insufficiency. Primary disease results in deficiencies of cortisol, aldosterone, and adrenal androgens, whereas central insufficiency causes only cortisol deficiency.

Diagnosis

The presentation of adrenal insufficiency may be acute or slowly progressive. Symptoms of acute adrenal crisis are nonspecific; therefore, one must be alert to the causes of adrenal insufficiency and the clinical settings in which they occur. Acute adrenal crisis most commonly follows discontinuation of long-term corticosteroid therapy, and patients are vulnerable for up to 1 year. Other settings associated with acute adrenal insufficiency include sepsis, trauma, surgery, autoimmune disease, adrenal hemorrhage/infarction, granulomatous disease (tuberculosis, sarcoidosis), AIDS, and, rarely, pituitary/hypothalamic disease. Look for unexplained weight loss, anorexia, weakness, fatigue, and orthostatic hypotension. Hyperpigmentation may be present due to elevated adrenocorticotropic hormone (ACTH) levels in primary adrenal insufficiency. Hyperkalemia, hyponatremia, hypoglycemia, and eosinophilia may be present.

A cosyntropin stimulation test establishes the diagnosis of adrenal insufficiency. ACTH and cortisol values are obtained at baseline and at 30 minutes and 60 minutes following administration of cosyntropin. A rise of serum cortisol ≥18 µg/dL (496.8 nmol/L) rules out adrenal insufficiency. These values may not apply to critically ill patients who have low concentrations of albumin and cortisol-binding globulin; in these patients, measure serum free cortisol concentrations. To distinguish primary adrenal insufficiency from central adrenal insufficiency, measure plasma ACTH and cortisol levels at 8 AM. ACTH is elevated >100 pg/mL (22 pmol/L) in primary adrenal insufficiency and is low or inappropriately normal in central adrenal insufficiency. Obtain a pituitary MRI scan in central insufficiency and a CT scan of the adrenal glands in primary adrenal insufficiency. The adrenal glands appear normal in the setting of autoimmune disease.

Therapy

If acute adrenal insufficiency is suspected, immediately obtain serum ACTH and cortisol levels. While awaiting results, give high-dose corticosteroids (dexamethasone is preferred, because it does not interfere with serum cortisol assays) and large-volume intravenous saline. For less critically ill patients, promptly administer oral corticosteroids for primary or central adrenal insufficiency; delay is potentially life-threatening. Fludrocortisone is required in primary but not central adrenal insufficiency; aldosterone production is controlled by the renin-angiotensin system and is intact in central adrenal insufficiency. Mild stress (e.g., fever, gastroenteritis) requires doubling or tripling the daily corticosteroid dose, and severe illness requires hospitalization for high-dose intravenous corticosteroid therapy. Oral corticosteroids used for daily replacement therapy are prednisone, hydrocortisone, and dexamethasone.

Follow-Up

Patients are advised to wear a medical alert bracelet stating their diagnosis. Patients need to understand and be able to articulate how to increase corticosteroids during minor illness. Adequacy of corticosteroid replacement is evaluated by looking for signs and symptoms of adrenal insufficiency (underreplacement) or Cushing syndrome (overreplacement). Adjust the mineralocorticoid dose based on the plasma renin activity or the patient's symptoms. Patients complaining of lightheadedness upon standing or who are orthostatic on examination may need more fludrocortisone, whereas patients with peripheral edema or increased blood pressure may need less.

Hyperadrenocorticism

Excess cortisol (hyperadrenocorticism, or *Cushing syndrome*) usually is secondary to exogenous corticosteroid ingestion. The most common endogenous cause is an ACTH-secreting pituitary tumor (Cushing disease); adrenocortical tumors and ectopic ACTH-secreting malignant tumors each account for 10% of endogenous cases (Table 1). When the syndrome is due to an ectopic ACTH-secreting tumor, symptoms of weight loss, muscle weakness, and profound hypokalemia may predominate. ACTH-dependent forms of Cushing syndrome result in bilateral adrenal enlargement.

Diagnosis

Exclude exogenous corticosteroid intake by any route. Seek indicators of corticosteroid excess, including change in menses, weight gain, history of recurrent or chronic infections, worsening diabetic control, or fractures. Look for abnormal fat distribution, particu-

Table 1. Differential Diagnosis of Endogenous Cushing Syndrome

Disease	Notes
ACTH-independent forms:	ACTH level <10 pg/mL (2.2 pmol/L); DHEAS levels tend to be below normal, except in adrenal carcinoma
Adrenal adenoma	Unilateral mass and small contralateral gland on CT
Adrenal carcinoma	Unilateral mass and small contralateral gland on CT; may observe elevated DHEAS levels
Bilateral macronodular adrenal disease	Large nodular glands on CT; more common after age 50
ACTH-dependent forms:	ACTH level >10 pg/mL (2.2 pmol/L)
Cushing disease	Bilateral adrenal hyperplasia with or without nodules; pituitary mass on MRI
Ectopic ACTH secretion	Bilateral adrenal hyperplasia; look for a lung cancer

ACTH = adrenocorticotropic hormone; CT = computed tomography; DHEAS = dehydroepiandrosterone sulfate.

larly in the supraclavicular and temporal areas, proximal muscle weakness, or wide purple striae. Also look for physical features that support a specific cause of Cushing syndrome, such as feminization or virilization and abdominal mass (adrenal tumor) or visual field losses (pituitary tumor). Examination of photographs over time can highlight otherwise subtle physical changes and provide an estimate of change over time.

To diagnose for hypercortisolism, obtain a 24-hour urine free cortisol measurement or overnight 1-mg dexamethasone suppression test. A 24-hour urine free cortisol level >3 times normal supports the diagnosis of Cushing syndrome. Inability to suppress serum cortisol following the overnight 1-mg dexamethasone suppression test also suggests the diagnosis. Obesity, alcohol abuse, kidney failure, and depression can cause false-positive results (pseudo–Cushing syndrome). An elevated 24-hour urine free cortisol measurement <3 times normal is likely due to pseudo–Cushing syndrome. If the test result is equivocal, perform confirmatory testing with another 24-hour urine free cortisol or dexamethasone suppression test.

In patients with unequivocal excess cortisol production, measure plasma ACTH to differentiate between ACTH-dependent (pituitary or ectopic) and ACTH-independent (adrenal) causes of Cushing syndrome. Basal ACTH levels <6 pg/mL (1.3 pmol/L) are found in adrenal forms of Cushing syndrome; levels >6 pg/mL (1.3 pmol/L) occur in ACTH-dependent disease. Undetectable ACTH levels may be spurious if the sample is not processed within 2 hours, due to the high susceptibility of ACTH to proteolysis.

Once the source of hypercortisolism (pituitary, adrenal, or ectopic) is biochemically determined, imaging studies are indicated. Obtain an adrenal CT scan to localize lesions in patients with suppressed ACTH values. In patients with nonsuppressed ACTH levels, obtain a pituitary MRI scan; if negative, consider expert consultation regarding how to further distinguish a pituitary from an ectopic source of ACTH. The most common ectopic ACTH-secreting tumors are small cell carcinoma of the lung, bronchial carcinoid tumor, pheochromocytoma, and medullary thyroid carcinoma. Begin the evaluation with a chest MRI or CT scan. If negative, obtain an abdominal CT or MRI scan to look for a pancreatic tumor or other mass. Consider nuclear medicine scanning to locate the source of ectopic ACTH, if other imaging is negative. Figure 1 summarizes the evaluation of suspected Cushing syndome.

Therapy

Surgical resection of an identified tumor (adrenal, pituitary, or ectopic) is the optimal therapy for Cushing syndrome. Pituitary radiation ("gamma knife") therapy can be used for patients with persistent or recurrent Cushing disease after transsphenoidal surgery or for those in whom pituitary surgery is contraindicated.

Drugs are used adjuvantly in patients undergoing surgery and as sole therapy for those with occult ectopic ACTH secretion or metastatic adrenal cancer to reduce cortisol production. Ketoconazole, mitotane, metyrapone, and aminoglutethimide reduce endogenous cortisol levels and reverse most signs and symptoms of Cushing syndrome. Steroidogenesis inhibitors may be needed as adjuncts to pituitary radiation therapy in patients with Cushing disease, because radiation therapy can take 2 to 5 years to ablate the tumor.

Follow-Up

Following surgery, some patients will require daily corticosteroid replacement until the hypothalamic-pituitary-adrenal axis has recovered (up to 1 year). Recovery should be assessed with serial cosyntropin stimulation tests. Monitor patients for the development of panhypopituitarism after pituitary irradiation or extensive pituitary resection. Ensure that patients with occult ectopic ACTH production undergo imaging surveillance every 6 months the first year then annually to localize the tumor. More than half of tumors are initially occult.

Hyperaldosteronism

Once thought to be a rare cause of hypertension, hyperaldosteronism (also called *aldosteronism*) has been recognized in up to 14% of unselected hypertensive patients. Depending on the cause, hyperaldosteronism is amenable to medical or surgical treatment.

Diagnosis

Consider the diagnosis of hyperaldosteronism in patients with difficult-to-control or worsening hypertension despite multiple antihypertensive agents, spontaneous hypokalemia, severe hypokalemia after institution of diuretic therapy, or hypertension at a young age. Hypokalemia results when hyperaldosteronism causes excess distal renal tubule exchange of sodium for potassium. In the presence of an elevated aldosterone and suppressed renin level, a 10 am upright plasma aldosterone concentration/plasma renin

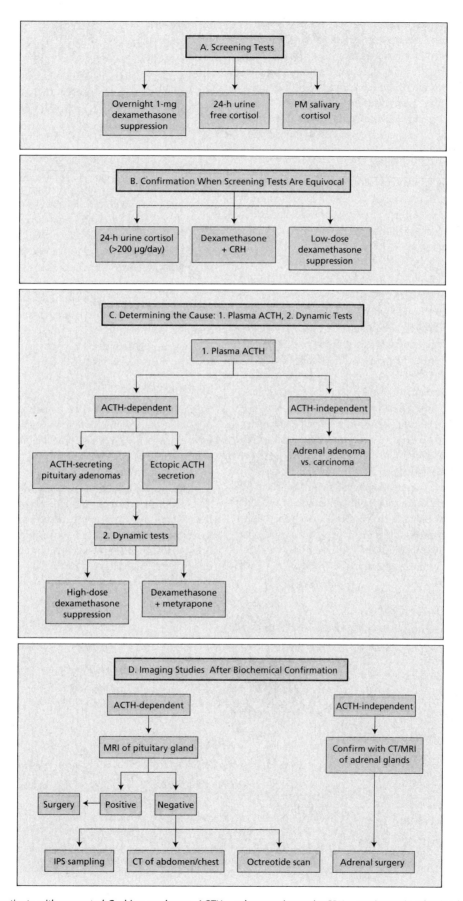

Figure 1. Evaluation of patients with suspected Cushing syndrome. ACTH = adrenocorticotropic; CRH = corticotropin-releasing hormone; IPS = inferior petrosal sinus.

activity (PAC/PRA) ratio >20 suggests primary hyperaldosteronism. Spironolactone, angiotensin-converting enzyme (ACE) inhibitors, angiotensin receptor blockers, diuretics, and β-blockers should be stopped prior to testing, because they can alter the levels of renin and aldosterone. If the screening PAC/PRA ratio is positive, a confirmatory test should be performed. One approach is 24-hour urine aldosterone testing after 3 days of dietary salt loading; if aldosterone secretion is not suppressed, hyperaldosteronism is confirmed.

Once hyperaldosteronism is confirmed, obtain a dedicated CT scan of the adrenal glands. Unilateral aldosteronoma (Conn syndrome) is the most common cause of primary hyperaldosteronism, followed by bilateral adrenal hyperplasia and idiopathic hyperaldosteronism (no adrenal abnormalities visualized).

Therapy

Adrenalectomy is the treatment of choice for a unilateral aldosterone-producing adrenal adenoma. Bilateral adrenal resection is not indicated for bilateral adrenal hyperplasia, due to the development of adrenal insufficiency. Hypokalemia usually resolves following surgery, but hypertension does not always resolve; long-standing hypertension results in permanent vascular changes, making normalization of blood pressure difficult.

Spironolactone is the treatment of choice for idiopathic hyperaldosteronism, bilateral adrenal hyperplasia, and nonsurgical candidates with unilateral disease. If additional antihypertensive medications are required to control blood pressure, low-dose thiazide therapy is usually effective in combination with spironolactone; calcium channel blockers or ACE inhibitors are used if additional antihypertensive therapy is indicated. A more selective mineralocorticoid receptor antagonist, eplerenone, can be used in patients unable to tolerate side effects from spironolactone, such as decreased libido, impotence, or gynecomastia. Dietary sodium restriction will decrease urinary potassium wasting and help potentiate the effect of antihypertensive therapy.

Follow-Up

Postsurgical patients should be monitored for hypoaldosteronism (hypotension and hyperkalemia) due to long-term suppression of the contralateral adrenal gland. Patients taking spironolactone or eplerenone require titration of medication to maximal effect on potassium concentration and blood pressure, as well as tapering of potassium supplementation.

Pheochromocytoma

Pheochromocytoma is a rare tumor of the adrenal gland that accounts for a small number of cases of secondary hypertension (0.1%-0.6%). Ten percent of pheochromocytomas are extra-adrenal, 10% are malignant, 10% recur, and 10% are asymptomatic. Up to 25% of pheochromocytomas are familial. These tumors are more likely to occur at a young age; to be bilateral, extra-adrenal, and malignant; and to recur. Genetic testing should be considered in suspected familial cases. Pheochromocytomas are paraganglioma tumors that arise in the chromaffin cells of the adrenal medulla. The tumors can produce, store, and secrete catecholamines (norepinephrine, epinephrine, and/or dopamine); most produce norepinephrine.

Diagnosis

Consider pheochromocytoma in patients with moderate-to-severe hypertension (sustained or paroxysmal) coupled with episodes of severe headache, sweating, and palpitations. Table 2 describes some important disorders in the differential diagnosis of pheochromocytoma.

Measure 24-hour urine metanephrine excretion or plasma free metanephrine level. Many medications can interfere with these tests, which are best performed and interpreted with the help of a specialist. Avoid plasma catecholamine measurement (high false-positive rates) and urine vanillylmandelic acid (requires a special diet prior to collection).

Table 2. Differential Diagnosis of Pheochromocytoma

Disease	Notes
Thyrotoxicosis (see Chapter 12)	Weight loss, tachycardia, tremor and suppressed serum TSH concentration, evaluate T_4 and/or T_3 levels.
Insulinoma	Whipple triad: neuroglycopenia (sympathetic symptoms alone are not enough), glucose <50 mg/dL (2.8 mmol/L) during the occurrence of symptoms, and prompt resolution of symptoms with administration of glucose.
Essential hypertension (see Chapter 41)	Labile blood pressure is quite common and is associated with normal levels of catecholamines and metanephrine.
Renovascular hypertension (see Chapter 41)	Paroxysmal hypertension can occur. Normal levels of metanephrines exclude pheochromocytoma.
Anxiety, panic attacks, and hyperventilation	Panic disorder is frequently confused with pheochromocytoma. Normal levels of metanephrines exclude pheochromocytoma.
Carcinoid syndrome	Typically presents with flushing, diarrhea, and cardiac-related symptoms. Symptoms are sometimes associated with eating. Elevated 24-hr urinary excretion of 5-hydroxyindole acetic acid is diagnostic.
Unexplained flushing spells	Diagnosis of exclusion. Signs and symptoms may be clinically indistinguishable from patients with pheochromocytoma, except that metanephrine levels are normal.

TSH = thyroid-stimulating hormone.

When the diagnosis of pheochromocytoma is biochemically confirmed, obtain a CT scan of the adrenal glands to localize the tumor. Intravenous contrast is contraindicated, as it can precipitate hypertensive crisis. If no adrenal abnormality is seen, obtain CT scans of the chest, abdomen, and pelvis to look for paragangliomas along the sympathetic chain.

Therapy

Surgical resection is the treatment of choice. Patients must receive full α-adrenergic blockade prior to surgery to avoid a hypertensive emergency during the procedure. Phenoxybenzamine is a long-acting irreversible nonselective α-blocker that is classically used for preoperative management, but shorter-acting selective α₁-adrenergic antagonists (e.g., terazosin, prazosin, doxazosin) also can be used. If needed, β-blockade can follow α-blockade for additional control of blood pressure and heart rate. β-Blockade prior to α-blockade is contraindicated due to the dangers of unopposed α-adrenergic activity.

Follow-Up

Screen patients for recurrence of preoperative symptoms, and monitor blood pressure. Perform 24-hour urine metanephrine collection after tumor resection to ensure normalization and if recurrence is suspected. Blood pressure does not always normalize following resection due to the long-term vascular effects of hypertension.

Adrenal Incidentaloma

Given the frequency of abdominal CT and MRI scanning, it is not surprising that adrenal nodules are incidentally noted on these images. In fact, 1% to 7% of patients are found to have adrenal "incidentalomas" when imaged for other conditions, and the incidence increases with age.

A careful history and physical examination should be performed on all patients with an incidentally discovered adrenal adenoma. Greater than 90% of incidentalomas are nonfunctional, but all patients should be screened for Cushing syndrome and pheochromocytoma. Patients with hypertension or spontaneous hypokalemia should be screened for hyperaldosteronism. If the patient is virilized (voice deepening, clitoral enlargement), adrenal androgen levels should be measured, along with dehydroepiandrosterone sulfate and testosterone levels.

The imaging characteristics of an adrenal nodule can indicate a higher risk of malignancy (metastatic disease or primary adrenal cancer). High lipid content is consistent with a benign adenoma, but high intranodular vascularity can indicate malignancy or pheochromocytoma. Irregular borders or intranodular necrosis are worrisome for malignancy. If the nodule is >4 cm, the risk of malignancy is approximately 25%, and surgical resection is recommended. If the nodule is <4 cm, the risk of malignancy is approximately 5%, and surgery is not recommended. To avoid hypertensive crisis, biopsy of an adrenal nodule should never be attempted until pheochromocytoma has been ruled out. If the patient has a history of malignancy, an incidentally noted adrenal nodule is likely to represent metastatic disease, especially if bilateral nodules are present.

Follow-up recommendations include annual testing over several years for hormonal functionality and repeat imaging (CT or MRI) two to three times over 2 years to assess for change in the size of nodule.

Book Enhancement

Go to www.acponline.org/essentials/endocrinology-section.html. In *MKSAP for Students 5*, assess your knowledge with items 22-27 in the **Endocrinology and Metabolism** section.

Bibliography

Chakera AJ, Vaidya B. Addison disease in adults: diagnosis and management. Am J Med. 2010;123:409-413. [PMID: 20399314]

Newell-Price J. Diagnosis/differential diagnosis of Cushing's syndrome: a review of best practice. Best Pract Res Clin Endocrinol Metab. 2009;23 (Suppl 1):S5-14. [20129193]

Young WF Jr. Clinical practice. The incidentally discovered adrenal mass. N Engl J Med. 2007;356:601-610. [PMID: 17287480]

Chapter 14

Osteoporosis

Mark D. Corriere, MD

Osteoporosis is a skeletal disorder characterized by compromised bone strength predisposing to an increased risk of fractures. Decreased bone strength occurs because peak bone mass is low, bone resorption is excessive, or bone formation is decreased during remodeling. All three mechanisms contribute to osteoporosis. The disease affects an estimated 44 million Americans or 55% of people aged 50 years or older. The prevalence of low bone mineral density is particularly high in the elderly, approaching 80% in women aged >80 years. Effective screening modalities and treatments are available.

Prevention

Prevention of bone loss should be attempted whenever a dual-energy x-ray absorptiometry (DEXA) T score is less than −1 (see Screening) or risk factors are present. Nonpharmacologic preventive measures include adequate daily calcium and vitamin D intake, regular exercise, and avoidance of tobacco and excessive alcohol use. Exercise should focus on weight-bearing activities (e.g., walking, jogging, stair climbing) and muscle strengthening (e.g., weight or resistance training). Excessive exercise may actually be counterproductive in the adolescent or young adult female patient, since this may lead to the "athlete's triad" of a restrictive eating disorder, amenorrhea, and osteoporosis. Reducing fall risk is particularly important for helping to prevent fracture in the frail elderly (see Chapter 40).

Several medications are approved by the FDA for treatment and/or prevention of osteoporosis. These medications should be considered in patients who have maximized nonpharmacologic measures, are at high risk for worsening bone loss, or have a high likelihood of future falls. The World Health Organization developed an algorithm to calculate a patient's 10-year probability of a hip fracture or major osteoporotic fracture (www.sheffield.ac.uk/FRAX/). The FRAX tool has been helpful in establishing fracture risk and identifying patients in the osteopenic range who should be treated with medications.

Screening

The goal of screening is to identify individuals at increased risk for osteoporosis who would benefit from lifestyle modification or pharmacologic treatment to prevent fractures. Modifiable risk factors include low calcium or vitamin D intake, inadequate physical activity, low BMI, cigarette smoking, and alcoholism. Nonmodifiable risk factors include increasing age, female sex, race (white or Asian), impaired mobility, and a family history of fragility fracture in a first-

degree relative. A fragility fracture is a spontaneous fracture or a fracture due to a fall from standing height or less.

All women aged ≥65 years and men aged ≥70 years should be screened regardless of risk factors. Several other specific populations also require screening (Table 1). Screening for osteoporosis should also be considered in a patient with a known secondary cause of osteoporosis (Table 2).

The screening modality of choice is a dual-energy x-ray absorptiometry (DEXA) scan. DEXA scans use x-rays at two different doses to create images used to estimate the mineral content of bone. Measurements are usually made in the spine and hip. The reliability of these sites allows for repeat serial measurements to monitor disease progression over time. Results of DEXA scans are provided as T and Z scores.

- T scores represent standard deviations from the mean bone mineral density of young healthy adults. T scores less than -2.5 are considered to be diagnostic of osteoporosis; scores between -1 and -2.5 define osteopenia.
- Z scores represent the number of standard deviations from the normal mean value for age- and sex-matched controls. Z scores are used in assessing osteoporosis risk in individuals aged <40 years. In individuals aged >40 years, abnormally low Z scores suggest the presence of a secondary cause of osteoporosis.

Diagnosis

The focused medical history in patients with osteopenia or osteoporosis includes daily calcium and vitamin D intake, physical

Table 1. Indications for Measurement of Bone Mineral Density

Women age ≥65 years and men age ≥70 years (regardless of risk factors)

Postmenopausal women age <65 years and men age <70 years who have at least one risk factor for osteoporosis (other than menopause in women)

Women or men who have fractures on presentation

Women or men who are considering therapy for osteoporosis and for whom bone mineral densitometry test results would influence this decision

Radiographic findings suggestive of osteoporosis or vertebral deformity

Corticosteroid therapy for more than 3 months

Primary hyperparathyroidism

Treatment for osteoporosis (to monitor therapeutic response)

Table 2. Selected Causes of Secondary Osteoporosis

Endocrine disorders: hyperparathyroidism, Cushing syndrome, hypogonadism, hyperthyroidism, prolactinoma, acromegaly, osteomalacia

Hematopoietic disorders: multiple myeloma, sickle-cell disease, thalassemia minor, leukemia, lymphoma, polycythemia vera

Connective tissue disorders: osteogenesis imperfecta, homocystinuria

Renal disease: chronic renal failure, renal tubular acidosis, hypercalciuria

Nutritional: malabsorption, total parenteral nutrition

Gastrointestinal disorders: gastrectomy, primary biliary cirrhosis, celiac disease

Medications: corticosteroids, anticonvulsants, heparin

Genetic: Turner syndrome, Klinefelter syndrome

Table 3. Optimal Calcium Requirements

Group	Optimal Daily Intake
Men	
25-65 years	1000 mg
>65 years	1500 mg
Women	
25-50 years	1000 mg
>50 years (postmenopausal)	1500 mg
>65 years	1500 mg
Pregnant and nursing	1200-1500 mg

Data from Optimal calcium intake. NIH Consens Statement. 1994;12:1-31. [PMID: 7599655]

activity, smoking, alcohol use, menstrual history, falls, and medication use. In patients without standard risk factors, the history should also review possible secondary causes.

Physical examination can provide critical information if osteoporosis is suspected. Height should be measured using a wall-mounted stadiometer and serial measurements followed for possible height loss. The spine should be assessed for evidence of kyphosis or vertebral fractures. Physical findings predictive of osteoporosis include frail appearance and poor proximal muscle strength demonstrated by difficulty rising from a chair without pushing off with the arms.

Reasonable screening laboratory tests include complete blood count, serum thyroid-stimulating hormone, calcium and phosphorus, creatinine, alanine aminotransferase, aspartate aminotransferase, alkaline phosphatase, erythrocyte sedimentation rate, serum testosterone in males, serum 25-hydroxyvitamin D (if vitamin D deficiency is suspected), and tissue transglutaminase antibodies (if celiac disease is suspected). In the absence of fractures, primary osteoporosis is associated with no abnormalities on laboratory testing.

In evaluating patients with low bone mass or fractures, causes other than osteoporosis should be entertained (Table 2).

Therapy

Nonpharmacologic Measures

Ensuring adequate oral calcium intake is an essential treatment for osteoporosis. The recommended daily calcium intake varies by age and sex (Table 3). It is most desirable to achieve oral calcium goals through regular dietary intake. Daily dietary calcium intake can be estimated by multiplying each serving of a dairy product (milk, yogurt, cheese) by 300 mg and then adding 250 mg, representing the average calcium intake from other foods. Calcium supplements (calcium carbonate or calcium citrate) are recommended for patients who do not routinely consume adequate amounts of daily dietary calcium. Calcium carbonate requires stomach acid for absorption and should be taken with meals. Calcium citrate does not require an acidic environment to be absorbed and is more appropriate for elderly patients who are taking acid-suppression medications.

Vitamin D is required for small intestinal absorption of calcium. Vitamin D deficiency is common and has been linked to decreased bone density. Several trials support the use of calcium and vitamin D in prevention and reversal of postmenopausal bone loss. Dietary sources of vitamin D include fortified foods such as milk, juice, and cereals. Supplementation is accomplished with multivitamins (most contain 200-400 IU of vitamin D), combined calcium/vitamin D preparations, or oral vitamin D repletion. The recommended vitamin D intake is 600-800 IU/day for all adults aged >50 years. Doses up to 2000 IU/day may be needed in certain patients to maintain a recommended 25-hydroxyvitamin D level of >30 ng/mL (74.9 nmol/L). Vitamin D levels also rise with adequate sun exposure.

Pharmacologic Therapy

Pharmacologic therapy is effective in reducing fracture risk in patients with or at risk for osteoporosis (Table 4). Therapy is begun in patients with a DEXA T score of less than -2.0, in patients with a DEXA T score of less than -1.5 if additional risk factors are present, or in any patient with a prior fragility, vertebral, or hip fracture.

Bisphosphonates are first-line agents. Bisphosphonate treatment results in a 30% to 60% decrease in fracture rates, with the greatest efficacy shown in the prevention of new vertebral fractures. Three oral bisphosphonates are currently available: alendronate, risedronate, and ibandronate. These drugs reduce the risk of fracture by preventing bone resorption. Oral bisphosphonates are taken on an empty stomach with at least 8 oz (237 mL) of water, and patients must remain upright for at least 30 minutes (60 minutes for ibandronate) to prevent pill-induced esophageal ulceration. Bisphosphonates are contraindicated in patients with chronic kidney disease or esophageal disease. Intravenous ibandronate (administered once every 3 months) and intravenous zoledronate (administered once yearly) also have FDA approval for the treatment of osteoporosis in postmenopausal women. Bisphosphonate therapy (mainly intravenous) in patients with metastatic cancer has been associated with osteonecrosis of the jaw. There are reports of atypical subtrochanteric or diaphyseal femur fractures in patients taking long-term bisphosphonates. Further studies are needed to determine if this is a clinically significant side effect. Alendronate, risedronate, and zoledronate all have FDA approval for treatment of osteoporosis in men.

Raloxifene is a selective estrogen receptor modulator. It has an estrogen agonist effect on bone and an antagonist effect in the

Table 4. Drug Therapy for Osteoporosis

Class/Agent	Notes
Oral bisphosphonates (alendronate, risedronate, ibandronate)	Decrease bone resorption by attenuating osteoclast activity. First-line treatment of osteoporosis. Increase bone mass; decrease vertebral and nonvertebral fractures. May cause esophageal irritation. Must take in morning without food and with 8 oz of water and not recline for 30-60 min.
Intravenous bisphosphonates (zoledronate, ibandronate)	Decrease bone resorption by attenuating osteoclast activity. First-line treatment of osteoporosis. Increase bone mass; decrease vertebral fracture, hip fracture, and nonvertebral fractures. Flu-like symptoms after first dose. Zoledronate is given every 12 mo and ibandronate every 3 mo.
Raloxifene	Selective estrogen receptor modulator. Suppresses osteoclasts and decreases bone resorption; estrogen antagonist in uterus and breast. Increases bone mass; decreases vertebral fractures; decreases risk of breast cancer; increases thromboembolic risk, increases vasomotor symptoms; increases risk of fatal stroke. Not recommended for pre-menopausal women or women using estrogen replacement.
Teriparatide	Recombinant parathyroid hormone. Stimulates bone formation. Increases bone mass; decreases vertebral and nonvertebral fracture rates. Treatment cannot exceed 18 mo. Contraindicated in patients with history of bone malignancy, Paget disease, hypercalcemia, or skeletal radiation.
Calcitonin	Decreases bone resorption by attenuating osteoclast activity. Increases bone mass slightly; decreases vertebral fracture rates. Decreases pain associated with vertebral fracture. Causes rhinitis. Not considered first-line treatment for osteoporosis.
Denosumab	Monoclonal antibody that inhibits the proliferation, differentiation, and maturation of preosteoclasts into active bone-resorbing cells. Decreases bone remodeling and increases bone mineral density. Not considered first-line therapy for osteoporosis. Long-term safety unknown.

breast and uterus and may be used in women who cannot tolerate bisphosphonate therapy. Side effects include increased risk of thromboembolism and increased vasomotor symptoms. The effect of raloxifene on bone mass is less than that of estrogen or alendronate, with efficacy in reducing the risk of vertebral but not hip fracture rates. Although estrogen is effective, it is no longer recommended for prevention or treatment of osteoporosis due to an overall unfavorable risk/benefit profile.

Teriparatide is the first FDA-approved osteoporosis medication that stimulates bone formation rather than decreasing bone resorption. It is indicated for treatment of men and women with severe osteoporosis who have failed or cannot take other osteoporosis medications. Teriparatide reduces vertebral fractures by 65% and nonvertebral fractures by 53%, a reduction that continues even after therapy is discontinued. The drug is given as a subcutaneous injection once daily for 18 months. Side effects include lightheadedness, nausea, arthralgias, leg cramps, and, rarely, an increase in postinjection calcium level. Teriparatide is ten times more expensive than other therapies for osteoporosis and cannot be continued beyond 18 months because of concern about a potential risk for osteosarcoma.

Calcitonin is an antiresorptive agent administered as a nasal spray. It is indicated for patients with bone pain from osteoporotic fractures or patients with contraindications to other therapies. Calcitonin is not a first-line agent, as other therapies are typically more effective.

Denosumab is a monoclonal antibody that blocks activation of osteoclasts, leading to decreased bone resorption and increased bone density. It is given as a subcutaneous injection once every 6 months. Denosumab has been shown to reduce the risk of vertebral, nonvertebral, and hip fractures in women with osteoporosis. It is FDA-approved for use in postmenopausal women with a history of osteoporotic fracture or multiple risk factors for fracture or who have failed or cannot take other osteoporosis med-

ications. Denosumab may lower serum calcium, particularly in patients with chronic kidney disease, and it should not be used in patients with hypocalcemia. The long-term safety profile of denosumab is unknown.

Follow-Up

Use DEXA scan to measure bone mineral density 12 to 24 months after initiating pharmacologic therapy and periodically thereafter. Look for percent improvements in the bone density value to determine treatment efficacy and the T score to assess current fracture risk. Consider possible secondary causes, poor adherence, and need for additional treatment in patients with continuing bone loss after 12 to 18 months of medical therapy.

Book Enhancement

Go to www.acponline.org/essentials/endocrinology-section.html. In *MKSAP for Students 5*, assess your knowledge with items 28-32 in the **Endocrinology and Metabolism** section.

Acknowledgment

We would like to thank Drs. Melissa A. McNeil and Janine M. Frank, who contributed to an earlier version of this chapter.

Bibliography

Nelson HD, Haney EM, Dana T, Bougatsos C, Chou R. Screening for osteoporosis: an update for the U.S. Preventive Services Task Force. Ann Intern Med. 2010;153:99-111. [PMID: 20621892]

Qaseem A, Snow V, Shekelle P, et al. Pharmacologic treatment of low bone density or osteoporosis to prevent fractures: a clinical practice guideline from the American College of Physicians. Ann Intern Med. 2008; 149:404-415. [PMID: 18794560]

Chapter 15

Approach to Abdominal Pain

Eric Hsieh, MD

Abdominal pain is a common symptom, accounting for 18% to 42% of hospital admissions. Although some patients have classic symptoms pointing to a particular diagnosis, in other patients the diagnosis is obscure. Pain in the abdomen is generally of visceral or peritoneal origin, originates from the abdominal wall, or is referred from other sites. Visceral pain is usually caused by stretching of the organ and is not associated with signs of peritoneal inflammation. In contrast, peritoneal pain is secondary to inflammation or irritation of the overlying peritoneum and is associated with tenderness, guarding, or rebound. Abdominal wall pain tends to be chronic and to be precisely located by the patient. Referred pain generally follows a dermatomal distribution and is not associated with underlying tenderness or signs of peritoneal inflammation.

Evaluation

The history and physical examination help develop a differential diagnosis (Table 1) and direct the relevant investigations. Important clues to the underlying diagnosis can be discovered through carefully characterizing the abdominal pain with respect to onset (acute or insidious), duration, nature (intermittent or constant), relation to eating, association with bleeding, and location. Pain that is acute in onset generally points to acute inflammatory, infectious, or ischemic causes. Upper abdominal pain is usually of gastric, hepatobiliary, or pancreatic origin, whereas pain in the lower abdomen originates from the hindgut and genitourinary organs. The origin of periumbilical pain is the midgut and pancreas. Hematemesis definitely points to an upper gastrointestinal etiology, but melena, maroon stools, hematochezia, or occult blood can be from either upper or lower gastrointestinal sources. General symptoms such as anorexia, nausea, or vomiting are insensitive in diagnosing abdominal pain. Associated medical problems can often suggest a diagnosis such as embolic or ischemic infarction due to cardiovascular disease, arrhythmia, or infective endocarditis. A history of multiple sexual partners, unprotected intercourse, or previous sexually transmitted disease highlights the possibility of pelvic inflammatory disease in women. The evaluation of abdominal pain is never complete until a physical examination, including pelvic and rectal examination, has been performed.

Acute Abdominal Pain

Acute abdominal pain is defined as pain lasting <1 week. The most common diagnoses are appendicitis, biliary disease, and nonspecific abdominal pain. Patients with acute abdominal pain, peritoneal signs, and hemodynamic instability require an urgent investigation and may need early surgical intervention. Obtain a chest radiograph and flat and upright abdominal radiographs in every patient with significant acute abdominal pain to exclude bowel obstruction or perforation (free peritoneal air localized under the diaphragm) or intrathoracic processes that can present as abdominal pain (e.g., pneumonia, pneumothorax, aortic dissection). In older patients, consider an electrocardiogram to exclude an atypical presentation of myocardial infarction.

Abdominal aortic aneurysms occur in 1% of all men aged >65 years. The pain is often of acute onset, radiating to the back. A pulsatile mass may be palpated in the abdomen. The mortality rate is greater than 50% with free rupture of an aneurysm, and affected patients frequently present with hemodynamic instability and cardiovascular collapse. Immediate treatment of patients with hemodynamic instability should include judicious fluid replacement, because overaggressive fluid resuscitation can worsen hemorrhage.

Upper Abdominal Pain

Biliary pain is the most common cause of acute abdominal pain among patients aged >50 years. Cholelithiasis should be suspected in patients with postprandial, right upper quadrant pain associated with ingesting fatty foods. Murphy sign (respiratory arrest on deep inspiration while palpating the right upper quadrant) suggests cholecystitis, and Charcot triad (pain, fever, jaundice) suggests cholecystitis or ascending cholangitis. Abdominal ultrasonography is the imaging modality of choice for cholelithiasis, with sensitivity and specificity both approaching 100%. Cholescintigraphy scans (e.g., hepatobiliary iminodiacetic acid [HIDA] scans) are an alternative to diagnose acute cholecystitis and can be used when ultrasonography is equivocal.

Peptic ulcer disease and gastritis commonly present as burning abdominal pain, but the pain may be vague or even cramping. In two-thirds of cases the pain is epigastric, with the remainder of cases involving pain in the upper right or upper left quadrant. Pain that radiates through to the back is unusual with peptic ulcer disease or gastritis and suggests pancreatitis or penetrating peptic ulcer disease; hematemesis or blood in the nasogastric aspirate excludes pancreatitis. Ingestion of food worsens gastric ulcer pain and improves duodenal ulcer pain, but this relationship is found in less than half of patients with confirmed peptic ulcer disease. The presence of peritoneal signs strongly suggests perforation and is supported by finding free air under the diaphragm on chest radiograph or upright abdominal radiograph.

Table 1. Differential Diagnosis of Acute Abdominal Pain

Disorder	Notes
Right Upper Quadrant (RUQ)	
Acute cholangitis (see Chapter 18)	RUQ pain, fever, jaundice. Bilirubin generally >4 mg/dL (68.4 mmol/L), AST and ALT may be >1000 U/L.
Pneumonia (see Chapter 57)	Cough, shortness of breath, chest or upper abdominal pain.
Acute viral hepatitis (see Chapter 24)	Jaundice; AST and ALT generally >1000 U/L.
Acute alcoholic hepatitis	Recent alcohol intake, fever. Leukocytosis, bilirubin generally >4 mg/dL (68.4 mmol/L), AST usually 2-3 times greater than ALT.
Fitz-Hugh–Curtis syndrome (gonococcal perihepatitis)	Pelvic adnexal tenderness, leukocytosis. Cervical smear shows gonococci.
Cholecystitis (see Chapter 18)	Epigastric and RUQ pain that radiates to right shoulder. Mildly elevated bilirubin, AST, and ALT. Ultrasonography shows thickened gallbladder and pericholecystic fluid.
Mid-Epigastric/Periumbilical	
Acute pancreatitis (see Chapter 19)	Mid-epigastric pain radiating to the back, nausea, vomiting. Elevated amylase and lipase. Usually secondary to gallstones or alcohol. Pain from penetrating peptic ulcer may present similarly.
Inferior myocardial infarction (see Chapter 3)	Chest/mid-epigastric pain, diaphoresis, shortness of breath. Elevated cardiac enzymes. Acutely abnormal electrocardiogram.
Perforating peptic ulcer (see Chapter 21)	Postprandial abdominal pain, weight loss, abdominal bruit (chronic presentation); pain out of proportion to tenderness on palpation.
Mesenteric ischemia	Possible anion gap metabolic acidosis. Abdominal plain films may show classic thumbprinting sign (acute presentation).
Small bowel obstruction	Colicky pain. Obstructive pattern seen on CT or abdominal series.
Aortic dissection/rupture	Elderly patient with vascular disease and sudden-onset severe pain that radiates to the back and lower extremity.
Diabetic ketoacidosis (see Chapter 10)	Blood glucose always elevated, anion gap always present.
Right Lower Quadrant (RLQ)	
Acute appendicitis	Mid-epigastric pain radiating to RLQ. Ultrasonography and CT may confirm diagnosis.
Ectopic pregnancy, ovarian cyst/torsion	RLQ or LLQ abdominal pain, nausea, fever; leukocytosis. Suspect in female with unilateral pain.
Pelvic inflammatory disease	May be RLQ or LLQ; fever; abdominal tenderness, uterine/adnexal tenderness, cervical motion tenderness; cervical discharge.
Nephrolithiasis	Right or left flank pain that may radiate to groin; hematuria.
Pyelonephritis (see Chapter 52)	Fever, dysuria, and pain in right or left flank that may radiate to lower quadrant. Urinalysis shows leukocytes and leukocyte casts.
Left Lower Quadrant (LLQ)	
Acute diverticulitis	Pain usually in LLQ but can be RLQ if ascending colon is involved. CT can diagnose complicated diverticular disease with abscess formation.
Toxic megacolon	Nonobstructive dilatation of transverse and descending colon. Systemic toxicity. Associated with inflammatory bowel disease and *Clostridium difficile* infection.

ALT = alanine aminotransferase; AST = aspartate aminotransferase.

Acute pancreatitis presents as acute epigastric pain, often radiating to the back. Vomiting occurs in >85% of cases; the absence of vomiting favors another diagnosis. Bending forward or lying curled up on one's side may relieve the pain, but many patients report no alleviating factors. The diagnosis of pancreatitis is confirmed by serum amylase (sensitivity 60%, specificity 99%) and serum lipase (sensitivity 90%-100%, specificity, 99%) concentrations that are at least three times the upper limits of normal. The degree of elevation does not correlate with severity of disease. Jaundice frequently accompanies gallstone pancreatitis, and a history of alcohol abuse supports alcoholic pancreatitis. Occasionally, patients may have flank ecchymoses from retroperitoneal bleeding (Grey-Turner sign). Perform ultrasonography to evaluate the biliary tract for stones. Obtain an abdominal CT scan, ideally with oral and intravenous contrast, when the diagnosis of acute pancreatitis is in question, to stage the severity, or to determine the presence of complications such as abscess or pseudocyst.

Central and Lower Abdominal Pain

Appendicitis is the most common cause of acute abdominal pain in patients aged <50 years. Despite the development of sophisticated diagnostic techniques and algorithms, appendicitis is missed in at least 20% of cases. The pain classically begins in the periumbilical region and migrates to the right lower quadrant and may be followed by nausea and vomiting. The diagnosis of appendicitis is doubtful if nausea and vomiting are the first signs of illness. Physical examination will reveal tenderness over McBurney point; abdominal rigidity and a positive psoas sign (pain elicited by extending the patient's right thigh while the patient is lying on his or her left side) increase the pretest probability of appendicitis. Leukocytosis and fever, although sensitive, are not specific for appendicitis. Abdominal CT with oral and intravenous contrast is the diagnostic test of choice in non-pregnant patients (sensitivity and specificity >92%, positive likelihood ratio = 18). Ultrasonography and plain abdominal radiography have poor sensitivity and specificity in the diagnosis of appendicitis.

Small bowel obstruction presents as central or generalized abdominal pain associated with vomiting or constipation. History of prior abdominal surgery, hyperactive bowel sounds, and abdominal distension increase the probability of small bowel obstruction. Abdominal radiography shows multiple dilated bowel loops with air fluid levels usually arranged in a stepladder pattern; this finding plus a lack of colonic gas is pathognomic. Strangulating small bowel obstructions are better visualized on CT. CT scans with contrast are also superior to plain radiographs in detecting complete small bowel obstruction, but early or partial obstruction may be missed by either modality. Other causes of small bowel obstruction include neoplasms, strictures, intussusception, and volvulus.

Acute colonic distension is most likely due to mechanical obstruction, toxic megacolon (a complication of inflammatory bowel disease or *Clostridium difficile* infection), and colonic pseudo-obstruction. Mechanical obstruction presents as crampy abdominal pain. On abdominal radiographs, dilated loops of small and large bowel and lack of gas in the distal colon or rectum suggest mechanical obstruction but can also be seen in pseudo-obstruction. Mechanical obstruction is most commonly due to tumors and sigmoid volvulus. Acute colonic pseudo-obstruction (Ogilvie syndrome) is characterized by dilatation of the cecum and right hemicolon in the absence of mechanical obstruction; the most common causes are trauma, infection, and cardiac disease (i.e., myocardial infarction, heart failure). Toxic megacolon presents as fever, tachycardia, and abdominal tenderness, and there is usually a history of bloody diarrhea. Abdominal films may show thumbprinting due to the presence of submucosal edema or thickening of the colonic wall.

Acute diverticulitis presents as left lower quadrant abdominal pain and tenderness to palpation. Patients may have a history of chronic constipation and intermittent low-grade abdominal pain prior to an acute attack. Abscess formation should be suspected if guarding, rigidity, or a tender fluctuant mass is present. Abdominal and pelvic CT with contrast is the test of choice.

Nonspecific abdominal pain is the third most common cause of acute abdominal pain presenting to the emergency department. It includes all causes of abdominal pain for which no specific surgical, medical, or gynecologic diagnosis can be made, including dyspepsia, constipation, irritable bowel syndrome (IBS), viral gastroenteritis, mesenteric adenitis, and dysmenorrhea.

Kidney stones, acute urinary obstruction, and urinary tract infection including pyelonephritis are common causes of abdominal pain. Pain due to a kidney stone is typically acute and colicky and may radiate from the flank to the groin, particularly as the stone travels down the ureter. Renal colic may be associated with hematuria and dysuria. Helical CT is the most sensitive and specific imaging study available for stones and also excels in making the diagnosis of nonrenal causes of flank pain.

Acute urinary obstruction presents as suprapubic discomfort and oliguria or anuria. It is common in older males, secondary to prostatic hypertrophy. Insertion of a catheter relieves the obstruction and pain. Testicular torsion may cause referred pain to the lower abdomen. Physical examination will classically reveal an asymmetrically high-riding testis. The cremasteric reflex (elevation of ipsilateral testis after stroking the skin of the upper thigh) is usually absent. Color Doppler ultrasonography can help to confirm the diagnosis (absent blood flow).

Women presenting with lower abdominal or pelvic pain must have a pelvic examination and a urine pregnancy test; pelvic inflammatory disease and ectopic pregnancy are often overlooked causes of lower abdominal pain. Ovarian cyst rupture, which is best diagnosed with ultrasonography, and endometriosis, which requires direct visualization of the implants for diagnosis, should also be considered in women with lower abdominal or pelvic pain.

Generalized Abdominal Pain

Diffuse abdominal pain is seen in acute peritonitis, ischemic small bowel, and small bowel obstruction. The most common cause of ischemic small bowel is a mesenteric arterial embolism originating from the heart (50%), followed by mesenteric arterial thrombosis (25%) and mesenteric venous thrombosis (10%). Initially, abdominal pain is poorly localized and is more severe than the findings suggested by abdominal palpation. Peritoneal signs may signify bowel infarction. Selective mesenteric angiography is the diagnostic study of choice.

Colonic ischemia, also called ischemic colitis, is much more common than mesenteric ischemia. Although an underlying cause often is not identified, colonic ischemia can occur in association with colonic hypoperfusion in the setting of aortic or cardiac bypass surgery, prolonged physical exertion, and any cardiovascular event associated with hypotension. Medications such as oral contraceptives, illicit drugs such as cocaine, vasculitides, and hypercoaguable states also are risk factors. Most patients with colonic ischemia are aged >60 years. Colonoscopy is the primary diagnostic procedure.

Abdominal pain can be a presenting feature of metabolic disorders such as diabetic and alcoholic ketoacidosis, adrenal crises, sickle cell crisis, porphyria, and familial Mediterranean fever. Vasculitides (Henoch-Schönlein purpura, systemic lupus erythematosus, polyarteritis nodosa) also should be considered in the differential diagnosis, particularly if the abdominal pain is associated with extra-abdominal manifestations such as rash, arthralgias, pleuritic pain, hematuria, or kidney failure.

Chronic Abdominal Pain

Abdominal pain is chronic if it has persisted for >3 months. Chronic abdominal pain is a common cause of ambulatory care visits; within this category, IBS is one of the most common causes of chronic abdominal pain. Abdominal wall pain is an often-overlooked cause of chronic pain and includes entities such as hernia and rectus sheath hematomas. The pain is precisely localized by the patient with one finger.

Irritable Bowel Syndrome

The pain of IBS is localized to the lower abdomen and may be associated with bloating, nausea, and diarrhea or constipation. Physical examination characteristically reveals only nonspecific tenderness over the sigmoid colon. IBS frequently coexists with other chronic conditions such as depression, fibromyalgia, and chronic pelvic pain syndrome. The pain of IBS often is exacerbated by psychological stress.

For many years, IBS has been considered a diagnosis of exclusion, but this approach leads to unnecessary additional tests. Recent clinical and epidemiologic studies have led to the development of symptom-based diagnostic criteria that can accurately discriminate IBS from other disorders. The Rome criteria (sensitivity approximately 48%, specificity 100%) and the Manning criteria (sensitivity 60%, specificity 80%) are used to diagnose IBS (Table 2). Diagnostic accuracy of the Manning criteria is better in women, in younger patients, and when more criteria are positive. Red flags that make the diagnosis of IBS unlikely and that should prompt an early investigation for other causes include onset of abdominal pain in older age, anorexia, weight loss, signs of malnutrition, and a recent change in bowel habits. IBS is recognized to have three major subtypes: diarrhea predominant, constipation predominant, and pain predominant. Alternating between diarrhea and constipation or changing from constipation predominance to diarrhea predominance (or vice versa) over time is not uncommon.

The management of IBS focuses on managing symptoms rather than on cure. Treatment is targeted at the predominant symptom and, therefore, the patient's subtype. Pharmacologic approaches include antispasmodic agents, bulking agents, antidiarrheal agents, tricyclic antidepressants, and the 5-hydroxytryptamine-3 (5HT3) receptor antagonist, alosetron (available only through an FDA-restricted program). Nonpharmacologic treatments for IBS include exercise, relaxation therapy, biofeedback, hypnotherapy, cognitive behavioral therapy, and psychotherapy. There currently are no data that dietary modification will improve IBS symptoms. However, if food triggers can be clearly identified, they should be eliminated or reduced from the patient's diet. Because psychiatric disorders are common in patients with IBS, screening patients for depression and anxiety is indicated, and any coexisting disorders should be treated.

Pancreatic Disease

Pancreatic disease is an important cause of chronic abdominal pain. The four cardinal findings characterizing chronic pancreatitis include pain (90% to 95% of cases), diabetes mellitus, steatorrhea, and pancreatic calculi (best detected on CT scan). Periods of pain may be irregular, with weeks to months of remission. One third to half of patients with pancreatitis may become pain-free, but this may take years. Pancreatic enzyme replacement is often ineffective for pain relief, and many patients require chronic opiates. Refractory pain in these patients sometimes necessitates sphincterotomy, stenting, or surgical resection, although evidence confirming the efficacy of these procedures is limited.

Age and tobacco smoking are the most important risk factors for pancreatic cancer. The most common symptom is constant epigastric pain that radiates to the back. Patients with tumors of the body and tail of the gland usually present with pain, because these tumors tend to be large when detected. The most common location of pancreatic cancers is in the head of the gland; these tumors often are accompanied by painless jaundice caused by obstruction of the common bile duct. Physical examination often reveals weight loss, jaundice, and abdominal tenderness. Occasionally, there is a nontender palpable gallbladder (Courvoisier sign) in a jaundiced patient; rarely, migratory thrombophlebitis is noted. Pancreatic protocol contrast-enhanced spiral CT is the most effective diagnostic and staging tool for pancreatic cancer, with sensitivity greater than 90%.

Table 2. Criteria for Diagnosis of Irritable Bowel Syndrome

Rome Criteria

≥3 mo of continuous or recurrent symptoms of abdominal pain or discomfort that is:	Relieved with defecation and/or Associated with a change in frequency of stool and/or Associated with a change in consistency of stool
and ≥2 of these 5 symptoms on >25% of occasions or days:	Altered stool frequency (>3 bowel movements daily or <3 bowel movements weekly) Altered stool form (lumpy/hard, loose/watery) Altered stool passage (straining, urgency, feeling of incomplete evacuation) Passage of mucus Bloating or feeling of abdominal distension

Manning Criteria

The presence of abdominal pain and ≥2 of these 6 symptoms:	Pain relief with defecation Looser stools at pain onset More frequent stools at pain onset Abdominal distentionMucus per rectum Feeling of incomplete evacuation

Book Enhancement

Go to www.acponline.org/essentials/gastroenterology-section .html. In *MKSAP for Students 5*, assess your knowledge with items 1-7 in the **Gastroenterology and Hepatology** section.

Acknowledgment

We would like to thank Dr. Priya Radhakrishnan, who contributed to an earlier version of this chapter.

Bibliography

Jacobs DO. Clinical practice. Diverticulitis. N Engl J Med. 2007;357:2057-2066. [PMID: 18003962]

Mayer EA. Clinical practice. Irritable bowel syndrome. N Engl J Med. 2008; 358:1692-1699. [PMID: 18420501]

Trowbridge RL, Rutkowski NK, Shojania KG. Does this patient have acute cholecystitis? JAMA. 2003;289:80-86 [published erratum appears in JAMA. 2009;302:739]. [PMID: 12503981]

Chapter 16

Approach to Diarrhea

Sarang Kim, MD

Diarrhea is traditionally defined as >200 g of stool per day. In clinical practice, diarrhea is defined as >3 loose stools per day. Diarrhea may occur due to a variety of mechanisms, such as presence of poorly absorbed solutes in the lumen of the gut (e.g., lactose), disruption of intestinal mucosal ion transport and subsequent water secretion (e.g., cholera), disruption in the mucosal barrier secondary to infection or inflammation (e.g., ulcerative colitis, *Clostridium difficile* infection), malabsorption of fat from pancreatic or bile salt insufficiency (e.g., chronic pancreatitis, obstructive jaundice), bowel resection, reduced mucosal surface area (e.g., celiac disease), injury from radiation treatment, bacterial overgrowth (e.g., surgical blind loop), intestinal ischemia (e.g., chronic mesenteric artery insufficiency), and disorders of motility (e.g., systemic sclerosis). Start the evaluation of patients with diarrhea by differentiating acute diarrhea from chronic diarrhea.

Acute Diarrhea

Acute diarrhea is diarrhea lasting <14 days. The most common cause is an infectious agent. Acute infectious diarrhea is transmitted predominantly through the fecal-oral route by ingestion of contaminated food or water. Diarrhea may result from ingestion of preformed bacterial toxins or from ingestion of bacteria that subsequently produce exotoxins and/or invade the gastrointestinal mucosa.

Diagnosis

The first step in evaluation of patients with acute diarrhea is to obtain a detailed history and physical examination to assess the severity, quality, and duration of diarrhea and to identify epidemiologic clues for potential diagnosis (Table 1). Ask patients about recent food ingestion, antibiotic use, travel, and sick contacts. Ingestion of preformed bacterial toxins results in nausea and vomiting followed by diarrhea within 12 hours. Bacteria that require colonization to produce symptoms may not cause diarrhea until 2 to 3 days after ingestion of contaminated food. Outbreaks of diarrhea in families, cruise ships, airplanes, day care centers, nursing homes, or schools are commonly associated with *Norovirus*. Traveler's diarrhea is most commonly caused by *Escherichia coli, Campylobacter, Shigella, Salmonella, Giardia,* and *Entamoeba,* although the exact causative agent will vary depending on area of travel and exposure risks. For hospitalized patients or those with recent antibiotic use, *C. difficile* infection should be considered, as disruption of the intestinal flora by antibiotics and decreased gastric acidity caused by proton pump inhibitors and H_2-receptor blockers are recognized risk factors for *C. difficile* infection. *C. difficile* infection is an inflammatory condition of the colon caused by the ingestion of the spore-forming, anaerobic, gram-positive bacillus. The inflammatory response is secondary to toxin-induced cytokines (toxins A and B) in the colon. Findings can range from watery diarrhea to ileus and life-threatening conditions (toxic megacolon, perforation, sepsis). Noninfectious causes of acute diarrhea include ischemic colitis, diverticulitis, and medications or ingestion of substances that can cause osmotic diarrhea (sorbitol, fructose, laxatives).

Because most episodes of diarrhea are self-limited, diagnostic testing generally is reserved for patients with severe diarrheal illness characterized by fever, blood in the stool, or signs of dehydration (weakness, thirst, decreased urine output, orthostasis) or patients with diarrhea lasting >7 days. For severe community-acquired or traveler's diarrhea, obtain stool cultures for *Salmonella, Shigella,* and *Campylobacter.* Routine stool culture cannot distinguish path-

Table 1. Causes of Infectious Diarrhea

Clues	Likely Causes
Contaminated food with rapid onset of symptoms	*Staphylococcus aureus* (potato salad, mayonnaise, ham); *Bacillus cereus* (fried rice); *Clostridium perfringens* (beef, poultry)
Contaminated food with delayed onset of symptoms	*Vibrio cholerae* (shellfish); enterotoxigenic *Escherichia coli* (salads, cheese, meats); enterohemorrhagic *E. coli* (ground beef, raw vegetables); *Salmonella* (beef, poultry, eggs, dairy); *Yersinia* (raw milk); *Campylobacter jejuni* (poultry, raw milk)
Travel history	*E. coli, Salmonella, Shigella, Campylobacter, Giardia, Entamoeba, Vibrio*
Blood in stool	*Campylobacter, Shigella,* Shiga toxin–producing *E. coli* (e.g., *E. coli* O157:H7)
Health care facility or antibiotic exposure	*Clostridium difficile*
Acute or chronic watery diarrhea in immunocompromised patient	*Cryptosporidium, Cyclospora, Isospora,* microsporidia, *Mycobacterium avium* complex
Outbreak in nursing home, day care center, or cruise ship	*Norovirus, Rotavirus*

ogenic *E. coli* from normal fecal flora. Therefore, in the setting of blood in the stool, test specifically for *E. coli* O157:H7 and Shiga toxin. If symptoms have persisted beyond 7 days, stool should be examined for ova and parasites. For health care–related diarrhea, test for *C. difficile* toxin. Fecal specimens collected after 3 days of hospitalization have a very low yield for standard bacterial pathogens, and routine stool culture is not indicated for inpatients with diarrhea unless there is evidence of a specific outbreak. In an immunocompromised patient, also test for *Mycobacterium avium* complex (MAC) by sending stool for acid-fast bacillus (AFB) stain and culture, as disseminated MAC infections often involve the gastrointestinal tract and cause diarrhea.

Therapy

Adequate hydration and avoidance of easily malabsorbed carbohydrates (lactose, sorbitol) often are sufficient treatments for otherwise healthy patients with acute noninflammatory diarrhea (i.e., diarrhea without pain, fecal blood or pus, or fever) that is most likely secondary to a transient infection. Empiric antibiotics (quinolones) often are appropriate for patients with acute traveler's diarrhea. Untreated traveler's diarrhea usually resolves in 3 to 5 days, but treatment can improve symptoms and shorten the course. Antidiarrheal agents should be avoided in patients with suspected inflammatory diarrhea (e.g., diarrhea due to ulcerative colitis, *C. difficile* infection, or Shiga toxin–producing *E. coli*) because of the association with toxic megacolon. Use oral metronidazole for mild to moderate *C. difficile* infection and oral vancomycin for severe infection or for patients who cannot tolerate or fail to respond to metronidazole.

Complications may occur after treatment of acute diarrhea. Chronic diarrhea may occur due to lactase deficiency after an acute diarrheal illness. Exacerbation of inflammatory bowel disease or irritable bowel syndrome may occur after acute infectious diarrhea. Reactive arthritis can occur after *Shigella, Salmonella,* and *Campylobacter* infections. Guillain-Barré syndrome is associated with *Campylobacter* and *Yersinia* infections. Hemolytic uremic syndrome (hemolytic anemia, thrombocytopenia, acute kidney injury) can occur with Shiga toxin–producing *E. coli* or *Shigella* infection. Relapse is common after initial treatment for *C. difficile* infection, occurring in up to 20% of patients. A first recurrence is treated the same way as the initial episode, based on disease severity. For later recurrences, prolonged courses of oral vancomycin can be used.

Chronic Diarrhea

Chronic diarrhea is diarrhea lasting >4 weeks. A patient-centered approach to evaluation focuses on attributes that are most appar-

Table 2. Causes of Noninfectious Diarrhea

Disorder	Clues or Risk Factors	Diagnosis
Inflammatory bowel disease (ulcerative colitis, Crohn disease)	Bloody diarrhea, tenesmus, weight loss, anemia, hypoalbuminemia	Colonoscopy with biopsy
Microscopic colitis	Chronic relapsing-remitting watery diarrhea	Normal colonoscopy, abnormal biopsy (includes collagenous colitis, lymphocytic colitis)
Irritable bowel syndrome (diarrhea-predominant)	No weight loss or alarm features	Chronic bloating, abdominal discomfort relieved by bowel movement
Celiac disease	Iron deficiency anemia, dermatitis herpetiformis	Anti–tissue transglutaminase antibodies, small bowel biopsy
Whipple disease	Arthralgia, neurologic or ophthalmologic symptoms	Polymerase chain reaction for *Tropheryma whippelii*, small bowel biopsy
Carbohydrate intolerance	Lactose or fructose intake, use of artificial sweeteners (sorbitol, mannitol)	Dietary exclusion, hydrogen breath test
Pancreatic insufficiency	Steatorrhea, chronic pancreatitis, pancreatic resection	Tests for excess fecal fat, CT scan showing pancreatic calcification
Small bowel bacterial overgrowth	Intestinal dysmotility (e.g., systemic sclerosis)	Duodenal aspirate for bacterial culture, response to empiric antibiotics
Common variable immune deficiency	Pulmonary disease, recurrent *Giardia* infection	Immunoglobulin assay
Medications	Acarbose, antibiotics, antineoplastic agents, magnesium-based antacids, metformin, misoprostol, NSAIDs, proton pump inhibitors, quinidine	Withhold suspected medications
Enteral feedings	Osmotic diarrhea	Modify enteral feeding
Bile acid malabsorption	Resection of <100 cm of distal small bowel	Empiric response to cholestyramine
Bile acid deficiency	Cholestasis, resection of >100 cm of small bowel	Tests for excess fecal fat
Radiation exposure	History of radiation therapy (may begin years after exposure)	Bowel imaging, characteristic biopsy findings
Dumping syndrome	Postprandial flushing, tachycardia	History of gastrectomy or gastric bypass surgery
Factitious diarrhea	Psychiatric history, history of laxative abuse	Low stool osmolarity

ent to the patient, including duration of the diarrhea, severity of symptoms, and stool characteristics (Table 2).

Diagnosis

Ask the patient about stool frequency and characteristics, association of diarrhea with food, medications, previous surgery, and prior radiation treatment. Ask specifically about fecal incontinence, as patients may not volunteer this symptom but instead report it as diarrhea; fecal incontinence is a common problem, especially in elderly patients. Diet history may reveal large quantities of indigestible carbohydrates (osmotic diarrhea) or intolerance to wheat products (celiac disease, Whipple disease). A patient's fixation on body image and weight loss may be a clue to laxative abuse. Frequent, high-volume, watery stools suggest a disease process affecting the small intestine. High-volume diarrhea that is exacerbated with eating and relieved with fasting or a clear liquid diet suggests carbohydrate malabsorption, whereas persistent or nocturnal diarrhea suggests a secretory process. The presence of persistent, severe or aching abdominal pain suggests an invasive process associated with inflammation or destruction of the mucosa. Skin findings, when present, may provide significant diagnostic clues. For example, flushing may indicate carcinoid syndrome; dermatitis herpetiformis (grouped, pruritic, erythematous papulovesicles on the extensor surfaces of the arms, legs, central back, buttocks, and scalp) may occur in patients with celiac disease; and erythema nodosum (Plate 2) or pyoderma gangrenosum (Plate 3) may suggest underlying inflammatory bowel disease. Bloody diarrhea typically indicates an invasive process with loss of intestinal mucosal integrity. An oily residue or evidence of undigested food in the toilet bowl is more suggestive of malabsorption.

Consider irritable bowel syndrome in patients with a long-standing history of abdominal pain and abnormal bowel habits (constipation, diarrhea, or variable bowel movements) in the absence of other defined illnesses. The presence of weight loss, blood in the stool, or nocturnal diarrhea almost always indicates that the patient does not have irritable bowel syndrome.

The number and variety of diagnostic tests available for patients with chronic diarrhea are extensive, and testing should be guided by information obtained from the history and physical examination. A complete blood count and chemistry panel can reveal anemia, leukocytosis, and electrolyte and nutritional status. Bacterial infections rarely cause chronic diarrhea in immunocompetent patients, but common infectious causes of acute diarrhea such as *Campylobacter* or *Salmonella* can cause persistent diarrhea in immunocompromised patients, as can *Cryptosporidium* infection. Infection should always be ruled out in patients with chronic diarrhea before proceeding with more extensive testing (Table 3).

Table 3. Common Diagnostic Tests for Diarrhea

Test	Condition	Characteristics
Fecal leukocytes	Infectious or inflammatory diarrhea	Poor sensitivity and specificity (limited usefulness)
Stool culture	Infectious diarrhea	Detects *Salmonella, Shigella, Campylobacter*; specify if needed to test for *E. coli* O157:H7
Stool ova and parasites	Infectious diarrhea	Microscopic examination for *Giardia, Entamoeba, Cryptosporidium, Cyclospora, Isospora,* microsporidia
Stool enzyme immunoassays	Infectious diarrhea	Detect Shiga toxins 1 and 2 and antigens for *Giardia, Entamoeba, Campylobacter, Cryptosporidium*
Qualitative fecal fat (Sudan stain)	Fat malabsorption	Sensitivity >90% for significant steatorrhea
Quantitative fecal fat (48- or 72-h collection)	Fat malabsorption	Values >10 g/24 h indicate fat malabsorption
Stool osmolarity	Factitious diarrhea	<250 mosm/kg (250 mmol/kg) suggests factitious diarrhea
Stool electrolytes (sodium, potassium)	Differentiate osmotic versus secretory diarrhea	Osmotic gap[a] >125 mosm/kg (125 mmol/kg) suggests osmotic diarrhea, <50 mosm/kg (50 mmol/kg) suggests secretory diarrhea
Stool magnesium	Magnesium-containing antacids, cathartics (factitious or iatrogenic diarrhea)	Spot magnesium sample >90 meq/L (37.1 mmol/L)
Stool pH	Carbohydrate malabsorption	pH <6.0 suggests carbohydrate malabsorption
C. difficile toxin enzyme immunoassay	*C. difficile* infection	Sensitivity 70%-80%, specificity >97% for toxins A and B
Anti–tissue transglutaminase, anti-endomysial antibodies	Celiac disease	Sensitivity 90%, specificity 98%; diagnosis confirmed by small bowel biopsy
Hydrogen breath test	Lactase deficiency	Lactose metabolized by bacterial flora in distal small intestine releases hydrogen, which is excreted by lungs
Duodenal aspirate	Small bowel bacterial overgrowth	Quantitative bacterial culture; responds to empiric antibiotic trial
Neuropeptide assays[b]	Neuroendocrine tumors	Useful if persistent diarrhea despite fasting

[a]Osmotic gap calculation: 290 − (2 × [Na + K]).

[b]Gastrin, vasoactive intestinal peptide, glucagon, somatostatin, pancreatic peptide, neurotensin, substance P, calcitonin, motilin, urine 5-hydroxyindoleacetic acid.

A fecal fat study is usually indicated for evaluating a patient with noninvasive diarrhea. However, test results are valid only if the patient ingests an adequate amount of dietary fat (>100 g/d). Any cause of diarrhea may mildly elevate fecal fat values (6-10 g/24 h), but values in excess of 10 g/24 h almost always indicate primary fat malabsorption.

The presence of fecal leukocytes or lactoferrin suggests an inflammatory process but rarely provides more specific clues about the cause of diarrhea. If infection is excluded in a patient with chronic inflammatory diarrhea, colonoscopy or flexible sigmoidoscopy with biopsies usually are required for diagnosis.

Measurement of stool electrolytes is valuable for only a subset of patients who remain a diagnostic challenge despite the exclusion of infectious, iatrogenic, and inflammatory causes of diarrhea. Stool electrolytes help differentiate osmotic from secretory diarrhea. If factitious diarrhea is suspected, a fresh liquid stool sample should be obtained for determination of total osmolarity and stool sodium and potassium concentrations, and the osmotic gap should be calculated.

Celiac disease (gluten-sensitive enteropathy) occurs in approximately 1 in 120 to 1 in 300 persons in the United States. Classic symptoms include steatorrhea and weight loss, but many patients have only mild or nonspecific symptoms that often result in erroneous diagnosis of irritable bowel syndrome. Laboratory tests that aid the diagnosis include anti–tissue transglutaminase and anti-endomysial antibodies (sensitivity 90%, specificity 98%); confirmation is by endoscopic small bowel biopsy showing intraepithelial lymphocytes, crypt hyperplasia, and partial to total villous atrophy.

Excessive bacterial colonization of the small bowel lumen may result in diarrhea and malabsorption. A clue to the presence of bacterial overgrowth is finding a low serum vitamin B_{12} level (bacteria bind vitamin B_{12} and cleave it from intrinsic factor) and a high serum folate level (intestinal bacteria synthesize folate). Common conditions that predispose patients to bacterial overgrowth include diabetes, systemic sclerosis, and surgically created blind loops (i.e., gastrojejunostomy). Although the gold standard is aspiration of duodenal luminal contents for quantitative culture at the time of upper endoscopy, many clinicians first attempt a trial of empiric antibiotics (e.g., amoxicillin-clavulanate, norfloxacin) to see if the patient's symptoms improve.

Therapy

Treatment of chronic diarrhea should be based on the underlying cause. Symptomatic therapy may be considered if a diagnosis is pending, if a diagnosis cannot be confirmed, or if the condition diagnosed does not have a specific treatment. Symptoms may be controlled with stool-modifying agents (e.g., fiber), opiate-based medications, bile acid–binding agents, and bismuth-containing medications.

Book Enhancement

Go to www.acponline.org/essentials/gastroenterology-section .html. In *MKSAP for Students 5*, assess your knowledge with items 8-13 in the **Gastroenterology and Hepatology** section.

Bibliography

Sellin JH. A practical approach to treating patients with chronic diarrhea. Rev Gastroenterol Disord. 2007;7 Suppl 3:S19-26. [PMID: 18192962]

De Bruyn G. Diarrhea in adults (acute). Am Fam Physician. 2008;78:503-504. [PMID: 18756660]

Chapter 17

Approach to Liver Chemistry Tests

Jonathan S. Appelbaum, MD

Up to 4% of asymptomatic persons have abnormal results on liver chemistry tests. Standard tests that evaluate liver injury include serum alanine aminotransferase (ALT), aspartate aminotransferase (AST), alkaline phosphatase (ALP), and bilirubin. Tests that reflect liver synthetic function include serum albumin and prothrombin time (PT). This chapter addresses the approach to patients with hepatocellular and cholestatic liver injury test patterns, abnormal liver synthetic function tests, and drug-induced liver injury.

Liver Injury Test Patterns

Hepatocellular injury most often results in an elevation of serum ALT and AST. ALT and AST are released from injured hepatocytes. AST is also released from other tissues (heart, skeletal muscle), whereas ALT is minimally produced in nonhepatic tissues. Thus, ALT elevations are more specific for diagnosing liver disease. In alcoholic liver disease, 70% of patients have AST levels that are twice as elevated as ALT levels.

Cholestatic injury (cholestasis) is indicated by an elevation of serum ALP and, possibly, bilirubin. Cholestasis (impaired flow of bile from the liver) may occur without jaundice because of the liver's capacity to continue to secrete bile sufficiently until injury to the bile ducts is significant. Profound disruption of the bile secretory mechanisms is likely to result in elevation of serum bilirubin, and therefore, jaundice. Bilirubin elevations may be due to increases in either conjugated (direct) or unconjugated (indirect) bilirubin. The predominance of unconjugated bilirubin may indicate overproduction (hemolysis) or impaired conjugation, which may be the result of a congenital defect (e.g, Gilbert syndrome). Hepatocyte dysfunction (hepatocellular injury) and impaired bile flow (cholestasis) are associated with conjugated hyperbilirubinemia (direct fraction >50%). ALP can be found in bone, intestine, placenta and other organs. To confirm that an elevated ALP is of liver origin, measure other bile duct enzymes (γ-glutamyl transpeptidase, 5'-nucleotidase), which will be elevated.

Liver Synthetic Function Tests

Serum albumin and PT reflect the liver's synthetic capacity. Serum albumin will decrease only after significant liver damage, so it is an insensitive test of early synthetic function. An elevated PT may indicate impaired hepatic production of clotting factors; however, these parameters may also be elevated in the setting of vitamin K deficiency (malnutrition, malabsorption), so PT is a nonspecific test of synthetic function.

Clinical Approach to Abnormal Liver Studies

In the patient without known liver disease, abnormal liver test results must be interpreted in the context of the clinical presentation and the pattern, degree, and duration of the biochemical abnormalities. Repeat the liver chemistry studies in asymptomatic patients to confirm any abnormal test results. Normal or minimally elevated liver chemistry tests do not exclude serious liver disease, such as hepatitis B or C. After confirming abnormal results, determine the pattern of liver study abnormality (hepatocellular, cholestatic, or mixed) to narrow the differential diagnosis. Next, it is important to determine whether the patient has symptoms of liver disease, which may be constitutional (malaise, listlessness, weight loss, nausea) or more specific (jaundice, right upper quadrant pain). The duration of liver test abnormalities can be determined through the history and laboratory records. Hepatocellular disorders present <6 months are considered acute forms of hepatitis, whereas hepatocellular abnormalities present >6 months are considered chronic forms of hepatitis (Table 1). Characteristics of cholestatic liver diseases are shown in Table 2.

Drug-induced Liver Disease

Most drug-induced liver injury results in hepatocellular injury and an acute hepatitis syndrome that may include jaundice. Cholestatic forms of liver injury are typical of hypersensitivity reactions and generally take longer to resolve than hepatitis syndromes. Patients who develop abnormal liver enzyme values while taking medications known to cause hepatotoxicity need to be evaluated carefully, because the enzyme elevation often is due to a previously undiagnosed primary liver disease rather than to the medication. Asymptomatic patients with mild liver enzyme abnormalities require only follow-up with repeated laboratory studies. However, symptomatic patients require prompt evaluation and discontinuation of the possible hepatotoxic drug.

Book Enhancement

Go to www.acponline.org/essentials/gastroenterology-section .html. In *MKSAP for Students 5* assess your knowledge with items 14-15 in the **Gastroenterology and Hepatology** section.

Bibliography

Pratt DS, Kaplan MM. Evaluation of abnormal liver-enzyme results in asymptomatic patients. N Engl J Med. 2000;342:1266-1271. [PMID: 10781624]

Table 1. Characteristics of Hepatitis

Disease	Liver Enzyme Pattern		Historical Features	Diagnostic Findings
	ALT	AST		
			Acute Hepatitis	
Hepatitis A	↑↑↑	↑↑	Fecal-oral exposure	Anti-HAV
Hepatitis B	↑↑↑	↑↑	Blood or body fluid exposure	Anti-HBc, anti-HBs
Hepatitis C	↑↑	↑	Recent injection drug use	HCV RNA (anti-HCV may be absent up to 3 mo after exposure)
Alcoholic hepatitis	↑	↑↑	Heavy alcohol use (binge, chronic)	Improvement with cessation of alcohol use; AST/ALT ratio >2, AST usually <500 U/L
Drug-induced hepatitis	↑↑↑↑	↑↑	History of medication use within 3 mo (often a drug previously associated with liver injury)	Absence of other diagnostic markers of liver disease
NAFLD	↑↑↑	↑↑↑	Late pregnancy, amiodarone	History of medication use
Ischemic hepatitis	↑↑↑↑	↑↑↑↑	Severe hypotension	Rapid improvement with resolution of hypotension
Acute liver failure	↑↑↑	↑	Ingestion of an associated agent, rapid progression from jaundice to encephalopathy (12-24 wk)	Signs of impaired hepatic synthetic function
			Chronic Hepatitis	
Hepatitis B	↑↑	↑	Blood or body fluid exposure, born in endemic area	HBsAg, may have HBV DNA
Hepatitis C	↑↑	↑	Injection drug use, blood transfusion prior to 1992, other parenteral exposure; born to infected mother	Anti-HCV, HCV RNA
NAFLD	↑↑	↑	Presence of metabolic syndrome (obesity, insulin resistance, hypertriglyceridemia)	Hepatic imaging shows fat
Alcoholic liver disease	↑	↑↑	Remote history of heavy alcohol use	Absence of other diagnostic markers of liver disease
Autoimmune hepatitis	↑↑	↑	More common in women	Positive antinuclear and anti–smooth muscle antibodies
Hemochromatosis	↑	↑	Arthritis, diabetes, family history	Elevated ferritin (>1000 ng/mL [1000 µg/L]) and iron saturation (>55%), presence of *HFE* gene mutations
Wilson disease	↑↑	↑↑	Young, movement disorders, psychiatric disease, Kayser-Fleischer rings	Hemolysis, low ALP, low ceruloplasmin
α_1-Antitrypsin deficiency	↑	↑	Lung disease	Low serum α_1-antitrypsin, liver biopsy

ALP = alkaline phosphatase; ALT = alanine aminotransferase; anti-HAV = antibody to hepatitis A virus; anti-HBc = antibody to hepatitis B core antigen; anti-HBsAg = antibody to hepatitis B surface antigen; anti-HCV = antibody to hepatitis C virus; AST = aspartate aminotransferase; ERCP = endoscopic retrograde cholangiopancreatography; HBsAg = hepatitis B surface antigen; HBV = hepatitis B virus; HCV = hepatitis C virus; NAFLD = nonalcoholic fatty liver disease.

Table 2. Characteristics of Cholestatic Liver Diseases

Disease	Liver Biochemistry Pattern		Historical Features	Diagnostic Evaluation
	ALP	Total Bilirubin		
Primary biliary cirrhosis	↑↑	↑	More common in women, fatigue, pruritus	Antimitochondrial antibodies (95% of cases), liver biopsy
Primary sclerosing cholangitis	↑↑	↑	More common in men, history of inflammatory bowel disease	ERCP, MRI, liver biopsy
Large bile duct obstruction	↑↑	↑	Pain, fever	Ultrasonography
Drug-induced cholestasis	↑↑	↑	History of medication use within 3 mo (often a drug previously associated with liver injury)	Improvement with cessation of medication
Infiltrative liver disease	↑↑		History of sarcoidosis or other granulomatous disease or cancer	CT, MRI, liver biopsy

ALP = alkaline phosphatase; ERCP = endoscopic retrograde cholangiopancreatography.

Chapter 18

Diseases of the Gallbladder and Bile Ducts

Nora L. Porter, MD

Gallstones are the most common cause of biliary disease in the United States. The incidence of gallstones increases with increasing age and is higher in women than in men. Ninety percent of gallstones in the United States are cholesterol stones. Cholesterol stones form when there is excess cholesterol relative to bile salts and lecithin in bile, resulting in cholesterol crystal precipitation. Risk factors for the formation of cholesterol stones include advancing age, estrogen (female gender, pregnancy, estrogen therapy), obesity, physical inactivity, American Indian or Mexican-American ancestry, impaired gallbladder emptying (total parenteral nutrition, biliary strictures), rapid weight loss (gastric bypass surgery), and medications (thiazide diuretics, ceftriaxone). The major risk factor for black pigment stones is the increased bilirubin seen in hemolytic disease, including sickle cell disease. Brown pigment stones form in the setting of biliary infection. Microlithiasis, or biliary sludge, can present similarly to gallstones.

Most patients with gallstones remain asymptomatic. When gallstones obstruct the cystic duct, symptoms of biliary colic develop. Prolonged obstruction can cause inflammation of the gallbladder (cholecystitis). Gallstones may migrate to the common bile duct (choledocholithiasis), where obstruction can lead to the more serious complications of cholangitis (infection of the biliary tree) and pancreatitis. Untreated acute cholecystitis can progress to perforation, gangrenous cholecystitis (especially in patients with diabetes), and acute cholangitis. In cholangitis, bacterial infection proximal to a bile duct obstruction may result in bacteremia and septic shock. Acalculous cholecystitis usually results from stasis of bile in the gallbladder, which causes inflammation and ultimately infection, often in critically ill patients. Biliary dyskinesia includes functional gallbladder dysmotility and biliary sphincter of Oddi dysfunction. Other chronic diseases that can affect the gallbladder and bile ducts include malignancy, primary biliary cirrhosis, and primary sclerosing cholangitis.

Prevention

As obesity and a sedentary lifestyle are major modifiable risk factors for gallstones, primary prevention includes counseling patients about the importance of eating a diet high in fiber and plant-based foods, increasing physical activity, and maintaining a normal body weight. In most patients with asymptomatic gallstones, the risk of developing symptoms or complications is less than the risk of surgery, so prophylactic cholecystectomy is not indicated. Populations at increased risk for developing complicated gallbladder disease or gallbladder cancer include Pima Indian women, patients with calcified (porcelain) gallbladders or with gallstones >3 cm, patients with sickle cell anemia, and organ transplant candidates. These at-risk individuals may be candidates for prophylactic cholecystectomy.

Diagnosis

No single sign or symptom is sensitive or specific enough to establish or rule out the diagnosis of biliary disease (Table 1). An appropriate history and physical examination, with selected laboratory and imaging studies, is required. Classic biliary colic is constant right upper quadrant abdominal pain that develops over ≤1 hour, radiates to the right scapula or shoulder, and subsides in several hours. In acute cholecystitis, the pain frequently starts in the epigastric area before localizing in the right upper quadrant. Pain lasting >6 hours, especially if accompanied by fever, chills, and diaphoresis, suggests cholecystitis. Nausea and vomiting are common. A history of jaundice, pruritus, acholic stools, and dark urine indicates biliary obstruction due to choledocholithiasis. The physical examination in biliary colic may be benign, although there may be right upper quadrant tenderness. A positive Murphy sign (inspiratory arrest when the gallbladder fossa is palpated during deep inspiration) has a 50% to 80% specificity for acute cholecystitis; infrequently, a tender right upper quadrant mass is palpable. Jaundice supports the diagnosis of choledocholithiasis and, in the presence of fever, cholangitis. Peritoneal signs point to a perforated or inflamed viscus.

Suspect acute gallstone cholecystitis or cholangitis in patients with leukocytosis. Mild increases in serum aminotransferase and bilirubin concentrations may be seen. A bilirubin concentration >4 mg/dL (68.4 mmol/L) is not a feature of cholecystitis and should prompt an evaluation for cholangitis. In cholangitis, serum alkaline phosphatase elevation is common, and more significant elevations in aminotransferase levels may be seen.

Acalculous cholecystitis, like acute gallstone cholecystitis, may present as fever, leukocytosis, and abnormal aminotransferase levels. Characteristic abdominal pain may be absent in critically ill or elderly patients.

Ultrasonography is the initial imaging modality of choice in suspected biliary disease. It is the most sensitive and specific test for detecting gallstones, has no risk, is widely available, and is relatively inexpensive (Table 2). Ultrasonography will demonstrate dilatation of the cystic or biliary duct if there is an obstructing stone. In acute cholecystitis, ultrasonography will show pericholecystic fluid and a thickened gallbladder wall; a sonographic Murphy sign further supports the diagnosis. Findings in acalculous cholecystitis are the same as in acute cholecystitis, but no gallstones or obstruction

Table 1. Differential Diagnosis of Acute Cholecystitis

Disorder	Notes
Acute cholecystitis	Epigastric and RUQ pain with Murphy sign. Bilirubin <4 mg/dL (68.4 mmol/L), unless complicated by choledocholithiasis; AST and ALT levels may be minimally elevated.
Biliary crystals (microlithiasis, sludge)	Typical biliary pain and no gallstones on imaging studies. Diagnosis made by aspiration of gallbladder bile from the duodenum or directly from the gallbladder during ERCP and microscopic examination. May cause pain, cholecystitis, or pancreatitis. Treated with cholecystectomy.
Biliary dyskinesia	Typical biliary pain, no gallstones on imaging studies, and a cholecystokinin-induced gallbladder ejection fraction <35%-40% on cholescintigraphy. Symptoms usually relieved with cholecystectomy.
Acute cholangitis	Charcot triad (RUQ pain, fever, jaundice) or Reynold pentad (Charcot triad plus shock and mental status changes). Bilirubin >4 mg/dL (68.4 mmol/L); AST and ALT levels may exceed 1000 U/L.
Acute pancreatitis	Mid-epigastric pain radiating to the back, nausea, and vomiting. Elevated serum amylase and lipase levels (amylase level more than two times normal). Vomiting and hyperamylasemia generally are more pronounced than in acute cholecystitis.
Pyelonephritis (right)	Costovertebral angle tenderness and evidence of urinary infection. Urinalysis helps to establish the diagnosis.
Peptic ulcer disease	RUQ or mid-epigastric pain. Free air on upright radiograph. Perforated ulcer can mimic acute cholecystitis.
Acute viral hepatitis	Prodromal syndrome and jaundice. AST and ALT levels generally >1000 U/L; bilirubin level generally >4 mg/dL (68.4 mmol/L) and often much higher.
Acute alcoholic hepatitis	Recent significant alcohol intake. RUQ pain, fever, and jaundice. Coagulopathy, leukocytosis; AST level usually two to three times greater than ALT level; bilirubin level generally >4 mg/dL (68.4 mmol/L).
Fitz-Hugh–Curtis syndrome (gonococcal perihepatitis)	RUQ pain and pelvic adnexal tenderness; leukocytosis. Cervical smear shows gonococci.

ALT = alanine aminotransferase; AST = aspartate aminotransferase; ERCP = endoscopic retrograde cholangiopancreatography; RUQ = right upper quadrant.

will be visualized. If ultrasonography is nondiagnostic, cholescintigraphy scans (e.g., hepatobiliary iminodiacetic acid [HIDA] scans) should be obtained; nonvisualization of the gallbladder suggests cholecystitis. Abdominal CT should be used when other studies are equivocal or when complications of cholecystitis (e.g., perforation, cholangitis, gangrenous cholecystitis) are suspected. If bile duct stones are suspected, magnetic resonance cholangiography is more sensitive than ultrasonography and is the preferred noninvasive imaging modality.

Symptoms of biliary dyskinesia are similar to those of biliary colic. Clinical diagnosis of biliary dyskinesia is suggested by abdominal pain that is moderate to severe, episodic but constant while present, ≥30 minutes in duration, and located in the epigastric area or right upper quadrant. Functional gallbladder dysmotility is diagnosed by finding a decreased cholecystokinin-induced gallbladder ejection fraction on cholescintigraphy. Sphincter of Oddi manometry may be required to diagnose sphincter of Oddi dysfunction.

Primary biliary cirrhosis (PBC) and primary sclerosing cholangitis (PSC) are chronic diseases of the bile ducts. PBC is a slowly progressive autoimmune liver disease that is more common in women and typically affects persons aged 30 to 65 years. Fatigue and pruritus are the most common presenting symptoms, and pruritus usually predates the development of jaundice, which can occur months to years thereafter. Most patients have antimitochondrial antibodies and elevated serum IgM and alkaline phosphatase levels; aminotransferase levels also may be elevated. PBC frequently is associated with other autoimmune disorders, such as hypothyroidism, Sjögren syndrome, sicca syndrome, and systemic sclerosis (scleroderma).

PSC is a chronic condition characterized by progressive bile duct inflammation and destruction and, ultimately, fibrosis of both the intrahepatic and extrahepatic bile ducts, which leads to cirrhosis. PSC is strongly associated with ulcerative colitis. The most common symptoms of PSC are pruritus and fatigue; as the disease progresses, most patients develop jaundice. PSC is associated with a markedly elevated alkaline phosphatase level and mildly elevated aminotransferase levels. The diagnosis of PSC depends on detecting multifocal strictures with beading of the bile ducts on cholangiographic imaging, usually endoscopic retrograde

Table 2. Imaging Studies for Acute Cholecystitis

Test	Notes
RUQ ultrasonography	Sensitivity 81%-98%, specificity 70%-98%. Sonographic Murphy sign (showing maximal tenderness directly over the visualized gallbladder) is >90% predictive of acute cholecystitis.
HIDA scan	Sensitivity 85%-97%, specificity 90%.
CT	Most useful to diagnose complications (perforation, cholangitis, gangrenous cholecystitis); expensive.
MRI or MRCP	Cystic duct obstruction is 100% predictive of acute cholecystis; gallbladder wall thickening is 69% sensitive. Extremely expensive; not universally available.

HIDA = hepatobiliary iminodiacetic acid; MRCP = magnetic resonance cholangiopancreatography; RUQ = right upper quadrant.

cholangiopancreatography (ERCP). Cholangiocarcinoma occurs in approximately 10% of patients with PSC. Cholangitis is a common complication of PSC.

Gallbladder cancer, the most common malignancy of the biliary tract, usually is diagnosed at an advanced stage and, therefore, has a very poor prognosis. Presenting symptoms include jaundice, weight loss, and anorexia and usually occur when the cancer is advanced and unresectable. The diagnosis can be made with ultrasonography, which may show an irregular, fixed polypoid lesion without acoustic shadowing.

Cholangiocarcinomas are rare tumors that arise from the biliary tract. Risk factors include PSC, ulcerative colitis, and intrahepatic bile duct stones. Patients usually present with painless jaundice, pruritus, and weight loss. MRI with magnetic resonance cholangiopancreatography is the diagnostic imaging modality of choice as it can also assist in staging.

Therapy

Surgery provides definitive management for most patients with symptomatic gallstone disease. In patients with uncomplicated cholecystitis, early cholecystectomy (within 24 to 48 hours) is associated with fewer complications and earlier hospital discharge. Compared with open cholecystectomy, laparoscopic cholecystectomy results in shorter hospital stays, less pain, and a more rapid recovery. When bile duct stones are suspected, intraoperative cholangiography should be performed at the time of the cholecystectomy. If this procedure is not available, postoperative ERCP with sphincterotomy is an alternative approach. In patients with severe cholangitis, sepsis, or gallstone pancreatitis, urgent ERCP is essential to remove obstruction and allow biliary drainage.

In most patients with gallstone disease, drug therapy is supportive until definitive surgery can be performed. Diclofenac provides pain relief in biliary colic and decreases the risk of developing acute cholecystitis. NSAIDs also are helpful in patients with acute cholecystitis with mild to moderate pain; patients with more severe pain may require narcotic analgesia. Treat patients with acute cholecystitis—especially those with fever, leukocytosis, or complications—and patients with cholangitis with broad-spectrum antibiotics (i.e., metronidazole plus ciprofloxacin or ampicillin-sulbactam). Ursodeoxycholic acid (a choleretic agent) may be used in selected patients who are unable or unwilling to undergo surgery. Ursodeoxycholic acid should be used only in a patient with cholesterol stones, a patent biliary tract, and a functioning gallbladder.

Treatment of acalculous cholecystitis is similar to treatment of acute cholecystitis, including the use of supportive therapy and antibiotics. As patients with acalculous cholecystitis often are too unstable for immediate surgical intervention, initial management usually is percutaneous cholecystostomy and drainage, with surgery deferred until the patient's other medical conditions have stabilized.

Treatment of functional gallbladder dysmotility is cholecystectomy. Treatment of sphincter of Oddi dysfunction is endoscopic sphincterotomy. This invasive procedure should be reserved for patients with severe symptoms who meet diagnostic criteria and in whom other diagnoses have been excluded.

PBC may be effectively treated with ursodeoxycholic acid, if the medication is used early in the disease. Pruritus can be managed with bile acid resins, such as cholestyramine. PSC is managed with liver transplantation at the point when complications of end-stage liver disease become apparent. Treatment for gallbladder cancer is surgical resection; most studies report a 5-year survival rate of 0 to 10%. Surgical resection is the only curative treatment for cholangiocarcinoma; however, even with successful resection, the 5-year survival rate is 20% to 35%.

Follow-Up

Most patients with asymptomatic gallstone disease should be followed for the development of symptoms. Patients with PBC or PSC should be screened for deficiencies of vitamins A, D, E, and K, and appropriate supplementation should be instituted. PSC-related complications include recurrent cholangitis, bile duct stones, large strictures, and cholangiocarcinoma. In some cases, dominant strictures can be managed with placement of endoscopic stents across the stricture.

Book Enhancement

Go to www.acponline.org/essentials/gastroenterology-section.html. In *MKSAP for Students 5*, assess your knowledge with items 16-19 in the **Gastroenterology and Hepatology** section.

Bibliography

Trowbridge RL, Rutkowski NK, Shojania KG. Does this patient have acute cholecystitis? JAMA. 2003;289:80-86. [PMID: 12503981]

Chapter 19

Acute Pancreatitis

Nora L. Porter, MD

Acute pancreatitis occurs when the pancreatic enzyme trypsinogen is prematurely activated to trypsin, which in turn activates pancreatic zymogens. The resulting pancreatic autodigestion leads to an inflammatory response that causes further pancreatic damage. Most cases of acute pancreatitis are mild and self-limited, but in severe cases, the inflammation may progress to a systemic inflammatory response that can lead to multiple organ failure and death. Repeated episodes of acute pancreatitis may result in chronic pancreatitis and pancreatic endocrine and exocrine insufficiency.

The most common etiology of acute pancreatitis in the United States is biliary obstruction due to gallstones; the second most common cause is alcohol abuse. Pancreatitis also may be caused by common medications such as sulfonamides, estrogens, valproic acid, thiazide diuretics, and furosemide. Other etiologies include very high serum triglyceride levels (>500 mg/dL [5.7 mmol/L]), hypercalcemia, sphincter of Oddi dysfunction, trauma, surgery, endoscopic retrograde cholangiopancreatography (ERCP), cystic fibrosis and other genetic disorders, and penetrating peptic ulcer. Other causes of acute pancreatitis can be classified as obstructive, toxic or drug-induced, infectious, or vascular. Approximately 10% of acute pancreatitis is idiopathic.

Prevention

The best preventive measures for pancreatitis involve avoidance of known etiologic agents and medical or surgical management of other precipitating factors. Avoiding diagnostic ERCP and, instead, using noninvasive magnetic resonance cholangiopancreatography (MRCP) decreases the risk of procedure-related pancreatitis. However, MRCP cannot replace ERCP for therapeutic drainage of the biliary system.

Diagnosis

The most common symptom of acute pancreatitis is abdominal pain. The pain may be epigastric or diffuse. It typically is sudden in onset, peaks in 30 minutes to a few hours, is moderate to severe and constant, and radiates to the back. The pain usually is not positional, although it may improve when sitting up or leaning forward. Nausea and vomiting are common; the pain of acute pancreatitis usually is not alleviated with vomiting. Fever also is common. Table 1 summarizes the differential diagnosis of pancreatitis.

Tachycardia is common due to pain and fever but should also prompt evaluation for hypovolemia. Abdominal tenderness (diffuse or epigastric), guarding, and distension are common in acute uncomplicated pancreatitis. Diminished bowel sounds may point to an associated ileus. Some physical findings may suggest a specific etiology. For example, jaundice suggests biliary obstruction, and eruptive xanthomas suggest hypertriglyceridemia. Evaluation should include consideration of complications. Large pseudocysts may be palpable and painful. Grey-Turner or Cullen sign (painless ecchymoses in the flank or periumbilical region, respectively) suggests retroperitoneal bleeding.

Table 1. Differential Diagnosis of Acute Pancreatitis (AP)

Disorder	Notes
Perforated viscus (see Chapter 15)	Very sudden onset (in AP, pain gradually increases over 30 min to 1 h). Intraperitoneal air present on x-ray.
Acute cholecystitis and biliary colic (see Chapter 18)	Pain tends to be located in epigastrium and right upper quadrant and radiates to right shoulder or shoulder blade (in AP, pain tends to radiate to the back). Ultrasonography shows thickened gallbladder and pericholecystic fluid.
Intestinal obstruction (see Chapter 15)	Colicky pain (versus constant pain in AP). Obstructive pattern seen on CT or abdominal series.
Mesenteric vascular occlusion (see Chapter 15)	Classic triad for chronic mesenteric ischemia: postprandial abdominal pain, weight loss, and abdominal bruit. Acute mesenteric ischemia is characterized by pain out of proportion to exam findings and metabolic acidosis.
Dissecting aortic aneurysm (see Chapter 1)	Sudden-onset pain that may radiate to lower extremity (in AP, pain gradually increases over 30 min to 1 h and does not radiate to lower extremity).
Myocardial infarction (see Chapter 3)	Include in differential diagnosis in all patients with upper abdominal pain.
Appendicitis (see Chapter 15)	Pain may start in epigastrium but eventually migrates to right lower quadrant. CT very helpful for diagnosis.
Diabetic ketoacidosis (see Chapter 10)	Blood glucose always elevated, anion gap always present (blood glucose may be elevated in severe AP but usually develops later in the clinical course, acidosis may be present in severe AP).

Table 2. Nonpancreatic Causes of Elevated Serum Amylase and Lipase Levels

Elevated Amylase	Elevated Lipase
Intestinal ischemia, obstruction, or radiation injury	Intestinal ischemia or obstruction
Parotitis	Duodenal ulcer
Ectopic pregnancy, salpingitis	Ketoacidosis
Kidney failure	Celiac disease
Anorexia nervosa	Macrolipasemia
Alcoholism	Head trauma, intracranial mass
Ketoacidosis	Kidney failure

Serum amylase and lipase levels are elevated in approximately one third of patients with acute pancreatitis. The degree of elevation of pancreatic enzymes does not correlate with disease severity. Elevation to at least three times the upper limit of normal is considered diagnostic but is not sensitive, as many patients with acute pancreatitis do not have enzyme levels that reach this threshold. Serum lipase is more specific than amylase and stays elevated up to 14 days following an episode of acute pancreatitis. However, neither elevated amylase nor elevated lipase is specific to acute pancreatitis (Table 2).

In addition to local complications, pancreatitis may cause significant systemic complications, including hypocalcemia, hyperglycemia, acute kidney injury, disseminated intravascular coagulation, and acute respiratory distress syndrome. Therefore, in all patients with acute pancreatitis, obtain a complete blood count, electrolytes, calcium, blood glucose, blood urea nitrogen (BUN), creatinine, prothrombin time, and partial thromboplastin time, as well as pulse oximetry or, in more critically ill patients, arterial blood gases (Table 3).

Chest and abdominal (flat and upright) radiographs may be obtained to exclude bowel perforation or obstruction. Abdominal ultrasonography is performed if gallstones are suspected. Use contrast-enhanced, thin-section CT of the abdomen in patients with moderate or severe pancreatitis or persistent fever and in those who do not improve clinically within 48 to 72 hours to confirm the diagnosis, exclude other intra-abdominal processes, grade the severity of pancreatitis, and diagnose local complications (pancreatic necrosis, pseudocyst, abscess). In acute interstitial pancreatitis, CT may show enlargement or irregular contour of the gland, peripancreatic inflammation, and fluid collections. Pancreatic necrosis is identified by areas of nonenhancement on a CT scan with contrast. MRI is used if there is a contraindication to intravenous radiocontrast.

Scoring systems such as the Ranson, Glasgow, and Acute Physiology and Chronic Health Evaluation II (APACHE II) scores are used to determine prognosis. However, these scoring systems lack sensitivity and specificity and should not supplant clinical findings such as third-space fluid loss or remote organ failure in determining risk. Serum C-reactive protein level correlates with the severity of acute pancreatitis but is not a sensitive early marker of severity. BMI >30 also is associated with more severe acute pancreatitis. Organ failure, the most important indicator of sever-

Table 3. Laboratory and Other Studies for Acute Pancreatitis (AP)

Test	Notes
Amylase	Cutoff values just above normal: sensitivity 90%, specificity 70%. Cutoff values three times the upper limit of normal: sensitivity 60%, specificity 99%.
Lipase	Cutoff values three times the upper limit of normal: sensitivity 90%-100%, specificity 99%.
AST/ALT	Elevated levels raise suspicion for biliary pancreatitis.
Triglycerides	Hypertriglyceridemia can cause AP.
Calcium	Hypercalcemia can cause AP. Hypocalcemia can be a complication of AP.
BUN and creatinine	Incidence of acute kidney injury: 4% in interstitial AP, 22% in noninfected necrotic AP, and 45% in infected necrotic AP.
Glucose	Hyperglycemia is a negative prognostic factor.
PT/PTT	May be elevated in AP complicated by DIC.
Abdominal and chest x-rays	Can exclude perforated viscous or obstructed bowel.
Abdominal ultrasonography	Evaluates for presence of gallstones.
CT	Test of choice to determine the presence of local complications.
Test for arterial hypoxemia	Pulse oximetry in mild cases of AP. Arterial blood gases in severe cases of AP.

ALT = alanine aminotransferase; AST = aspartate aminotransferase; BUN = blood urea nitrogen; DIC = disseminated intravascular coagulation; PT = prothrombin time; PTT = partial thromboplastin time.

ity, is defined by the presence of shock (systolic blood pressure <90 mm Hg), pulmonary insufficiency (arterial P_{O_2} <55 mm Hg [7.3 kPa]), acute kidney injury (serum creatinine >2 mg/dL [176.8 mmol/L]), or gastrointestinal bleeding (>500 mL/24 h). Most patients with multiple organ system involvement have pancreatic necrosis involving 30% to 50% of the pancreas, often with infection; these patients have very high mortality.

At least 80% of patients with chronic pancreatitis have abdominal pain, which characteristically is constant midepigastric pain that radiates to the back and is exacerbated by food. Acute exacerbations of pain may occur. Destruction of exocrine pancreatic tissue may result in malabsorption leading to steatorrhea and weight loss. Destruction of insulin-producing β-cells may lead to diabetes mellitus; concurrent destruction of glucagon-producing α-cells increases the risk of hypoglycemia in patients with diabetes. In chronic pancreatitis, pancreatic calcifications can be seen on abdominal radiograph and CT scans. CT scans also may show pancreatic atrophy or ductal dilatation in the pancreas. Patients with chronic pancreatitis should be evaluated for diabetes and deficiencies of fat-soluble vitamins.

Therapy

Therapy for acute pancreatitis depends on disease severity. Mild acute interstitial pancreatitis is usually self-limited and is treated with bowel rest and intravenous hydration. Oral intake is withheld until there is clear clinical improvement. In more severe cases, when it is anticipated that patients will be unable to receive oral nourishment for a few weeks, nutritional support may be required. Jejunal enteral feeding is preferred but may be contraindicated in patients with bowel obstruction, in which case parenteral nutrition is provided. Compared to intravenous feeding, early jejunal enteral feeding may decrease the risk of complications, particularly infections. Use of nasogastric suction is limited to patients with refractory vomiting due to ileus.

There is no specific drug therapy for acute pancreatitis. Provide symptomatic treatment, including narcotic analgesics for pain and antiemetics for nausea and vomiting. Treat documented infections (cholangitis, abscess, infected pseudocyst) with antibiotics. Prophylactic antibiotics reduce morbidity and mortality in necrotizing pancreatitis. Patients with evidence of pancreatic necrosis on CT scan should have percutaneous fine-needle aspiration with Gram stain and culture of the aspirated fluid to determine if infection is present and to guide choice of antibiotics. Empiric treatment with imipenem, fluoroquinolones, or cephalosporins is used pending results of cultures. Patients with interstitial (non-necrotizing) pancreatitis without evidence of infection do not require antibiotics.

ERCP is indicated if there is evidence of biliary obstruction, including cholelithiasis, choledocholithiasis, bile duct dilatation, or elevated liver enzymes. Stone extraction with biliary sphincterotomy improves mortality, decreases the risk of cholangitis and biliary sepsis, and may prevent further attacks of acute biliary pancreatitis. Surgical debridement is indicated for infected pancreatic necrosis and pancreatic abscess. Pancreatic pseudocysts that fail to resolve may need surgical drainage. Cholecystectomy is indicated in patients with biliary pancreatitis to prevent recurrence.

Pancreatic pseudocysts and abscesses may present several weeks after an episode of acute pancreatitis. A pseudocyst is a collection of pancreatic fluid with a fibrous, nonepithelialized lining. Pseudocysts usually take at least 4 weeks to form and resolve spontaneously. They are usually asymptomatic; symptoms of pain or obstruction result from compression of adjacent structures. Symptomatic pseudocysts require drainage (percutaneous, endoscopic, or surgical). Pancreatic abscess (infected pseudocyst) presents with worsening abdominal pain, fever, and leukocytosis. Treatment includes antibiotics and drainage.

Follow-Up

Acute pancreatitis typically is a self-limited condition that does not recur if the precipitating factor is removed. Patients with alcohol abuse should be advised to abstain from alcohol or referred for counseling and appropriate treatment. Hypertriglyceridemia is controlled with a combination of diet and triglyceride-lowering medications. Hypercalcemia requires evaluation and appropriate medical or surgical management to lower serum calcium levels. If a specific drug precipitated the pancreatitis, discontinue its use and substitute another as needed.

Book Enhancement

Go to www.acponline.org/essentials/gastroenterology-section.html. In *MKSAP for Students 5*, assess your knowledge with items 20-22 in the **Gastroenterology and Hepatology** section.

Bibliography

Gupta K, Wu B. In the clinic. Acute pancreatitis. Ann Intern Med. 2010; 153:ITC51-5. [PMID: 21041574]

Chapter 20

Gastroesophageal Reflux Disease

Shalini Reddy, MD

Gastrointestinal reflux disease (GERD) is a highly common disorder characterized by symptoms of heartburn and regurgitation. GERD is multifactorial and results from increased esophageal exposure to gastric acid. Defects in the lower esophageal sphincter (LES) and the antireflux barrier located at the gastroesophageal junction contribute to prolonged exposure to acid. Esophageal acid exposure is also increased when normal esophageal acid clearance is impaired. Normal acid clearance occurs through peristalsis and neutralization by saliva and alkaline esophageal secretions. Examples of extraesophageal conditions that impair acid clearance include systemic disorders such as systemic sclerosis (scleroderma) and cigarette smoking. Although acid exposure is central to the pathogenesis of GERD, inappropriate, non-physiologic relaxation of the LES is the most important etiologic factor in the development of reflux. Anatomic anomalies such as hiatal hernias are more commonly found in patients with GERD than in the unaffected population. The major complication of GERD is Barrett esophagus, which can progress to esophageal adenocarcinoma. Other potential complications include esophagitis and chronic bleeding, with resultant iron deficiency anemia.

Diagnosis

The diagnosis of GERD is suggested by symptoms of heartburn and regurgitation that occur after meals; are aggravated by recumbency, bending, or physical exertion; and are relieved by antacids. Patients with classic symptoms rarely require confirmatory testing. Response to a 4-week trial of empiric proton pump inhibitor (PPI) therapy has a 75% sensitivity and 55% specificity when compared to

pH probe testing, the gold standard for diagnosing GERD. Up to 33% of patients have extra-esophageal manifestations of GERD. Extra-esophageal manifestations include wheezing, shortness of breath, chronic cough and hoarseness, chest pain, choking, halitosis, and sore throat. Physical examination findings are less prominent but may include wheezing, signs of pharyngeal irritation, and dental erosions.

Patients who require additional testing include those who do not respond to empiric PPI therapy or have alarm symptoms. Weight loss, bleeding, dysphagia, odynophagia, anemia, and long-standing symptoms all raise concern about significant complications of GERD and should prompt further diagnostic testing, including upper endoscopy. GERD associated with dysphagia may represent a complication of long-term acid reflux (stricture, ulceration, adenocarcinoma) and requires evaluation with upper endoscopy. GERD that presents atypically or is unresponsive to empiric therapy also warrants the consideration of alternative diagnoses, such as infectious esophagitis, medication-induced esophagitis (e.g., alendronate, NSAIDs, iron, potassium supplements, doxycycline), esophageal motility disorders, esophageal cancer, nonulcer dyspepsia, peptic ulcer disease, cardiac disease, and biliary disease (Table 1).

The gold standard for diagnosing GERD is 24-hour pH monitoring, which establishes whether there is increased esophageal exposure to acid. Upper endoscopy should be used when visualization of the esophagus is desired (e.g., when there is concern for esophagitis, stricture, cancer, or Barrett esophagus). Barium studies should not be used, because they are neither sensitive nor specific for GERD. *H. pylori* testing is not indicated in patients with

Table 1. Differential Diagnosis of Gastroesophageal Reflux Disease (GERD)

Condition/Disease	Notes
Achalasia	Dysphagia for liquids and solids; also may be associated with chest pain. Heartburn/chest pain in achalasia is not due to reflux but to fermentation of retained esophageal contents or esophageal muscle spasm.
Coronary artery disease (CAD; see Chapter 3)	Chest pain in CAD may be clinically indistinguishable from chest pain associated with GERD. CAD should be ruled out in patients with CAD risk factors before evaluating GERD as a cause.
Diffuse esophageal spasm	Dysphagia for liquids and solids; also may be associated with chest pain; may be coincident with GERD
Esophageal cancer	Dysphagia for solids (initially) and liquids (later), weight loss; often in patients with long-standing GERD; usually incurable by the time it presents clinically
Infectious esophagitis	Dysphagia/odynophagia; often in immunocompromised patients with candidal, CMV, or HSV esophagitis
Medication-induced esophagitis	Dysphagia/odynophagia; history of offending pill ingestion
Peptic ulcer disease (see Chapter 21)	Pain or distress centered in the upper abdomen, relieved by food or antacids
Biliary disease (see Chapter 18)	Epigastric or right upper quadrant pain, jaundice, acholic stools, dark urine, abnormal liver tests

CMV = cytomegalovirus; HSV = herpes simplex virus.

GERD. Esophageal manometry is neither sensitive nor specific in the diagnosis of GERD.

Therapy

Behavior modification is an important adjunct to pharmacologic or surgical therapy, although the therapeutic benefits have not been vigorously studied. The effects of behavioral therapy on the eradication of GERD symptoms are modest. Smoking cessation, raising the head of the bed, avoiding recumbency after eating, and sleeping in the left lateral decubitus position may be helpful. Patients should be counseled to limit or avoid the consumption of alcohol, fatty foods, chocolate, peppermint, tomato juice, citrus juices, onions, and garlic. Theophylline, nitrates, anticholinergic agents, calcium channel blockers, α-adrenergic antagonists, and diazepam may all induce GERD. If possible, the elimination of offending medications that can cause esophagitis may improve symptoms.

Treatment aims to eliminate symptoms, heal esophagitis, prevent complications, and maintain remission. Antacids are appropriate for the rapid but brief relief of reflux symptoms. Approximately 20% of patients achieve adequate symptom control with antacids. Prescription-strength H_2-receptor antagonists (ranitidine, famotidine, nizatidibine) are first-line therapy for mild or intermittent symptoms of uncomplicated GERD; these medications have a 50% to 60% efficacy. Cimetidine may be less effective and has greater potential to interact with other medications. Tolerance to H_2-receptor antagonists may develop with long-term use.

For patients with endoscopically proven erosive esophagitis or GERD symptoms at least twice weekly, an over-the-counter PPI such as omeprazole is first-line therapy; this treatment brings relief in >80% of patients. PPI doses should be titrated to achieve symptom control. All PPI drugs (omeprazole, esomeprazole, lansoprazole, pantoprazole, rabeprazole) are equally effective in equivalent doses. PPI therapy usually is given once daily before meals, usually before breakfast. Optimal duration of therapy for GERD is unknown, but GERD symptoms often recur after acid-suppression therapy is stopped; therefore, many patients require long-term maintenance therapy. Growing data show that long-term use of PPI drugs may result in decreased bone density or increased pulmonary or gastrointestinal infections.

Surgical intervention with a Nissen fundoplication is an option for patients who wish to avoid lifelong medication, but it is not likely to improve symptoms that were unresponsive to PPI therapy.

Patients should undergo pH probe testing to document GERD and manometry to exclude major motor disorders prior to surgery.

Follow-Up

Patients with alarm symptoms such as dysphagia, odynophagia, bleeding, weight loss, early satiety, choking, anorexia, or frequent vomiting require endoscopy. These symptoms may be indicative of cancer, stricture, or ulceration. Because the presence of Barrett esophagus (a premalignant condition) increases the risk for esophageal adenocarcinoma, screening is recommended for patients who have had symptoms for >5 years and for patients at high risk for developing esophageal adenocarcinoma. Such patients include those who are aged >50 years, have a family history of esophageal cancer, or have had symptoms for >13 years. The detection of intestinal metaplasia on esophageal biopsy indicates the presence of Barrett esophagus. The risk of adenocarcinoma in patients with Barrett esophagus is 30 to 40 times that of the general population. Once Barrett esophagus is diagnosed, repeat endoscopy with biopsy is recommended every 6 months to 3 years. Acid suppression and surgical therapy have not been shown to decrease the risk of progression to cancer. The presence of low-grade or high-grade dysplasia requires more intensive management. In patients with low-grade dysplasia, ablative photodynamic therapy can lead to the regeneration of squamous mucosa in some individuals. For patients with high-grade dysplasia, the risks and benefits of esophagectomy or endoscopic ablative therapy must be weighed against the risk and benefits of intensive endoscopic surveillance for adenocarcinoma, which is then treated with esophagectomy.

Book Enhancement

Go to www.acponline.org/essentials/gastroenterology-section.html. In *MKSAP for Students 5*, assess your knowledge with items 23-24 in the **Gastroenterology and Hepatology** section.

Acknowledgment

We would like to thank Dr. Brown J. McCallum, who contributed to an earlier version of this chapter.

Bibliography

Wilson JF. In the clinic. Gastroesophageal reflux disease. Ann Intern Med. 2008;149:ITC2-1-15; quiz ITC2-16. [PMID: 18678841]

Chapter 21

Peptic Ulcer Disease

Karen Szauter, MD

A peptic ulcer is an ulcer of the mucous membrane of the alimentary tract caused by gastric acid. Gastric acid is made by parietal cells in the stomach. Parietal cells have three stimulant receptors for gastric acid production: gastrin, acetylcholine, and histamine. Gastric acid production is inhibited by somatostatin and prostaglandins. Excessive gastric acid can cause peptic ulceration, esophagitis (in patients predisposed to reflux), and steatorrhea. Steatorrhea results from acid inactivation of pancreatic lipase, which aids in fat digestion. Gastric defenses include a mucous and bicarbonate layer, an epithelial barrier function, and adequate blood flow. Gastric acid aids in absorption of various nutrients (iron, vitamin B_{12}), defends against food-borne illnesses, and prevents small intestinal bacterial overgrowth.

The most common causes of peptic ulcer disease (PUD) are *Helicobacter pylori* infection and NSAIDs, which together account for >90% of PUD. *H. pylori* expresses a host of factors that contribute to its ability to colonize the gastric mucosa and cause mucosal injury. NSAIDs likely cause ulcers by inhibiting the prostaglandin-mediated gastrointestinal release of the protective mucous and bicarbonate layer and through a direct toxic mucosal effect.

If neither *H. pylori* infection nor NSAID use is documented in a patient with PUD, consider other causes of PUD, including Crohn disease, gastric acid hypersecretory states (Zollinger-Ellison syndrome), malignancy, viral infections (cytomegalovirus), and drugs (cocaine). See Table 1 for additional entities in the differential diagnosis of PUD.

Prevention

Cigarette smoking, alcohol consumption, corticosteroid administration, and psychological stress are not currently thought to be independent risk factors for the development of peptic ulcers in the absence of *H. pylori* infection or NSAID use. Although lifestyle modification for other health reasons may be advisable, there is no evidence that modification of diet or tobacco, alcohol, or caffeine use is helpful in PUD prevention. In patients who require NSAIDs for other health reasons, concomitant use of misoprostol or a proton pump inhibitor (PPI) can reduce the incidence of ulcer complications. Prophylactic treatment is recommended for high-risk NSAID users, including patients with a prior history of ulcers, those taking prednisone or anticoagulants, and patients aged >65 years.

Diagnosis

Most patients with PUD do not have pain at diagnosis; the ulcers usually are detected during an evaluation for potential ulcer-related complications, such as overt or obscure bleeding. When symptoms are present, they include dyspepsia or a nonspecific, gnawing epigastric pain. Other presentations include bleeding, perforation (sometimes with penetration into adjacent organs), and gastric outlet obstruction. The most common complication of PUD is gastrointestinal bleeding, which occurs in approximately 15% of cases. Bleeding may manifest as hematemesis, melena, or hematochezia; occult bleeding manifesting as iron deficiency anemia is less common. Patients with perforation from PUD often present with sudden, severe abdominal pain and hemodynamic compromise. Affected patients may be febrile, hypotensive, and tachycardic; bowel sounds may be absent, and abdominal examination may show guarding and rebound tenderness. The ulcer may penetrate into the pancreas, manifesting additionally with acute pancreatitis. Imaging often reveals free intraperitoneal air. Gastric out-

Table 1. Differential Diagnosis of Peptic Ulcer Disease

Disorder	Notes
Irritable bowel syndrome (see Chapter 15)	Bloating, change in bowel habits, cramping; absence of weight loss, bleeding, anemia, or relief with acid-suppressive agents
Gastric cancer	Weight loss, early satiety, anemia, occult gastrointestinal bleeding
Dyspepsia (see Chapter 22)	Pain, fullness, or bloating often related temporally to eating and unaffected by bowel movements; normal upper endoscopy
Biliary colic (see Chapter 18)	Pain (usually right upper quadrant, intermittent); may be associated with fever
Pancreatitis (see Chapter 19)	Pain (mid-epigastric, with radiation to the back), nausea, vomiting; may be secondary to penetrating peptic ulcer
Gastroesophageal reflux disease (see Chapter 20)	Heartburn, dysphagia, extra-esophageal manifestations (chronic cough, laryngitis, asthma)
Intolerance to medications	Ingestion of bisphosphonates, NSAIDs, or antibiotics; symptoms abate with discontinuation of the medications

let obstruction is a rare complication of PUD, typically from ulceration in the prepyloric region or pyloric channel. Patients with obstruction present with progressive nausea, vomiting, early satiety, and weight loss.

Upper endoscopy (esophagogastroduodenoscopy) is used to establish the diagnosis of PUD. Endoscopy is indicated for patients aged >45 years with new-onset epigastric abdominal pain and for patients with abdominal pain and unexplained weight loss, gastrointestinal bleeding, microcytic anemia, or recurrent vomiting. Younger patients with mild to moderate epigastric pain and no other associated symptoms can be treated empirically with a PPI and forego endoscopy. However, endoscopy is indicated in these patients if symptoms persist after an adequate PPI trial. Upper endoscopy is contraindicated in patients with perforation; these patients require emergent surgical consultation.

Endoscopy allows for both diagnostic and therapeutic interventions. Biopsies of the gastrointestinal mucosa provide important information about underlying inflammatory changes as well as evidence for the presence of *H. pylori* infection, gastric cancer, or MALT (mucosa-associated lymphoid tissue) lymphoma. For ulcers with associated gastrointestinal bleeding, endoscopy provides the option for direct visualization and management of the underlying cause.

Testing for *H. pylori* is indicated in patients with active PUD (Table 2). The most commonly used endoscopic tests include histologic assessment and the rapid urease test. The sensitivity of the rapid urease test can be reduced up to 25% in patients who have taken a PPI within 2 weeks or bismuth or antibiotic therapy within 4 weeks of the endoscopy; histology is the endoscopic test of choice in such patients. Non-endoscopic studies include serum antibody tests, the urea breath test, and stool examination for *H. pylori* antigens. The sensitivity of the urea breath test and stool antigen test, like that of the rapid urease test, are reduced by medications that affect urease production; therefore, PPI therapy, bismuth, and antibiotic therapy should be held for the intervals previously noted. The urea breath test and stool antigen test can be used to confirm *H. pylori* eradication; confirmatory tests should be done at least 4 weeks after completion of therapy.

Patients with refractory or recurrent ulcer disease, ulcers located in the distal duodenum, or ulcers and watery diarrhea should be evaluated for a gastrinoma. Gastrinomas are tumors that secrete an excess and unregulated amount of gastrin that, in turn, stimulates the parietal cells, leading to excess acid production. The acid leads to peptic ulcer formation and watery diarrhea—a clinical syndrome termed *Zollinger-Ellison syndrome*. The diagnosis is made by identification of a serum gastrin level >1000 pg/mL (1000 ng/L). Information about family history of PUD or evidence of other endocrine tumors should also be obtained, as gastrinomas are associated with multiple endocrine neoplasia (MEN) I syndrome (hyperparathyroidism, pancreatic islet cell tumor, pituitary adenoma).

Therapy

The mainstay of PUD treatment is to identify and manage the contributing factors and to reduce gastric acid to promote ulcer healing. For patients on NSAID treatment, stopping the drug or decreasing the dose is essential. Continued use of PPI therapy is recommended if ongoing treatment with NSAIDs is needed. Alternatively, misoprostol can be used along with NSAIDs to prevent ulcer complications; however, side effects of misoprostol (diarrhea) may limit long-term adherence. Four to six weeks of treatment with a PPI is recommended. For gastric or duodenal ulcers associated with *H. pylori*, treatment includes a PPI and antibiotics. A variety of drug combinations and dosing schedules have been tested, but current recommendations support the use of a PPI with amoxicillin, clarithromycin, and metronidazole. Other regimens include bismuth, tetracycline, metronidazole, and a PPI. It is likely that recommendations will continue to evolve as resistant strains of *H. pylori* are recognized.

Surgery for PUD usually is reserved for patients whose disease fails to respond to medical therapy or for patients with life-threatening complications. The surgery typically involves a vagotomy with a drainage procedure but depends on the urgency, indication, and baseline anatomy.

Follow-Up

Follow-up for patients with PUD is determined by the location of the ulcer, the underlying cause, and associated symptoms.

Table 2. Tests for Detection of *Helicobacter pylori*

Test	Comments
Non-endoscopic studies	
Serum antibody test	Sensitivity 88%-94%, specificity, 74%-88%. Provides evidence of current or previous infection. Remains positive after successful therapy and is not recommended to document eradication of infection.
Stool antigen test	Sensitivity 94%, specificity, 92%. Useful for diagnosis or follow-up testing. False-negative results may occur with recent use of proton pump inhibitor, bismuth, or antibiotics (4 wk). H_2-Blocker use does not interfere with test.
Urea breath test	Sensitivity 90%-96%, specificity 88%-98%. Useful for diagnosis or follow-up testing. False-negative results may occur from medications (as above). Must fast for 6 h prior to testing and stop H_2-blocker for 24 h prior to testing.
Endoscopic studies	
Biopsy	Sensitivity 93%-96%, specificity, 98%-99%. Requires upper endoscopy. Staining of biopsy provides evidence of *H. pylori* infection. Requires adequate sampling of tissue for optimal sensitivity.
Rapid urease test	Sensitivity 88%-95%, specificity 95%-100%. Requires upper endoscopy and biopsy. False-negative results may occur from medications (as above).

Ongoing treatment with a PPI is not recommended once an adequate treatment regimen has been completed and the patient is free of symptoms. Uncomplicated duodenal ulcers in asymptomatic patients do not require endoscopic follow-up. All patients with *H. pylori*–associated ulcers should undergo follow-up testing to ensure that the organism is eradicated; persistence of *H. pylori* infection requires a second treatment course with an alternative antibiotic regimen.

Patients with complicated duodenal ulcers (bleeding, perforation, obstruction) or with large gastric ulcers should undergo follow-up endoscopy to ensure healing. Gastric ulcers associated with *H. pylori* infection or with worrisome features (e.g., irregular borders) should be reassessed to verify healing and biopsied to confirm the absence of gastric cancer. Patients should be educated about symptoms of PUD, signs of gastrointestinal bleeding, and medications associated gastrointestinal symptoms.

Book Enhancement

Go to www.acponline.org/essentials/gastroenterology-section.html. In *MKSAP for Students 5*, assess your knowledge with items 25-26 in the **Gastroenterology and Hepatology** section.

Acknowledgment

We would like to thank Dr. Brown J. McCallum, who contributed to an earlier version of this chapter.

Bibliography

Malfertheiner P, Chan FK, McColl KE. Peptic ulcer disease. Lancet. 2009; 374:1449-1461. [PMID: 19683340]

Chapter 22

Dyspepsia

Chad S. Miller, MD

Dyspepsia is chronic or recurrent discomfort in the upper mid-abdomen (epigastrium) usually accompanied by fullness, early satiety, bloating, or nausea. The etiology and pathophysiology of dyspepsia are unclear; the disorder may be multifactorial. Potential causes or contributing factors include dysmotility, visceral hypersensitivity, *Helicobacter pylori* infection, acid peptic disease (damage from gastric acid and pepsin activity), food or drug intolerance, central nervous system dysfunction, and psychosocial factors. *Functional dyspepsia* refers to symptoms of dyspepsia for 3 months with no significant abnormalities found by endoscopy. Patients with features of dyspepsia that have not had testing to exclude other conditions are said to have *uninvestigated dyspepsia*. It is estimated that dyspepsia affects close to 25% of the general population and accounts for approximately 2% to 5% of primary care visits.

Diagnosis

The Rome III criteria are used to diagnose functional dyspepsia. The patient must have symptoms for 3 months and no evidence of structural disease with upper endoscopy. The predominant symptom(s) must be one or more of the following: bothersome postprandial fullness, early satiety, epigastric pain, or epigastric burning. If the predominant symptom is heartburn or acid regurgitation, the diagnosis of functional dyspepsia is excluded, because the patient most likely has gastroesophageal reflux disease (GERD). Medications should be thoroughly evaluated for potential dyspeptic side effects; NSAIDs are the most common offenders. If the patient has pain that improves with defecation, irritable bowel syndrome should be considered. Finally, if the patient has dysphagia, esophageal etiologies should be pursued. Table 1 summarizes the differential diagnosis of dyspepsia.

Once a diagnosis of functional dyspepsia is established, the Rome criteria can be used to classify a patient by symptom category:

- Ulcer-like dyspepsia: predominant symptom is epigastric pain or burning
- Dysmotility-like dyspepsia: predominant symptom is epigastric discomfort associated with postprandial fullness, early satiety, bloating, or nausea
- Unspecified (nonspecific) dyspepsia: patients who do not fit into the previous two categories

Classifying patients into symptom subgroups can help guide therapy. For example, patients with ulcer-like functional dyspepsia have been shown to respond better to treatment with proton pump inhibitors (PPIs), compared to patients with dysmotility-like functional dyspepsia. A promotility agent such as metoclopramide may have efficacy in the dysmotility-like group.

Not all patients presenting with dyspepsia need urgent endoscopy. Many, especially those aged <55 years, can be treated empirically without endoscopy. Despite the relatively low yield of endoscopy in patients with dyspepsia, the procedure is recommended for patients 55 or older who have new-onset symptoms, because the incidence of gastrointestinal malignancy is higher. Other alarm features that warrant urgent endoscopy include unintentional weight loss, unexplained iron deficiency anemia, progressive dysphagia, odynophagia, persistent vomiting, a palpable abdominal mass, jaundice, or a family history of proximal gastrointestinal cancer.

Table 1. Differential Diagnosis of Dyspepsia

Disorder	Notes
Functional dyspepsia	No evidence of structural disease with endoscopy; up to 60% of epigastric pain
Gastroesophageal reflux disease (see Chapter 20)	Heartburn or acid regurgitation; 2%-29% of epigastric pain
Peptic ulcer disease (see Chapter 21)	Pain or distress centered in the upper abdomen; ulcerative lesions visualized with endoscopy; 7%-25% of epigastric pain
Gastric or esophageal cancer	Alarm features present; 1%-3% of epigastric pain
Medication side effect	Examples: NSAIDs, erythromycin, digitalis, bisphophonates, potassium supplements; 2%-8% of epigastric pain
Biliary disease (see Chapter 18)	Jaundice, dark urine, abnormal liver tests; <5% of epigastric pain
Pancreatitis (see Chapter 19)	Nausea/vomiting, pain radiating to the back, elevated amylase and lipase
Irritable bowel syndrome	Symptoms of bowel dysfunction (diarrhea or constipation) associated with abdominal pain or discomfort in the absence of alarm features

Therapy

Potential offending medications (e.g., NSAIDs, bisphophonates) should be stopped or changed to different agents. If medications cannot be changed, a PPI can be added. Although endoscopy is required for definitive diagnosis of functional dyspepsia, patients aged <55 years without alarm features can be treated empirically. A noninvasive "test and treat" approach for *H. pylori* is recommended, using a urea breath test or stool antigen assay. If the patient tests positive, eradication of *H. pylori* may relieve symptoms. However, it is important to note that randomized controlled trials provide conflicting results as to the efficacy of *H.*

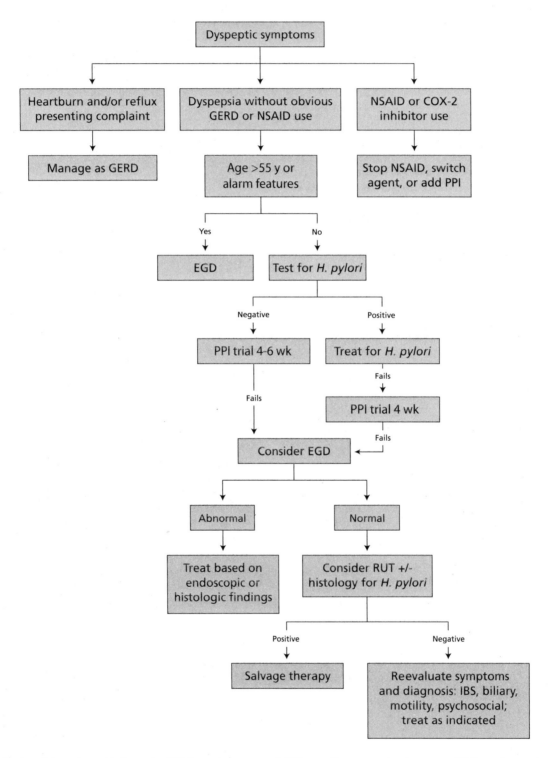

Figure 1. Evaluation of the patient with dyspepsia. COX-2 = cyclooxygenase-2; EGD = esophagogastroduodenoscopy; GERD = gastroesophageal reflux disease; *H. pylori* = *Helicobacter pylori*; IBS = irritable bowel syndrome; PPI = proton pump inhibitor; RUT = rapid urease test. Adapted from Talley NJ; American Gastroenterological Association. American Gastroenterological Association medical position statement: evaluation of dyspepsia. Gastroenterology. 2005;129:1754. [PMID: 16285970] Copyright 2005, Elsevier.

pylori eradication in improving symptoms of functional dyspepsia. Typical treatment might include a PPI, bismuth subsalicylate, metronidazole, and tetracycline for 7 to 10 days. If the patient does not test positive for *H. pylori,* a trial of a PPI is warranted. If symptoms persist after 4 weeks of PPI therapy, consider endoscopy for further evaluation (Figure 1).

For patients diagnosed with functional dyspepsia, consider a 4- to 6-week trial of acid-suppression therapy, especially for those with ulcer-like dyspepsia. For patients with dysmotility-like symptoms, consider a prokinetic such as metoclopramide. Note, however, that metoclopramide has significant side effects; the drug typically is reserved for patients with severe, recalcitrant symptoms and is used only for short durations.

Patients aged >55 years or patients with alarm features should always be evaluated with upper endoscopy. Treatment will ultimately depend on endoscopic or histologic findings.

Follow-Up

Patients treated for *H. pylori* should undergo a urease breath test or stool antigen assay to confirm eradication. Patients who continue to have symptoms despite appropriate diagnostic investigations and therapy are difficult to manage. Reassessment of symptoms and potential offending agents is appropriate. Psychiatric illness, especially depression, may need to be considered.

Book Enhancement

Go to www.acponline.org/essentials/gastroenterology-section.html. In *MKSAP for Students 5*, assess your knowledge with items 27-28 in the **Gastroenterology and Hepatology** section.

Acknowledgment

We would like to thank Dr. Brown J. McCallum, who contributed to an earlier version of this chapter.

Bibliography

Camilleri M. Functional dyspepsia: mechanisms of symptom generation and appropriate management of patients. Gastroenterol Clin North Am. 2007;36:649-664, xi-xx. [PMID: 17950442]

Chapter 23

Approach to Gastrointestinal Bleeding

Warren Y. Hershman, MD

Gastrointestinal bleeding is classified as acute or chronic and as originating from either the upper gastrointestinal tract (proximal to the ligament of Treitz) or the lower gastrointestinal tract. Patients with acute gastrointestinal bleeding typically present with melena (black, tarry, foul-smelling stools), hematochezia (bright red or maroon-colored stools), or hematemesis (vomiting blood or coffee ground–like material). In other patients, occult bleeding may be identified by fecal occult blood testing, the presence of iron deficiency anemia, or symptoms due to blood loss or anemia (fatigue, dyspnea, syncope, angina). Management begins with assessment and stabilization of the patient's hemodynamic status. Subsequent interventions focus on identifying and controlling the source of bleeding and preventing a recurrence.

Differential Diagnosis

Upper Gastrointestinal Bleeding

The most common causes of upper gastrointestinal (UGI) bleeding requiring hospitalization are peptic ulcer, esophageal varices, Mallory-Weiss tears, gastric erosions, and erosive esophagitis. Peptic ulcer disease accounts for approximately 50% of all acute UGI bleeding. Patients taking aspirin or NSAIDs or who have *Helicobacter pylori* infection are at increased risk for ulcers and ulcer-related bleeding. *H. pylori* attaches to gastric epithelial cells and releases toxins that can cause mucosal injury and initiate an inflammatory response. NSAIDs block the enzyme cyclooxygenase and interfere with production of prostaglandins that play a central role in the defense and repair of gastric epithelium. Hospitalized patients with severe comorbid conditions and patients who use anticoagulants also are at increased risk for ulcer-related bleeding. Esophageal or gastric varices account for 5% to 30% of acute UGI bleeding; variceal bleeding often is brisk and can lead to hemodynamic instability. Bleeding due to portal hypertension is less likely to resolve spontaneously and is associated with a higher mortality rate than UGI bleeding due to other causes. Mallory-Weiss tears are mucosal lacerations near the gastroesophageal junction. The classic history of vomiting and/or retching followed by hematemesis suggests this diagnosis but is noted in only a minority of patients. Erosive esophagitis and gastric erosions are more likely to present as small-volume bleeding or occult blood loss. Erosive esophagitis usually is associated with symptoms of gastroesophageal reflux disease. Gastric erosions tend to develop in patients who use NSAIDs, have heavy alcohol intake, or are severely ill with other medical illnesses.

Lower Gastrointestinal Bleeding

The most common causes of acute, severe lower gastrointestinal (LGI) bleeding are colonic diverticula, angiectasis (also known as angiodysplasia), colitis (e.g., due to inflammatory bowel disease, infection, ischemia, or radiation therapy), and colonic neoplasia. Bleeding from a colonic diverticulum typically is acute and painless. Bleeding stops spontaneously in approximately 80% of patients but recurs in 10% to 40% of patients. Angiectasis is most common among the elderly and usually presents as chronic or occult blood loss, but it can also cause acute painless, hemodynamically significant bleeding. Ischemic colitis is due to a temporary interruption in mesenteric blood flow and typically occurs in older individuals with significant cardiac and peripheral vascular disease; patients present with abdominal pain. Acute small bowel (mesenteric) ischemia should be suspected in patients who have risk factors for embolism or thrombosis and who present with sudden-onset, severe abdominal pain that, in the early stage, is out of proportion to the physical examination findings. Although the stool is often positive for occult blood, brisk bleeding rarely is associated with early-stage acute small bowel ischemia. Perianal disease also may present as LGI bleeding. Hemorrhoids probably are the most common cause of minor LGI bleeding. They usually are associated with straining on bowel movement. Anal fissures typically present as intermittent, severe pain on defecation and, like hemorrhoids, may also cause a small amount of bright red blood on the toilet paper or in the toilet. Fissures and hemorrhoids can be diagnosed by direct rectal examination or by anoscopy. Gastrointestinal bleeding should not be attributed solely to hemorrhoids or fissures until other causes have been excluded. Colon cancer must always be considered in patients who are aged >50 years or who have a recent change in bowel movements, constitutional symptoms, anemia, or a family or personal history of cancer or polyps. Bleeding from a colonic polyp or carcinoma usually is occult or small volume.

Immediate Assessment

The first step in the management of acute gastrointestinal bleeding is hemodynamic stabilization. This begins with measuring the blood pressure and heart rate and checking for postural changes in these measures. It is advisable to wait 2 minutes before measuring supine vital signs and to wait 1 minute after the patient stands before measuring upright vital signs. The presence of either severe postural dizziness on attempting to stand (dizziness that prevents the patient from standing) or a postural pulse increment of ≥30/min upon standing provides a sensitive and specif-

Table 1. Common Causes of Gastrointestinal Bleeding

Cause	Notes
Upper Gastrointestinal Tract	
Gastric and duodenal ulcers	Dyspepsia, *Helicobacter pylori* infection, NSAID use, anticoagulation, severe medical illness
Variceal bleeding	Stigmata of chronic liver disease on examination and evidence of portal hypertension or risk factor for cirrhosis (heavy alcohol use, viral hepatitis)
Mallory-Weiss tear	Retching prior to hematemesis
Esophagitis	Heartburn, regurgitation, dysphagia; usually small-volume or occult bleeding
Gastroduodenal erosions	NSAID use, heavy alcohol use, severe medical illness; usually small-volume or occult bleeding
Esophageal or gastric cancer	Progressive dysphagia, weight loss, early satiety, abdominal pain; usually small-volume or occult bleeding
Lower Gastrointestinal Tract	
Diverticula	Painless, self-limited hematochezia
Angiectasis	Chronic blood loss or acute painless hematochezia in elderly; frequently involves upper gastrointestinal tract in addition to colon
Colonic polyp	Usually asymptomatic; stool positive for occult blood
Colon cancer	Age >50 y and usually asymptomatic; change in bowel pattern or microcytic anemia
Ischemic colitis	Risk factors for atherosclerosis and evidence of vascular disease in elderly; abdominal pain
Acute small bowel (mesenteric) ischemia	Severe abdominal pain out of proportion to physical findings; atherosclerotic or embolic risk factors; anion gap metabolic acidosis; bleeding a late finding
Hemorrhoids	Intermittent mild rectal bleeding associated with straining on bowel movement
Infectious colitis	Bloody diarrhea, fever, urgency, tenesmus; exposure history
Inflammatory bowel disease	History of condition and bloody diarrhea, tenesmus, abdominal pain, fever
Meckel diverticulum	Painless hematochezia in young patient; normal esophagogastroduodenoscopy and colonoscopy

ic indication of large-volume (630-1150 mL) blood loss but may be insensitive to smaller amounts. The presence of supine tachycardia (pulse >100/min) and supine hypotension (systolic blood pressure <95 mm Hg) are specific but not sensitive indicators of blood loss.

Two large-caliber intravenous catheters are inserted to allow volume replacement with normal saline and, if necessary, blood products. The goals of volume resuscitation are to restore normal intravascular volume and prevent complications from red blood cell loss, including myocardial infarction, heart failure, and stroke. There is no absolute hemoglobin value that determines when transfusions are appropriate. The decision to transfuse should incorporate an assessment of the patient's age and comorbidities, amount of ongoing blood loss, stability of vital signs, and adequacy of tissue perfusion.

While the hemodynamic status is being stabilized, a focused history and physical examination can suggest specific causes for the bleeding and can provide prognostic information (Table 1). Particular attention should be paid to:

- Nature, amount, and duration of the bleeding and whether it is ongoing
- Character and frequency of stool output
- Presence or absence of abdominal pain and other symptoms, such as fever, diarrhea, retching prior to hematemesis, recent weight loss, or change in bowel habits
- Complications from bleeding, such as chest pain, dyspnea, or oliguria

- Medications and ingestions, such as the use of aspirin, NSAIDs, anticoagulants, and alcohol
- Conditions predisposing to bleeding, including abdominal or pelvic radiation, previous bleeding episodes, and abdominal surgery
- Stigmata of chronic liver disease and previous episodes of variceal bleeding
- Comorbid conditions that increase the risk of a poor outcome, such as diabetes and cardiopulmonary, kidney, or neurologic disease
- Vital signs and postural changes and findings on skin, cardiopulmonary, abdominal, and digital rectal examinations

Evaluation and Management

Initial studies include a complete blood count, blood type and crossmatch, INR and partial thromboplastin time (PTT), serum electrolytes, blood urea nitrogen (BUN), creatinine, aminotransferase levels, and an electrocardiogram (Table 2). Although an isolated elevation of the BUN or elevated BUN-to-creatinine ratio suggests a UGI source of blood loss, neither finding reliably discriminates between UGI and LGI bleeding. In acute, severe bleeding, the initial hematocrit often is an unreliable indicator of the volume of blood loss; it can take 24 to 72 hours before the hematocrit reveals the true reduction in oxygen-carrying capacity.

Clinical risk factors are used to assess the patient's risk for rebleeding and mortality. These include: increased age, large-vol-

Table 2. Management Considerations for Acute Gastrointestinal Bleeding

Consideration	Notes
Hemodynamic stabilization	Two large-bore IV access sites or central venous access: resuscitation with IV fluids and blood products. Endotracheal intubation prior to endoscopy to prevent aspiration in patients who have ongoing UGI bleeding and altered level of consciousness.
Initial laboratory studies	CBC, blood type and crossmatch, coagulation profile, serum electrolytes, blood urea nitrogen, serum creatinine
Electrocardiogram	In all patients aged >50 y and all patients with underlying cardiac disease or features of ischemia
Gastric and duodenal ulcers (see Chapter 21)	Intravenous PPI and endoscopic therapy[a] (for high-risk lesions) reduces risk of recurrent bleeding. If ineffective, consult surgery or interventional radiology. After stabilization, therapy for *Helicobacter pylori* (for patients found to be infected).
Variceal bleeding (see Chapter 25)	Prophylactic antibiotics for all patients (to prevent spontaneous bacterial peritonitis). First-line therapy: endoscopic band ligation or sclerotherapy and octreotide. Second-line therapy: TIPS, balloon tamponade.
Colonic bleeding (diverticulosis, angiectasis)	First-line therapy: colonoscopy and endoscopic therapy.[a] Second-line therapy (when endoscopy not feasible for persistent or recurrent bleeding): arteriography (vasopressin infusion or embolization). Third-line therapy: exploratory laparotomy and segmental colectomy.

CBC = complete blood count; IV = intravenous; PPI = proton pump inhibitors; TIPS = transjugular intrahepatic portosystemic shunt; UGI = upper gastrointestinal bleeding.
[a]Endoscopic therapy incorporates injection therapy (epinephrine, sclerosing agents), thermal techniques (probes, argon plasma coagulation), and mechanical modalities (clips). The type of lesion and the presence or absence of ongoing bleeding determine which technique is used.

ume bleeding (as indicated by hemodynamic instability), significant comorbidities (diabetes, liver failure, heart failure, chronic kidney disease), and endoscopic characteristics. Obtain early consultation with a gastroenterologist and a surgeon for high-risk patients.

After hemodynamic stabilization, the next step is to distinguish UGI bleeding from LGI bleeding. Although melena and hematemesis generally are associated with UGI bleeding and hematochezia is more often a sign of LGI bleeding, these distinctions are not absolute. Melena indicates that blood has been present in the gastrointestinal tract for at least 14 hours, but some patients with melena have bleeding distal to the ligament of Treitz, and 10% to 15% of patients with hematochezia may have UGI bleeding. Therefore, in patients with hematochezia and large-volume blood loss, exclude a UGI bleeding source with nasogastric tube aspiration of gastric contents or endoscopy. The presence of blood or coffee ground–like material on gastric lavage indicates ongoing or recent UGI bleeding and the need for upper endoscopy. Negative nasogastric tube lavage is reliable only if the aspirate contains bile (a yellow or green fluid that tests positive for bile with a urine dipstick), indicating passage of the tube beyond the pylorus into the duodenum. If the nasogastric aspirate contains bile but no blood, it is appropriate to proceed to colonoscopy (Table 2).

Most gastrointestinal bleeding is self-limited. Emergent diagnostic studies usually are required only for patients with persistent, rapid bleeding or for those who are hemodynamically unstable. For most patients with UGI bleeding, esophagogastroduodenoscopy (upper endoscopy) should be performed within the first 24 hours of admission. Endoscopy identifies the bleeding source with considerable accuracy, provides important prognostic information, and allows for immediate treatment for many patients. Variceal or ulcer-related bleeding with specific features (i.e., adherent clot, nonbleeding visible vessel, or active bleeding) has a higher risk for recurrent bleeding, need for surgery, and mortality. Endoscopic therapy reduces morbidity and mortality in these patients. In patients with a bleeding peptic ulcer, the use of intravenous proton pump inhibitor therapy has been shown to

reduce the risk of recurrent hemorrhage following endoscopic hemostasis (Table 2). If bleeding persists despite endoscopic therapy, further options include endoscopic retreatment, angiographic embolization, and surgery. Surgery should be reserved for patients who have persistent bleeding that is unresponsive to medical and endoscopic therapy.

When LGI bleeding is suspected, colonoscopy is recommended within the first 48 hours of admission. Colonoscopy may identify a bleeding diverticulum (responsible for 24%-50% cases of LGI bleeding) and permit endoscopic treatment with epinephrine and/or electrocautery; colonoscopy may also help identify other causes of bleeding, such as vascular angiectasis. Surgery is reserved for refractory bleeding; ideally, when the site is known, a segmental resection can be done rather than a subtotal colectomy. Ischemic colitis, which accounts for between 1% and 19% of episodes of LGI bleeding, results from a sudden temporary reduction in mesenteric blood flow. Colonoscopy reveals a well-defined segment of cyanotic or ulcerated mucosa. CT, which is increasingly used to make the diagnosis, shows a segmental colitis. Most episodes of ischemic colitis resolve spontaneously with supportive care, such as intravenous fluids and pain control. In contrast, acute small bowel (mesenteric) ischemia is associated with a high mortality and requires an aggressive early approach to management, often involving angiography or laparotomy.

Ongoing rectal bleeding without an identifiable source despite upper endoscopy and colonoscopy can be evaluated with a technetium 99m pertechnetate–labeled red blood cell scan or angiography. Tagged red cell scanning is positive in 45% of patients with active bleeding and has an overall accuracy for localizing the bleeding of 78%. It can detect ongoing bleeding occurring at a rate of 0.1 to 0.5 mL/min. This is often the first radiologic test performed, as it is much more sensitive than angiography in detecting bleeding, but it is not very specific. Visualization of the bleeding site (usually a diverticulum or vascular angiectasis) by angiography necessitates a bleeding rate of at least 1 mL/min, but the advantage of angiography is the ability to provide selective embolization to control bleeding. Barium studies have low sensitivity and may interfere with subsequent testing; these tests are not done in the setting of acute gastrointestinal bleeding.

Patients aged <40 years at low risk for colorectal cancer who present with small-volume, self-limited hematochezia may not require colonoscopy. If the bleeding consists of blood on toilet paper or a few drops of blood in the stool, a bleeding hemorrhoid is the most likely cause. Patients with pain on defecation may have an anal fissure. These patients often can forego colonoscopy if a digital rectal examination and anoscopy confirm a benign anorectal process and there are no other concerning features, such as constitutional symptoms, anemia, blood in the stool, change in bowel habits, or family history of colorectal polyps or cancer.

Obscure Gastrointestinal Bleeding

Obscure gastrointestinal bleeding refers to recurrent or persistent bleeding from the gastrointestinal tract without an obvious source on endoscopic studies. In many instances, the bleeding site is in the UGI or colon but is not recognized. Some causes, such as a Dieulafoy lesion (an abnormal submucosal artery that protrudes through the gastric mucosa), produce brisk but intermittent bleeding. Cameron lesions are erosions or ulcerations in the herniated sac of patients with a hiatal hernia. Cameron lesions are relatively common and often are incidental findings on upper endoscopy, but they may present as acute or chronic gastrointestinal bleeding. Gastric antral vascular ectasia (GAVE) is an uncommon cause of gastrointestinal bleeding. It is commonly referred to as a "watermelon stomach" because of the characteristic striped appearance of the gastric vascular malformations on endoscopy. Meckel diverticulum is a congenital anomaly that is located near the ileocecal valve. It often contains heterotopic gastric mucosa that can ulcerate and bleed. Technetium 99m pertechnetate has an affinity for gastric mucosa, and the Meckel scan identifies the heterotopic mucosa. Meckel diverticulum tends to cause bleeding in children and should be considered in younger patients presenting with gastrointestinal bleeding of obscure origin.

The evaluation of gastrointestinal bleeding of obscure origin usually begins with repeat endoscopy directed at the most likely site. If repeat endoscopy is unrevealing in a patient who is not actively bleeding, examination should focus on the small intestine, using such tests as enteroscopy or capsule endoscopy.

Book Enhancement

Go to www.acponline.org/essentials/gastroenterology-section.html. In *MKSAP for Students 5*, assess your knowledge with items 29-33 in the **Gastroenterology and Hepatology** section.

Bibliography

Barkun AN, Bardou M, Kuipers EJ, et al; International Consensus Upper Gastrointestinal Bleeding Conference Group. International consensus recommendations on the management of patients with nonvariceal upper gastrointestinal bleeding. Ann Intern Med. 2010;152: 101-113. [PMID: 20083829]

Chapter 24

Hepatitis

Carlos Palacio, MD

Hepatitis can be acute or chronic. The laboratory hallmark of acute hepatitis is elevated serum aminotransferase levels; the clinical course ranges from asymptomatic disease to fulminant hepatic failure. Chronic hepatitis is an inflammatory process that persists >6 months and can progress to cirrhosis. Histologically, hepatitis is characterized by inflammatory cell infiltration involving the portal areas or the parenchyma, often with associated necrosis; significant fibrosis may be seen in chronic hepatitis.

Viral hepatitis is caused by infection with any of at least five distinct viruses, of which the most commonly identified in the United States are hepatitis A virus (HAV), hepatitis B virus (HBV), and hepatitis C virus (HCV). HAV is transmitted through the fecal-oral route, spreading primarily through close personal contact with an HAV-infected person. HBV is transmitted through exposure to the blood or body fluids of an infected person (e.g., injection drug use, sexual contact, maternal-newborn transmission). HCV, also transmitted parenterally, is the most prevalent blood-borne infection in the United States. All three viruses can cause an acute illness characterized by nausea, malaise, abdominal pain, and jaundice. HBV and HCV also can produce a chronic infection that is associated with an increased risk for chronic liver disease and hepatocellular carcinoma. Hepatitis D virus (HDV; also called *delta hepatitis*) depends on the presence of hepatitis B surface antigen (HBsAg) for its replication and, therefore, cannot survive on its own. In an HBV-infected patient, HDV infection may present as an acute hepatitis (in which case it is a coinfection) or an exacerbation of preexisting chronic hepatitis (in which case it is a superinfection). Patients with a history of injection drug use are at greatest risk for acquiring HDV infection. Hepatitis E virus (HEV) is most likely to occur in residents of or recent travelers to underdeveloped nations; it is transmitted via the fecal-oral route. Pregnant woman with acute HEV infection are at greatest risk for developing severe hepatitis or liver failure.

Prevention

Administer hepatitis A vaccine to adults whose departure to endemic areas for HAV is >2 weeks away. These areas include Africa, Central and South America, the Middle East, and Asia (see www.cdc.gov/travel/default.aspx for relevant countries). If departure is <2 weeks away, immunoglobulin should be administered alone or in combination with the vaccine. Immunoglobulin ensures passive immunity for several months. Other risk groups that benefit from hepatitis A immunization include men who have sex with men (MSM), illicit drug users (oral and injection), persons with occupational risks (i.e., sewage handlers, persons working with non-

human primates), and persons with clotting factor disorders or chronic liver disease.

It is now universal practice to provide hepatitis B vaccine to all newborns. However, persons who were born before the onset of universal vaccination should be offered vaccination, especially if they are at risk of being exposed. Such persons include all children and adolescents who did not get the vaccine when they were younger. Other people who should be vaccinated include MSM and others with high-risk sexual behavior, current or recent injection drug users, persons with chronic liver disease or with end-stage kidney disease on hemodialysis, health care workers and public safety workers exposed to blood or potentially infectious body fluids, household or sexual contacts of HBV carriers, clients and staff members of institutions for persons with developmental disabilities, travelers to countries endemic for HBV, and any adult seeking protection from HBV infection.

Administer hepatitis A immunoglobulin as postexposure prophylaxis (within 2 weeks of exposure) to household, sexual, and day care contacts of persons with confirmed cases of hepatitis A and to individuals who have consumed HAV-contaminated products. Administer hepatitis B immunoglobulin as postexposure prophylaxis, along with hepatitis B vaccine, for exposure to HBV-positive blood, sexual exposure to an HBV-positive person, or household exposure to a person with acute hepatitis B. There is no passive or active immunization for HCV.

Screening

Screen all pregnant women and persons at high risk for hepatitis B. The benefit of screening high-risk patients for hepatitis C is unknown. Risk factors for hepatitis C include injection drug use, receipt of blood products before 1992, and needle-stick exposure to HCV-positive blood. Other potential exposures that may warrant screening for hepatitis C include high-risk sexual exposures, tattoos, body piercing, and non-injection illicit drug use. Screen patients with unexplained acute or chronic hepatitis for hepatitis B and C. Consider anti-HDV testing in patients with acute or chronic hepatitis B who are injection drug users or immigrants from HCV-endemic areas.

Diagnosis

Hepatitis A accounts for approximately half of all cases of acute hepatitis in the United States. Hepatitis A typically is associated with abrupt onset of constitutional symptoms, such as fatigue, anorexia, malaise, nausea, and vomiting. Low-grade fever and right

Table 1. Serologic Diagnosis of Hepatitis B Infection

Test	Acute Hepatitis	Inactive Carriers	Chronic Hepatitis	Prior Exposure	Prior Vaccination
HBsAg	Positive	Positive	Positive	Negative	Negative
Anti-HBc	Positive (IgM)	Positive	Positive	Positive	Negative
Anti-HBs	Negative	Negative	Negative	Positive	Positive
HBV DNA	Positive	Negative	Positive	Negative	Negative
HBeAg	Positive	Negative	Positive or negative	Negative	Negative
Anti-HBe	Positive or negative	Positive	Positive or negative	Positive or negative	Negative

anti-HBc = antibody to hepatitis B core antigen; anti-HBe = antibody to hepatitis B e antigen; anti-HBs = antibody to hepatitis B surface antigen; HBeAg = hepatitis B e antigen; HBsAg = hepatitis B surface antigen; HBV = hepatitis B virus.

upper quadrant pain often are present as well. Skin, sclera, or urine color changes are particularly helpful findings. Approximately 50% of patients with hepatitis A have no identifiable source for their infection, so the absence of classic risk factors cannot exclude the diagnosis. Physical examination often reveals jaundice, hepatomegaly, and abdominal tenderness. Confirm the diagnosis with serologic testing, specifically IgM antibody to HAV. In most patients, IgM antibody is detectable by the time a person is symptomatic and becomes undetectable by 6 months. The IgG antibody indicates prior infection and immunity; there is no chronic state of hepatitis A. Hepatitis A is almost always self-limited but can rarely cause fulminant hepatic failure; therefore, test all patients with unexplained acute liver failure for hepatitis A.

Hepatitis B accounts for approximately one third of cases of acute viral hepatitis in the United States and approximately 15% of cases of chronic viral hepatitis. Symptoms of acute hepatitis B are similar to those of acute hepatitis A; however, approximately 70% of patients have anicteric or subclinical acute infection. Approximately 30% to 40% of patients with acute hepatitis B have no risk factors identified. A characteristic pattern of serologic tests usually is seen in acute hepatitis B (Table 1). During the course of acute infection, a "window period" exists when HBsAg levels have fallen but antibody to HBsAg (anti-HBs) has not yet become detectable; diagnosis is then based on the presence of antibody to hepatitis B core antigen (anti-HBc [IgM]). Test patients with evidence of chronic liver disease for chronic hepatitis B. Also test patients with glomerulonephritis, polyarteritis nodosa, or cryoglobulinemia, as these are extrahepatic manifestations of chronic hepatitis B. Serologic assays can distinguish between chronic hepatitis B and the inactive carrier state (Table 1). Obtain a liver biopsy to determine the grade and stage of liver injury in chronic hepatitis B, as well as to exclude additional causes of liver injury. Although rare, acute liver failure can occur in acute hepatitis B, and all patients with unexplained acute liver failure should have serologic testing.

Hepatitis C usually manifests as chronic liver disease, because the acute infection is usually asymptomatic. Test patients with chronic liver disease for anti-HCV antibody. Consider testing patients with extrahepatic complications of hepatitis C, including cryoglobulinemia, glomerulonephritis, and porphyria cutanea tarda. A positive antibody test indicates only exposure, not immunity; therefore, HCV RNA must be measured to confirm ongoing infection. Up to 40% of patients with chronic hepatitis C have normal aminotransferase levels and this finding cannot exclude the diagnosis. There is poor correlation between viral load and hepatic histology. For those with detectable viral loads, HCV genotype should be obtained in any patient being considered for therapy, because genotype affects likelihood of treatment response and duration of therapy. Consider liver biopsy to evaluate the severity of disease, although this is not essential before initiating treatment.

Consider anti-HDV antibody testing in patients with acute or chronic hepatitis B who are injection drug users or immigrants from HDV-endemic areas. This test currently is available in reference laboratories. HEV infection can be confirmed by the presence of HEV antibodies.

Differential Diagnosis

Important conditions that can mimic viral hepatitis include alcoholic liver disease, drug- and toxin-induced liver injury, autoimmune hepatitis, and, occasionally, metabolic liver diseases (Table 2). Acute alcoholic hepatitis is diagnosed by finding hepatic inflammation in a patient with recent heavy alcohol consumption. Inflammation is indicated by modest elevation of the serum aspartate aminotransferase (AST) concentration; the AST value usually is <400 U/L and approximately twice the serum alanine aminotransferase (ALT) value. Patients may present with leukocytosis, jaundice, hepatomegaly, and right upper quadrant pain suggesting acute viral infection.

Any drug can cause liver injury through such mechanisms as the formation of protein adducts that disrupt cell membranes, an immunologic response, or the generation of injurious free radicals. Drug-induced liver injury may be either dose-dependent and predictable or idiosyncratic. There are many idiosyncratic hepatotoxins, but a few have become known for their "signature" patterns of hepatotoxicity (Table 3).

Autoimmune hepatitis is more common in women and usually presents in adulthood. Approximately 50% of patients are asymptomatic. The remainder of patients may have malaise, rash, and arthralgias. Findings on physical examination may include only hepatomegaly. Other findings include jaundice or signs of hepatic decompensation, such as ascites or encephalopathy. The presence of other autoimmune disorders may also be a clue to the diagnosis. In most cases, serum aminotransferases are elevated, ranging from mild increases to values >1000 U/L. Hyper-

Table 2. Differential Diagnosis of Viral Hepatitis

Disorder	Notes
Alcoholic liver disease	Common cause of chronic hepatitis and cirrhosis. History of excessive alcohol consumption. AST/ALT ratio >2. Improvement with alcohol cessation.
Autoimmune hepatitis	Typically women (90%); acute hepatitis in 25% of patients; other autoimmune disorders may be present. Test for ANA, ASMA, and elevated immunoglobulins; characteristic liver biopsy.
Drug-induced chronic hepatitis	Typically women and elderly but may affect men and women of all ages; history of drug consumption. Improvement with drug discontinuation.
Hemochromatosis	Most common genetic liver disease; iron overload usually not evident until midlife; cardiac dysfunction, diabetes, and arthritis. Elevated fasting serum iron, transferrin saturation, and ferritin. Quantitative hepatic iron index on liver biopsy and HFE genotyping assist with diagnosis.
Nonalcoholic fatty liver disease	Perhaps most common cause of chronic hepatitis in United States. Spectrum of liver disease ranges from steatosis to steatohepatitis to cirrhosis. Associated with diabetes mellitus, obesity, dyslipidemia, and insulin resistance.
Other metabolic liver disease	Wilson disease: rare; most cases diagnosed before age 40 y; may present as speech or gait difficulties; low serum ceruloplasmin, elevated urine copper, and Kayser-Fleischer rings on slit-lamp examination; quantitate hepatic copper for diagnosis. α_1-Antitrypsin deficiency: serum α_1-antitrypsin and phenotyping; PAS-positive inclusions in liver biopsy specimen.

ALT = alanine aminotransferase; ANA = antinuclear antibody; anti-HBc = antibody to hepatitis B core antigen; ASMA = anti–smooth muscle antibody; AST = aspartate aminotransferase; PAS = periodic acid–Schiff stain.

Table 3. Signature Pattern of Drug-induced Hepatotoxicity

Signature Pattern	Specific Agents
Acute liver injury	Acetaminophen, isoniazid
Chronic liver injury	Nitrofurantoin, minocycline, methyldopa
Fibrosis and cirrhosis	Methotrexate, vitamin A
Jaundice	Erythromycin, amoxicillin-clavulanate, chlorpromazine, estrogens
Hypersensitivity (rash, fever, and multi-organ failure)	Phenytoin
Fatty liver	Amiodarone, tamoxifen, valproic acid, didanosine

bilirubinemia may occur with a normal or near-normal serum alkaline phosphatase level. Certain autoantibodies may be elevated, including anti–smooth muscle antibody, antinuclear antibody, and, rarely, anti–liver-kidney microsomal antibody type 1 (anti-LKM1). In addition, serum IgG and IgM are elevated.

Nonalcoholic fatty liver disease consists of variable degrees of fat accumulation, inflammation, and fibrosis in the absence of significant alcohol intake. It is possibly the most common form of liver disease in the United States. Nonalcoholic fatty liver disease is most commonly seen in patients with underlying consequences of obesity, including insulin resistance, hypertension, and/or hyperlipidemia. The diagnosis usually is made when patients with characteristic clinical risk factors are found to have mildly to moderately elevated serum aminotransferase concentrations. Imaging with ultrasonography, CT, or MRI can confirm the presence of steatosis.

Hereditary hemochromatosis is a common genetic disorder in white persons, characterized by excessive iron deposition in tissues, especially the liver, heart, pancreas, and pituitary gland. The iron overload can lead to cirrhosis, heart disease, and diabetes mellitus. The gene mutations leading to phenotypic hereditary hemochromatosis are the C282Y mutation and H63D mutation of the HFE gene. Initial evaluation involves fasting transferrin saturation and serum ferritin measurements. A fasting transferrin saturation >50% in women and >60% in men strongly suggests the diagnosis of hemochromatosis.

Wilson disease is a rare autosomal recessive disorder. It is characterized by the reduced excretion of copper into the bile secondary to a transport abnormality, leading to the pathologic accumulation of copper in the liver and other tissues, particularly the brain. Patients may present with fulminant disease characterized by elevated serum aminotransferase concentrations in the setting of hemolytic anemia.

α_1-Antitrypsin deficiency affects the liver, lungs, and skin. Disease in the liver is the result of abnormal accumulation of a variant protein in hepatocytes, which can be identified as inclusions with periodic acid–Schiff staining. The disease can manifest in early childhood or in adulthood and is associated with an increased risk of cirrhosis and hepatocellular carcinoma.

Therapy

In patients with acute hepatitis, be alert to the development of asterixis or any subtle changes in neurologic or mental status (e.g., somnolence). Such clinical findings signal the onset of encephalopathy, which defines the patient as having fulminant hepatic failure (a rare complication of acute hepatitis A and B). A patient suspected of being at high risk for development of fulminant hepatic failure should be transferred to a liver transplantation center for an expedited liver transplant evaluation.

All patients with acute or chronic viral hepatitis are counseled to avoid alcohol and acetaminophen and to eat a balanced, nutritionally adequate diet. Criteria for hospitalization in acute viral hepatitis include inability to maintain oral hydration and symptoms or signs of liver failure.

The treatment for hepatitis A is primarily supportive. No conclusive data show that bed rest or inactivity affects the course of hepatitis A.

Antiviral drug therapy is used in selected patients with chronic hepatitis B to reduce likelihood of progression to cirrhosis and hepatocellular carcinoma. The goals of therapy in chronic hepatitis B are suppression of viral replication, conversion from HBeAg-positive to HbBeAg-negative status, and mitigation of hepatic inflammation as evidenced by a reduction in serum liver enzyme concentrations. An additional goal is sustained suppression of viral replication, indicated by lack of recurrent HBV DNA after antiviral therapy is discontinued. There are six approved therapies for chronic, replicative hepatitis B: interferon (standard and pegylated), lamivudine, adefovir, entecavir, and telbivudine. The advantages of interferon are limited duration of therapy, lack of resistance, and high response rate. Interferon alfa is administered subcutaneously and is associated with frequent side effects, including flu-like symptoms, myelotoxicity, depression, and exacerbation of autoimmune conditions. Pegylated interferon allows for less frequent administration than standard interferon and is more efficacious. Patients with advanced liver disease or decompensated cirrhosis should not be given interferon therapy, because they may be at risk for decompensation of liver disease and infection. Other contraindications include severe preexisting bone marrow suppression and severe depression. In such patients, the oral agents are used; however, disadvantages of these agents are limited ability to achieve sustained suppression of viral replication, cost, and propensity for drug resistance.

Therapy for hepatitis C consists of the combination of pegylated interferon and ribavirin. The ideal candidate for therapy is the patient with detectable virus, some indication of hepatic inflammation (elevated liver tests or inflammation on liver biopsy), and no contraindication to therapy. The goal of therapy is to achieve a sustained virologic response, which is defined as undetectable HCV beyond 6 months after the end of treatment. The most important variable affecting the response rate is the genotype of the virus. Patients infected with genotype 1 have an approximately 45% sustained response rate if treated for 48 weeks. Patients with genotypes 2 and 3 have a sustained virologic response rate in excess of 80% and require only 24 weeks of therapy; in addition, the dosage of ribavirin can be reduced in these patients. Ribavirin can be associated with hemolytic anemia. Because most patients with chronic hepatitis C never develop cirrhosis, there is controversy about the treatment of patients with persistently normal aminotransferase levels and minimal histologic evidence of hepatitis.

Patients with alcoholic hepatitis should abstain from alcohol. The Maddrey Discriminant Function (DF) score, which helps to identify patients whose short-term survival is improved by corticosteroid therapy, is calculated as follows:

$$DF = 4.6 \text{ (prothrombin time [s] − control prothrombin time [s]) + serum bilirubin (mg/dL)}$$

Patients with a DF score greater than 32 have a >50% short-term (30-day) mortality risk. Such patients are candidates for therapy with prednisone.

Treatment of drug-induced liver injury is primarily supportive and involves withdrawal of the suspected offending agent. However, there are a few specific antidotes, including N-acetylcysteine for acetaminophen intoxication and L-carnitine for valproic acid overdose. Treatment for autoimmune hepatitis consists of prednisone alone or, more commonly, in combination with azathioprine. Treatment can be discontinued once remission is achieved. There is no definitive treatment for nonalcoholic fatty liver disease. Reduction of underlying risk factors is essential, including weight loss, exercise, and aggressive control of plasma glucose, lipids, and blood pressure. Treatment of Wilson disease is directed at reducing copper overload with the use of copper chelators (penicillamine, trientine) or agents that reduce copper absorption (zinc). Treatment of hereditary hemochromatosis involves therapeutic phlebotomy to extract excess iron or to prevent accumulation of iron before symptomatic overload occurs. Although there is no treatment for hepatic disease due to α_1-antitrypsin deficiency, liver transplantation is an option for patients who develop hepatic decompensation.

Follow-Up

Patients on antiviral therapy must have regular laboratory and clinical monitoring to assess response to treatment and development of side effects. Among patients with hepatitis C who develop cirrhosis, the risk for hepatocellular carcinoma is approximately 5% per year. Patients with established chronic hepatitis B must be monitored for the development of cirrhosis or hepatocellular carcinoma. Although cirrhosis seems to be the greatest risk factor for hepatocellular carcinoma in hepatitis B, 30% to 50% of cases occur without cirrhosis. Therefore, screening every 6 to 12 months with ultrasonography and serum alpha-fetoprotein is generally recommended for patients with chronic hepatitis B or cirrhosis due to hepatitis B or C. Patients with cirrhosis due to hepatitis B or C should be screened for the presence of esophageal varices by upper endoscopy.

Book Enhancement

Go to www.acponline.org/essentials/gastroenterology-section.html. In MKSAP for Students 5, assess your knowledge with items 35-40 in the Gastroenterology and Hepatology section.

Bibliography

Brundage SC, Fitzpatrick AN. Hepatitis A. Am Fam Physician. 2006;73: 2162-2168. [PMID: 16848078]

Jou JH, Muir AJ. In the clinic. Hepatitis C. Ann Intern Med. 2008;148: ITC6-1-ITC6-16. [PMID: 18519925]

Shiffman ML. Management of acute hepatitis B. Clin Liver Dis. 2010;14: 75-91; viii-ix. [PMID: 20123442]

Chapter 25

Cirrhosis

Mark J. Fagan, MD

Cirrhosis is a pathologic state of the liver characterized histologically by extensive fibrosis and regenerative nodules. Liver fibrosis begins with the activation of hepatic stellate cells, which produce excess extracellular matrix proteins, including type I collagen. Failure to degrade the increased interstitial matrix leads to progressive fibrosis. In general, cirrhosis is irreversible. A variety of toxic, infectious, and inflammatory insults to the liver may result in cirrhosis (Table 1). Patients with cirrhosis may present with symptoms related to either hepatocyte dysfunction (jaundice, coagulopathy) or increased portal venous pressure (ascites, edema, spontaneous bacterial peritonitis, bleeding esophageal varices, hepatic encephalopathy, hypersplenism).

Prevention

Counsel patients who consume hazardous amounts of alcohol to stop or reduce their intake of alcohol. Alcohol cessation is effective in reducing the risk of cirrhosis. Also counsel patients with chronic hepatitis B or C to avoid alcohol, because concomitant alcohol use increases the risk for cirrhosis. Antiviral treatment may reduce the risk of cirrhosis in some patients with hepatitis B or C. Administer hepatitis B vaccine to nonimmune patients with risk factors for hepatitis B (see Chapter 24).

Screening

Screen patients for hazardous drinking using validated questionnaires such as the CAGE or AUDIT instrument (see Chapter 31). Test patients with risk factors for chronic hepatitis B or C (see Chapter 24). Screen first-degree relatives of patients with hereditary hemochromatosis for evidence of iron overload.

Diagnosis

Patients with cirrhosis may be asymptomatic for years before developing evidence of hepatocyte dysfunction or portal hypertension. Patients may report a change in skin, sclera, or urine color due to jaundice, and they may develop pruritus related to cholestasis. The relative estrogen excess of the cirrhotic state may lead to symptoms of decreased libido, erectile dysfunction, or amenorrhea.

Table 1. Differential Diagnosis of Cirrhosis

Disorder	Notes
Chronic exposure to drugs or toxins	Exposure history most commonly alcohol but may be medications (methotrexate, amiodarone, high-dose vitamin A) or chemicals (hydrocarbons). Long-term TPN can lead to cirrhosis.
Chronic viral hepatitis	Etiology most commonly hepatitis B or C. Diagnosis by typical viral hepatitis serology.
Autoimmune hepatitis	Typically young women with fatigue and jaundice and, later, aminotransferase elevations; hypergammaglobulinemia and other autoimmune diseases may be present. Look for specific autoantibodies (ANA, ASMA).
Primary biliary cirrhosis	Typically women in their 50s who are often asymptomatic at diagnosis (incidental finding of elevated alkaline phosphatase); otherwise, fatigue and pruritus. AMA typically positive (>90%).
Primary sclerosing cholangitis	Typically men in their late 30s who are asymptomatic (incidental finding of elevated alkaline phosphatase), particularly in patients with established ulcerative colitis. Diagnosis usually by endoscopic cholangiography.
Nonalcoholic fatty liver disease	Typically obese, diabetic women with hyperlipidemia. Liver ultrasonography shows fatty infiltration. May require liver biopsy to identify steatohepatitis.
Hereditary hemochromatosis	Typically men; early findings include arthralgia and aminotransferase elevations; later findings may include diabetes, skin darkening, impotence, and heart failure. Diagnosis suggested by elevated transferrin saturation and ferritin and confirmed by hemochromatosis gene test.
Wilson disease	Variable presentation (fatigue, anorexia, abdominal pain, tremor, poor coordination, spastic dystonia, psychiatric conditions). Diagnosis suggested by low serum ceruloplasmin, elevated serum free copper levels, and Kayser-Fleischer rings on slit-lamp examination.
α_1-Antitrypsin deficiency	Typical presentation in first months of life, with jaundice and elevated aminotransferase levels. Some present in late childhood or early adolescence with hepatosplenomegaly and evidence of portal hypertension. Diagnosis by serum α_1-antitrypsin and phenotyping.
Cryptogenic cirrhosis	Typical clinical features of cirrhosis, but no obvious cause after extensive evaluation.

AMA = antimitochondrial antibody; ANA = antinuclear antibody; ASMA = anti–smooth muscle antibody; TPN = total parenteral nutrition.

Decreased hepatic production of clotting factors may lead to abnormal bleeding. Portal hypertension may cause esophageal varices, which may lead to hematemesis or melena. Patients may report weight gain, increased abdominal girth, or ankle swelling related to ascites and edema. Family members may report changes in the patient's behavior or mental status characteristic of hepatic encephalopathy.

Take a thorough history, including a detailed alcohol history. Question patients about risk factors for hepatitis C infection, such as intravenous drug use, blood transfusion prior to 1992, having a sexual partner who uses intravenous drugs, or incarceration. Similarly, ask patients about risk factors for hepatitis B infection, such as birth in an endemic country, having multiple sex partners, or intravenous drug use. Inquire about other diseases that may result in cirrhosis, such as right-sided heart failure, and about risk factors for nonalcoholic fatty liver disease (obesity, diabetes, hyperlipidemia). Ask about the use of medications associated with increased risk for cirrhosis, such as methotrexate, amiodarone, and high-dose vitamin A. A family history of liver disease should prompt a consideration of genetic diseases that cause cirrhosis, such as hemochromatosis, α_1-antitrypsin deficiency, or Wilson disease.

Jaundice usually is first noticed in the conjunctiva, with more severe degrees apparent in other mucous membranes or the skin. Spider angiomata, thought to be the result of an increased ratio of serum estradiol to testosterone, may be found over the face, neck, shoulders, and upper thorax. The lesions blanch with pressure and refill from the center outward. Palmar erythema, gynecomastia, and testicular atrophy are thought to be related to the same hormonal effects. The breath may have a characteristic odor (fetor hepaticus) caused by the presence of dimethyl sulfide due to portosystemic shunting. The liver may be palpable or reduced in size, and the spleen may be palpable due to engorgement from portal hypertension. Bulging flanks, flank dullness, shifting dullness, or a fluid wave suggests ascites. Of these findings, flank dullness has the highest sensitivity (84%) and fluid wave has the highest specificity (90%). Patients with ascites may have a palpable umbilical hernia. The presence of leg edema in patients with cirrhosis increases the likelihood that ascites is present. Rarely, portal hypertension causes markedly dilated abdominal wall veins (caput medusae). Impaired mental status, confusion, agitation, hyperreflexia, or asterixis (the inability to maintain a fixed posture) suggests hepatic encephalopathy. Other physical examination findings in cirrhosis include parotid enlargement, Dupuytren contracture, clubbing, axillary hair loss, and white nails.

Although liver biopsy is the definitive method of establishing a diagnosis of cirrhosis, laboratory tests and imaging studies, in combination with physical examination findings, can be used to estimate the likelihood of cirrhosis (Table 2). In clinical practice, liver biopsy is generally not performed if the history, physical examination, laboratory tests, and imaging studies strongly suggest cirrhosis. The serum albumin level, prothrombin time, total and direct bilirubin levels, and aminotransferase levels are useful in assessing hepatic function. Thrombocytopenia suggests hypersplenism due to portal hypertension.

Use the history, along with laboratory tests, to establish the cause of cirrhosis. Alcoholic liver disease and chronic hepatitis C, the two most common causes of cirrhosis in the United States, are diagnosed from the history and the presence of antibody to hepatitis C virus, respectively. Chronic hepatitis B, a less common cause of cirrhosis in the United States, is indicated by the presence of hepatitis B surface antigen. In parts of the world with a high prevalence of chronic hepatitis B (sub-Saharan Africa, China, Southeast Asia), hepatitis B is an important and vaccine-preventable cause of cirrhosis.

Chronic cholestatic liver diseases such as primary biliary cirrhosis (PBC) and primary sclerosing cholangitis (PSC) can cause cirrhosis. PBC is a slowly progressive autoimmune liver disease that is five times more common in women than in men and usually affects those between 30 and 65 years of age. Fatigue and pruritus are the most common presenting symptoms, and other autoimmune disorders such as hypothyroidism, Sjögren sicca syndrome, and systemic sclerosis (scleroderma) may coexist. In PBC, the alkaline phosphatase is usually markedly elevated, and more than 90% of patients have antimitochondrial antibodies. PSC is a chronic condition characterized by progressive bile duct inflammation and destruction and, ultimately, fibrosis of both the intrahepatic and extrahepatic bile ducts, leading to cirrhosis. PSC is strongly associated with ulcerative colitis and, like PBC, is associated with markedly elevated alkaline phosphatase. In contrast to PBC, PSC is not associated with antimitochondrial antibodies.

Autoimmune hepatitis can vary in severity from subclinical illness to fulminant hepatic failure and is associated with elevated gamma globulin levels as well as antinuclear, anti–smooth muscle, and anti–liver-kidney microsomal antibodies. The disease is more common in women. Approximately 50% of patients are asymptomatic and are diagnosed as a result of incidental findings on screening tests.

Nonalcoholic fatty liver disease (NAFLD) consists of variable degrees of fat accumulation, inflammation, and fibrosis in the liver in the absence of significant alcohol intake. NAFLD is increasingly recognized as possibly the most common form of liver disease in the United States. NAFLD in the absence of inflammation is more common in women than in men and occurs in 60% of obese patients. Nonalcoholic steatohepatitis (NASH) is an extreme form of NAFLD characterized by the presence of inflammation that is indistinguishable from alcohol steatohepatitis. The prevalence of NASH is difficult to determine but may occur in about 20% of obese patients; 2% to 3% of patients with NASH also have cirrhosis. Other common associations include type 2 diabetes mellitus and hyperlipidemia.

Consider hereditary causes of cirrhosis in patients with a family history of liver disease. Hereditary hemochromatosis can be associated with diabetes, skin hyperpigmentation, pseudogout, and cardiomyopathy. A serum transferrin saturation ≥60% in men and ≥50% in women has 90% sensitivity for identifying patients homozygous for the hemochromatosis gene. Wilson disease, an autosomal recessive disorder affecting copper transport, is associated with neuropsychiatric symptoms and cirrhosis. A very low serum ceruloplasmin level strongly suggests the diagnosis. α_1-Antitrypsin deficiency affects the liver and lungs (emphysema). Liver disease is the result of abnormal accumulation of a variant protein in hepatocytes, which can be identified as inclusions with periodic acid–Schiff staining. The diagnosis is confirmed by a low serum α_1-antitrypsin level.

Table 2. Laboratory and Other Studies for Cirrhosis

Test	Notes
Tests for Diagnosis	
AST/ALT ≤1	Sensitivity 44%, specificity, 94%
Platelets <100,000	Sensitivity 38%, specificity 97%; suggests presence of splenomegaly
PT, bilirubin, albumin	Measures of liver function
Liver ultrasonography	Sensitivity 71%-100%, specificity 88%; compare to liver histology
Abdominal CT	Sensitivity 84%, specificity 100%; based on caudate lobe–right lobe ratio >0.65
Abdominal MRI	Sensitivity 93%, specificity 92%; based on enlargement of hilar periportal space as sign of early cirrhosis
Serum-ascites albumin gradient	Sensitivity 97%, specificity 91%; gradient >1.1 compatible with cirrhosis
Tests to Determine Etiology	
Viral hepatitis studies	HBsAg, anti-HBs, anti-HBc, anti-HCV antibody
Alkaline phosphatase	Increased in PSC and PBC
Antimitochondrial antibody	Positive in PBC (>90% of cases)
Antinuclear antibody	Positive in autoimmune hepatitis and PBC
Anti–smooth muscle antibody	May be positive in autoimmune hepatitis
Anti–LKM antibody	May be positive in autoimmune hepatitis
Total protein, globulin	May be elevated in autoimmune hepatitis, viral hepatitis, and PBC
Iron studies	Transferrin saturation and ferritin increased in hemochromatosis
GGT	Elevated GGT may be only abnormality in NASH
Ceruloplasmin	Decreased in Wilson disease
α_1-Antitrypsin	Decreased in α_1-antitrypsin deficiency
Tests to Detect Complications	
α-Fetoprotein	Levels >500 ng/mL (500 μg/L) highly suggest HCC
Abdominal ultrasonography	Screening for HCC; gold standard for detection of ascites
Ascitic fluid granulocyte count	Count >250/μL (250 x 10⁶/L) suggests SBP
Serum electrolytes	Abnormal in cirrhosis due to diuretic therapy for ascites or alcoholism
Serum BUN, creatinine	Elevated in hepatorenal syndrome
Upper endoscopy	Used to document (and treat) varices
Serum ammonia	Elevated serum ammonia may be helpful in unusual presentations of hepatic encephalopathy

ALT = alanine aminotransferase; anti-HBc = antibody to hepatitis B core antigen; anti-HBs = antibody to hepatitis B surface antigen; HCV = hepatitis C virus; anti–LKM antibody = anti–liver-kidney microsomal antibody; AST = aspartate aminotransferase; BUN = blood urea nitrogen; GGT = gamma-glutamyl transpeptidase; HBsAg = hepatitis B surface antigen; HCC = hepatocellular carcinoma; NASH = nonalcoholic steatohepatitis; PBC = primary biliary cirrhosis; PSC = primary sclerosing cholangitis; PT = prothrombin time; SBP = spontaneous bacterial peritonitis.

In patients with ascites, diagnostic paracentesis is an important tool for identifying the cause and determining if infection (spontaneous bacterial peritonitis [SBP]) is present. Thirty percent of patients with SBP do not have fever, and 40% do not have abdominal pain. Abdominal paracentesis is indicated in patients with newly identified ascites and in situations associated with an increased risk for SBP (hospital admission, signs of infection, clinical deterioration, gastrointestinal bleeding). Samples should be sent for albumin and protein concentrations, cell count, Gram stain, and culture. Bleeding complications from paracentesis are uncommon, even when the INR is prolonged, so that pre-paracentesis plasma or platelet transfusions are not necessary. Calculate the serum-ascites albumin gradient to differentiate among causes of ascites. A gradient ≥1.1 indicates that the ascites is due to portal hypertension; a gradient <1.1 indicates that another process is present, such as nephrotic syndrome, tuberculosis, or cancer. An ascitic fluid granulocyte count >250/μL (250 x 10⁶/L) is compatible with infection. Patients with an ascitic fluid protein concentration <1 g/dL (10 g/L) are at increased risk for developing SBP.

Thirty to fifty percent of patients with portal hypertension will bleed from varices, and mortality from variceal bleeding is 30% to 50%. Patients with cirrhosis should undergo upper endoscopy to search for esophageal varices (Table 2).

Therapy

The goals of therapy for cirrhosis are to slow the progression of the underlying liver disease, prevent further injury to the liver, prevent and treat complications (esophageal varices, ascites, hepatic encephalopathy, hepatocellular carcinoma), and evaluate the patient for liver transplantation. Protein-calorie malnutrition and hypermetabolism are common in patients with cirrhosis, and nutritional assessment is important. Alcoholic patients should receive folate and thiamine supplementation, and patients with ascites should have dietary sodium restriction (<2 g/day). Abstinence from alcohol is critically important to reduce further liver injury. Vaccinate nonimmune patients against hepatitis A and B, and administer pneumococcal and yearly influenza vaccines.

Nonselective β-blockers (propranolol, nadolol) are effective for primary prophylaxis of bleeding from high-risk varices and for secondary prophylaxis following an episode of variceal bleeding. The dose is titrated to produce a 25% reduction in resting heart rate. Endoscopic variceal band ligation or sclerotherapy is indicated for primary and secondary prophylaxis in patients with contraindications to or intolerance of β-blockers. Patients who rebleed despite variceal banding may be considered for alternative treatments such as a transjugular intrahepatic portosystemic shunt (TIPS) procedure or portosystemic shunt surgery. TIPS creates a low-resistance channel between the hepatic vein and the intrahepatic portion of the portal vein using angiographic techniques. The channel is kept open by an expandable metal stent. Thirty percent of patients will develop hepatic encephalopathy following TIPS.

Diuretics and sodium restriction are the mainstays of treatment for ascites. Combination diuretic therapy with spironolactone plus furosemide is most effective; in one trial, this combination controlled ascites in 90% of patients. The drugs can be given together in once-daily dosing. Refractory ascites can be treated with repeat large-volume paracentesis. When >5 L of ascitic fluid is removed, intravenous albumin is administered to reduce the risk for hemodynamic instability, hyponatremia, or worsening kidney function. TIPS is an alternative when repeat large-volume paracentesis is impractical or ineffective.

SBP commonly develops in hospitalized patients with ascites and an ascitic fluid protein <1.0 g/dL (10 g/L), variceal bleeding, or prior SBP. Patients with an ascitic fluid neutrophil count >250/μL (250 x 10^6/L) should be treated for SBP initially with antibiotics active against *Enterobacteriaceae*, *Streptococcus pneumoniae*, and enterococcus. Patients with ascitic fluid neutrophil counts < 250/μL (250 x 10^6/L) but with risk factors for SBP benefit from short-term antibiotic prophylaxis (i.e., trimethoprim-sulfamethoxazole, ciprofloxacin, norfloxacin) directed at the common organisms causing SBP. It is uncertain whether long-term antibiotic prophylaxis of SBP is superior to intermittent prophylaxis during hospitalizations.

Hepatorenal syndrome is the development of kidney failure in patients with portal hypertension, ascites, and normal renal tubular function. Vigorous diuretic therapy, large-volume paracentesis without volume expansion, and gastrointestinal bleeding may precipitate hepatorenal syndrome. Other causes of kidney failure should be excluded, particularly SBP. Failure to improve following withdrawal of diuretics and administration of 1 to 1.5 L of normal saline is indicative of hepatorenal syndrome. Dialysis is indicated for patients with significant volume overload or severe electrolyte abnormalities. Albumin and vasopressin or norepinephrine may improve renal arterial blood flow, but almost all patients will require liver transplantation.

The treatment of hepatic encephalopathy begins with a search for precipitating causes such as hypovolemia, electrolyte and acid-base disturbances, gastrointestinal bleeding, infections (including SBP), and medication effects. Lactulose is the mainstay of drug treatment to lower serum ammonia levels and prevent or treat hepatic encephalopathy. The lactulose dose is titrated to produce two to three soft stools per day. For patients who do not respond to lactulose, nonabsorbable antibiotics such as neomycin or rifaximin can be added.

Patients with cirrhosis are at increased risk for hepatocellular carcinoma, although the magnitude of the risk varies with the cause of cirrhosis. With chronic hepatitis C, hepatocellular carcinoma generally occurs only in patients who have progressed to cirrhosis. In chronic hepatitis B, hepatocellular carcinoma can occur even without cirrhosis. Ultrasonography is the recommended screening test, performed every 6 to 12 months. The beneficial impact of screening on hepatocellular carcinoma-specific mortality has been best established for patients with chronic hepatitis B.

Liver transplantation is the definitive treatment for patients with end-stage liver disease and complications such as variceal bleeding, ascites, or hepatic encephalopathy. Some patients with cirrhosis and hepatocellular carcinoma can also be treated with liver transplantation. The MELD (Model for End-Stage Liver Disease) scoring system uses the patient's bilirubin, creatinine, and INR to prioritize transplant candidates. Contraindications to liver transplantation include cardiopulmonary disease that constitutes prohibitive risk for surgery, non-skin malignancy outside of the liver within 5 years of evaluation or not meeting oncologic criteria for cure, and active substance abuse.

Follow-Up

Follow-up issues for patients with cirrhosis include counseling about substance abuse, monitoring for complications (bleeding, ascites, SBP, hepatic encephalopathy, hepatorenal syndrome), monitoring for medication side effects, screening for hepatocellular carcinoma, and assessing for liver transplantation. Cessation of substance abuse is critical for reducing further liver damage from toxins such as alcohol and to permit consideration for liver transplantation. Instruct patients to report any symptoms suggestive of cirrhotic complications, such as melena, weight gain, increased abdominal girth, edema, abdominal pain, change in mental status, or decreased urine output. For patients taking diuretics, careful monitoring of the BUN, creatinine, and electrolytes is important to detect potential volume depletion, hyperkalemia, hypokalemia, or hyponatremia.

Book Enhancement

Go to www.acponline.org/essentials/gastroenterology-section.html. In *MKSAP for Students 5* assess your knowledge with items 42-45 in the **Gastroenterology and Hepatology** section.

Bibliography

Garcia-Tsao G, Bosch J. Management of varices and variceal hemorrhage in cirrhosis. N Engl J Med. 2010;362:823-832. [PMID: 20200386]

Ginès P, Schrier RW. Renal failure in cirrhosis. N Engl J Med. 2009; 361:1279-1290. [PMID: 19776409]

Chapter 26

Inflammatory Bowel Disease

Susan T. Hingle, MD

nflammatory bowel disease (IBD) is a group of inflammatory conditions of the colon and small intestine. Two distinct disorders account for the majority of IBD: ulcerative colitis and Crohn disease. Ulcerative colitis is characterized by diffuse mucosal inflammation that is limited to the colon and extends proximally and continuously from the anus. Crohn disease is characterized by focal, asymmetric, transmural lesions and by skip lesions, rather than continuous disease. Rectal sparing is common in Crohn disease. As many as 10% of patients cannot be shown to have either Crohn disease or ulcerative colitis and are considered to have indeterminate colitis.

The pathophysiology of IBD appears to involve an imbalance between pro-inflammatory mediators (interleukin 1β, tumor necrosis factor, thromboxane A_2) and anti-inflammatory mediators (prostaglandin E_2, interleukin 10), resulting in an inflammatory response. Immunoregulatory cytokines also appear to be imbalanced in patients with IBD.

The cause and pathogenesis of IBD are unclear, although several epidemiologic associations and risk factors have been identified. There is no gender predilection for IBD; men and women are at similar risk. There is a bimodal age distribution for presentation, with the first and largest peak in the third decade of life and a second, smaller peak between age 50 and age 80 years. The incidence is highest in northern climates (Scandinavia, northern Europe, North America) and lowest in southern climates and underdeveloped regions (Asia, Africa, South America).

Both genetic and environmental factors appear to play a role in development of IBD. IBD is more common in those of Jewish descent. There also is a familial tendency for IBD. From 10% to 25% of patients with IBD have an affected first-degree relative, and twin studies show a higher concordance for identical twins than for fraternal twins. Numerous environmental factors also have been studied, including cigarette smoking, diet, oral contraceptives, NSAIDs, and infections. It is likely that the interplay between genetics and environment is responsible for development of IBD.

Diagnosis

Patients with ulcerative colitis generally present with bloody diarrhea associated with rectal urgency, discomfort, and cramping. Patients have profound tenesmus (feelings of urgency and incomplete evacuation), which is secondary to proctitis. Inflammation of the rectum can cause constipation to be a more prominent manifestation than diarrhea. Weight loss secondary to the inflammatory disease itself or to chronic diarrhea is common. Physical examination findings can range from mild lower abdominal tenderness to life-threatening nonobstructive colonic dilatation with systemic toxicity (toxic megacolon).

In Crohn disease, large-volume diarrhea can occur; diarrhea is associated with both small- and large-bowel disease, whereas hematochezia is almost always a sign of colonic disease. The transmural nature of Crohn disease results in three distinct types

Table 1. Extraintestinal Manifestations of Inflammatory Bowel Disease (IBD)

Manifestation	Notes
Peripheral arthritis	Type 1 affects large joints of arms and legs (elbows, wrists, knees, ankles); symptoms often migratory and correlate with active bowel disease. Type 2 is symmetric and affects small joints; unrelated to bowel disease activity.
Sacroiliitis	Pain and stiffness in lower spine and sacroiliac joints; may present before IBD symptoms.
Ankylosing spondylitis (see Chapter 94)	Rare complication; seen more in CD than UC.
Osteoporosis	More common in women with CD; related to IBD and therapy. Periodic screening is important.
Erythema nodosum (Plate 2)	Tender, red nodules over shins and ankles; more common in UC and women; related to IBD disease activity.
Pyoderma gangrenosum (Plate 3)	Papules and pustules coalesce to form deep, chronic ulcers, often on shins and ankles; more common in UC; related to IBD disease activity.
Aphthous stomatitis	Small ulcers between gums and lower lip or along tongue; related to IBD disease activity.
Uveitis	Pain, blurry vision, photosensitivity, redness of eye. An ophthalmologic emergency.
Scleritis	Deep pain, redness of sclera. An ophthalmologic emergency.
Primary sclerosing cholangitis (see Chapter 24)	Severe inflammation and scarring of bile ducts; more common in UC and men. Jaundice, nausea, pruritus, weight loss. May be complicated by cholangiocarcinoma and/or colon cancer.

CD = Crohn disease; UC = ulcerative colitis.

Table 2. Differences Between Ulcerative Colitis and Crohn Disease

Characteristic	Ulcerative Colitis	Crohn Disease
Pathology		
Granulomas	No	Yes
Fissures	No	Yes
Transmural inflammation	No	Yes
Continuous disease	Yes	No
Crypt abscesses	Yes	No
Clinical presentation	Diarrhea (prominent), hematochezia, weight loss, fever	Abdominal pain (prominent), diarrhea, inflammatory masses, fever, weight loss
Laboratory findings		
Anti–Saccharomyces cerevisiae antibody	10% of cases	60% of cases
Perinuclear anti-neutrophil cytoplasmic antibody	75% of cases	10% of cases
Smoking	Alleviates symptoms	Risk factor for disease
Colon cancer risk	High risk	High risk

of lesions: inflammatory, fistulizing, and fibrostenotic. Inflamed tissue causes a secretory diarrhea and protein-losing enteropathy, as well as steatorrhea from fat malabsorption. Fistulae are abnormal connections between the bowel and adjacent organs. Fistulae around the anus (perianal fistulae) may drain fecal material, whereas those through the skin (enterocutaneous fistulae) may seep bowel contents. Feces may pass through fistulae to the vagina (rectovaginal fistulae), and fistulae to the bladder (enterovesical fistulae) may cause pneumaturia or recurrent urinary tract infections. Fistulae connecting to abscesses may drain pus. Patients with intestinal strictures present with signs of obstruction. Strictures may be secondary to severe inflammation or to fibrosis of the bowel and are relieved only by surgical resection.

Approximately 10% to 20% of patients with IBD have extraintestinal manifestations at some point in the course of disease. The musculoskeletal, dermatologic, ocular, and hepatobiliary systems may be involved (Table 1).

Approximately two thirds of patients with ulcerative colitis but only 15% to 20% of patients with Crohn disease are positive for perinuclear anti-neutrophil cytoplasmic antibody (p-ANCA). Approximately half of patients with Crohn disease have anti–Saccharomyces cerevisiae antibody (ASCA), compared to 5% of patients with ulcerative colitis. Therefore, measuring serum p-ANCA and ASCA is reasonably reliable for the diagnosis of Crohn disease or ulcerative colitis. In patients with Crohn disease, an upper gastrointestinal barium study with small bowel follow-through is helpful in determining the extent of involvement, and presence of strictures (demonstrating string signs) and fistulae. Colonic disease may be seen on barium enema. In patients with ulcerative colitis, abdominal radiography can be useful to diagnose toxic megacolon. Diagnosis of both ulcerative colitis and Crohn disease is made by colonoscopy and confirmed with biopsy. Table 2 lists essential differences between ulcerative colitis and Crohn disease. Table 3 summarizes the differential diagnosis of IBD.

Therapy

Medical therapy for IBD is based on the location and severity of disease. The goal of medical therapy is to achieve and maintain clinical remission. Induction therapy is a short course of therapy used to control active disease; induction usually requires higher and/or more frequent doses than are used after the disease is brought under control. Maintenance therapy is used long term to prevent relapse. Five classes of drugs are available to treat IBD: 5-aminosalicylates, antibiotics, corticosteroids, immunomodulators, and biologic agents (Table 4).

Mild ulcerative colitis is treated with the 5-aminosalicylates. Moderate disease often requires steroids for induction therapy and immunomodulators, (azathioprine, 5-mercaptopurine) for maintenance therapy. Severe ulcerative colitis requires intravenous corticosteroids, immunomodulators, and biologic agents. Medically refractory ulcerative colitis can be treated surgically with colectomy, which is considered curative.

Mild to moderate Crohn disease (no fever, weight loss, or abdominal pain) is treated with the 5-aminosalicyates, topical budesonide, or metronidazole. Patients with moderate to severe Crohn disease (fever, weight loss, dehydration, abdominal pain) receive oral corticosteroids for induction therapy but require immunomodulators for maintenance therapy. Biologic agents also may be helpful. Severe to fulminant (steroid-refractory) disease is treated with intravenous corticosteroids and biologic agents. Cyclosporine also may be effective. Patients with fistulae respond well to infliximab and azathioprine.

There generally is no viable medical therapy for fibrostenotic stricturing disease that leads to bowel obstruction. Limited small bowel or ileocolic resection or bowel-sparing small bowel stricturoplasties are the only therapy. Recurrence of disease at the sites of previous surgery is common; therefore, surgery is not a preferred strategy for inflammatory Crohn disease. Metronidazole following surgery reduces the incidence of severe relapses, and 6-mercaptopurine is modestly effective for decreasing both endoscopic and clinical recurrences in patients with Crohn disease.

Table 3. Differential Diagnosis of Inflammatory Bowel Disease

Disease	Notes
Bacterial enteritis (see Chapter 16)	Acute-onset diarrhea with fever, chills, hematochezia, and/or pus in stool; positive stool culture (*Camplylobacter, Shigella, Salmonella, Escherichia coli, Yersinia*)
Protozoan enteritis (see Chapter 16)	Acute diarrhea caused by *Entamoeba* or *Giardia; Entamoeba* may cause hepatic abscess and RUQ pain; history of travel or drinking untreated water; stool antigens detected by ELISA
Clostridium difficile infection (see Chapter 16)	Watery stool, lower abdominal cramping, fever, leukocytosis; recent antibiotic use, hospitalization, or stay in long term-care facility; *C. difficile* toxin in stool
Irritable bowel syndrome (see Chapter 15)	Altered bowel movements with pain; no nocturnal symptoms, fever, weight loss, or hematochezia; normal colonoscopy
Celiac disease	Abdominal pain, bloating, diarrhea; anti–tissue transglutaminase, anti-endomysial, and anti-gliadin antibodies; avoidance of gluten-containing foods is curative
Microscopic colitis	Abdominal pain, bloating, chronic watery diarrhea; normal colonoscopy but abnormal biopsy with 2 subtypes (lymphocytic, collagenous); chronic NSAID use implicated in >50% of cases
Lactose intolerance (see Chapter 16)	Abdominal pain, bloating, diarrhea after lactose ingestion
Diverticulitis (see Chapter 15)	LLQ pain, fever, diarrhea; abdominal CT shows inflamed diverticula
Ischemic colitis (see Chapter 15)	Abdominal pain, diarrhea, hematochezia; elderly patients with vascular disease; imaging of mesenteric vessels confirms diagnosis
Infectious proctitis	Tenesmus, diarrhea, hematochezia; history of receptive anal intercourse; positive bacterial or viral cultures (*Neisseria, Chlamydia, Treponema,* HSV)

ELISA = enzyme-linked immunosorbent assay; HSV = herpes simplex virus; LLQ = left lower quadrant; RUQ = right upper quadrant.

Table 4. Drug Therapy for Inflammatory Bowel Disease

Drug	Indication	Side Effects/Adverse Effects
5-Aminosalicylates (sulfasalazine, olsalazine, balsalazide, mesalamine); oral, rectal	UC: induction and maintenance; CD (weak): induction and maintenance	Interstitial nephritis (rare), diarrhea (olsalazine)
Antibiotics (metronidazole, ciprofloxacin)	CD: perianal and colonic disease	Metronidazole: peripheral neuropathy, metallic taste, Antabuse effect with alcohol consumption; Ciprofloxacin: arthropathy, seizure
Corticosteroids		
Corticosteroid (oral, intravenous, rectal)	UC/CD: Induction only	Acne, truncal obesity, osteoporosis, osteonecrosis, diabetes, hypertension, cataracts, infection
Topical budesonide	CD: Ileal and right colonic induction only	Minimal effects
Immunomodulators		
Methotrexate	CD: Induction and maintenance	Bone marrow suppression, hepatotoxicity, pulmonitis
6-Mercaptopurine, azathioprine	UC/CD: Steroid-sparing and maintenance	Pancreatitis, fever, infection, leukopenia, hepatotoxicity, lymphoma
Cyclosporine	UC: Steroid-refractory only	Hypertension, nephrotoxicity, neurotoxicity
Biologic agents (infliximab, adalimumab)	UC/CD: Induction and maintenance; fistulae	Infusion reaction, tuberculosis reactivation, demyelination, infection, heart failure, lymphoma

CD = Crohn disease; UC = ulcerative colitis.

Follow-Up

Smoking should be avoided in all patients but particularly patients with Crohn disease. Patients with sclerosing cholangitis may benefit from therapy with ursodeoxycholic acid, which has been shown to reduce the risk of colon cancer in this setting. Colon cancer screening recommendations include colonoscopy every 1 to 2 years beginning 8 years after diagnosis. Unlike sporadic colorectal cancer that develops primarily from colonic polyps, IBD-associated colon cancer can arise from flat dysplastic mucosa, which is not readily detectable from underlying inflammatory tissue; therefore, multiple random biopsies are performed. Patients with biopsies positive for dysplastic changes are encouraged to consider prophylactic colectomy.

Book Enhancement

Go to www.acponline.org/essentials/gastroenterology-section.html. In *MKSAP for Students 5*, assess your knowledge with items 46-49 in the **Gastroenterology and Hepatology** section.

Acknowledgment

We would like to thank Dr. Brown J. McCallum, who contributed to an earlier version of this chapter.

Bibliography

Kornbluth A, Sachar DB; Practice Parameters Committee of the American College of Gastroenterology. Ulcerative colitis practice guidelines in adults: American College Of Gastroenterology, Practice Parameters Committee. Am J Gastroenterol. 2010;105:501-523; quiz 524 [published erratum appears in Am J Gastroenterol. 2010;105:500]. [PMID: 20068560]

Lichtenstein GR, Hanauer SB, Sandborn WJ; Practice Parameters Committee of American College of Gastroenterology. Management of Crohn's disease in adults. Am J Gastroenterol. 2009;104:465-483; quiz 464, 484. [PMID: 19174807]

Chapter 27

Test Interpretation

D. Michael Elnicki, MD

One of the most interesting and exciting aspects of medicine is the search for a diagnosis to explain a patient's symptoms. The clinician starts with a medical history and physical examination and uses the findings to order diagnostic tests to confirm clinical suspicions. To use test results in an evidence-based fashion, the clinician needs to ask a series of questions:

- Is there valid evidence that the test is accurate?
- Does the test accurately distinguish between patients with the disease in question and those without the disease?
- Does the test apply to this patient?

Evaluating Tests

For the evidence supporting the use of a new test to be valid, the assessment of the test should follow certain steps. First, the study subjects should be recruited in a systematic fashion from a population that is appropriate for the disease being studied. All subjects should receive the reference ("gold standard") test. The gold standard test is not necessarily perfect but represents the current practice standard. The results of the new test are compared with the gold standard. Importantly, the results of the two tests (the gold standard and the new test) are assessed independently. That is, the investigators are blinded to the results of one test when evaluating the results of the other to avoid bias in their decisions. For example, knowing the result of a patient's angiogram could bias the interpretation of a nuclear medicine study.

Test Characteristics

Quantifiable terms are used to describe the accuracy of tests. *Sensitivity* and specificity describe test results for patients with and without a disease. Sensitivity is the proportion of patients with the disease who have a positive test; specificity is the proportion of patients without the disease who have a negative test. As illustrated in Figure 1, these proportions can be expressed as:

$$Sensitivity = a/(a + c)$$

$$Specificity = d/(b + d)$$

Sensitivity and specificity do not change as disease prevalence changes. Note that this assertion can be checked by multiplying the values of a and c by 10 (see Figure 1).

A highly sensitive test is very useful in excluding a disease when test results are negative. The mnemonic SNOUT is used to refer to this concept (i.e., a SeNsitive test, when negative, rules OUT

disease). Conversely, a highly specific test is very useful in establishing the presence of a disease when test results are positive. The mnemonic SPIN refers to this concept (i.e., a SPecific test, when positive, rules IN disease).

As with anything that is measured, sensitivity and specificity cannot be determined absolutely, so some uncertainty remains. For this reason, the precision of sensitivity and specificity often is expressed in terms of 95% confidence intervals (95% CI). A way to conceptualize 95% CI is that if an experiment were performed 100 times, 95 times out of 100 the measured outcome value would fall within these parameters. For example, if a nuclear medicine scan has a sensitivity of 84% (95% CI, 76%-92%) for the diagnosis of a disease, a clinician can be 95% confident that the actual sensitivity of the scan is between 76% and 92%.

Positive predictive value refers to the proportion of patients with a positive test result who do have the disease. *Negative predictive value* refers to the proportion of patients with a negative test result who do not have the disease. As illustrated in Figure 1, these proportions can be expressed as:

$$Positive\ predictive\ value = a/(a + b)$$

$$Negative\ predictive\ value = d/(c + d)$$

For a specific prevalence of disease, positive and negative predictive values are the same as posttest probability. However, as the dis-

DISEASE

		Positive	Negative
TEST	Positive	18 a	20 b
	Negative	2 c	60 d

Sensitivity = a/(a + c)
Specificity = d/(b + d)
Positive predictive value = a/(a + b)
Negative predictive value = d/(c + d)

Figure 1. Test characteristics.

ease prevalence in a population changes, the positive and negative predictive values will change as well. Again, this assertion can be checked by multiplying the values of a and c by 10 (see Figure 1).

A *likelihood ratio* (LR) determines how much the results of a given test will increase or decrease the pretest probability of a disease. Therefore, LRs are the most useful way to individualize tests to specific patient scenarios. A positive LR (LR+), used when a test is positive, is expressed as:

$$LR+ = \text{sensitivity}/(1 - \text{specificity})$$

The negative LR (LR−), used after a negative test, is expressed as:

$$LR− = (1 − \text{sensitivity})/\text{specificity}$$

To illustrate these concepts, consider this case example:

A clinician is evaluating a new test to screen for hemochromatosis, a relatively common genetic disease involving iron storage. The clinician knows that the prevalence of hemochromatosis in the study population is 20% (when screening, prevalence is equal to the pretest probability of disease). The clinician appropriately selects 100 patients, and all undergo liver biopsy (the gold standard test). The new screening test characteristics are: sensitivity = 90%, negative predictive value = 0.97, specificity = 75%, and positive predictive value = 0.47. A patient from this population (that with a disease prevalence of 20%) with a positive test will have a posttest probability of having hemochromatosis of 47%, whereas someone with a negative test will have a posttest probability of 3%. To use these data in a population with a different prevalence of disease, however, the clinician would need to use the LRs (i.e., LR+ = 3.6, LR− = 0.13) to determine the effect of the test on the likelihood of disease.

LRs between 0.5 and 1 and between 1 and 2 do not change probability significantly. Some easy positive LRs to remember are 2, 5, and 10, which increase disease probability by 15%, 30%, and 45%, respectively. Negative LRs of 0.5, 0.2, and 0.1 decrease disease probability by 15%, 30%, and 45%, respectively. Larger pos-

itive LRs and smaller negative LRs are more apt to affect clinical decisions.

Using LRs requires that the chance of a disease being present be expressed in terms of pretest odds, or:

$$\text{Pretest odds} \times \text{LR} = \text{posttest odds}$$

Therefore, probabilities need to be converted to odds. These conversions can be done using the following equation:

$$\text{Odds} = \text{probability}/(1 − \text{probability})$$

For example, if a patient's pretest probability of disease is 0.2, the pretest odds would then be $0.2/(1 − 0.2) = 0.25$. To convert back to probability, the following equation is used:

$$\text{Probability} = \text{odds}/(\text{odds} + 1)$$

In the above example, the probability is $0.25/(0.25 + 1) = 0.2$. These calculations can be easily performed using widely available online medical calculators.

Many test outcomes are continuous variables that clinicians arbitrarily divide into normal and abnormal values; the level at which abnormal is defined is the cutpoint. Some common examples of continuous variables are troponin and prostate specific antigen (PSA) concentrations. Increasing the cutpoint for abnormal decreases the number of false-positive test results but at the price of increasing false-negative results (less sensitive but more specific). Decreasing the cutpoint has the opposite effect (more sensitive but less specific). The receiver operator characteristic (ROC) curve shown in Figure 2 demonstrates how increasing sensitivity (moving up the y axis) can decrease specificity (moving across the x axis). In the example shown, changing the cutpoint for abnormal from 4 to 2 increases the specificity from 70% to 90% but decreases the sensitivity from 90% to 70%. For the test shown, a cutpoint of 3 is best, as this maximizes both sensitivity and specificity at 80%.

A test with both good sensitivity and specificity will "crowd" the upper left margins of the ROC curve. This concept is partic-

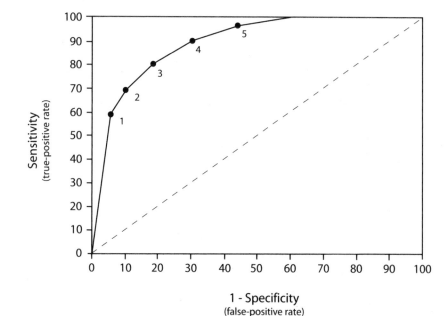

Cutpoint	Sensitivity	Specificity
1	60	95
2	70	90
3	80	80
4	90	70
5	95	60

Figure 2 Receiver operator characteristic curve.

ularly valuable when comparing two tests. The test with the greatest overall accuracy will have the largest area under the ROC curve. A perfect test (100% sensitive and 100% specific) would have an area of 1.0, so a good test might have an area of 0.9, whereas one that is less good would have an area of 0.8.

Applying Results to Patients

Before applying test results to patient care, and ideally before ordering a test, a clinician must estimate the pretest probability that a patient has a condition or disease. The pretest probability of disease is based on demographic variables and history and physical examination findings. When screening large asymptomatic populations, the prevalence of disease often is used as the pretest probability. For many symptomatic conditions, pretest probabilities in varying populations have been calculated and published. For example, a 50-year-old man with atypical angina has a pretest probability of coronary artery disease that is >60%, but a 30-year-old woman with the same chest pain has a <15% chance of having coronary artery disease (see Chapter 3). Knowing pretest probability can dramatically affect testing strategy. The sensitivity and specificity of history and physical examination findings have been studied and published (http://jama.ama-assn.org/cgi/collection/rational_clinical_exam?notjournal=jama,amajnls) and can assist clinicians in estimating the likelihood of conditions. Constellations of findings can be grouped to give an overall estimate of pretest probability that is more precise than any single element of the history or physical examination; these groups of findings are referred to as clinical prediction tools (see Chapter 51, **Table 2** for an example of a clinical prediction tool used in the diagnosis of pharyngitis). An evidence-based estimate can guide clinicians on the utility of further testing, since a very low or very high pretest probability may not change significantly regardless of a test's result.

Using LRs, clinicians can assign probabilities of disease to patients based on test results. At some point, however, a clinician needs to apply clinical judgment and test results to patient care decisions. The threshold for offering or withholding treatment will vary based on consequences of the disease and the risks of treatment. A clinician may be comfortable with a degree of uncertainty when the risk of significant morbidity or mortality is low. For example, one might withhold antibiotics for pharyngitis with a 10% risk of streptococcal infection, since the risk of serious complications is <1%. Conversely, a disease with significant risk of mortality would prompt further testing. To illustrate, consider this case example:

A 55-year-old man presents to an emergency department with chest pain consistent with atypical angina. The patient's pretest probability of significant coronary artery disease is calculated to be 65%. A nuclear imaging stress test (sensitivity 82%, specificity 60%) is read as negative (LR– = 0.3). The patient's physician calculates the posttest probability as 35% and orders a cardiac catheterization (the gold standard), which reveals multivessel coronary artery disease.

In some cases, the diagnosis can be made easier by sequential testing. If two tests are independent, the posttest probability after the first test can become the pretest probability for the second. This is the premise behind Bayes theorem, which quantifies successive probabilities as testing unfolds and allows a precise estimate of certainty before treatment is started or a diagnosis is excluded. A strategy often employed for sequential testing is the initial use of a noninvasive, sensitive test followed by a more specific (and often more invasive) confirmatory test if the first test is positive (e.g., PSA measurement followed by prostate biopsy). Sequential testing is used to move a clinician toward a treatment threshold—the point at which the clinician acts on the clinical information that has been gathered thus far. For a serious disease such as multivessel coronary artery disease, the clinician needs to be very certain; for patients with chest pain, the clinician might need a posttest probability of <2%-5% to feel comfortable excluding a diagnosis of a potentially lethal condition.

As medical technology continues to advance at a rapid rate, clinicians will increasingly be confronted with new diagnostic tests. Various factors including cost, availability, and risks will compete in the clinical decision-making process. However, having a solid working knowledge of evidence-based clinical practices will enable clinicians to more easily assess new tests and appropriately apply them to patient care.

Book Enhancement

Go to www.acponline.org/essentials/general-internal-medicine-section.html. In *MKSAP for Students* 5, assess your knowledge with items 1-5 in the **General Internal Medicine** section.

Bibliography

Akobeng AK. Understanding diagnostic tests 1: sensitivity, specificity and predictive values. Acta Paediatr. 2007;96:338-341. [PMID: 17407452]

Akobeng AK. Understanding diagnostic tests 2: likelihood ratios, pre- and post-test probabilities and their use in clinical practice. Acta Paediatr. 2007;96:487-491. [PMID: 17306009]

Akobeng AK. Understanding diagnostic tests 3: receiver operating characteristic curves. Acta Paediatr. 2007;96:644-647. [PMID: 17376185]

Chapter 28

Health Promotion, Screening, and Prevention

L. James Nixon, MD

The periodic health examination includes counseling to maintain health, screening for disease, and immunizing against future disease. All physicians should be familiar with the principles of preventive health care. Details of screening procedures are provided in disease-specific chapters.

In general, interventions that address personal health practices have a greater potential to improve health than does screening for disease. As an example, a periodic health examination with a young woman is an opportunity to discuss healthy lifestyle choices, including dietary intake of saturated fats, exercise and activity levels, substance use (tobacco, alcohol) and its effects, psychosocial stresses, environmental risks (seat belts, sun exposure), safe sexual practices, and contraception.

Although the value of the periodic health examination has been the subject of debate, a recent systematic review demonstrated that it improved delivery of some preventive services and decreased patient worry. This is in addition to evidence showing the effectiveness of brief, primary care–based interventions for changing identified risk behaviors, such as smoking and risky alcohol use. The "5 A's" model can be a useful framework for brief patient counseling geared toward changing identified risk behaviors (see Chapter 31, **Table 3**).

Primary prevention is the prevention of disease before its onset. Examples include immunizing patients against disease and reminding patients to wear seatbelts. Secondary prevention measures include most forms of screening, during which asymptomatic patients with risk factors for disease or preclinical disease are identified and managed. Examples include mammography for early detection of breast cancer and colonoscopy to screen for colon cancer. Tertiary prevention includes treating a disease with the goal of restoring the patient to previous level of health, minimizing the negative effects of disease, and preventing complications. An example is treating a patient after a myocardial infarction with cholesterol-lowering drugs to prevent a second cardiovascular event.

Principles of Screening

The goal of screening is to prevent or delay the development of disease by early detection. Early detection may result in diagnosis at a more treatable stage or before the disease has caused complications. The following principles of screening are widely accepted:

- Screen for a clinically important disease (common and associated with substantial morbidity or mortality).
- Screen for a disease that has an asymptomatic period during which the disease can be detected.

- Use an effective and acceptable screening method, that is, one that is accurate, readily available, affordable, and acceptable to both patient and provider.
- Screen for a disease for which there is an acceptable and efficacious treatment.
- Early treatment is more beneficial than treatment once the patient is symptomatic.

Bias

When determining whether a particular screening test meets these criteria, be aware of certain biases that have the potential to make a screening test appear to perform better than it actually does.

Lead-time bias is the artificial increase in survival time introduced with every screening test by simply diagnosing the disease earlier without necessarily increasing overall life expectancy. For example, the lead-time bias associated with prostate cancer screening is estimated at 5 to 10 years.

Length bias occurs with every screening test, because screening is less likely to detect rapidly progressive diseases than to detect slowly progressive, more indolent diseases. It will always appear that cancer detected by screening will have better outcomes than cancer detected by signs or symptoms. For example, lung cancer detected by spiral CT appears to have doubling times nearly twice as long as lung cancer detected by routine chest radiography.

An extreme form of length-biased sampling is *overdiagnosis*, in which the disease is so indolent that it probably would never have been detected during the screened person's lifetime had it not been for screening. For such a person, early detection and associated treatment can only do harm, yet the person seems to benefit because he or she is "cured."

Screening Guidelines

Screening guidelines change due to availability of new evidence, and recommendations vary depending on the organization. One source for screening recommendations followed by many is the U.S. Preventive Services Task Force (USPSTF) (Table 1). An excellent resource for other recommendations or for updates to screening guidelines is the National Guidelines Clearinghouse (www.guidelines.gov).

This section focuses on conditions for which screening currently is recommended. There are certain conditions for which the USPSTF recommends against screening, as the potential harm from follow-up testing or therapeutic interventions outweighs any potential benefit. These conditions include carotid artery stenosis,

Table 1. Recommended Interventions for Preventive Care[a]

Screening

Height and weight (periodically)

Blood pressure

Alcohol and tobacco use

Depression (if appropriate follow-up is available)

Diabetes mellitus (patients with hypertension or dyslipidemia)

Dyslipidemia (total and HDL cholesterol): men and women aged ≥20 y who have cardiovascular risk factors

Colorectal cancer screening (men and women aged 50-75 y)

Mammogram every 1 to 2 y for all women aged ≥40 y; evaluation for *BRCA* testing in high-risk women only

Pap test (at least every 3 y until age 65 y)

Chlamydial infection (sexually active women aged ≤25 y and older at-risk women)

Routine voluntary HIV screening (patients aged 13-64 y)

Bone mineral density test (women aged ≥65 y and at-risk women aged 60-64 y)

AAA screening (one time in men aged 65-75 y who have ever smoked)

Substance Abuse Counseling

Tobacco cessation counseling

Alcohol misuse: brief office-based behavioral counseling; alcohol abuse: referral for specialty treatment

Dietary and Exercise Counseling

Behavioral dietary counseling in patients with hyperlipidemia, risks for CHD, and other diet-related chronic disease

Regular physical activity (at least 30 min/d most days of the week)

Intensive counseling/behavioral interventions for obese patients

AAA = abdominal aortic aneurysm; *BRCA* = breast cancer susceptibility gene; CHD = coronary heart disease; HDL = high-density lipoprotein.
[a]Based on recommendations from the U.S. Preventive Services Task Force.

coronary artery disease in low-risk patients, testicular cancer, and ovarian cancer. There are other conditions for which the USPSTF indicates there is insufficient evidence to recommend for or against screening. These conditions include hypothyroidism, glaucoma, and skin cancer.

Cancer

Cancers for which there is good evidence that screening is beneficial include breast, colon, and cervical. Screening for human papillomavirus (HPV) infection in conjunction with routine Pap smear has been proposed as a method to improve detection of cervical cancer based on evidence that cervical cancer is linked to HPV infection. At present, the USPSTF has indicated that the evidence is insufficient to recommend either for or against routine screening for HPV infection. Prostate cancer is common, but evidence regarding efficacy of screening is still lacking. The American Cancer Society recommends examination of the thyroid, testicles, ovaries, lymph nodes, oral region, and skin during periodic health examinations. However, the USPSTF recommends against screening for testicular, ovarian, pancreatic, and bladder cancers because of lack of evidence showing benefit.

Obesity

The periodic physical examination should include height and weight measurements. Patients with a BMI >25 (overweight) or

>30 (obese) should receive counseling regarding weight loss and lifestyle modification.

Depression

In general, screening for depression should be conducted in clinical practices where accurate diagnosis, effective treatment, and follow-up are available. A two-question screen for abnormal mood and anhedonia ("Over the past 2 weeks, have you felt down, depressed, or hopeless?" and "Over the past 2 weeks, have you felt little interest or pleasure in doing things?") is likely as effective as longer screening instruments.

Fall Prevention

Falls are a common cause of morbidity and mortality among persons aged >70 years. A minimum assessment includes inquiring about a history of falls and assessing risk for future falls. Although little direct evidence links fall screening with reduction of adverse outcomes in screened populations, screening in all at-risk populations is warranted given the combination of disease burden, available screening tools ("Get Up and Go" test), and available risk-intervention strategies.

Abdominal Aortic Aneurysm

One-time screening for abdominal aortic aneurysm (AAA) with ultrasonography is recommended for all men aged 65 to 75 years who have ever smoked. Data from randomized clinical trials indicate that identification and repair of AAAs that are >5 cm reduces AAA-related mortality in older men.

Dyslipidemia

Screening for dyslipidemia should begin between the ages of 20 and 35 years in men and between the ages of 20 and 40 years in women. Patients who have other risk factors for coronary vascular disease or who have a suspected heritable familial lipid disorder should be screened at an earlier age. Usual screening consists of a fasting lipid panel, although the combination of serum total cholesterol and high-density lipoprotein cholesterol can be used as a screening test in non-fasting patients who may not return for a fasting blood test. Repeat lipid screening every 5 years or when the patient's risk profile changes.

Osteoporosis

The USPSTF recommends routine screening for osteoporosis in all women aged ≥65 years and in women aged 60 to 64 years who are at increased risk for osteoporotic fractures. This recommendation is based on good evidence that bone density measurements accurately predict the risk for fractures in the short-term, and that treating asymptomatic women with osteoporosis reduces their risk for fracture. Women at increased risk for low bone density include those with a smoking history, physical inactivity, prolonged hyperthyroidism, celiac sprue, a family history of osteoporosis, and inadequate calcium intake. The evidence is not as strong for men, but screening may be indicated in men with certain risk factors (long-term corticosteroid use, androgen deprivation). The most widely used and validated screening test for osteoporosis is dual-energy x-ray absorptiometry.

Type 2 Diabetes Mellitus

Although there is no direct evidence that screening for diabetes reduces adverse outcomes, screening for diabetes is recommended by the USPSTF in patients with hypertension, dyslipidemia, and other coronary artery disease risk factors. In these patients, the added presence of diabetes may increase cardiovascular risk to a level worthy of interventions that have been shown to reduce coronary artery disease events. The American Diabetes Association recommends screening all adults aged >45 years for diabetes every 3 years, citing the rationale that one third of all people with diabetes may be undiagnosed and that early diagnosis may prevent complications. Also consider screening younger adults with risk factors for type 2 diabetes (family history, obesity, gestational diabetes, polycystic ovary syndrome, high-risk ethnic group), with repeat screening every 3 years. Appropriate screening tests include fasting plasma glucose concentration, oral glucose tolerance test, and hemoglobin A_{1c} level. All abnormal tests must be repeated on a subsequent day.

Sexually Transmitted Disease

All sexually active women aged <25 years should undergo screening for chlamydial infection with polymerase chain reaction assay from a cervical swab or urine sample; this recommendation is based on evidence that screening reduces the incidence of pelvic inflammatory disease by 50%. The USPSTF also recommends screening all sexually active women for gonorrhea infection if they are at increased risk (defined by young age or having other indi-

vidual or population-based risk factors). Additionally, any male or female deemed to have risk behaviors (new or multiple sexual partners, history of a sexually transmitted disease, history of sex work, inconsistent condom use) should be screened for chlamydial infection, syphilis, and gonorrhea. Screening for herpes simplex virus infection is not recommended.

HIV Infection

The Centers for Disease Control and Prevention now recommends routine voluntary screening for HIV infection in all patients aged 13 to 64 years, unless the prevalence of undiagnosed HIV infection in the screened population is documented to be <0.1%. Targeted screening should still continue in high-risk patients, including all patients initiating treatment for tuberculosis and patients seeking treatment for sexually transmitted diseases.

Coronary Artery Disease

Routine screening for coronary artery disease in asymptomatic persons without cardiovascular risk factors is not recommended. Screening electrocardiograms (ECGs) are not recommended, because abnormalities of the resting ECG are rare, are not specific for coronary artery disease, and do not predict subsequent mortality from coronary disease. Exercise testing may identify persons with coronary artery disease, but two factors limit routine testing in asymptomatic adults. First, the prevalence of significant coronary artery disease is low in this population, rendering the predictive value of a positive exercise test low (i.e., false-positive results are common). Second, abnormalities of exercise testing do not accurately predict major coronary events in asymptomatic persons. There may still be a role for screening for coronary artery disease, however, in patients with diabetes prior to beginning an exercise program and in selected asymptomatic persons whose occupations may affect public safety or who engage in high-intensity physical activity. The role of coronary artery calcium (CAC) scoring by CT is still evolving. In 2007, a report of the American College of Cardiology Foundation Clinical Expert Consensus Task Force concluded that it may be reasonable to consider use of CAC measurement in patients whose estimated 10-year risk of coronary events is 10% to 20%. This conclusion is based on the possibility that such patients might be reclassified to a higher risk status based on high CAC score, and subsequent patient management may be modified.

Hypertension

Early detection of hypertension is essential in reducing the likelihood of target organ damage. Cure of some secondary forms of hypertension (e.g., primary aldosterone excess) is more likely if the duration of elevated blood pressure is short. Screen at every office visit, using the correctly sized blood pressure cuff. The average of two readings on two different occasions is used to classify the stage of hypertension.

Immunization

Most vaccines are safe and can be administered in the presence of a recent mild illness, including low-grade fever. Immunization recommendations change frequently; for up-to-date information regarding current recommendations, two excellent Web sites are www.cdc.gov/vaccines and www.needletips.org.

Influenza

In 2010, the U.S. Advisory Committee on Immunization Practices (ACIP) expanded the recommendation for influenza vaccination to include all persons aged ≥6 months. The trivalent inactivated virus vaccine is given intramuscularly and is appropriate for all groups, including pregnant women. The intranasal live attenuated vaccine is approved for patients aged 2 to 49 years but should be avoided in pregnant women and in patients with diabetes, immunosuppression, and certain other chronic conditions. Persons with allergy to eggs or with a history of Guillain-Barré syndrome should not receive either vaccine.

Pneumococcal Infection

Pneumococcal vaccination is associated with substantial reductions in morbidity and mortality among the elderly and high-risk adults and, therefore, is recommended for all adults aged ≥65 years and for adults with other risk factors (asthma, diabetes, cirrhosis, asplenia). Patients who receive an initial vaccine at age <65 years should receive a second dose after 5 years. One-time revaccination also is recommended in 5 years for patients with chronic kidney disease, asplenia, malignancy, or immunosuppression.

Tetanus, Diphtheria, and Pertussis

Booster tetanus-diphtheria toxoid (Td) vaccinations are recommended every 10 years. Booster Td vaccination also should be given to any patient presenting with a wound who has received fewer than 3 doses of vaccine, whose vaccination status is unknown, or whose last vaccination was >10 years ago for a clean minor wound or >5 years ago for a more significant wound.

The ACIP recommends routine administration of a single dose of combined tetanus, diphtheria, and acellular pertussis (Tdap) vaccine for adults aged 19 to 64 years to replace one Td booster. This vaccine can be given as early as 2 years after the last Td vaccine to provide the added pertussis protection. Subsequent vaccinations should be with the usual Td vaccine. As with other inactivated vaccines and toxoids, pregnancy is not considered a contraindication for Tdap vaccination.

Measles, Mumps, and Rubella

Adults born before 1957 generally are considered immune to measles and mumps but not necessarily to rubella. Persons born after 1956 require measles, mumps, and rubella (MMR) vaccination unless there is documentation of prior administration, physician-confirmed disease, or laboratory evidence of immunity to all three diseases. It is important to ensure that women who are considering pregnancy have positive antibody titers for rubella. As with all live virus vaccines, women who are known to be pregnant should not receive the MMR vaccine, and pregnancy should be avoided for 4 weeks following vaccination. MMR vaccination also should be avoided in immunocompromised patients.

Human Papillomavirus

The ACIP recommends routine HPV vaccination of females aged 9 to 26 years who have not been previously vaccinated or who have not completed the full series of either the bivalent or quadrivalent HPV vaccine, regardless of sexual activity. In 2010, the ACIP stated that the quadrivalent vaccine may be given to males aged 9 to 26 years to reduce their likelihood of acquiring genital warts.

Hepatitis A

Hepatitis A vaccination is now routinely recommended in children. In addition, international travelers, persons relocating to areas of poor sanitation, day care staff, food handlers, military personal, illicit drug users, men who have sex with men, persons with clotting factor disorders, and persons with hepatitis B and/or hepatitis C infection or other chronic liver disease should be vaccinated if not already immune. The safety of hepatitis A vaccine in pregnancy has not been established.

Hepatitis B

Children are routinely vaccinated against hepatitis B virus (HBV). All adolescents and young adults not immunized in childhood and those at increased risk for infection (e.g., health care workers) should be immunized. Postvaccination testing is recommended only for those who are at occupational risk or are receiving hemodialysis. To decrease the risk of perinatal HBV transmission, all pregnant women are tested for hepatitis B surface antigen during an early prenatal visit. The hepatitis B vaccine is safe for pregnant women.

Varicella

Varicella vaccination (live attenuated virus) should be considered for any adult not previously immunized, particularly those working in high-risk environments (e.g., schools), and for women who could become pregnant. Women who are known to be pregnant should not receive the varicella vaccine, and pregnancy should be avoided for 3 months following vaccination. Varicella vaccination also should be avoided in immunocompromised patients.

Zoster

Zoster vaccination is recommended for adults aged ≥60 years to prevent shingles and to reduce the incidence of postherpetic neuralgia. As patients can have a second herpes zoster outbreak, zoster vaccination is indicated irrespective of a history of shingles. The vaccine is a live virus and is contraindicated in immunocompromised adults.

Meningococcal Infection

A single dose of meningococcal conjugate vaccine (MCV4) is recommended for young adults, particularly those living in dormitories. Others who should receive meningococcal immunization include patients with asplenia or terminal complement deficiency and persons traveling to areas of the world where meningococcal infection is endemic. The safety of MCV4 administration during pregnancy is unknown.

Book Enhancement

Go to www.acponline.org/essentials/general-internal-medicine-section.html. In *MKSAP for Students 5*, assess your knowledge with items 6-13 in the **General Internal Medicine** section.

Bibliography

Boulware LE, Marinopoulos S, Phillips KA, et al. Systematic review: the value of the periodic health evaluation. Ann Intern Med. 2007;146:289-300. [PMID: 17310053]

Chapter 29

Approach to Syncope

Gretchen Diemer, MD

Syncope is a common symptom in adults, with a lifetime prevalence of almost 40%. Syncope is defined as a sudden, transient loss of consciousness and postural tone caused by global cerebral hypoperfusion, followed by spontaneous recovery. Presyncope is the sensation of impending syncope, without loss of consciousness. Syncope accounts for up to 3% of emergency department visits and 6% of all hospital admissions. It is more common in women than in men. Syncope from cardiac causes has a higher morbidity and mortality. A major purpose of the evaluation of a patient with syncope is to distinguish cardiac from noncardiac causes.

Diagnosis

In most cases, the cause of syncope is established by a combination of a history and physical examination and simple diagnostic studies. The history and physical examination focus on a search for precipitating causes and associated symptoms. Causes of syncope can be divided into three main groups: cardiac causes, neurocardiogenic causes, and orthostatic hypotension (Figure 1). The history should distinguish true syncope from falls without loss of consciousness, stroke or transient ischemic attack (TIA), trauma-related loss of consciousness, intoxication, and hypoglycemia. Seizure often is mistaken for syncope, but generalized tonic-clonic movements, loss of continence, tongue biting, and postictal confusion are rare in syncope. Tonic posturing can be seen in both syncope and seizure.

The history and physical examination identify a cause of syncope in 45% of cases. In general, brain imaging, electroencephalography, and carotid Doppler ultrasonography play a small role in the workup of syncope. Hospital admission is appropriate when the cause of syncope is unknown or if the risk of illness or death from presumed cardiac disorders is high. Table 1 summarizes a differential diagnosis of syncope.

Cardiac Causes

Cardiac causes of syncope can be divided further into arrhythmias, structural heart disease, and ischemic heart disease. These conditions account for 15% of all cases of syncope. Patients with underlying cardiac disease and syncope have a 5-year mortality of approximately 50%, so it is important to identify these individuals.

Arrhythmias cause approximately 15% of cardiac syncope. Syncope with no warning or prodrome should raise the suspicion of an arrhythmia. Palpitations can occur in both tachycardia- and bradycardia-associated disorders, although syncope can occur without presyncopal palpitations. Ventricular tachycardia, atrial arrhythmia, and bradyarrhythmia can cause syncope. Atrial tachyarrhyth-

mia is more likely to cause palpitations and lightheadedness than syncope. Ischemic heart disease and systolic heart failure are risk factors for ventricular tachycardia. Syncope also may be associated with long (>3 seconds) sinus pauses and advanced heart block. Regardless of heart rate, arrhythmias cause syncope by reducing cardiac output and reducing cerebral perfusion. Male sex, age >54 years, and syncope lasting only a few seconds are predictive of cardiac arrhythmia. Syncope without warning or in a supine position also should raise concern for arrhythmia. Patients who sustain facial or head injuries as a result of syncope also should be evaluated for potential arrhythmia. A family history of syncope or sudden death suggests long QT syndrome. Physical examination may reveal an abnormal heart rate or rhythm but typically is normal.

Important structural cardiac causes include aortic stenosis, hypertrophic obstructive cardiomyopathy, and, less commonly, mitral stenosis. Syncope associated with these conditions usually is exertional and is caused by an inability to increase cardiac output in response to exercise and the associated decrease in systemic vascular resistance. More than 25% of patients with hypertrophic obstructive cardiomyopathy will have syncope from dynamic outflow obstruction during exertion; these patients also are predisposed to ventricular tachycardia. Physical examination should focus on listening for murmurs of aortic stenosis, mitral stenosis, or hypertrophic obstructive cardiomyopathy.

Pulmonary hypertension, particularly in the setting of an acute rise in pressure from a pulmonary embolism, can cause transiently decreased cardiac output and syncope. A careful examination revealing signs of right-sided heart failure (elevated central venous pressure, peripheral edema, and a normal pulmonary examination) suggests elevated pulmonary pressure.

Syncope rarely is the sole presenting symptom of an acute coronary syndrome. Hospitalization and evaluation for acute coronary syndrome rarely is indicated unless additional clues suggest active myocardial ischemia.

Diagnostic testing is based on the pretest probability for a particular cause of the syncope (Table 2). Unless a clear noncardiac cause can be established, a 12-lead resting electrocardiogram (ECG) should be obtained; however, a normal ECG does not rule out a cardiac cause unless it is obtained during an episode of presyncope or syncope. The ECG may reveal arrhythmias, a prolonged QT interval, a high-degree atrioventricular block, a delta wave (preexcitation syndrome), or evidence of structural heart disease (left ventricular hypertrophy, ST-segment elevation, Q waves suggesting current or previous ischemic heart disease). If the cause of syncope is unexplained from the initial evaluation, continuous telemetry may be useful to screen for paroxysmal arrhythmias. If

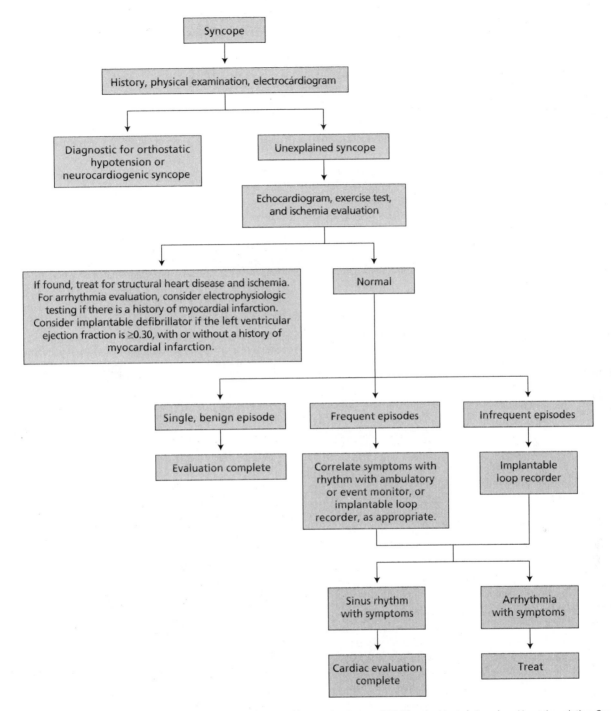

Figure 1. Evaluation of syncope. Reproduced with permission from Strickberger SA, Benson DW, Biaggioni I, et al; American Heart Association Councils on Clinical Cardiology, Cardiovascular Nursing, Cardiovascular Disease in the Young, and Stroke; Quality of Care and Outcomes Research Interdisciplinary Working Group; American College of Cardiology Foundation; Heart Rhythm Society; American Autonomic Society. AHA/ACCF Scientific Statement on the evaluation of syncope. Circulation. 2006;113:317. [PMID: 16418451]. Copyright 2006, American Heart Association, Inc.

symptoms are frequent, 24-hour electrocardigraphic monitoring may be useful to exclude arrhythmia as a cause of symptoms. If symptoms are infrequent, an event monitor or loop recorder should be used. If structural heart disease is suspected, an echocardiogram is indicated. If syncope occurs during exercise, a graded exercise test may reveal useful information.

Neurocardiogenic Causes

Neurocardiogenic syncope is a broad term referring to a syndrome of either increased parasympathetic tone or decreased sympathetic tone resulting in transient loss of consciousness. Approximately one third of syncope will be "reflex mediated," or neurocardiogenic. Patients with neurocardiogenic syncope usually are younger and have presyncopal symptoms, such as lightheadedness, nausea,

Table 1. Differential Diagnosis of Syncope

Disorder	Notes
Carotid sinus hypersensitivity	Syncope precipitated by pressure on the carotid sinus (tight collar, sudden turning of head). Generally can be diagnosed by history. Carotid massage may be confirmatory.
Situational syncope	Syncope that occurs in association with specific activities (micturition, cough, swallowing, defecation). Generally can be diagnosed by history alone.
Psychiatric disorder (e.g., anxiety, depression, conversion disorder)	A high incidence (24%-35%) of psychiatric disorders has been reported in patients with syncope.
Orthostatic hypotension	Syncope occurs on assuming the upright position. May be due to hypovolemia, drugs, or disorders of the autonomic nervous system (idiopathic hypotension, Shy-Drager syndrome).
Cerebrovascular disease	Invariably is associated with neurologic signs and symptoms. Carotid Doppler ultrasonography is not indicated, because ischemia of the anterior cerebral circulation rarely causes syncope.
Seizure disorder	Typically have a history of a seizure disorder or have seizure activity during an episode. Additional findings include blue face or absence of pallor during the episode, frothing at the mouth, tongue biting, disorientation, postictal muscle aching and somnolence, age <45 y, and duration of unconsciousness >5 min. Diaphoresis or nausea before the event and postsyncopal orientation argue against seizure.
Obstruction to left ventricular outflow (see Chapter 7)	May be related to exercise or associated with angina or heart failure. Can be diagnosed by physical examination or echocardiography. Specific causes include aortic stenosis, hypertrophic cardiomyopathy, mitral stenosis, myxoma, pulmonic stenosis, pulmonary embolism, and pulmonary hypertension.
Bradyarrhythmia (see Chapter 4)	May be associated with symptoms of near-syncope (transient) or signs of diminished cardiac output (persistent). Can be diagnosed by electrocardiography, 24-hour electrocardiographic monitoring, or electrophysiologic studies. Includes both sinoatrial and atrioventricular node dysfunction, which may be drug-induced (β-blockers, calcium channel blockers, antiarrhythmic drugs).
Tachyarrhythmia (see Chapter 5)	May be associated with palpitations. Ventricular arrhythmias causing syncope typically occur in the setting of structural heart disease or with a family history of sudden cardiac death (long QT syndrome, Brugada syndrome). 24-Hour electrocardiographic monitoring or electrophysiologic studies may be required to document arrhythmia.

warmth, diaphoresis, or blurred vision. These presyncopal warning symptoms, if lasting >10 seconds, are highly sensitive for the diagnosis of neurocardiogenic syncope. Patients with neurocardiogenic causes of syncope do not have increased mortality compared to the general population. The physical examination typically is unrevealing.

Vasogal syncope is the most common cause of neurocardiogenic syncope. Vasovagal syncope occurs due to sudden vasodilation and bradycardia, with resultant hypotension and cerebral hypoperfusion. In these patients, a sudden sympathetic surge may activate mechanoreceptors in the left ventricle and stretch receptors in the great vessels. Such stimulation may result in inappropriately increased vagal tone. Vasovagal syncope precipitated by a specific trigger is referred to as *situational syncope*. Common triggers include micturition, defecation, cough, fear, pain, phlebotomy, and prolonged standing. Eliciting the exact circumstances surrounding the event usually reveals the trigger. Patients with vasovagal syncope often give a history of previous episodes.

Carotid sinus hypersensitivity is a similar cardiac reflex provoked by carotid sinus massage or other factors that place direct pressure on the carotid sinus, such as a tight shirt collar. The association of presyncope or syncope with shaving or turning one's head to the side is consistent with carotid sinus hypersensitivity.

Patients with a history suggestive of neurocardiogenic syncope who are deemed at low risk may require no further evaluation. If the history suggests carotid sinus hypersensitivity, carotid sinus massage with monitoring can be attempted in patients without bruits or cerebrovascular disease and when other causes of syncope

have been excluded. The massage attempts to reproduce index symptoms with a characteristic heart rate and blood pressure response. In patients with recurrent syncope and in those with a single episode who are at high risk based on their occupation (e.g., pilots), a tilt table test can be useful; in this test, the patient is passively moved from the supine position to the head-up position (between 60 and 90 degrees). The tilt table test provides a diagnosis in up to 60% of cases when done with pharmacologic stimulation; however, the poor sensitivity, specificity, and reproducibility of the test must be considered when interpreting the results.

Orthostatic Hypotension

Syncope with a change in posture or prolonged standing suggests orthostatic hypotension. Orthostatic hypotension is defined as a systolic blood pressure decrease of ≥20 mm Hg or diastolic pressure decrease of ≥10 mm Hg within 3 minutes of standing. Causes include hypovolemia, disorders of the autonomic nervous system, and drug effect (especially in elderly patients).

A careful history should be obtained, looking for reasons for volume loss, such as vomiting, diarrhea, bleeding, or limited oral intake. Adrenal insufficiency also can contribute to orthostasis. The physical examination is directed at identifying signs of hypovolemia and orthostatic blood pressure changes.

Drugs particularly prone to producing orthostatic syncope include vasodilatory antihypertensive medications and preload-reducing agents, such as diuretics, nitrates, and α-blockers. β-Blockers impair the compensatory increase in heart rate with posi-

Table 2. Laboratory and Other Studies for Unexplained Syncope

Test	Notes
12-Lead electrocardiography	Perform in all patients with unexplained syncope. Arrhythmias, conduction defects predisposing to complete heart block, and evidence of structural heart disease may be documented. Yields a diagnosis in approximately 5% of patients in whom the initial history and physical examination are nondiagnostic.
Routine blood tests	Not recommended, as they rarely yield diagnostic information not suggested by the history and physical examination. Blood testing yields a diagnosis in approximately 0.5% of patients in whom the initial history and physical examination are nondiagnostic.
Echocardiography	Should be performed in patients with syncope and clinically suspected heart disease or with exertional syncope. Can diagnose and quantify obstructive lesions and can identify abnormalities that provide a substrate for malignant arrhythmias (i.e., cardiomyopathy, valvular heart disease, and pulmonary hypertension). Yields a diagnosis in approximately 0% of patients in whom the initial history and physical examination are nondiagnostic.
Stress testing	Recommended in patients with exercise-associated syncope and patients whose clinical evaluation suggests the presence of ischemic heart disease.
Ambulatory (24-h) electrocardiographic monitoring	Indicated in patients whose symptoms suggest arrhythmia, patients with known or suspected heart disease, and patients with abnormal ECGs. Ambulatory (24-h) electrocardiographic monitoring correlates symptoms with an arrhythmia in only 4% of patients. Increasing the duration of monitoring (i.e., to 48 or 72 h) increases the number of arrhythmias detected but not the diagnostic yield.
Implantable loop recorders	Indicated in patients with recurrent, unexplained syncope. Long-term follow-up (median, 17 mo) led to diagnosis of the cause of syncope in 41% of patients, compared to 7% of patients assigned to conventional evaluation.
Invasive electrophysiologic studies	Performed in patients with structural heart disease and syncope that remains unexplained after appropriate evaluation. The diagnostic yield in patients without organic heart disease is 10%.
Tilt table test	Poor sensitivity, specificity, and reproducibility; despite its limitations, the tilt table test is the only diagnostic tool available for determining susceptibility to neurocardiogenic syncope.

ECG = electrocardiogram.

tional changes and are common causes of orthostasis in the elderly. Autonomic neuropathy can impair the blood pressure response to a change in position; diabetes is a common cause of autonomic neuropathy, but other conditions (alcoholic polyneuropathy, multiple system atrophy) can produce similar symptoms. Multiple system atrophy is a heterogeneous degenerative disorder that can be associated with parkinsonism, ataxia, and autonomic nervous system impairment.

Therapy

Treatment of syncope is directed at the underlying cause, with the goal of preventing recurrence and decreasing morbidity and mortality. Structural cardiac disease and arrhythmias are covered elsewhere and will not be discussed in this section. Pacemakers or implantable cardioverter-defibrillators can improve outcomes for some of these conditions.

If neurocardiogenic syncope is suspected, isometric muscle contraction to increase systemic vascular resistance and decrease venous pooling of blood at the onset of impending syncope may be useful. Prophylactic fluid loading prior to high-risk situations (e.g., prolonged standing) also may be helpful. All patients should be educated regarding the pathophysiology of situational syncope and avoidance strategies. As a last resort, the placement of a pacemaker for neurocardiogenic syncope has been shown to reduce recurrence in up to 70% of cases.

If orthostatic hypotension is diagnosed as the cause of syncope, volume expansion is recommended to increase intravascular volume. For patients with chronic orthostatic hypotension unre-

lated to acute volume loss, liberalized salt and fluid intake is appropriate. For syncope refractory to these measures, compression stockings or abdominal binders may decrease venous pooling. Additional treatment steps include elimination of drugs associated with orthostatic hypotension, including α- and β-blockers and anticholinergic agents, if possible. If orthostatic hypotension or neurocardiogenic syncope is insufficiently addressed by nondrug approaches, the addition of mineralocorticoids (to increase plasma volume by renal sodium retention) and α-adrenergic receptor agonists (to increase peripheral vascular tone) may be successful. Alternative agents may include NSAIDs and caffeine. In elderly patients on antihypertensive medications, dose modification can be useful in resolving symptoms of syncope or presyncope.

Book Enhancement

Go to www.acponline.org/essentials/general-internal-medicine-section.html. In *MKSAP for Students 5*, assess your knowledge with items 14-18 in the **General Internal Medicine** section.

Acknowledgment

We would like to thank Dr. Lawrence I. Kaplan, who contributed to an earlier version of this chapter.

Bibliography

Parry SW, Tan MP. An approach to the evaluation and management of syncope in adults. BMJ. 2010;340:c880. doi: 10.1136/bmj.c880. [PMID: 20172928]

Chapter 30

Depression

Karen E. Kirkham, MD

Depressive disorders are the most common psychiatric disorders. In the United States, 16% of adults are affected by depression at some point during their lifetime. Depression is second only to hypertension as the most commonly encountered condition in primary care offices. Only about half of patients with depression receive treatment, despite the evidence that treatment improves quality of life. The spectrum of depressive disorders ranges from mild to severe and from brief to lifelong. Depression can occur alone or coexist with other mood or psychiatric disorders, impairing social and occupational functioning. The detrimental effects of depression on quality of life and daily function match those of heart disease and exceed those of diabetes mellitus and arthritis.

Demographic and socioeconomic risk factors for depression include older age (an independent risk factor, especially when associated with neurologic conditions), female sex, unemployment, poverty, low level of education, alcohol dependence, nonmarried status, and stressful life events. Medical risk factors include previous personal or family history of depression or other psychiatric disorder, postpartum state, and chronic disease (diabetes, dementia, coronary artery disease, cancer, stroke). Recent evidence has identified depression as an independent risk factor for increased mortality in patients with coronary artery disease, cancer, and stroke.

The biologic basis for depression involves imbalances in norepinephrine, serotonin, and/or dopamine in the prefrontal cortex, basal ganglia, hippocampus, and cerebellum. Serotonergic pathways are believed to function largely in mood, whereas norepinephrine is likely involved with drive and energy state. Both systems function in appetite, sleep regulation, and anxiety. Depression is strongly linked with stress, and stress systems in the brain are largely mediated by changes in norepinephrine transmission. There also is evidence of a genetic component, with elevated rates of depression in those with first-degree relatives affected by depression and high rates of concordance among twins. No genes that provide increased susceptibility or resistance to depression have been identified to date.

Prevention

Identifying and counseling asymptomatic persons at higher risk for depression can prevent or mitigate the severity of the disorder. Inquire about chronic disease, previous episodes of depression, recent stressful events, a family history of depression, and postpartum stress; offer counseling to asymptomatic adults with any of these risk factors. Antepartum counseling helps prevent postpartum depression in women with previous episodes of major depression, premenstrual dysphoric disorder, or psychosocial stress or inadequate social support during pregnancy.

Screening

Routine screening is recommended for all adults. The presence of risk factors or medical conditions associated with depression should further heighten the clinician's application of screening for depressive disorders. A simple two-question screening tool has been shown to have a sensitivity of 96% and a specificity of 57%, similar to longer instruments studied. The questions are:

- "Over the past 2 weeks, have you felt down, depressed, or hopeless?"
- "Over the past 2 weeks, have you felt little interest or pleasure in doing things?"

An affirmative answer to one or both questions from a patient with depressed mood or anhedonia should precipitate a full diagnostic assessment for mood disorders using case-finding tools. The nine-item Patient Health Questionnaire (PHQ-9) is a validated patient self-report tool that assists with both diagnosis and evaluation of severity. The PHQ-9 is easy to score and is available in English and Spanish. Other validated screening instruments that are commonly used include the Beck Depression Inventory, Geriatric Depression Scale (GDS), and Edinburgh Postnatal Depression Scale (EPDS). Women should be screened 4 to 6 weeks after giving birth using the EPDS, which has been well validated in this population and is available in multiple languages. The GDS is the best tool for screening elderly patients for depression, because it takes into account the patient's level of cognition as well as visual deficits that are common in older age.

Diagnosis

The diagnosis of clinical depression is based on patient history and exclusion of alternative diagnoses (Table 1); there are no additional tests that can confirm the diagnosis. Physicians skilled in clinical interviewing are more likely to recognize depression. The interview must establish whether the patient meets established criteria for major depression, dysthymia, or a different psychiatric condition, as well as assess for substance abuse. Depressed mood and anhedonia are cardinal symptoms, and the presence of either is highly sensitive but not specific for major depression; hence, patients are evaluated with a structured instrument based on the DSM-IV criteria to assess symptoms of specific mood disorder syndromes. A structured approach sequences questions for maximum

Table 1. Differential Diagnosis of Major Depressive Disorder

Disorder	Notes
Major depressive disorder	Depressed mood or loss of interest or pleasure in almost all activities. In addition, symptoms must occur nearly every day for ≥2 wk, and a total of five DSM-IV symptoms must be present.
Dysthymia	Characterized by depressed mood or anhedonia at least half the time for ≥2 y, accompanied by two or more vegetative or psychological symptoms and functional impairment.
Minor/subsyndromal depression	An acute depression that is less symptomatic than major depression and causing less impairment in social or occupational functioning.
Situational adjustment reaction with depressed mood	Subsyndromal depression with a clear precipitant. Usually resolves with resolution of the acute stressor and without medication.
Bipolar disorder	Characterized by one or more manic or mixed episodes, usually accompanied by major depressive disorder.
Seasonal affective disorder	A subtype of major depression occurring with seasonal change, typically fall or winter onset, and resolving with seasonal remission.
Premenstrual dysphoric disorder	Characterized by depressed mood, anxiety, and irritability during the week before menses, resolving with menses.
Grief reaction	Major depression may be transiently present in normal grief, although sadness without the complete syndrome is more common. Pervasive and generalized guilt and persistent vegetative signs and symptoms should raise concern for major depression.
Dementia	Characterized by impairment of memory, judgment, and other higher cortical functions; usually has an insidious onset. Assess mental status or perform neuropsychiatric testing if diagnosis is uncertain.
Hypothyroidism	Characterized by features that overlap with depression, including fatigue, decreased cognitive function, and depressive symptoms. Laboratory testing (elevated TSH level) confirms the diagnosis.
Medication effect	Symptoms may have a temporal relationship to medication initiation (corticosteroids, interferon, propranolol, levodopa, oral contraceptives).

TSH = thyroid-stimulating hormone.

efficiency (average administration time is 1 to 5 minutes) and is facilitated with instruments such as the PHQ-9, to establish the diagnosis of depression, and the Primary Care Evaluation of Mental Disorders (PRIME-MD) or Symptom-Driven Diagnostic System for Primary Care (SDSS-PC), to differentiate major depression from other psychiatric disorders. These tools have an additional benefit compared with other screening modalities, in that they assess a spectrum of psychiatric disorders in addition to the principle mood disorders. The diagnosis of depression is confirmed if patients have ≥2 weeks of anhedonia and/or depressed mood plus three or four more symptoms, for a total of at least five symptoms. Up to 72% of depressed patients also present with moderate to severe anxiety. The major symptoms of depression can be recalled by the mnemonic SIG-E-CAPS (Table 2).

After a loved one dies, a person may experience symptoms of anger or bitterness over the death, a sense of disbelief in accepting the death, recurrent feelings of intense longing for the deceased person, preoccupation with thoughts about the person (including intrusive thoughts related to the death), and a feeling that life is empty and the future has no meaning without the person who has died. When these symptoms persist for ≥6 months after the death of a loved one, they are defined as *complicated grief*. Depression persisting for ≥2 weeks longer than 2 months after a loved one's death should be considered for treatment. Treatment improves some symptoms of depression but does not reduce the intensity of grief.

Once the diagnosis of major depression has been established, it is critical to assess symptom severity, functional impairment, and

Table 2. SIG-E-CAPS Mnemonic for Major Symptoms of Depression

Sleep changes (increased or decreased)

Interest in previously pleasurable activities (decreased)

Guilt

Energy (decreased)

Cognition or concentration (decreased)

Appetite (increased or decreased)

Psychomotor agitation or retardation

Suicidal ideation or preoccupation with death

suicide risk. The PHQ-9 uses a Likert scale for each symptom of depression and has been validated for initial severity assessment and follow-up response to treatment. Depressed patients must be asked about suicidal thoughts, intent, and plans. Such questioning does not increase the likelihood of committing suicide and is effective in detecting patients at risk for carrying out a planned suicide. Patients with suicidal ideation but without a plan or intent are begun on treatment, and suicidal ideation is closely monitored. Patients with a suicide plan are emergently referred to a psychiatrist or for hospitalization and psychiatric assessment, depending on the clinical situation. Operationally, the "No Harm Contract" is a verbal or written agreement, in which the patient at risk for suicide is asked to agree not to harm or kill him/herself for a particular period of time. Such contracting may be the community

Table 3. Frequently Prescribed Antidepressants

Agent	Advantages	Disadvantages
SSRIs		
Citalopram	Few drug interactions; safe in cardiovascular disease	
Escitalopram	Few drug interactions	
Fluoxetine	Effective for OCD, GAD, bulimia, PMDD. Long half-life (good for missed doses, poor adherence)	Long half-life (can lead to accumulation); affects cytochrome P-450 system and drug interactions are common
Paroxetine	Effective for panic disorder, GAD, PTSD, OCD, social phobia	Highest risk (class D) in pregnancy; affects cytochrome P-450 system and drug interactions are common; weight gain
Sertraline	Few drug interactions; effective for panic disorder, PTSD, OCD, social phobia, PMDD; safe in cardiovascular disease	
SNRIs		
Venlafaxine	Effective for anxiety spectrum disorders; few drug interactions	Nausea; can exacerbate hypertension
Duloxetine	Effective in pain conditions and GAD	Nausea
Serotonin Antagonist (and Noradrenergic Enhancement)		
Mirtazapine (tetracyclic)	Facilitates improved sleep; few drug interactions	Weight gain; sedation.
Tricyclic Antidepressant		
Nortriptyline	Drug levels can be monitored; analgesic effect	Anticholinergic side effects (dry mouth, sedation, weight gain); cardiac toxicity with overdose
Norepinephrine and Dopamine Reuptake Inhibitor		
Bupropion	Effective in smoking cessation; less sexual side effects than SSRIs; less weight gain; lowest risk (class B) in pregnancy Seizure risk	

GAD = generalized anxiety disorder; OCD = obsessive compulsive disorder; PMDD = premenstrual dysphoric disorder; PTSD = posttraumatic stress disorder; SNRI = selective serotonin-norepinephrine reuptake inhibitor; SSRI = selective serotonin reuptake inhibitor.

standard in many settings, but there is no evidence to suggest it impacts morbidity or mortality in such patients.

It is important to screen for a history of manic episodes (unusually high energy, euphoria, hyperactivity, hypersexuality, intense drug use, spending sprees, or other manifestations of impaired judgment). The Mood Disorders Questionnaire (MDS) is a formal tool used in defining a history of possible bipolar disorder. Should a patient with undiagnosed bipolar disorder be treated for depressive disorder alone, frank mania may be unmasked.

A physical examination at the time of a patient interview does not increase the diagnostic accuracy and may be normal. Symptomatic patients may appear anxious or exhibit poor eye contact, depressed mood, decreased psychomotor activity, or tearfulness. In severe depression, affect is blunted or flat, and delusions may be present. In select cases, tests should be performed to exclude conditions associated with depression, such as hypothyroidism, anemia, and vitamin B_{12} deficiency. Consultation with a mental health professional should be considered when there is diagnostic uncertainty, particularly as to the presence of possible bipolar disorder.

Therapy

In patients with mild to moderate depression, psychotherapy and pharmacotherapy are equally effective. In patients with severe depression, a combination of psychotherapy and antidepressant drug therapy is more effective than either treatment alone. Of the different psychotherapy modalities, cognitive behavioral therapy (CBT), interpersonal therapy, and problem-solving therapy have the greatest evidence of benefit. CBT focuses on recognizing unhelpful patterns of thinking and reacting that lead to emotional distress, then modifying or replacing these patterns with more realistic or helpful ones. Multifaceted approaches that include readily accessible care, patient education, reminders, reinforcement, counseling, and additional supervision by a member of the care team are the most effective in improving adherence.

Initially, patients with major depression, dysthymic disorder, or both are started on single-agent antidepressant drug therapy. The choice of agent depends on tolerance, safety, cost, side effect profile, and evidence of previous effectiveness in the patient or a first-degree relative who has been treated for depression (Table 3). Rates of withdrawal from clinical trials suggest that second-generation antidepressants (e.g., selective serotonin reuptake inhibitors [SSRIs], serotonin and norepinephrine reuptake inhibitors [SNRIs], selective serotonin and norepinephrine reuptake inhibitors [SNRIs], selective serotonin and norepinephrine reuptake inhibitors) are better tolerated than tricyclic antidepressants (TCAs) and have less potential overdose lethality, whereas monoamine oxidase inhibitors (MAOIs) have a longer list of restrictions and interactions, making them the least commonly prescribed category of antidepressants. Recent clinical practice guidelines from the American College of Physicians recommend second-generation antidepressants as first-line therapy in acute major depression, noting that existing evidence does not support the choice of one agent over another on the basis of efficacy. In mild to moderate depression, St. John's wort is as effective as other antidepressant agents and rarely has side effects. For patients on second-generation antidepressants with incomplete response, increasing the dose of the drug is reasonable. A recent good-quality study provided evidence that switching to sustained-release bupropion, sertraline (an SSRI), or extended-release venlafaxine (an SNRI) resulted in remission in a quarter of such patients. Combining MAOIs with SNRIs or TCAs is contraindicated, because it may trigger the serotonin syndrome (triad of mental status changes, autonomic hyperactivity, and neuromuscular abnormalities). There is mixed evidence on the efficacy and effectiveness of second-generation antidepressants in the treatment of dysthymia. Also, of note, studies show that coexisting anxiety responds equally well to second-generation antidepressants.

The goal of treatment is to achieve complete remission within 6 to 12 weeks; once remission is achieved, treatment should continue for 4 to 9 months (maintenance drug therapy). The duration of treatment will be longer if the precipitating event or other stressors persist, if there is a history of previous depressive episodes, or if depression existed for a long time before starting therapy. Up to 50% of patients will experience recurrent symptoms and will require long-term maintenance pharmacotherapy.

Counsel patients about antidepressant drug therapy to improve adherence, and educate patients about the nature of their illness, the use of medications, strategies for coping, and the risks and benefits of treatment. Provide educational materials appropriate for the patient's health literacy skills, culture, and language. Specific points of emphasis should include the importance of taking the medication daily, the anticipated 2- to 4-week delay before noticing any improvement in symptoms, the need to continue the medication even if feeling better, and potential side effects. Common side effects should be discussed, and patients should be encouraged to be in contact should side effects occur. Common adverse reactions to anticipate are sexual dysfunction (decreased libido, anorgasmia, delayed ejaculation), weight gain, nausea/vomiting, sedation, or agitation, depending on the specific antidepressant used and the patient's individual response. Regarding sexual dysfunction, bupropion is associated with the lowest incidence, whereas paroxetine (an SSRI) is associated with the highest incidence.

It is important to consider whether involving a mental health professional will improve morbidity and mortality in patients with depressive disorders. Referral to a psychiatrist is advisable for patients with significant suicidal or homicidal ideation, psychotic symptoms (delusions, disorganized speech, hallucinations, catatonia), substance abuse, suspected bipolar disorder, or inadequate response to standard treatments (two or more antidepressants). Some of these patients may require hospitalization, whereas others may require more complex management than is practical for the primary care physician to provide.

Follow-Up

Patients must be monitored at regular intervals during initiation of treatment, titration to remission, and maintenance. Therapy discontinuation as a result of drug side effects is common and occurs in up to 50% of patients; counseling helps prevent discontinuation. Patients should be seen 2 weeks and 4 weeks after initiating therapy (to assess for adherence, adverse drug reactions, and suicide risk) and again at 6 to 8 weeks (to assess for response to therapy). At this latter visit, patients should complete a formal questionnaire (e.g., PHQ-9) to assess symptom severity; a ≥50% decrease in symptom score is considered evidence of a response to treatment. After severity assessment, patients can be classified as having a complete or partial response or no response. Patients with a complete response should continue on the same therapy for an additional 4 to 9 months.

Treatment options for patients with a partial response include using a higher dose of the same agent, switching to an agent from a different class, or adding psychotherapy. For some side effects (insomnia, agitation), atypical antidepressants (e.g., trazodone, mirtazapine) may be helpful alone or at low doses at bedtime, in combination with a second-generation antidepressant. Bupropion can be helpful in patients with particularly low energy levels related to the depression. Patients with no response are switched to a different category of drug or to psychotherapy. Any change in therapy requires periodic follow-up as previously outlined. Once patients achieve remission, they are monitored regularly and receive continued counseling about medication adherence and risk of symptom recurrence.

Book Enhancement

Go to www.acponline.org/essentials/general-internal-medicine-section.html. In *MKSAP for Students 5*, assess your knowledge with items 19-22 in the **General Internal Medicine** section.

Acknowledgment

We would like to thank Dr. Hugo A. Alvarez, who contributed to an earlier version of this chapter.

Bibliography

Fancher TL, Kravitz RL. In the clinic. Depression. Ann Intern Med. 2010;152:ITC51-15; quiz ITC5-16. [PMID: 20439571]

Chapter 31

Substance Abuse

Mark Allee, MD

Alcohol Abuse

Alcoholism is defined by a spectrum of alcohol-related problems, including a craving or compulsion to drink, a loss of control, physical dependence, and alcohol tolerance. *Alcohol abuse* is a pattern of drinking that results in personal or legal problems; *alcohol dependence* indicates physiologic addiction and maladaptive behavior. At-risk or hazardous drinking has been demonstrated to lead to injuries from falls, depression, memory problems, liver disease, cardiovascular disease, cognitive changes, and sleep problems. Alcohol dependence is best understood as a chronic disease, with peak onset by age 18 years. The spectrum of alcohol abuse can be defined by a patient's drinking patterns (Table 1).

Screening

Alcoholism may be difficult to diagnose. Patients often present with complaints that may be attributable to other medical conditions or associated only with the consumption of alcohol. These problems might include depression, insomnia, injuries, gastroesophageal reflux disease, uncontrolled hypertension, and important social problems. It is useful to inquire about recurrent legal or marital problems, absenteeism or loss of employment, and committing or being the victim of violence.

The U.S. Preventive Services Task Force (USPSTF) recommends screening all adults and adolescents for alcohol abuse with either directed questioning or use of a standardized tool. The most frequently used screening tool is the CAGE questionnaire, which is a brief interviewer-administered test designed to screen for alcoholism or covert problem drinking. The test includes four questions:

- Have you ever felt that you should Cut down on your drinking?
- Have people Annoyed you by criticizing your drinking?
- Have you ever felt bad or Guilty about your drinking?
- Have you ever taken a drink first thing in the morning (an "Eye-opener")?

Table 1. Spectrum of Alcohol Abuse

Condition	Notes
Moderate drinking	Men, ≤2 drinks per day. Women, ≤1 drink per day. Patients aged >65 y, ≤1 drink per day.
At-risk drinking	Men, >14 drinks per week or >4 drinks per occasion.[a] Women, >7 drinks per week or >3 drinks per occasion.[a]
Hazardous drinking	At risk for adverse consequences from alcohol.
Harmful drinking	Alcohol is causing physical or psychological harm.
Alcohol abuse	One or more of the following events in a year:
	• Recurrent alcohol use resulting in failure to fulfill major role obligations
	• Recurrent alcohol use in hazardous situations
	• Recurrent alcohol-related legal problems
	• Continued use despite social or interpersonal problems caused or exacerbated by alcohol use
Alcohol dependence	Three or more of the following events in a year:
	• Alcohol tolerance
	• Increased amounts to achieve effect
	• Diminished effect from same amount
	• Withdrawal
	• Great deal of time spent obtaining alcohol, using it, or recovering from its effects
	• Important activities given up or reduced because of alcohol
	• Drinking more or longer than intended
	• Persistent desire or unsuccessful efforts to cut down or control alcohol use
	• Use continues despite knowledge of having a psychological problem caused or exacerbated by alcohol

[a]Both criteria represent alcohol consumption above the levels recommended by the National Institute on Alcohol Abuse and Alcoholism.

Table 2. Modified Alcohol Use Disorders Identification Test (AUDIT)

	0 Points	1 Point	2 Points	3 Points	4 Points
How often did you have a drink containing alcohol in the past year?	Never	≤1 per month	2-4 per month	2-3 per week	≥4 per week
How many drinks did you have on a typical day when you were drinking in the past year?	0-2	3-4	5-6	7-9	≥10
How often did you have 6 or more drinks on one occasion in the past year?	Never	<1 per month	Monthly	Weekly	Daily or almost daily

With a cutoff of two positive answers, the CAGE questionnaire is useful (positive likelihood ratio = 6.9, negative likelihood ratio = 0.33) for detecting alcohol abuse or dependence in primary care settings; the tool may be less accurate in women and blacks. The CAGE questionnaire has less utility in identifying persons with hazardous use of alcohol (i.e., drinking that confers risk of physical or psychological harm).

The World Health Organization developed the AUDIT (Alcohol Use Disorders Identification Test) screening tool, which has the best operating characteristics for identifying at-risk drinking. The AUDIT uses 10 questions, including current use pattern, and takes longer to administer than the CAGE questionnaire. A modification of the AUDIT, AUDIT-C, is reduced to three questions and still performs relatively well (Table 2). With a cutoff of four points, the AUDIT has a sensitivity of 86% and a specificity of 78% for identifying at-risk drinking and/or alcohol abuse or dependence. The AUDIT is sensitive enough to detect hazardous as well as harmful drinking, both in primary care settings and in hospitals. The CAGE questionnaire is better at identifying lifetime alcohol abuse and dependence, but the AUDIT is preferred for the detection of hazardous and harmful drinking.

In the United States, 1 in 10 women has a drinking problem, which often is hidden. Women are more likely than men to develop long-term sequelae of alcohol abuse. With women, there is an increased risk of violence, sexual assault, and unplanned pregnancy. Persons aged >65 years represent the fastest growing segment of the United States population, and practitioners may miss alcoholism in this group by thinking of it as a young person's disease. Age-related complications and illnesses (falls, cognitive decline, depression) might present as similar symptoms. The average senior takes 2 to 7 prescription medications, so there is an increased risk of a drug-alcohol interaction. Fortunately, seniors are more likely to participate in and complete a treatment program when identified as having an alcohol problem.

There are no specific laboratory tests to screen for alcohol use. The main objective of the clinical evaluation is to look for physical and behavioral effects of alcohol, such as liver disease, pancreatitis, seizure disorder, and mood disorder. Abnormal laboratory studies, including elevated serum aminotransferases (sensitivity 30%-50%, specificity 80%) and macrocytic anemia (sensitivity 30%-50%, specificity 80%), although supportive of alcohol use, do not make the diagnosis.

Therapy

Alcoholism can be treated but not cured. Nonpharmacologic intervention is rooted in behavioral treatment for the patient with at-risk alcohol use. Abstinence is essential to the maintenance of a successful treatment program. A patient is encouraged to set drinking goals (*I will start on this date; I will cut down by this many drinks; I will stop drinking by this date*), to use a diary to observe patterns of drinking, and to avoid situations that lead to alcohol use. A patient cannot do this alone and will need support from a counselor.

Several studies have shown that the brief intervention counseling strategy is effective for up to 1 year. A brief intervention is a 10- to 15-minute session during which the patient receives feedback and advice, sets goals, and has follow-up assessments. The goal is to move the patient along the path of behavior change. Brief interventions need to be motivational, with the practitioner offering empathetic listening and autonomy for decisions. Brief intervention counseling is used longitudinally in the outpatient setting and, therefore, lacks benefit in a hospital setting.

Detoxification consists of forced abstinence with treatment of alcohol withdrawal. Contraindications to ambulatory detoxification include acute or chronic medical or psychiatric illness that would require hospitalization or that would be complicated by alcohol withdrawal, pregnancy, history of seizures or delirium tremens, inability to follow up daily, and no reliable contact person. These patients should be hospitalized for alcohol detoxification. Intoxicated patients should be observed until intoxication has resolved or admitted if a responsible adult is not available. Withdrawal symptoms generally begin 6 to 24 hours after alcohol intake is substantially reduced or stopped. Delirium tremens, a rare complication of withdrawal characterized by fever, profound confusion, and hallucinations, usually does not occur before the second to third day of abstinence. Clinicians should identify the severity of withdrawal and factors that may predict the onset of serious complications. The 10-item Clinical Institute Withdrawal Assessment Scale for Alcohol, Revised can be used to measure symptom severity and to help provide guidance in the course of treatment. Benzodiazepines are first-line therapy for patients who require alcohol withdrawal treatment or prophylaxis. Patients with alcohol withdrawal syndrome who are treated with benzodiazepines have fewer complications, including a lower incidence of seizures and delirium tremens. Longer-acting agents (chlordiazepoxide, diazepam) may be more effective in preventing seizures but can pose a risk of excess sedation in the elderly and in patients with liver disease. Patients with a history of seizures should receive a prophylactic long-acting benzodiazepine on a fixed schedule, even if they are asymptomatic during the acute alcohol withdrawal period. β-Blockers and clonidine can control tachycardia and hypertension, and haloperidol can treat agitation and hallucinosis. However, β-blockers have been associated with a greater incidence of delirium and neuroleptic medications have been associated with a greater incidence of seizures during withdrawal.

For long-term management, a multidisciplinary approach may be necessary. Alcoholics Anonymous has been shown to be helpful in maintaining abstinence; the organization provides fellowship and a support group to the patient. Unfortunately, Alcoholics Anonymous outpatient programs are inferior to inpatient alcohol treatment. Cognitive behavioral therapy is conducted by a mental health practitioner. With this treatment approach, patients learn skills to cope with situations that perpetuate drinking. Spousal involvement has been shown to improve the completion of the behavioral program.

Naltrexone, an opioid receptor antagonist, is effective for short-term treatment of alcohol dependence and should be coadministered with psychosocial support. Naltrexone can be used in patients who are still actively drinking and in cases when abstinence may be difficult. The drug reduces the frequency of relapse and the number of drinking days by attenuating craving and blocking the reinforcing effects of alcohol. Naltrexone is contraindicated in patients with active hepatitis and opioid dependence. The most common side effects are headache and nausea.

Disulfiram, an aldehyde dehydrogenase inhibitor, leads to the accumulation of acetaldehyde if alcohol is consumed, resulting in flushing, headache, and emesis. Administration of disulfiram under supervision of another person improves abstinence and adherence to therapy. Patients who use disulfiram must avoid all alcohol-containing products, including mouthwash and cold medications. Disulfiram interferes with the metabolism of several medications (e.g., phenytoin, sertraline) and should be used cautiously in patients with liver disease.

Acamprosate, a synthetic compound resembling homotaurine (a γ-aminobutyric acid analogue), and has been successful in decreasing drinking days, enhancing abstinence, and helping to prevent withdrawal symptoms. The main side effect is diarrhea. Acamprosate is contraindicated in patients with kidney disease. Further information about alcohol abuse can be found at www.niaaa.nih.gov.

Drug Use

Although alcohol is the most commonly abused substance, illicit and legal drug use remains an important medical problem. Marijuana, cocaine, and opioid substances (including prescription drugs) are among the more frequently used drugs. The USPSTF does not recommend for or against routine screening for drug abuse. Patients may be less likely to volunteer information on drug use (as opposed to alcohol use) given the potential legal ramifications. There are no formal screening tests for drug use, so a careful history is critical. Most authorities recommend that patients be considered at risk for drug abuse based on positive responses to questions about quantity and frequency of use, with the understanding that any use of illicit drugs should be considered at-risk behavior. When there is a heightened clinical suspicion, urine toxicology testing may play a confirmatory role. Some clinicians have adapted the CAGE questionnaire to assess drug dependency.

Certain medical problems may arise from the use of injected illicit drugs, including HIV infection, hepatitis C, and infective endocarditis. A history focused on the route of drug administration and coexisting medical problems is needed. High-risk patients should be screened with serologic testing for relevant diseases.

With cocaine use, the most serious health concerns associated with acute intoxication are myocardial infarction, unstable angina, uncontrolled hypertension, and seizures. β-Blockers should be avoided in patients using cocaine, because the unopposed α-adrenergic stimulation may increase the vascular tone, thus worsening the cardiovascular effects. In the acute setting, benzodiazepines, vasodilators, calcium channel blockers, and labetalol are the safest and most effective agents to treat hypertension or chest pain. Withdrawal from cocaine can produce dysphoria, sleep disturbance, anxiety, and depression. The symptoms of anxiety and depression suggest a role for antidepressants, but these agents have a delayed onset of action and may be useful only after the period of withdrawal is over. Benzodiazepines are used to terminate seizures related to acute drug toxicity; chronic antiseizure treatment is necessary only if seizures persist following detoxification.

All amphetamines cause an adrenergic syndrome from release of catecholamines, thus producing tachycardia, hyperthermia, agitation, hypertension, mydriasis, and acute psychosis. Myocardial ischemia, seizures, intracranial hemorrhage, stroke, and kidney failure can result. Overdose of the recreational drug "ecstasy" (3,4-methylenedioxymethamphetamine) is associated with bruxism, jaw clenching, and hyponatremia due to elevated antidiuretic hormone concentration, which may result in seizures, cerebral edema, and death in some users. Fulminant hepatic failure has been reported. Treatment is supportive, with a focus on correcting the hyponatremia and using benzodiazepines to manage extreme agitation.

Opioids can depress the respiratory drive and cause sedation, requiring respiratory support with mechanical ventilation and naloxone to reverse the opioid effects. Opioid withdrawal syndrome is characterized by pupillary dilation, lacrimation, rhinorrhea, piloerection, anorexia, nausea, vomiting, and diarrhea. Opioid detoxification has three goals: initiating abstinence, reducing withdrawal, and retaining the patient in treatment. Pharmacologic treatment of withdrawal often involves substituting a long-acting agent for the abused drug and then gradually tapering its dosage. The desirable qualities for outpatient medications include administration by mouth, low potential for abuse and overdose, and low incidence of side effects.

β-Blockers and clonidine reduce autonomic manifestations of opioid withdrawal, but use of a long-acting, orally active opioid (methadone, buprenorphine) is preferred by most patients. This approach is associated with higher rates of retention within a treatment program and lower rates of illicit drug abuse. Methadone and buprenorphine both have a long half-life, allowing a once-daily dosing schedule. Methadone is used to treat acute withdrawal symptoms and may be used as maintenance therapy for weeks to years. Methadone dosage is titrated to balance sedation and patient discomfort. Buprenorphine may be preferred over methadone because it is a partial opioid agonist that has superior ability in reducing withdrawal symptoms, and its combination with naloxone allows for less abuse potential and respiratory depression in overdose. Buprenorphine is restricted to qualified physicians who have received training and a waiver to practice medication-assisted opioid addiction therapy.

Table 3. The "5 A's" of Behavior Change Counseling

Assess	Ask about/assess health risks and factors affecting choice of behavior change.
Advise	Give clear, specific, and personalized behavior change advice.
Agree	Select appropriate treatment goals and methods based on patient interest and willingness to change.
Assist	Aid the patient in achieving agreed-upon goals with use of social/environmental support and adjunctive medical treatments when appropriate (including pharmacotherapy).
Arrange	Schedule follow-up contacts to provide ongoing support and referral as needed.

Patients may benefit from referral to a formal drug treatment center that addresses motivation, teaches coping skills, provides reinforcement, improves interpersonal functioning, and fosters compliance with pharmacotherapy. One study demonstrated higher retention in the treatment program and fewer opioid-positive urinalyses in patients receiving methadone and psychosocial and other services compared with patients receiving methadone alone. Patients with moderate to severe withdrawal symptoms, poor social support, or substantial medical or psychiatric conditions should be referred to specialized outpatient or inpatient programs. The U.S. Public Health Service has advocated use of the "5 A's" construct in behavioral counseling interventions (Table 3).

Book Enhancement

Go to www.acponline.org/essentials/general-internal-medicine-section.html. In *MKSAP for Students 5*, assess your knowledge with items 23-27 in the **General Internal Medicine** section.

Bibliography

Leikin JB. Substance-related disorders in adults. Dis Mon. 2007;53:313-335. [PMID: 17645897]

Saitz R. Clinical practice. Unhealthy alcohol use. N Engl J Med. 2005; 352:596-607. [PMID: 15703424]

Chapter 32

Approach to Low Back Pain

Rosa Lee, MD

Low back pain is a common symptom in adults, with a lifetime prevalence approaching 80%. Most low back pain is of musculoskeletal origin and will resolve within a 2- to 6-week period. However, in some patients, back pain may be recurrent or chronic, leading to significant disability. Rarely, low back pain may be related to a serious systemic illness. Evaluation is focused on looking for evidence of either neurologic involvement or systemic disease as the cause of the low back pain.

Prevention

Regular aerobic physical activity and maintenance of fitness and normal body weight may decrease the likelihood of low back pain, although there is no direct evidence to support this. Specific interventions to prevent low back pain in the workplace, such as educational interventions and the use of lumbar mechanical supports, have been studied in several randomized clinical trials but have not demonstrated any significant benefits.

Diagnosis

An appropriately directed history and physical examination is the first step in the evaluation of low back pain, with the goal of categorizing the pain as one of the following: nonspecific low back pain, back pain that may be associated with radiculopathy or spinal stenosis, or back pain that may be caused by specific spinal pathology (Table 1).

The most common cause of low back pain in adults is nonspecific musculoskeletal pain, although the precise biologic rationale for the symptoms is unknown. The history and physical examination should look for the precise mechanism of injury, although often there is not an identifiable precipitant. Musculoskeletal pain frequently is described as an ache or a cramp, with radiation across the back in a belt-like fashion. Musculoskeletal pain often will radiate to the proximal thigh or hip, but rarely further. Neurologic deficits are not observed in acute nonspecific musculoskeletal pain.

Low back pain due to disk herniation results in radicular pain that follows a dermatomal distribution and extends below the knee. Pain exacerbation with Valsalva, defecation, or cough suggests disk herniation. Since 95% of all disk herniations occur at L4-L5 or L5-S1, careful attention should be paid to these nerve roots. Pain radiating to the anterolateral leg and great toe with weakness in the ankle and dorsiflexion of the great toe is consistent with L5 nerve impingement from the L4-L5 disk. Pain radiating to the posterior leg with weakness in ankle plantar flexion and a decreased ankle jerk reflex suggests S1 nerve impingement from L5-S1 disk herniation. The straight leg raise test, in which the examiner passively raises the patient's leg off the table 30 to 70 degrees while the patient is in a supine position, will pull on the nerve, sending an "electric shock" sensation from the hip down to the ankle on the affected side. This test has a high sensitivity (91%; negative likelihood ratio = 0.28) but a low specificity (26%; positive likelihood ratio = 1.3) for lumbar disk herniation. The crossed straight leg raise test, in which the examin-

Table 1. Differential Diagnosis of Low Back Pain

Disorder	Notes
Degenerative joint disease	Common radiologic abnormality that may or may not be related to symptoms.
Degenerative disk disease with herniation	Common cause of nerve root impingement and radicular symptoms. Disk bulging is a common incidental finding on lumbar spine MRI in asymptomatic patients.
Spinal stenosis	Most common in elderly patient presenting with severe leg pain and pseudoclaudication aggravated by walking or standing.
Ankylosing spondylitis	Usual onset before age 40 years. Patients typically present with chronic low back pain that worsens with rest and improves with activity. Associated with decreased spinal range of motion.
Osteomyelitis (see Chapter 55)	Associated with probable previous or ongoing source of infection and constitutional symptoms.
Metastatic cancer	Most commonly from prostate, breast, or lung cancer; can cause cord compression. Look for overflow incontinence, saddle anesthesia, and leg weakness.
Intra-abdominal visceral disease	Gastrointestinal (peptic ulcer, pancreatitis), genitourinary (nephrolithiasis, pyelonephritis, prostatitis, pelvic infection, tumor), or vascular (abdominal aortic aneurysm, aortic dissection).
Osteoporosis with compression fracture (see Chapter 12)	Osteoporotic compression fracture accounts for approximately 4% of back pain complaints.
Psychosocial distress	An exacerbating factor that may delay recovery.

Table 2. "Red Flags" in the Evaluation of Low Back Pain[a]

Key Features on History/Physical Examination	Possible Cause	Imaging	Additional Studies
History of cancer with new onset of low back pain	Cancer	MRI	ESR
Unexplained weight loss, failure to improve after 1 month; age > 50 y		Lumbosacral plain radiography	ESR
Multiple risk factors present		Plain radiography or MRI	ESR
Fever; injection drug use; recent infection	Vertebral infection	MRI	ESR and/or CRP
Urinary retention; motor deficits at multiple levels; fecal incontinence; saddle anesthesia	Cauda equina syndrome	Emergent MRI	None
History of osteoporosis; use of corticosteroids; older age	Vertebral compression fracture	Lumbosacral plain radiography	None
Morning stiffness; improvement with exercise; alternating buttock pain; awakening due to back pain during the second part of the night; younger age	Ankylosing spondylitis	Anterior-posterior pelvis plain radiography	ESR and/or CRP, HLA-B27
Back pain with leg pain in an L4, L5, or S1 nerve root distribution; positive straight-leg raise test or crossed straight-leg raise test	Herniated disk	None	None
Radiating leg pain; older age (pseudoclaudication a weak predictor)	Spinal stenosis	None	None
Symptoms present > 1 month		MRI	Consider EMG/NCV

CRP = C-reactive protein; EMG = electromyography; ESR = erythrocyte sedimentation rate; NCV = nerve conduction velocity.
Adapted with permission from Chou R, Qaseem A, Snow V, et al; Clinical Efficacy Assessment Subcommittee of the American College of Physicians; American College of Physicians; American Pain Society Low Back Pain Guidelines Panel. Diagnosis and treatment of low back pain: a joint clinical practice guideline from the American College of Physicians and the American Pain Society [erratum in Ann Intern Med. 2008;148(3):247-248]. Ann Intern Med. 2007;147(7):481. [PMID: 17909209] Copyright 2007, American College of Physicians.

er passively lifts the unaffected leg, reproducing pain in the affected leg, has a higher specificity (88%; positive likelihood ratio = 2.4) but is less sensitive (29%; negative likelihood ratio = 0.8).

Back pain due to spinal stenosis is more common in elderly patients and typically presents as severe bilateral leg pain. The pain is described as *pseudoclaudication*, because it is similar to the claudication of peripheral vascular disease. Unlike claudication, which occurs with exertion and is relieved with rest, pseudoclaudication may be worsened with prolonged standing or walking downhill (lumbar extension) and is alleviated by lying down or with hip and lumbar flexion when sitting. In patients with progressive neurologic deficits due to spinal stenosis, physical examination findings may include numbness and decreased motor strength in the distal lower extremities bilaterally.

Certain "red flags" in a patient's presentation suggest a systemic illness or more serious spinal pathology as the cause of back pain (Table 2) and may warrant early imaging and referral. Although these findings are very sensitive, they are not specific and do not automatically warrant a more exhaustive evaluation. The evaluation depends on the patient's description of the pain, associated symptoms, and elements in the patient's past medical history. Rapidly progressive neurologic deficits should alert the clinician to potential spinal cord compression, which is a surgical emergency. Bilateral lower extremity weakness with bowel and/or bladder dysfunction, decreased anal sphincter tone, and perineal sensory loss (saddle anesthesia), raise concern for cauda equina syndrome, which is compression of sacral nerves from a tumor or central herniated disk. A previous history of cancer, unexplained weight loss, age >50 years, pain that wakes the patient from sleep, or pain that is slowly progressive increases the likelihood of cancer. A history of injection drug use or chronic immunosuppression and the presence of fever, chills, night sweats, or weight loss sug-

gest infection (osteomyelitis, septic diskitis, epidural abscess). A history of trauma or risk factors for osteoporosis (prolonged corticosteroid use, advanced age) raise suspicion for vertebral compression fracture. In a patient with atherosclerotic disease and hypotension, a leaking abdominal aortic aneurysm is a consideration, whereas ripping or tearing low back pain raises the rare possibility of aortic dissection with extension into a renal artery. Morning stiffness, pain that is alleviated with exercise, onset of symptoms before age 40 years, slow onset of pain, and pain lasting longer than 3 months suggest ankylosing spondylitis.

The most important factor predicting the course of acute or chronic back pain is the presence of psychosocial distress. Low back pain associated with pain and weakness in a nondermatomal distribution raises concern for psychosocial issues exacerbating the patient's symptoms. Physical examination findings suggesting that psychosocial distress may be causing or exacerbating low back pain include nondermatomal distribution of pain, increase in pain with passive rotation of the spine, increase in pain on axial loading (i.e., when the examiner applies a few pounds of pressure to the top of the patient's skull), and discrepancy in straight leg test results between the supine and sitting positions or with distraction.

Most patients with low back pain do not require imaging at the time of presentation; however, patients with history or physical examination findings suggesting potentially serious underlying systemic illness or fracture require imaging for further evaluation. Plain radiographs of the lumbar and sacral spine are most useful to evaluate for vertebral fractures when such pathology is suspected, but radiography otherwise adds little to a patient's evaluation. MRI is most useful for the evaluation of systemic illness, infection, and cord compression or cauda equina syndrome and is required emergently when these conditions are suspected. Imaging for nonspecific musculoskeletal pain is not recommended, as there is poor correlation between a patient's symptoms and imaging findings. In asymptomatic patients, a bulging disk can be seen in 60% of MRI studies, with true herniation present in 30%, so careful correlation between imaging studies and the patient's history and physical examination is necessary to prevent further unnecessary diagnostic and therapeutic maneuvers. In patients with low back pain due to suspected disk herniation or spinal stenosis, MRI is recommended only if the patient is a potential candidate for surgery or other interventions, such as epidural corticosteroid injection for radiculopathy. Laboratory studies, including a complete blood count, urinalysis, and erythrocyte sedimentation rate, also are highly sensitive but not specific in systemic illness, especially infections. Additional diagnostic studies including electromyography and nerve conduction velocity tests rarely are indicated in the initial evaluation of low back pain.

Therapy

Conditions that lead to rapid and potentially irreversible loss of neurologic function, such as spinal cord compression due to tumor or infection, are surgical emergencies that require immediate treatment. The greatest predictor of prognosis is pretreatment neurologic status. Treatment for spinal cord compression includes surgical decompression and, in cases of metastatic disease, radiation therapy. When cord compression is suspected, high-dose corticosteroids are given immediately for pain relief and to prevent further loss of neurologic function. Surgical therapy also may be considered in patients with severe or progressive neurologic deficits secondary to disk herniation.

Most cases of acute low back pain are self-limited. Up to 90% of cases of acute low back pain should resolve with conservative treatment by 6 weeks. Multiple systematic reviews have shown that bed rest is ineffective and can prolong low back pain. Early mobilization and continuation of normal activity is most beneficial, although back-specific exercise should not begin until there is resolution of acute pain. There is no evidence that any specific exercise program is more beneficial, but general exercise and weight control will help prevent future episodes of low back pain. Patients with chronic or subacute low back pain may benefit from physical therapy, chiropractic manipulation, massage, yoga, or acupuncture, although there are conflicting data on the effectiveness of these modalities.

First-line medication therapy is analgesia with acetaminophen or NSAIDs. Muscle relaxants and opioid analgesics have not been shown to be more effective than NSAIDs, and both may have central nervous system side effects and addiction potential. Therefore, they are not recommended as first-line therapy for low back pain. A short course of a muscle relaxant or opioid analgesic should be considered only in a patient with acute low back pain who has not responded to a first-line analgesic. Opioids should not be used long-term to treat chronic back pain. Anticonvulsants, such as gabapentin, have demonstrated small short-term benefits in treating radiculopathy. Systemic corticosteroid therapy has not been shown to improve acute or chronic low back pain. Corticosteroid injection therapy has shown mixed results for the treatment of lumbar radiculopathy due to disk herniation. Although some studies have shown moderate short-term improvement in symptoms, there has been no demonstrated long-term benefit of

corticosteroid injections for this condition. Currently, there is very little evidence to support the use of corticosteroid injections in the treatment of spinal stenosis and nonspecific low back pain.

Follow-Up

Patients with acute low back pain should have a scheduled follow-up office visit or telephone call at 2 to 4 weeks to determine whether recovery is consistent with the natural history of the condition. If recovery is delayed, consider reevaluation for more serious underlying causes of back pain. If no cause is found, the patient should be reexamined for possible psychosocial factors that may be exacerbating symptoms. Psychosocial factors that predict risk for chronic disability include depression, somatiform disorders, and job dissatisfaction. It may be appropriate to consider consultation with a back specialist when patients with nonspecific low back pain do not respond to standard noninvasive therapy. In general, decisions about consultation should be individualized and based on assessment of the patient's symptoms and response to interventions and the availability of specialists with relevant expertise. For patients with back pain due to radiculopathy or spinal stenosis, published guidelines suggest referral for surgery after a minimum of 3 months to 2 years of failed nonsurgical interventions. Failure is defined as progressive neurologic deficits and severe pain that is not responsive to conservative treatment. Surgical treatment for radiculopathy due to a herniated lumbar disk involves diskectomy. Spinal stenosis may be surgically treated with decompressive laminectomy. Both surgical treatments have shown moderate short-term benefits compared to nonsurgical interventions. However, in both cases, there is no evidence of long-term benefits from surgical treatment. Current guidelines from the American College of Physicians and the American Pain Society recommend that decision-making about surgical treatment for these conditions includes a discussion between the physician and patient about the benefits and risks of surgical treatment.

Book Enhancement

Go to www.acponline.org/essentials/general-internal-medicine-section.html. In *MKSAP for Students 5*, assess your knowledge with items 28-31 in the **General Internal Medicine** section.

Acknowledgment

We would like to thank Dr. Lawrence I. Kaplan, who contributed to an earlier version of this chapter.

Bibliography

Chou R, Qaseem A, Snow V, et al; Clinical Efficacy Assessment Subcommittee of the American College of Physicians; American College of Physicians; American Pain Society Low Back Pain Guidelines Panel. Diagnosis and treatment of low back pain: a joint clinical practice guideline from the American College of Physicians and the American Pain Society [published erratum appears in Ann Intern Med. 2008;148:247-248]. Ann Intern Med. 2007;147:478-491. [PMID: 17909209]

Wilson JF. In the clinic. Low back pain. Ann Intern Med. 2008;148:ITC5-1-ITC5-16. [PMID: 18458275]

Chapter 33

Approach to Cough

Patrick C. Alguire, MD

Acute Cough

Acute cough is one of the most common presenting complaints in ambulatory practice. Acute cough lasts <3 weeks and usually is self-limited; subacute cough lasts 3 to 8 weeks. Common causes of acute cough include viral upper respiratory tract infections, bacterial sinusitis, rhinitis due to allergens or environmental irritants, acute tracheobronchitis, pneumonia (viral or bacterial), influenza, exacerbation of chronic pulmonary disease or left ventricular failure, malignancy, aspiration or foreign body, medication reaction (ACE inhibitors), and, less commonly, pulmonary embolism.

Viral upper respiratory tract infection is the most common cause of acute cough; however, acute viral airway infection can result in protracted bronchial hyperreactivity, with secondary cough lasting weeks to months. Airway cough receptors are located in the larynx, trachea, and bronchi, and cough in the setting of rhinitis, rhinosinusitis, and pharyngitis is attributed to reflex stimulation from postnasal drainage or throat clearing. Specific viruses most often associated with cough are those that produce primarily lower respiratory tract disease (i.e., influenza B virus, influenza A virus, parainfluenza virus 3, respiratory syncytial virus) as well as viruses that produce upper respiratory tract symptoms (i.e., coronavirus, adenovirus, rhinovirus). Viral rhinitis or rhinosinusitis is characterized by rhinorrhea, sneezing, nasal congestion, and postnasal drainage with or without fever, headache, tearing, and throat discomfort. The chest examination in these patients is normal. Most viral causes of cough are treated symptomatically. There is no evidence to support the use of most over-the-counter and prescription antitussive medications. However, some studies have shown that NSAIDs, with or without an antihistamine, decrease cough severity.

Viral influenza is characterized by the sudden onset of fever and malaise, followed by cough, headache, myalgia, and nasal and pulmonary symptoms. Clinical criteria for diagnosis of influenza include temperature ≥37.7°C (100.0°F) and at least one of the following symptoms: cough, pharyngitis, or rhinorrhea. A diagnosis of influenza can be established by analysis of viral cultures of secretions or from results of several rapid diagnostic tests (immunofluorescence, polymerase chain reaction, enzyme immunoassays). Anti-influenza drugs shorten the duration of illness by about 1 day and allow return to normal activities 12 hours sooner. To obtain this benefit, influenza must be diagnosed and treatment must be initiated within 48 hours of symptom onset. Because of the emergence of resistance, the Centers for Disease Control and Prevention no longer recommend amantadine or rimantadine for prophylaxis or treatment. Historically, neuraminidase inhibitor resistance was uncommon (<1%). However, in 2008-2009, resistance to oselta-

mivir increased significantly. Consequently, treatment guidelines are now based on the predominant circulating strain. Unlike vaccination, antiviral chemoprophylaxis provides immediate protection and may be useful in persons who have not been vaccinated or who are not expected to respond to a vaccine, or until vaccine-induced immunity becomes effective (about 2 weeks after vaccination). However, antiviral chemoprophylaxis is expensive and can be associated with side effects and emergence of resistant strains; therefore, annual immunization is the preferred strategy to prevent infection. Chemoprophylaxis should be restricted to residents in an assisted-living facility during an influenza outbreak, persons who are at higher risk for influenza-related complications and who have had recent household or other close contact with a person with laboratory-confirmed influenza, and health care workers who have had recent close contact with a person with laboratory-confirmed influenza. H1N1 virus ("swine flu") is an emerging influenza A virus. Symptoms (cough, fever, rhinorrhea) are similar to those occurring in seasonal influenza, as is the mode of spread, including person-to-person transmission. This virus is susceptible to neuraminidase inhibitors but resistant to both amantadine and rimantadine. Oseltamivir and zanamivir are the drugs of choice for chemoprophylaxis of influenza- and H1N1-exposed high-risk adults.

Bordetella pertussis, Mycoplasma pneumoniae, and *Chlamydophila pneumoniae* are nonviral causes of uncomplicated acute bronchitis and cough in adults, accounting for 5% to 10% of total cases. Because Gram stain and culture of sputum do not reliably detect *M. pneumoniae, C. pneumoniae,* or *B. pertussis,* these tests and other diagnostic tests are not recommended. Routine antibiotic treatment of acute bronchitis does not have a consistent effect on the duration or severity of illness or on potential complications and is not recommended. The one uncommon circumstance for which evidence supports antibiotic treatment is suspicion of pertussis. Unfortunately, no clinical features allow clinicians to distinguish adults with persistent cough due to pertussis. Therefore, clinicians should limit treatment for suspected pertussis to adult patients with a high probability of pertussis (cough lasting >6 weeks or cough during a documented outbreak of *B. pertussis*). The diagnostic gold standard is recovery of bacteria in culture or by polymerase chain reaction. Antimicrobial therapy for suspected pertussis in adults is recommended primarily to decrease shedding of the pathogen and spread of disease, because antibiotic treatment does not appear to improve resolution of symptoms if it is initiated beyond 7 to 10 days after the onset of illness.

Pneumonia is the third most common cause of acute cough illness and the most serious; therefore, the primary diagnostic objective when evaluating acute cough is to exclude the presence of pneumonia. The absence of abnormalities in vital signs (i.e., heart rate ≥100/min [negative likelihood ratio = 0.7], respiration rate ≥28/min [negative likelihood ratio = 0.8], oral temperature ≥37.8°C [100.0°F; negative likelihood ratio = 0.7]) or on chest examination (i.e., crackles [negative likelihood ratio = 0.8], diminished breath sounds [negative likelihood ratio = 0.8]) sufficiently reduces the likelihood of pneumonia to the point where further diagnostic testing is unnecessary.

Asthma is a consideration in patients presenting with an acute cough illness. However, in the setting of acute cough, the diagnosis of asthma is difficult to establish unless there is a reliable previous history of asthma and episodes of wheezing and shortness of breath in addition to the cough. This is because transient bronchial hyperresponsiveness and associated abnormal results on spirometry are common to all causes of uncomplicated acute bronchitis. Postinfectious airflow obstruction on pulmonary function testing or bronchoprovocation testing (e.g., methacholine challenge) may be present up to 8 weeks after an acute bronchitis episode, making the distinction from asthma difficult. Inhaled short-acting β-agonists should be used in patients with cough and wheezing but are of unclear benefit in those with acute cough without wheezing.

Acute exacerbation of chronic bronchitis and bronchiectasis presents as an abrupt increase from baseline in cough, sputum production, sputum purulence, and shortness of breath (discussed later).

Classes of cough medications include antitussive agents, expectorants, mucolytic agents, antihistamines, and nasal anticholinergic agents. The main indications for therapy are sleep disruption, painful cough, and debilitating cough. Elderly patients are most vulnerable to the adverse effects of antitussive agents, including confusion, nausea, and constipation. In addition, the effect of placebo appears to be almost equal to that of antitussive agents in randomized trials. Recent systematic reviews indicate that no single antitussive agent is clearly superior in treating acute cough in adults. Among antitussive agents, codeine was no more effective than placebo, and evidence was mixed for dextromethorphan. Evidence suggests a benefit with guaifenesin. The combination of dexbrompheniramine and pseudoephedrine was associated with significantly less severe cough compared with placebo but caused more dizziness and dry mouth (Table 1).

Hemoptysis is defined as coughing up blood from the lower respiratory tract and may be associated with either acute or chronic cough syndromes. The most commonly encountered causes of hemoptysis in ambulatory patients are infection (bronchitis or pneumonia) and malignancy. Elevated pulmonary pressure from left-sided heart failure or pulmonary embolism may cause hemoptysis, although hemoptysis alone is not sufficiently sensitive or specific to diagnose pulmonary embolism. In up to 30% of patients, the cause is not identified (cryptogenic hemoptysis). A diagnosis of cryptogenic hemoptysis should not be made until the patient has undergone thorough evaluation. All patients with hemoptysis should undergo chest radiography. Factors that increase the risk of malignancy include male sex, age >40 years, a smoking history >40 pack-years, and symptoms lasting >1 week. These patients should be referred for chest CT and fiberoptic bronchoscopy, even if the chest radiograph is normal.

Chronic Cough

Chronic cough lasts >8 weeks. Clinical evaluation of chronic cough includes a careful history and physical examination focusing on common causes. All patients should undergo chest radiography. Smoking cessation and discontinuation of ACE inhibitors should be recommended for 4 weeks before additional workup (Figure 1). The cause(s) of cough may be determined by observing which therapy eliminates the symptoms associated with cough. Because cough may be caused by more than one condition, a second or third intervention should be added in the event of partial initial response.

Upper airway cough syndrome (UACS), asthma, and gastroesophageal reflux disease (GERD) are responsible for approximately 90% of cases of chronic cough in patients who are nonsmokers, have a normal chest radiograph, and are not taking an ACE inhibitor. The patient's description of the cough, the timing of the cough (e.g., when lying down), and the presence or absence of sputum production all have no predictive value in the evaluation of chronic cough. Chronic cough is due to more than one condition in most patients.

UACS refers to a recurrent cough that occurs when mucous from the nose drains down the oropharynx and triggers cough receptors. The diagnosis is confirmed when drug therapy eliminates the discharge and cough. Most patients with UACS have symptoms or evidence of one or more of the following: postnasal drainage, frequent throat clearing, nasal discharge, cobblestone appearance of the oropharyngeal mucosa, or mucus dripping

Table 1. Drug Therapies for Viral Upper Respiratory Tract Infection

Agent	Notes
Proven effective in randomized trials	
Naproxen	Reduces headache, myalgia, malaise, and cough
Dexbrompheniramine/pseudoephedrine	Reduces sneezing and nasal mucus/reduces congestion and nasal resistance
Ipratropium nasal spray	Reduces rhinorrhea and sneezing; high cost benefit
Guaifenesin	Reduces cough
Possibly effective (mixed trial results)	
Dextromethorphan	Reduces cough
β-Agonist inhaler	Reduces cough; may be more effective in patients with bronchial hyperresponsiveness and wheezing

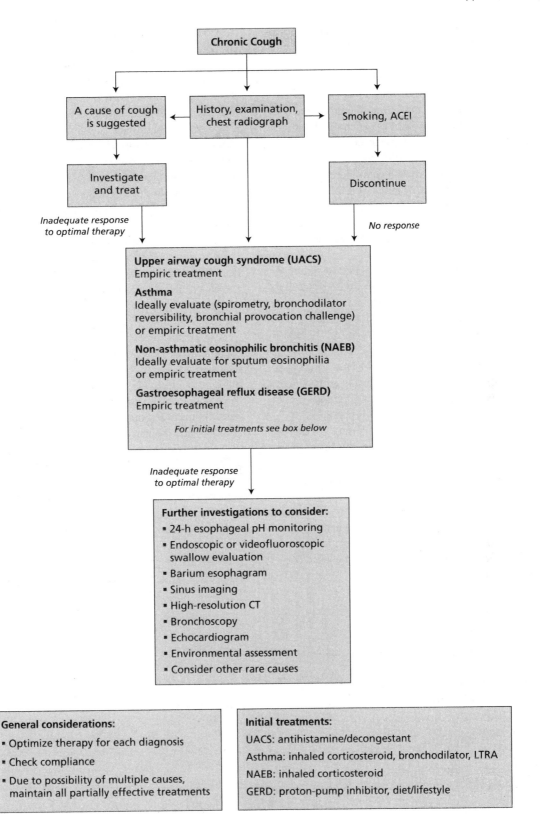

Figure 1. Evaluation of chronic cough. LRTA = leukotriene receptor antagonist.

down the oropharynx. First-generation antihistamines, in combination with a decongestant, are the most consistently effective form of therapy for patients with UACS not due to sinusitis. Additionally, the avoidance of allergens and the daily use of intranasal corticosteroids or cromolyn sodium are recommended for patients with allergic rhinitis. When the cause of a chronic cough is unclear, the American College of Chest Physicians recommends initial treatment with a first-generation antihistamine/decongestant combination to treat UACS. Patients who do not respond to empiric therapy should undergo sinus imaging to diagnose "silent" chronic sinusitis.

Cough-variant asthma is suggested by the presence of airway hyper-responsiveness and is confirmed when cough resolves with asthma medications. Cough-variant asthma (cough is the predominant symptom) occurs in up to 57% of patients with asthma. If the diagnosis is uncertain, bronchoprovocation testing should be considered. A negative test result is 100% sensitive in ruling out asthma, but a positive test result is less helpful because it is not specific for asthma; other conditions, such as COPD, can be associated with a positive test result. The treatment of cough-variant asthma is the same as for asthma in general, but the maximum symptomatic benefit may not occur for 6 to 8 weeks in cough-variant asthma.

Although GERD can cause cough by aspiration, the most common mechanism is a vagally mediated distal esophageal-tracheobronchial reflex. There is nothing about the character or timing of chronic cough due to GERD that distinguishes it from other causes of cough. Up to 75% of patients with GERD-induced cough may have no other GERD symptoms. The most sensitive (96%) and specific (98%) test for GERD is 24-hour esophageal pH monitoring; however, a therapeutic trial with a proton pump inhibitor is recommended before invasive testing. Symptom relief may not occur until 3 months after treatment is begun.

In patients with chronic cough who have normal findings on chest radiography, normal spirometry results, and a negative methacholine challenge test, the diagnosis of nonasthmatic eosinophilic bronchitis (NAEB) should be considered. NAEB is confirmed as a cause of chronic cough by the presence of airway eosinophilia (obtained by sputum induction or bronchial lavage during bronchoscopy) and improvement with treatment. Patients with NAEB should be evaluated for possible occupational exposure to a sensitizer. First-line treatment of NAEB is inhaled corticosteroids and avoidance of responsible allergens.

Cough with sputum is the hallmark symptom of chronic bronchitis. Treatment is targeted at reducing sputum production and airway inflammation by removing environmental irritants, particularly cigarettes. Ipratropium bromide can decrease sputum production, and systemic corticosteroids and antibiotics may be helpful in decreasing cough during severe exacerbations. Bronchiectasis, a type of chronic bronchitis, causes a chronic or recurrent cough characterized by voluminous (>30 mL/day) sputum production with purulent exacerbations. Chest radiography and high-resolution CT results may be diagnostic, showing thickened bronchial walls in a "tram line" pattern. Bronchiectasis should be treated with antibiotics selected on the basis of sputum culture and with chest physiotherapy.

Although most patients who smoke have a chronic cough, these are not the patients who commonly seek medical attention for cough. After smoking cessation, cough has been shown to resolve or markedly decrease in 94% to 100% of patients. In 54% of these patients, cough resolution occurred within 4 weeks of smoking cessation.

Cough due to ACE inhibitors is a class effect, not dose related, and may occur a few hours to weeks or months after a patient takes the first dose of an ACE inhibitor. The diagnosis of ACE inhibitor–induced cough can be established only when cough disappears with elimination of the drug. The median time to resolution is 26 days. Substituting an angiotensin receptor blocker for the ACE inhibitor also can eliminate an ACE inhibitor–induced cough.

Book Enhancement

Go to www.acponline.org/essentials/general-internal-medicine-section.html. In *MKSAP for Students 5*, assess your knowledge with items 32-36 in the **General Internal Medicine** section.

Bibliography

Dudha M, Lehrman SG, Aronow WS, Butt A. Evaluation and management of cough. Compr Ther. 2009;35:9-17. [PMID: 19351100]

Chapter 34

Smoking Cessation

Patrick C. Alguire, MD

Nicotine is a naturally occurring alkaloid found primarily in tobacco and most commonly consumed via cigarette smoking. The half-life of nicotine is about 2 hours; the principle metabolite of nicotine, cotinine, has a half-life of up to 20 hours. Nicotine stimulates α4β2 nicotinic acetylcholine receptors and, like other highly addicting drugs, increases dopamine release in the nucleus accumbens and prefrontal cortex, producing a pleasurable effect. The central nervous system effects of nicotine are related to both blood level and rate of increase at nicotinic acetylcholine receptors. Cravings for nicotine are stimulated by low levels of central nervous system dopamine during periods of smoking abstinence. During these periods, people who smoke experience a loss of the euphoric effects of nicotine and may also develop withdrawal symptoms (insomnia, irritability, anxiety, shaking, hunger, difficulty concentrating).

Smoking is the most common cause of avoidable death in the United States; 400,000 people die each year from tobacco-related diseases. Cigarettes are a known risk factor for coronary artery disease, COPD and other pulmonary diseases, aerodigestive cancers, genitourinary cancers, peptic ulcer disease, and complications of pregnancy. People who quit smoking before age 50 years have half the risk of dying within the next 15 years compared with those who continue to smoke. The excess risk of death from coronary artery disease drops by 50% in the first year of abstinence and continues to decline thereafter. In patients with peripheral arterial disease, smoking cessation is associated with improved walking distance, decreased pain, and improved bypass graft patency. Ten years after smoking cessation, the excess risk of lung cancer decreases steadily to 30% to 50% of that of persons who continue to smoke. In people with sustained abstinence from smoking, forced expiratory volume in 1 second declines 72 mL over 5 years compared with 301 mL in people who continue to smoke. Within 5 to 15 years, stroke risk is reduced to that of a person who does not smoke. Smoking cessation also results in a 50% reduction in bladder cancer. Up to 70% of people who smoke would like to quit, but only 5% to 8% can quit without therapy and usually only after several attempts.

Therapy

Smoking status should be determined in all patients. The U.S. Public Health Service suggests asking all patients two questions: "Do you smoke?" and "Do you want to quit?" The advice of physicians alone can improve the smoking cessation rate by 2.5%, resulting in an overall cessation rate of 10.2%. Although even brief interventions can be effective, high-intensity counseling (>10 minutes) is more likely to be successful. There is no apparent advantage of group therapy over individual therapy or gradual cessation over abrupt cessation. Some patients may benefit from self-help information (pamphlets, DVDs, Web sites), but the magnitude of benefit is small. The addition of self-help materials to personal counseling or drug treatment does not result in added benefit. Telephone counseling (i.e., a system of individual help that includes consistent support and reminders provided over the telephone) can be particularly beneficial. Whether initiated by a physician or by the patient, telephone counseling is equally effective in helping patients who want to quit to succeed in quitting. An example of a telephone counseling system is the National Smoking Cessation hotline (1-800-QUITNOW). There is insufficient evidence to support alternative therapies for smoking cessation, such as acupuncture, aversive therapy, and hypnosis.

The U.S. Public Health Service clinical practice guideline on smoking cessation recommends brief interventions for tobacco use and dependence (Table 1). For patients who are unwilling to quit, the "5 R's" are recommended as a motivating technique to move patients from the precontemplation stage of behavior change (*I don't want to quit*) to contemplation (*I am concerned but not ready to quit now*) or preparation (*I am ready to quit*).

Behavioral counseling is most efficacious when combined with pharmacotherapy, including nicotine replacement products (Table 2). All delivery systems of nicotine replacement therapy increase quit rates by alleviating symptoms of withdrawal. Nicotine replacement therapy is available over the counter (gum, patch, lozenge) and by prescription (inhaler, nasal spray, sublingual tablet). There is no

Table 1. Five-Step Brief Intervention for Smoking Cessation

The 5 A's: For Patients Willing to Quit	The 5 R's: To Motivate Patients Unwilling to Quit
Ask about tobacco use	Encourage patient to think of **R**elevance of quitting smoking to their lives
Advise to quit	Assist patient in identifying the **R**isks of smoking
Assess willingness to make a quit attempt	Assist the patient in identifying the **R**ewards of smoking cessation
Assist in quit attempt	Discuss with the patient **R**oadblocks or barriers to attempting cessation
Arrange follow-up	**R**epeat the motivational intervention at all visits

Table 2. Commonly Used Pharmacologic Therapies for Smoking Cessation

Agent	Mechanism	Effectiveness	Initial Prescription	Advantages	Disadvantages
Nicotine gum[a]	Prevents nicotine withdrawal	Increases cessation rates about 1.5-2 times at 6 mo.	2 mg (1 piece) whenever urge to smoke, up to 30 pieces/d. Continuous use for >3 mo not recommended.	Less expensive than other forms of nicotine replacement. Chewing replaces smoking habit. No prescription required.	Some patients find the taste unpleasant.
Nicotine patch (24 h)[a,b]	Prevents nicotine withdrawal	Increases cessation rates about 1.5-2 times at 6 mo.	Most patients: 21-mg patch for 4-8 wk (remove and replace every 24 h), then 14-mg patch for 2-4 wk, followed by 7-mg patch for 2-4 wk.	Less expensive than other forms of nicotine replacement. No prescription required.	Can cause skin irritation.
			Adults weighing <100 lb (45.5 kg), smoking fewer than 10 cigarettes/d, and/or with cardiovascular disease: 14-mg patch for 4-8 wk, then 7-mg patch for 2-4 wk.		
Nicotine spray[a]	Prevents nicotine withdrawal	Increases cessation rates about 1.5-2 times at 6 mo.	0.5 mg (1 spray) in each nostril 1-2 times/h whenever urge to smoke, up to 5 doses (10 sprays)/h or 40 doses (80 sprays)/d. Initially, encourage use of at least 8 doses (16 sprays)/d, the minimum effective dose. Recommended duration of therapy is 3 mo.	Some patients prefer this delivery method.	More expensive than other forms of nicotine replacement. Requires a prescription. Safety not established for use >6 mo.
Nicotine inhaler[a]	Prevents nicotine withdrawal	Increases cessation rates about 1.5-2 times at 6 mo.	24-64 mg (6-16 cartridges)/d for up to 12 wk, followed by gradual reduction in dosage over a period up to 12 wk.	Some patients prefer this delivery method.	More expensive than other forms of nicotine replacement. Requires a prescription. Use >6 mo not recommended.
Nicotine lozenge[a]	Prevents nicotine withdrawal	Increases cessation rates about 1.5-2 times at 6 mo.	1 lozenge every 1-2 h during weeks 1-6, then lozenge every 2-4 h during weeks 7-9, then 1 lozenge every 4-8 h during weeks 10–12. Patients who smoke within 30 min of waking require 4-mg lozenge; those who have first cigarette later in the day require 2-mg lozenge. Recommended duration of therapy is 12 wk.	Some patients prefer this delivery method.	Some patients find the taste unpleasant. Side effects include nausea, dyspepsia, and mouth tingling. Avoid acidic beverages (juice, soda) 15 min before use.
Bupropion	Unclear	Increases cessation rates about 2 times at 1 y.	Begin 1-2 wk before quit date; start with 150 mg once daily for 3 days, then 150 mg twice daily through end of therapy (7-12 wk maximum).	Some antidepressant activity; may be a good option for patients with a history of depression.	Requires a prescription. Can interact with other drugs. Safety in pregnancy is unclear. Associated with hypertension. Avoid in patients with seizure disorder or at risk for seizure; also avoid in patients with eating disorders.
Varenicline	Reduces cravings via nicotine receptor agonist	Increases cessation rates >3.5 times and almost 2 times over bupropion at 12 wk.	Begin 0.5 mg once daily on days 1-3, then 0.5 mg twice daily on days 4-7, then 1 mg twice daily through end of therapy (12 wk). Consider additional 12 wk of therapy to prevent relapse.	No hepatic clearance. No clinically significant drug interactions reported.	Requires a prescription. Associated with hypertension. Side effects include drowsiness, fatigue, nausea, sleep disturbance, constipation, and flatulence. Safety in pregnancy is unclear. Avoid in patients with kidney disease.

[a]Avoid nicotine replacement in patients with recent myocardial infarction, arrhythmia, or unstable angina. Safety of nicotine replacement in pregnancy is unclear.
[b]Several formulations of patches are available. Dosing guidelines are for patches designed to stay in place for 24 h and that come in doses of 21 mg, 14 mg, and 7 mg. Clinicians should check prescribing information on nicotine patches that come in other doses or that are designed for use <24 h/d.

Wilson JF. In the clinic. Smoking cessation. Ann Intern Med. 2007;146:ITC2-1-ICT2-16. [PMID: 17283345]

evidence that one form of replacement is more effective or safer than another, and decisions should be based on patient preference, side effects, and cost. In severely nicotine-addicted patients, combining a nicotine patch with another form of replacement (gum, inhaler, nasal spray, or lozenge) produced better results than the use of a single product. Nicotine replacement therapy is contraindicated in patients with a history of recent myocardial infarction, severe angina, or life-threatening arrhythmia; replacement appears to be safe in patients with chronic stable angina. Nicotine replacement is likely safer than smoking for pregnant women but is recommended only after failure of behavioral programs. Unlike other nicotine replacement therapies, nicotine gum has been shown to delay the weight gain associated with smoking cessation.

When used as sole pharmacotherapy, bupropion doubled the odds of cessation compared with placebo, but its mechanism of enhancing smoking abstinence is unknown. Like nicotine gum, bupropion has been shown to delay the weight gain associated with smoking cessation. Bupropion provides a better 1-year quit rate (30%) than nicotine replacement therapy (16%); combination bupropion and nicotine replacement therapy may be superior to monotherapy. Contraindications to bupropion include history of a seizure disorder, situations that lower seizure threshold (alcohol or benzodiazepine withdrawal), and recent monoamine oxidase inhibitor use. Bupropion is a category B drug for pregnancy (no evidence of risk in humans).

Varenicline has a higher affinity for the $\alpha 4 \beta 2$ nicotinic receptor than nicotine, blocking nicotine binding and stimulating receptor-mediated activity. Varenicline therapy reduces the cravings felt by smokers who quit. Varenicline given for 12 weeks increased the odds of long-term smoking cessation approximately threefold compared with placebo. When compared directly with bupropion or a nicotine patch, varenicline was more effective. There are no well-controlled studies of varenicline in pregnant women (the drug is category C for pregnancy); therefore, the use of varenicline is considered only when the potential benefits outweigh the potential risks to the fetus. In 2009, the FDA required boxed warnings on varenicline and bupropion, noting the risk for serious neuropsychiatric symptoms, including changes in behavior, hostility, agitation, depressed mood, suicidal thoughts and behaviors, and attempted suicide.

Book Enhancement

Go to www.acponline.org/essentials/general-internal-medicine-section.html. In *MKSAP for Students 5*, assess your knowledge with items 37-40 in the **General Internal Medicine** section.

Bibliography

Wilson JF. In The Clinic. Smoking Cessation. Ann Intern Med. 2007; 146:ITC2-1-ITC2-16. [PMID: 17283345]

Chapter 35

Obesity

L. James Nixon, MD

Obesity results from an imbalance of energy intake versus energy expenditure and a disturbance in the factors that regulate the feedback process. The causes of obesity are multifactorial and can be considered in terms of the biopsychosocial model; biologic factors (genetic, metabolic factors, comorbidities, medications), psychological factors (eating behaviors, activity habits, health knowledge), and social factors (socioeconomic status, food policy) all contribute to the current obesity epidemic. Obesity is linked with many illnesses, including structural (obstructive sleep apnea, osteoarthritis), metabolic (diabetes mellitus, nonalcoholic steatohepatitis, hypertension), and atherosclerotic (coronary, cerebral, and peripheral vascular disease).

Obesity affects >30% of Americans and currently is the second leading cause of preventable deaths. Compared with persons with a normal BMI, patients who are overweight have a 20% to 40% higher risk of death; the mortality risk is increased twofold to threefold in those who are obese. The best treatment for obesity is prevention. Obese patients require education about the health risks of obesity, treatment goals, and lifestyle interventions to achieve those goals. Some patients may require the addition of counseling about drug therapy or surgery to achieve weight goals.

Prevention

One goal for internists is to identify and counsel persons at risk for obesity. This approach, if successful, is ideal because it avoids the pitfalls associated with trying to treat obesity once it occurs. Inquire about a family history of obesity; obesity is influenced by both genetic and environmental factors. Also ask about exercise and television viewing habits; persons with a more sedentary lifestyle are at greater risk for obesity. A medication history can provide important information, as many drugs are associated with weight gain (corticosteroids; certain antipsychotic, antidepressant, anticonvulsant, and antidiabetic drugs). Also ask about any recent weight gain; a gain of >0.45 to 0.90 kg (1-2 lb) per year is a red flag for risk of future weight gain. Counsel patients who plan to stop smoking that they are at increased risk for weight gain. Other life events associated with increased risk for weight gain include pregnancy and short-term disability after surgery or injury. Additional risk factors for obesity include lower socioeconomic status and race/ethnicity (Hispanic, black, Polynesian).

Counsel at-risk patients to exercise regularly; a minimum of 30 minutes of moderate physical activity 5 or more days per week is ideal, although there is benefit from any form of physical exercise (e.g., taking stairs instead of an elevator). Beneficial dietary changes include controlling energy intake by using small portion sizes. Also counsel patients to reduce dietary fat intake, increase dietary fiber, drink fewer sugar-sweetened beverages, and eat breakfast to lower the risk of becoming overweight.

Educate patients about the adverse health effects of weight gain; this is particularly important for patients who have children. The rate of childhood obesity is increasing, and >50% of overweight children will become overweight adults. Internists have a role in preventing childhood obesity, because the children of overweight adults are more likely to become overweight themselves. Internists can also help by advising pregnant women about the risk that excessive weight gain poses to their health and the health of their unborn child, as intrauterine imprinting can affect long-term control of body weight. Higher maternal weight increases the risk for childhood weight above the 95th percentile and for the metabolic syndrome.

Screening

Measure height, weight, and waist circumference at each visit, and calculate BMI (i.e., weight in kilograms divided by height in meters squared). *Overweight* is defined as a BMI of 25 to 29.9; *obesity* is a BMI ≥30. Obesity is further divided into class I (BMI = 30-34.9), class II (BMI = 35-39.9), and class III (BMI >40). BMI has good correlation with health risks associated with obesity and excess body fat, such as diabetes, heart disease, osteoarthritis, gallbladder disease, gastroesophageal reflux disease (GERD), and certain cancers (breast, endometrium, prostate, colon, kidney, gallbladder).

Abnormal waist circumference (>102 cm [40 in] for males or >88 cm [35 in] for females) is a measure for central obesity, which is a surrogate estimate for visceral fat. Visceral fat is a more metabolically active fat that releases free fatty acids into the portal system, contributing to hyperlipidemia, hyperinsulinemia, and atherogenesis. In adults with a BMI of 25.0 to 34.9, an abnormal waist circumference is associated with a greater risk than that determined by BMI alone. For adults with a BMI >34.9, this measurement is less helpful. The coexistence of metabolic risk factors for both type 2 diabetes and coronary heart disease (i.e., abdominal obesity, hyperglycemia, dyslipidemia, and hypertension) defines the metabolic syndrome (see Chapter 11).

Diagnosis

Assess all patients identified as overweight, obese, or having an abnormal waist circumference for obesity-associated conditions, including hypertension, metabolic syndrome, endocrine disorders (hypothyroidism, diabetes, Cushing syndrome), and polycystic ovary disease (Table 1). In all patients with a BMI >25.0, obtain a fasting blood glucose measurement, serum creatinine level, and fasting lipid profile (high-density lipoprotein cholesterol, triglycerides, and low-density lipoprotein cholesterol levels) to assess for comorbidities. A sleep study may be indicated to confirm sleep apnea in patients with somnolence, hypertension, plethora, or a history of snoring.

Therapy

Help patients with a high BMI and/or increased central obesity to develop a plan to prevent further weight gain and, ultimately, reduce body weight. Initial steps include addressing modifiable risk factors for obesity and setting goals for gradual, sustainable weight loss. A 10% reduction in body weight is associated with significant risk reduction. Although rates for weight loss vary, a reasonable goal is to lose 0.22 to 0.45 kg (0.5-1.0 lb) per week.

Weight loss can be achieved through alterations in both diet and physical activity level. Behavioral interventions generally involve self-monitoring of food intake, learning about and controlling stressors that trigger eating, slowing food intake during meals, learning about portion size and nutrient content of foods (meal planning), setting realistic goals, behavioral contracting, increasing physical activity, and establishing a supportive social network.

Reducing energy intake is essential for weight loss. At reduced energy intake under controlled conditions, diet composition is less important than calorie restriction. Calorie-restricted diets generally fall into three major categories: balanced low-calorie diets, low-fat diets, and low-carbohydrate diets. Low-carbohydrate diets produce slightly greater weight loss compared with other diets and may have a slightly more favorable effect on glucose control, blood lipids, and blood pressure. Increased intake of high-fiber foods may enhance satiety, as may diets higher in protein. Very-low-calorie diets (<800 kcal/d) are difficult to administer and can be associated with a higher incidence of adverse effects; they are not recommended for routine use.

Increasing energy expenditure through increased physical activity also is crucial for weight loss. Advise patients to engage in 30 to 60 minutes of moderate physical activity 5 or more days a week (e.g., walking or other comparable activities). Once a lower weight is achieved, exercise is particularly helpful in maintaining weight loss. Sustained weight loss requires lifestyle changes, so consider referring obese patients to behavioral specialists, such as clinical psychologists or trained dietitians (Figure 1).

When lifestyle changes are ineffective in helping patients to lose excess weight, the addition of drug therapy may be helpful. Drug therapy generally is tried before surgical intervention. Drug therapy generally is considered for patients with a BMI ≥30.0 or for patients with a BMI ≥27.0 and comorbidities (hypertension, diabetes, heart failure, coronary artery disease, obstructive sleep apnea, osteoarthritis). Criteria for success with drug therapy include weight loss >2 kg (4 lb) at 4 weeks, >5% weight loss at 6 months, and sustained weight loss (>5%) at 1 year. Orlistat (a drug that blocks lipase and, thus, fat absorption in the intestine) is available without a prescription and is the only weight loss drug available in the U.S. for long-term use; however, the FDA has recently added a warning about rare cases of liver toxicity. Orlistat use often is limited by abdominal discomfort and increased frequency of defecation. Sibutramine (a nonamphetamine appetite suppressant) was voluntarily withdrawn from the U.S. market as a result of postmarketing data that indicated an increased risk of heart attack and stroke in sibutramine-treated patients with cardiovascular disease. Diethylpropion, benzphetamine, phendimetrazine, and phentermine are noradrenergic sympathomimetic drugs that are available for short-term use as appetite suppressants; they may increase blood pressure. The American College of Physicians clinical guidelines for management of obesity include fluoxetine and bupropion as alternate drugs for the treatment of obesity. The data supporting the use of these drugs for the treatment of obesity are equivocal; the drugs are not approved by the FDA for this indication. Exenatide, an injected drug that improves glycemic control by mimicking the action of the hormone incretin, is associated with weight loss among users. The weight loss may be related to delayed gastric emptying causing patients to feel full faster and longer. Exenatide is approved by the FDA for use only in patients with diabetes. There is limited efficacy and safety information about the use of over-the-counter herbal preparations for weight loss. Ephedra-containing compounds have been removed from the market because of safety concerns.

Consider bariatric surgery for obese patients (BMI ≥35 plus serious obesity-related medical comorbidities, BMI ≥40 without comorbidities) who have not achieved weight loss despite lifestyle attempts and drug therapy. Surgery also may be recommended to patients with progressive obesity, such as patients who have gained

Table 1. Differential Diagnosis of Obesity

Disorder	Notes
Hypothalamic injury	Headache, endocrine dysfunction, and hypothalamic symptoms. Order brain MRI or head CT.
Cushing syndrome (see Chapter 13)	Central obesity, hypertension, plethora, and striae. Measure urine cortisol.
Polycystic ovary syndrome (see Chapter 37)	Oligomenorrhea, hirsutism, increased LH/FSH ratio, high testosterone level, low SHBG level, and insulin resistance.
Drug-induced obesity	Antipsychotics, antidepressants, antiepileptics, corticosteroids, serotonin antagonists, and antidiabetic drugs.
Hypothyroidism (see Chapter 12)	High TSH level, low thyroxine level, lethargy, cold intolerance, and bradycardia. Weight gain often is due to fluid retention.

FSH = follicle-stimulating hormone; LH = luteinizing hormone; SHBG = sex hormone–binding globulin; TSH = thyroid-stimulating hormone.

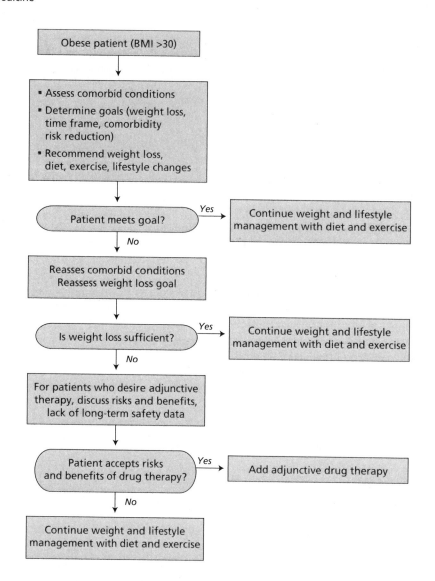

Figure 1. Medical management of obesity. Adapted with permission from Snow V, Barry P, Fitterman N, Qaseem A, Weiss K; Clinical Efficacy Assessment Subcommittee of the American College of Physicians. Pharmacologic and surgical management of obesity in primary care: a clinical practice guideline from the American College of Physicians. Ann Intern Med. 2005;142:526-531. [PMID: 15809464]

>5 kg (11 lb) per year before age 30 years. Bariatric surgery produces long-term weight loss that can be >25% of body weight at 1 year; after surgery, lost weight is regained slowly, if at all. The most common procedures target either early satiety (adjustable gastric banding) or a combination of early satiety and mild malabsorption (Roux-en-Y gastric bypass). After bariatric surgery, many patients have significant improvement or resolution of obesity-related diseases, including diabetes, hypertension, sleep apnea, and hyperlipidemia, and recent studies suggest a decreased overall mortality up to 29%. Referral for bariatric surgery should not be done lightly, however. The operative mortality in most studies ranges from 0.1% to 1%. Complications after gastric banding include nausea and vomiting, band erosion, stomal obstruction, and severe GERD. Gastric bypass complications include nutritional deficiencies (vitamin B_{12}, folate, iron, micronutrients), marginal ulcers, stomal stenosis, gallstones, infections, vomiting, and dumping syndrome. Bariatric surgery also is associated with pulmonary embolism.

Follow-Up

Schedule follow-up visits to monitor weight loss and comorbid conditions in all obese patients. Use ongoing office visits or ongoing behavioral therapy to reinforce or boost weight loss programs, as the recidivism rate is high for obesity. Generally, the more support the patient receives, the more successful the weight loss effort.

Book Enhancement

Go to www.acponline.org/essentials/general-internal-medicine-section.html. In *MKSAP for Students 5*, assess your knowledge with items 41-44 in the **General Internal Medicine** section.

Bibliography

Eckel RH. Clinical practice. Nonsurgical management of obesity in adults. N Engl J Med. 2008;358:1941-1950. [PMID: 18450605]

Chapter 36

Approach to Involuntary Weight Loss

Danelle Cayea, MD
Bruce Leff, MD

nvoluntary weight loss is defined as the loss of >5% of total body weight over a 6-month period or >10% over a 1-year period. Involuntary weight loss is common and may be associated with significant illness, malnutrition, decline in physical function, reduced quality of life, and a twofold increase in mortality.

Terminology used to describe weight loss is confusing and betrays an incomplete understanding of the underlying pathophysiology of involuntary weight loss. Classic definitions of involuntary weight loss are derived from two syndromes first described in starving children (kwashiorkor and marasmus), both of which are reversible with feeding. However, many adults with involuntary weight loss fail to respond to feeding. In adults, involuntary weight loss may result from several types of conditions that may overlap:

- Wasting, or *starvation*, is weight loss that occurs without an underlying inflammatory condition and may respond to increased calorie intake.
- Sarcopenia is age-related muscle loss that occurs without other precipitating causes.
- Cachexia is weight loss associated with an underlying inflammatory condition and characterized by increased cytokine production and possible muscle wasting; cachexia is associated with several chronic diseases (e.g., cancer, AIDS, COPD).
- Protein-energy malnutrition is characterized by weight loss, reduced mid upper arm circumference, and laboratory evidence of reduced dietary intake of protein and calories.
- Failure to thrive is weight loss and decline in physical and/or cognitive functioning associated with signs of hopelessness and helplessness.

Differential Diagnosis

Although few well-designed studies have been conducted on the causes of involuntary weight loss in adults, those studies have been relatively consistent in the proportion of patients reported with various causes. Approximately 50% to 70% of patients have a physical cause, 10% to 20% have a psychiatric cause, and 15% to 25% have no specific cause determined after a thorough evaluation and long-term follow-up (Table 1). Of note, the studies on which these proportions are based involved primarily referred inpatient populations, and some of the studies were performed at a time when body imaging techniques were less robust than today. Thus, it is reasonable to expect that among outpatient populations, the causes of involuntary weight loss may be different.

The most common physical cause of involuntary weight loss is cancer. Weight loss may be the presenting feature of cancer before other symptoms emerge. The second most common physical cause is nonmalignant gastrointestinal disease, including peptic ulcer disease, inflammatory bowel disease, malabsorption, oral disorders, dysphagia, and gallbladder disease. A broad spectrum of conditions accounts for the remainder of physical causes, including endocrine disorders (especially thyroid disorders and diabetes mellitus), infections (tuberculosis, HIV infection), and chronic conditions that cause increased energy expenditure, such as late-stage heart failure, COPD, and movement disorders (tardive dyskinesia, Parkinson disease). Kidney and liver disease may induce weight loss by causing nausea and decreased appetite.

Many medications can cause weight loss, especially among the elderly, by causing anorexia, dysgeusia (distortion of the sense of taste), or nausea. Such drugs include digoxin, ACE inhibitors, NSAIDs, selective serotonin reuptake inhibitors, cholinesterase inhibitors, anticholinergic agents, theophylline, and dopaminergic agents (L-dopa, metoclopramide). Additionally, polypharmacy can cause dysgeusia and anorexia.

Several psychiatric disorders are associated with weight loss, the most common being depression. Weight loss associated with dementia may precede the diagnosis of the underlying cognitive disorder. Eating disorders (anorexia) and substance abuse disorders (alcoholism) also cause weight loss. Socioeconomic and functional factors may cause or exacerbate weight loss; examples include difficulty in obtaining food because of functional disabilities, lack of financial resources, or social isolation.

Evaluation

Involuntary weight loss may be identified by patient self-report. However, because a substantial proportion of patients who report weight loss may not have experienced it, use documented weight measurements or objective evidence of weight loss, such as a change in how clothes fit or corroboration by a trusted observer, before pursuing an evaluation. Then, confirm that changes in total body water are not the cause of weight loss. Dramatic weight changes can occur with gain or loss of total body water, which occur more quickly and erratically than changes in lean body mass.

Although the differential diagnosis of weight loss is wide ranging, it is clear from the literature that a carefully performed history and physical examination, followed by targeted use of diagnostic studies, is likely to reveal the cause. An often-overlooked clinical pearl is that the chief complaint frequently points to a specific cause. Look for information suggesting chronic disease (cancer, gastrointestinal disease, endocrine disorder, infection, severe cardiopulmonary disorder). Patients with weight loss and an increased

Table 1. Differential Diagnosis of Involuntary Weight Loss (IWL)

Cause	Percentage of Patients with IWL
Cancer	16%-38%
Gastrointestinal disorder	10%-18%
Endocrine disorder	~5%
Infection	~5%
Pulmonary disorder	6%
Medication effect	2%-9%
Cardiovascular disorder	~9%
Kidney disorder	4%
Neurologic disorder	2%-7%
Depression	9%-18%
Undetermined	5%-26%

appetite may be more likely to have increased calorie loss (type 2 diabetes, malabsorption) or energy expenditure (hyperthyroidism). Take a careful medication history, with particular emphasis on medications known to affect appetite or to be temporally related to weight loss. Assess for affective and cognitive disorders; standard depression screening tools (based on DSM-IV criteria) and the Mini–Mental State Examination are helpful in this regard. Obtain a history of dietary practices, dietary intake, and use of nutritional supplements. Inquire about living environment, functional status, dependency, caregiver status, alcohol or substance abuse, social support, and resources. It is important to question relatives and caregivers.

Initial diagnostic testing is limited to basic studies unless the history and physical examination suggest a specific cause (Table 2). The following studies should be obtained in most patients: complete blood count (CBC); erythrocyte sedimentation rate or C-reactive protein; serum chemistry tests, including calcium level, kidney and liver function tests, and thyroid-stimulating hormone level; urinalysis; chest radiography; and stool occult blood test. Among patients with a completely normal baseline evaluation, later diagnosis of a serious organic disorder is rare, and watchful waiting may be the preferred approach (Table 3). In patients with gastrointestinal symptoms or abnormalities on CBC or liver tests, obtain an upper gastrointestinal series, abdominal ultrasonography, abdominal CT, or esophagogastroduodenoscopy, as appropriate. Indiscriminate imaging of the thorax and abdomen with CT or MRI in the absence of supporting findings on history, physical examination, or laboratory studies is not helpful. Truly occult malignancy is not common.

It may be difficult to establish a definitive diagnosis for weight loss, and perhaps a quarter of patients will not have a diagnosis after an appropriate initial evaluation. For such patients, careful

Table 2. Laboratory and Other Studies for Involuntary Weight Loss (IWL)

Test	Notes
CBC	Anemia is present in 14% of patients with a physical cause of weight loss.
Electrolytes, blood urea nitrogen, creatinine, glucose, liver tests	The combination of decreased albumin level and elevated alkaline phosphatase level has a sensitivity of 17% and specificity of 87% for cancer. Adrenal insufficiency is associated with electrolyte disturbances in 92% of patients.
ESR	Mean ESR is increased (49 mm/h) in patients with neoplasia compared with patients with a psychiatric or unknown cause of IWL (19 mm/h and 26 mm/h, respectively).
Thyroid-stimulating hormone (TSH)	Look for "apathetic" hyperthyroidism.
Chest radiography	A useful test overall in patients with a physical cause of IWL.
HIV antibody	HIV antibody testing is indicated if risk factors are present.
Upper GI radiography series, EGD, abdominal ultrasonography, or abdominal CT	Upper GI has the highest yield in disclosing a pertinent abnormality beyond basic screening tests among patients with a physical cause of weight loss if GI symptoms are present. Among patients diagnosed with cancer, the most useful follow-up tests include: • Patients with only an isolated abnormality on CBC: abdominal CT, abdominal ultrasonography, and endoscopy • Patients with only an isolated abnormality in liver tests: abdominal ultrasonography and abdominal CT • Patients with normal liver tests and CBC: upper endoscopy and abdominal CT

CBC = complete blood count; EGD = esophagogastroduodenoscopy; ESR = erythrocyte sedimentation rate; GI = gastrointestinal.

Table 3. Clinical Prediction Rule for Malignancy as a Cause of Isolated Weight Loss

Test or Feature	Points[a]
Age >80 y	+1
Serum albumin >3.5 g/dL (35 g/L)	-2
Leukocyte count >12,000/µL (12×10^9/L)	+1
Serum alkaline phosphatase >300 U/L	+2
Serum lactate dehydrogenase >500 U/L	+3

[a]A score of <0 indicates a low probability for malignancy (positive likelihood ratio = 0.07), a score of 0-1 indicates an intermediate probability (positive likelihood ratio = 1.2), and a score >1 indicates high probability (positive likelihood ratio = 28).
Adapted with permission from Hernández JL, Matorras P, Riancho JA, González-Macías J. Involuntary weight loss without specific symptoms: a clinical prediction score for malignant neoplasm. QJM. 2003;96:649-55. [PMID: 12925720]

reevaluation over time is appropriate; if serious disease is present, the cause is likely to become evident within 3 to 6 months. If a cause cannot be established over time, the prognosis is favorable.

Treatment

Once a specific diagnosis is made, treatment should alleviate weight loss in most cases. If weight loss continues, the putative diagnosis may not be correct or completely responsible. Consider medication and lifestyle changes for some patients. Change or eliminate medications that may be associated with anorexia and/or temporally related to weight loss. Address issues of social isolation and poor eating environment, if applicable. Ensure that oral health is adequate and that the patient has access to food and is able to eat it. Address personal and ethnic food preferences in the promotion of oral dietary intake. Assist those who need help with eating by seeking to improve functional status and making certain that patients obtain help to eat. Eliminate restrictive diets, where appropriate.

The proven benefit of oral nutritional supplementation for weight loss is limited. In fact, the amount of regular food intake is sometimes decreased by the use of oral nutritional supplements.

However, nutritional supplementation may be useful when access to calories is an issue due to functional impairments. Appetite stimulants often are recommended but are of limited benefit in patients not responding to treatment of the primary cause of weight loss or if the cause is unknown. Appetite-stimulant therapy has been studied mainly in patients with AIDS or cancer cachexia. In these patients, certain agents (e.g., megestrol acetate, human growth hormone) have been shown to promote weight gain. However, a survival benefit has never been demonstrated, quality of life benefits are modest, and in some trials patients who received such agents have experienced an increase in mortality.

Book Enhancement

Go to www.acponline.org/essentials/general-internal-medicine-section.html. In *MKSAP for Students 5*, assess your knowledge with items 45-48 in the **General Internal Medicine** section.

Bibliography

Vanderschueren S, Geens E, Knockaert D, Bobbaers H. The diagnostic spectrum of unintentional weight loss. Eur J Intern Med. 2005;16:160-164. [PMID: 15967329]

Chapter 37

Disorders of Menstruation and Menopause

Sara B. Fazio, MD

Disorders of menstruation are common and range from the complete absence of menstrual blood flow (amenorrhea) to irregular or heavy bleeding (abnormal uterine bleeding). The normal menstrual cycle depends on a tightly regulated system that includes the central nervous system, hypothalamus, pituitary gland, ovaries, uterus, and vaginal outflow tract. Disorders of menstruation can result from disruption at any level of the system (Table 1).

The menstrual cycle is regulated by the pituitary-hypothalamic axis. The hypothalamus secretes gonadotropin-releasing hormone (GnRH) in a pulsatile fashion, stimulating release of follicle-stimulating hormone (FSH) and leuteinizing hormone (LH) from the pituitary gland. FSH causes the development of multiple ovarian follicles, which in turn release estradiol. Estradiol inhibits FSH release, allowing only one or two dominant follicles to survive, and stimulates LH secretion. LH promotes progesterone production, which then causes a surge of LH secretion 34 to 36 hours before follicle rupture and ovulation. Once this occurs, progesterone is produced by ovarian granulose cells (the corpus luteum) for approximately 14 days; which then involutes unless pregnancy is established. Estrogen functions to increase the thickness and vascularity of the endometrial lining, whereas progesterone increases its glandular secretion and vessel tortuosity. The cyclical withdrawal of estrogen and progesterone results in endometrial sloughing and menstrual bleeding.

Amenorrhea

Primary amenorrhea is the absence of menarche in females aged ≥16 years. Secondary amenorrhea is the cessation of menstruation for 3 cycle intervals or 6 consecutive months in females who were previously menstruating regularly. Table 2 lists common tests used in the evaluation of primary and secondary amenorrhea.

Primary Amenorrhea

Approximately 50% of primary amenorrhea is caused by chromosomal disorders associated with gonadal dysgenesis and depletion of ovarian follicles. Turner syndrome is the most common disorder in this category and is classically associated with a 45,XO genotype. It is characterized by a lack of secondary sex characteristics, growth retardation, webbed neck, and frequent skeletal abnormalities. Hypothalamic hypoandrogenism accounts for approximately 20% of primary amenorrhea and includes both structural and functional hypothalamic disorders, such as developmental defects of cranial midline structures, tumors, and infiltrative disorders.

Less common causes of primary amenorrhea include developmental disorders (Müllerian agenesis, imperforate hymen) and defects of the cervix or vagina. Such patients have normal secondary sex characteristics. Patients with androgen insensitivity syndrome (testicular feminization) have some female secondary sex characteristics but an absence of or minimal pubic and axillary hair, a shallow vagina, and often a labial mass (testes). Endocrine abnormalities such as prolactin excess, thyroid disease, and polycystic ovary syndrome (PCOS), although more commonly associated with secondary amenorrhea, also cause primary amenorrhea.

Patients with primary amenorrhea should be examined for the presence of an intact uterus and vaginal outflow tract, secondary sex characteristics, and signs of hyperandrogenism. If evidence of characteristic developmental disorders is present, karyotyping should be considered. Primary ovarian failure of any cause can be diagnosed by an elevated serum FSH level. A low or normal FSH level warrants measurement of serum prolactin and thyroid-stimulating hormone (TSH) levels as well as brain imaging to exclude structural disease.

Secondary Amenorrhea

Secondary amenorrhea is much more common than primary amenorrhea. All previously menstruating women who present with amenorrhea should be tested for pregnancy, the most common cause. Premature ovarian failure may occur as a result of surgical oophorectomy, chemotherapy, radiation, or autoimmune destruction of ovarian tissue.

Diagnosis of secondary ovarian failure is made by an elevated FSH level. In such patients, vaginal bleeding will not occur with a progesterone challenge, because estrogen levels are low; however, bleeding will occur after estrogen priming followed by a progesterone challenge, demonstrating the integrity of the uterine lining and outflow tract. The presence of bleeding following a progesterone challenge suggests a serum estradiol level >40 pg/mL (146.8 pmol/L) and obviates the need for estradiol measurement. Absence of bleeding following a progesterone challenge indicates either insufficient circulating estrogen or an anatomic abnormality that prohibits blood flow, such as Asherman syndrome (endometrial scar tissue development after dilation and curettage).

PCOS affects 6% of women of childbearing age and typically presents as oligomenorrhea and signs of androgen excess (hirsutism, acne, alopecia [occasionally]). The cause is not fully understood but involves abnormal gonadotropin regulation, with subsequent overactivity of the ovarian androgen pathway. Insulin resistance is an important feature of the disorder, as is increased

Table 1. Differential Diagnosis of Amenorrhea

Disorder	Present in Primary Amenorrhea?	Present in Secondary Amenorrhea?	LH	FSH	E$_2$	Notes
Hypothalamus						
Hypothalamic amenorrhea	Yes	Yes	↓ or normal	↓ or normal	↓	Exercise, weight loss, stress, and chronic illness.
Hypogonadotropic hypogonadism	Yes	Yes	↓ or normal	↓ or normal	↓	Anosmia may be present.
Hypothalamic tumor	Yes	Yes	↓ or normal	↓ or normal	↓	Brain imaging indicated.
Pituitary						
Hypogonadotropic hypogonadism	Yes	Yes	↓ or normal	↓ or normal	↓	
Pituitary tumor (prolactinoma)	Yes	Yes	↓ or normal	↓ or normal	↓	Prolactin may be elevated; brain imaging.
Pituitary infection or infiltration	Yes	Yes	↓ or normal	↓ or normal	↓	
Sheehan syndrome	No	Yes	↓ or normal	↓ or normal	↓	After delivery; can be acute or insidious.
Ovary						
Gonadal dysgenesis	Yes	Yes	↑	↑	↓	45,XO karyotype
Pure gonadal dysgenesis	Yes	Yes	↑	↑	↓	46,XX or 46,XY karyotype
Premature ovarian failure	No	Yes	↑	↑	↓	Autoimmune syndromes
Polycystic ovary syndrome	Yes	Yes	↑ or normal	Normal	Normal	Hyperandrogenism, oligomenorrhea since menarche.
Ovarian tumor	No	Yes	↓	↓	↑ or normal	Look for acute virilization.
17α-Hydroxylase deficiency	Yes	No	↑	↑	↓	Sexual infantilism
Uterus						
Müllerian agenesis	Yes	No	Normal	Normal	Normal	May have cyclical pelvic pain.
Asherman syndrome	No	Yes	Normal	Normal	Normal	History of dilation and curettage (uterine synechiae).
Other						
Adrenal tumor	No	Yes	↓	↓	↑ or normal	Hyperandrogenism
Thyroid disease	Yes	Yes	Normal	Normal	Normal	
Testicular feminization	Yes	No	↑	↑ or normal	↑	XY karyotype

↑ = elevated; ↓ = decreased; DHEA = dehydroepiandrosterone sulfate; E$_2$ = estradiol; FSH = follicle-stimulating hormone; LH = luteinizing hormone.

BMI, although only 50% of affected women are obese. PCOS is characterized by mildly elevated testosterone and dehydroepiandrosterone sulfate (DHEAS) levels and an LH/FSH ratio >2:1. Diagnosis requires two of the following: ovulatory dysfunction, laboratory or clinical evidence of hyperandrogenism, and ultrasonographic evidence of polycystic ovaries. If the evaluation does not support a diagnosis of PCOS and evidence of androgen excess is present, other causes must be excluded, including an ovarian or adrenal androgen-producing tumor (associated with serum testosterone levels >150-200 ng/dL [5.0-6.9 nmol/L]), congenital adrenal hyperplasia (elevated DHEAS and 17-hydroxyprogesterone levels), and Cushing syndrome (elevated serum cortisol level, abnormal dexamethasone suppression test). In the absence of findings suggesting Cushing syndrome (hypertension, large purple striae, dorsocervical fat pad, centripetal obesity, easy bruising), routine laboratory testing generally is not needed.

Androgen-secreting tumors most often are associated with virilization, including hirsutism, acne, clitoromegaly, male-pattern balding, and deepening of the voice.

Hyperprolactinemia is a frequent cause of secondary amenorrhea and is commonly related to medications. Drugs that reduce central catecholamine and dopamine production or release can cause hyperprolactinemia; tricyclic antidepressants, phenothiazines, and metoclopramide are among the most common causes. Primary hypothyroidism is associated with increased levels of hypothalamic thyrotropin-releasing hormone, which stimulates prolactin production. Tumors that secrete prolactin or that compress the pituitary stalk will lead to hyperprolactinemia. If the prolactin level is elevated and medication and hypothyroidism are excluded, brain imaging is warranted. Generally, a prolactin-producing adenoma is associated with serum prolactin levels >200 ng/mL (200 μg/L), whereas hyperprolactinemia caused by drugs

Table 2. Laboratory and Other Studies for Amenorrhea

Test	Notes
β-hCG	Use to confirm or exclude pregnancy.
Follicle-stimulating hormone (FSH)	Ovarian failure or menopause is present when serum FSH levels are >20 mU/mL. Perform karyotyping in all patients aged <30 y with elevated FSH levels.
Prolactin	Serum prolactin levels can be elevated by stress, breast examination, and food intake; repeat analysis on a fasting morning sample before performing cranial imaging. Hypothyroidism, phenothiazine, tricyclic antidepressants, metoclopramide, reserpine, and methyldopa can cause hyperprolactinemia. Values >200 ng/mL (200 µg/L) suggest pituitary tumor.
Thyroid-stimulating hormone	Hypothyroidism and, less commonly, hyperthyroidism are associated with menstrual cycle abnormalities and infertility.
Testosterone, DHEAS	May be helpful in a patient with hirsutism and acne. Total serum testosterone levels >200 ng/dL (6.9 nmol/L) and DHEAS levels more than three times the upper limit of normal suggest tumor (although no tumor is found in most cases).
17-Hydroxyprogesterone	Beneficial in screening for congenital adrenal hyperplasia.
Estradiol	Decreased in hypothalamic and pituitary amenorrhea and in ovarian failure. Serum estradiol should always be assessed with serum FSH. Most useful in evaluating primary amenorrhea.
Luteinizing hormone (LH)	Normal levels are 5-20 mU/mL (5-20 U/L), with midcycle peak three times the base level. The level is <5 mU/mL (5 U/L) in hypogonadotropic states (hypothalamic or pituitary dysfunction) and >20-40 mU/mL (20-40 U/L) in hypergonadotropic states (postmenopausal, ovarian failure). Serum LH measurement is not needed to diagnose PCOS.
DEXA	May be required to evaluate amenorrhea in a patient who is estrogen deficient.
Brain MRI	Necessary to rule out hypothalamic or pituitary mass, infection, or infiltration; critical to consider in the setting of primary amenorrhea with hypogonadotropic hypogonadism.

β-hCG = β subunit of human chorionic gonadotropin; DEXA = dual-energy x-ray absorptiometry; DHEAS = dehydroepiandrosterone sulfate; PCOS = polycystic ovary syndrome.

and other nonpituitary tumor causes usually is associated with prolactin levels <150 ng/mL (150 µg/L). Hypothalamic amenorrhea involves disordered gonadotropin release, which may occur as a result of a tumor or an infiltrative lesion (lymphoma, sarcoidosis) but more commonly is functional. The usual causative factors are stress, significant loss of body weight or fat, excessive exercise, or some combination thereof. Diagnosis is one of exclusion.

The initial evaluation of a patient with secondary amenorrhea should consist of serum FSH, TSH, and prolactin measurements; if signs of androgen excess are present, a serum testosterone and plasma DHEAS level should be obtained. When amenorrhea is associated with low or inappropriately normal FSH levels, secondary causes (PCOS, androgen or prolactin excess, hypothyroidism) must be ruled out. If FSH, TSH, and prolactin levels are normal, the next step is to perform a progesterone challenge test to determine if there is an adequate circulating level of estrogen; absent withdrawal bleeding following progesterone challenge should prompt serum estradiol measurement and evaluation of the uterine outflow track with ultrasonography, MRI, or hysterosalpingography. If a functional cause is suspected, moderation of exercise, improvement in nutrition, and/or attention to stress factors may be helpful. Because lack of adequate estrogen predisposes to osteoporosis, it is important to initiate adequate estrogen and progesterone replacement until causative factors are resolved and menstruation can return to normal.

Abnormal Uterine Bleeding

Abnormal uterine bleeding is bleeding that is excessive or scanty or occurs outside the normal menstrual cycle. Similar to amenor-

rhea, the diagnosis is best approached in anatomic terms and can be further categorized by patient age (Table 3). Pregnancy always must be considered. Implantation, ectopic pregnancy, threatened or missed abortion, and gestational trophoblastic disease all can cause abnormal bleeding. In women of all ages, consider anatomic lesions of the uterus, including endometrial polyps, uterine leiomyomata (fibroids), and endometrial hyperplasia or carcinoma (particularly in peri- or postmenopausal women). Cervical polyps and cervical neoplasia commonly present as abnormal uterine bleeding, although typically with intermenstrual bleeding. All patients should have a speculum examination to assess for visible lesions, a Pap smear, and a bimanual examination to assess for structural abnormalities. Ultrasonography may be necessary to detect endometrial polyps or submucosal leiomyomata and can assess the endometrial thickness. The latter is particularly important in a peri- or postmenopausal woman with abnormal uterine bleeding, because an endometrial biopsy may be warranted if the endometrium is >4-5 mm in thickness or is heterogeneous. Risk factors for endometrial carcinoma include chronic unopposed estrogen (as seen in chronic anovulatory states), obesity, age >45 years, nulliparity, and tamoxifen use.

Anovulation is the most common cause of abnormal uterine bleeding. Estrogen is produced by FSH stimulation of the ovary, but because ovulation does not occur, progesterone is never produced and the uterine lining builds up. This eventually leads to discoordinate menstrual bleeding, often presenting as bleeding at intervals shorter than the typical cycle length (metrorrhagia) or extended periods of heavy blood loss (menorrhagia). It is common for patients at extremes of the menstrual cycle (puberty and perimenopause) to be anovulatory. The most common cause of anovulatory bleeding in reproductive-aged women is PCOS.

Table 3. Causes of Abnormal Uterine Bleeding by Age

Cause	Diagnostic Clues
Menarche to Teenage Years	
Pregnancy	Irregular or absent periods
Anovulation	Cycle length falls outside normal range or varies by ≥10 d
Stress	Physical or mental
Bleeding disorder	Other sources of abnormal bleeding (gums, nose)
Infection (cervical, vaginal)	Postcoital bleeding and/or vaginal discharge
Teens to 40s	
Pregnancy	Irregular or absent periods
Malignancy (uterine, cervical, vaginal, vulvar)	Postcoital bleeding and/or vaginal discharge
Infection (cervical, vaginal)	Postcoital bleeding and/or vaginal discharge
Polyps (cervical, endometrial)	Dysmenorrhea
Adenomyosis, leiomyomata	Dysmenorrhea
Anovulation	Irregular periods
Bleeding disorder	Other sources of abnormal bleeding (gums, nose)
Endocrine disorder	Signs of hypothyroidism, diabetes mellitus, hyperprolactinemia, or polycystic ovary syndrome
Ovarian or adrenal tumor	New-onset virilization or hirsutism
Perimenopausal	
Anovulation	Irregular periods
Endometrial hyperplasia and polyps, leiomyomata	Dysmenorrhea
Malignancy (uterine, cervical, vaginal, vulvar)	Postcoital bleeding and/or vaginal discharge
Postmenopausal	
Malignancy (uterine, cervical, vaginal, vulvar)	Postcoital bleeding and/or vaginal discharge
Atrophy of vaginal mucosa	Vaginal dryness, dyspareunia
Estrogen replacement therapy	Estrogen withdrawal bleeding

Anovulatory bleeding may precede amenorrhea in functional hypothalamic disorders. Endocrine causes also must be considered in patients with abnormal uterine bleeding. Prolactin excess initially will cause anovulation. Menorrhagia may be reported in women with hypothyroidism. Cushing syndrome commonly causes menstrual irregularities, likely secondary to cortisol suppression of GnRH.

Systemic illness, coagulopathy, and medication effect also should be considered as potential causes of abnormal uterine bleeding. Cirrhosis reduces the ability of the liver to metabolize estrogen and decreases clotting factor production. Kidney failure interferes with estrogen clearance and is associated with abnormalities in platelet function. In adolescents with menorrhagia, up to 20% have an inherited bleeding disorder, most commonly von Willebrand disease.

Hormone therapy can correct anovulatory bleeding. Options include combination oral contraceptives, cyclic progestins, or a progestin-containing intrauterine device. In most cases, regularity of menstrual flow can be reestablished, and control of heavy blood loss can be achieved. In patients who are at risk for endometrial hyperplasia or carcinoma, a biopsy should be obtained before initiating hormone therapy. NSAIDs inhibit endometrial prostaglandins and decrease blood flow.

Menopause

Menopause refers to cessation of ovarian function. Because one-third of the lifespan of most women encompasses the postmenopausal period, physicians who care for these women must recognize the effects of estrogen deficiency. Because the postmenopausal period encompasses one third of the life span of most women, physicians must recognize the effects of estrogen deficiency in women. Elements that should be addressed in the history include timing of change in menstrual cycle, presence of hot flashes or night sweats, and fluctuations in mood. Patients should be asked about symptoms of urinary incontinence, vaginal dryness, and changes in sexual function or desire. Examination should include evaluation for height loss and kyphosis (signs of osteoporosis), breast examination (given increased incidence of breast cancer with advancing age), and evidence of vulvar or vaginal atrophy. Because the diagnosis of menopause can be made by history and physical examination without laboratory confirmation, serum FSH measurement is only indicated if the diagnosis is unclear or if the patient requires confirmation for reassurance.

Osteoporosis is a direct effect of estrogen loss at any age. Premenopausal women have less heart disease than men (in the absence of other risk factors), but this relative protection is lost at menopause. The role of hormone replacement therapy has become increasingly controversial. Although clearly controlling many of the symptoms of menopause (vasomotor instability, vaginal dryness) and reducing the risk of osteoporotic fractures, recent research has suggested a higher frequency of cardiac events in the first 5 years of hormone replacement therapy. In addition, studies have demonstrated a small but statistically significant increase in breast cancer in women taking estrogen. Thus, the approach to management of menopausal symptoms has become more individualized and involves an assessment of risks and benefits; if estrogen is prescribed, it should be used at the lowest dose and for the shortest duration possible to treat menopausal symptoms (typically ≤2 years). Estrogen still remains the most effective treatment for vasomotor instability (hot flashes), reducing the severity and frequency of symptoms by 70%, usually within 1 month. Contraindications to hormone replacement therapy include unexplained vaginal bleeding or a history of venous thromboembolism, liver disease, coronary artery disease, stroke, breast cancer, or endometrial cancer.

Serotonin and norepinephrine reuptake inhibitors (most notably venlafaxine), serotonin reuptake inhibitors, clonidine, gabapentin, and black cohosh all may be helpful in controlling vasomotor symptoms in select patients. Soy preparations have minimal efficacy. Vaginal atrophy can be treated with lubricants or localized vaginal estrogen preparations, which have little systemic absorption and are the most effective. Patients should be educated about risk reduction for coronary artery disease. Bone density testing should be offered to all women aged >65 years as well as woman aged >50 years who are at increased risk for osteoporosis based on risk factor assessment.

Patients at the perimenopause frequently experience irregular bleeding secondary to anovulation. Shortened intermenstrual cycles (more frequent bleeding), longer duration of bleeding, episodes of heavy bleeding, or menstruation after ≥6 months of amenorrhea warrants further evaluation. In general, pelvic ultrasonography should be performed on all perimenopausal women with irregular bleeding. If the endometrial lining is <4 mm in thickness, an endometrial biopsy may occasionally be deferred. Postmenopausal bleeding almost always requires endometrial evaluation with both ultrasonography and biopsy. Although the most common cause is endometrial atrophy, the possibility of endometrial carcinoma must be excluded. Referral to a gynecologist generally is recommended in the context of abnormal peri- or postmenopausal bleeding and always in a patient who experiences bleeding while taking noncyclical estrogen replacement or tamoxifen.

Book Enhancement

Go to www.acponline.org/essentials/general-internal-medicine-section. In *MKSAP for Students 5*, assess your knowledge with items 49-54 in the **General Internal Medicine** section.

Bibliography

Col NF, Fairfield KM, Ewan-Whyte C, Miller H. In the clinic. Menopause. Ann Intern Med. 2009;150:ITC4-1-15; quiz ITC4-16. [PMID: 19349628]

Chapter 38

Common Dermatologic Disorders

Robert Jablonover, MD

In the United States, up to 60% of dermatologic disorders are treated by primary care physicians. Skin complaints account for approximately 5% of internal medicine visits.

Evaluation

A detailed and targeted history is obtained, including location of skin lesions, time of onset and evolution (acute or chronic), and any systemic symptoms, such as fever. Rash accompanied by fever is common with disseminated infections (viral or bacterial), drug reactions, collagen vascular diseases, and vasculitis. External factors (new medications, foods, soaps, detergents) and occupational, environmental, and sun exposures should be investigated. A detailed history of previous treatments may clarify altered natural progression of skin disorders.

It is imperative to inspect the entire skin and mucosal surfaces. Patients should be undressed, wearing only a hospital gown. Natural lighting is preferable. Skin palpation can help appreciate texture, depth, and tenderness of lesions. Learning how to describe skin lesions is critical to correctly communicate relevant findings. Several attributes of skin lesions are paramount, including location, color, border, type (Table 1), and arrangement.

Common Skin and Nail Infections

Bacterial Infections

The most common skin infections seen in the outpatient setting are cellulitis, folliculitis, and impetigo. These infections are increasingly caused by community-acquired methicillin-resistant *Staphylococcus aureus* (MRSA).

Cellulitis is a rapidly spreading deep (dermis) subcutaneous-based infection. The infection most often is caused by *Staphylococcus aureus* or group A streptococci and is characterized by a well-demarcated area of warmth, swelling, tenderness, and erythema (Plate 4), possibly accompanied by lymphatic streaking and/or fever and chills. Risk factors for lower-extremity cellulitis include eczema, tinea pedis, onychomycosis, skin trauma, chronic leg ulcers, type 2 diabetes mellitus, and edema. Cellulitis is a clinical diagnosis; cultures usually are not necessary and seldom are positive. Treatment is based on the risk of MRSA infection and the severity of illness (Table 2). Risk factors for MRSA infection include recent close contact with persons having a similar infection, recent antibiotic use, recent hospitalization, hemodialysis, illicit injection drug use, diabetes, and previous MRSA colonization or infection.

Folliculitis is a pustular skin infection arising from hair follicles and typically affecting the beard, pubic area, axillae, and thighs (Plate 5). Causes include *S. aureus* and, less frequently, group A streptococci. The infection often resolves spontaneously; therefore, systemic antibiotics should not be used routinely. Folliculitis often is effectively treated with local application of heat and a topical antibiotic (mupirocin, clindamycin).

Furuncles or "boils" (infection of the hair follicle) and skin abscesses (pus collections in the dermis and deeper tissues) are acute, tender, pus-containing nodules that commonly appear on the neck or in the axillae or groin but may occur at any skin site; furuncles and abscess nearly always are caused by *S. aureus*.

Table 1. Dermatologic Lexicon[a]

Description	Definition	Examples
Macule	Flat skin lesion <1 cm in diameter	Freckle
Patch	Flat skin lesion >1 cm in diameter	Tinea versicolor
Papule	Raised skin lesion <0.5 cm in diameter	Acne
Plaque	"Plateau-like" elevated lesion >0.5 cm in diameter	Psoriasis
Nodule	Raised sphere-like lesion >0.5 cm in diameter and depth; called a *cyst* when filled with liquid or keratin	Erythema nodosum
Vesicle	Blister filled with clear fluid <0.5 cm in diameter	Varicella
Bulla	Blister filled with clear fluid >0.5 cm in diameter	Poison ivy
Pustule	Vesicle filled with pus	Folliculitis
Crust (scab)	Dried pus, blood, and serum from breakage of vesicles, bullae, or pustules	Herpes zoster (shingles)
Scale	Dry, whitish, and flaky stratum corneum	Seborrheic dermatitis

[a]Other common terms include *induration* (dermal thickening), *lichenification* (epidermal thickening), *atrophy* (loss of epidermal or dermal tissue), *wheal* (dermal edema), *comedone* (acne lesion), *ulcer* (loss of epidermal tissue and some dermis), *erosion* (superficial loss of epidermis), and *fissure* (linear opening in epidermis).

Table 2. Antibiotic Therapy for Cellulitis

Disease Severity	Antibiotic Choices
Mild uncomplicated cellulitis at low risk for MRSA (oral treatment)	Dicloxacillin, a first-generation cephalosporin, clindamycin or a macrolide (if allergic to penicillin), a fluoroquinolone (moxifloxacin, levofloxacin, if intolerant to previous agents)
Mild uncomplicated cellulitis at risk for MRSA infection (oral treatment)	Trimethoprim-sulfamethoxazole,[a] clindamycin, doxycycline
Moderate to severe cellulitis with systemic manifestations and low risk for MRSA (parenteral treatment)	A semisynthetic penicillin (nafcillin), a cephalosporin (cefazolin), clindamycin (if allergic to penicillin), a fluoroquinolone, a macrolide (clarithromycin, azithromycin), an oxazolidinone (linezolid), vancomycin, daptomycin, tigecycline
Moderate to severe cellulitis with systemic manifestations and high risk for MRSA (parenteral treatment)	Clindamycin, vancomycin, linezolid, daptomycin, tigecycline

MRSA = methicillin-resistant *Staphylococcus aureus*.
[a]Trimethoprim-sulfamethoxazole is not recommended for nonpurulent cellulitis, because the likely pathogen (group A streptococcus) is resistant in most cases.

Furuncles frequently arise from a staphylococcal folliculitis. Warm compresses to facilitate drainage may be appropriate for small furuncles. Incision and drainage is the treatment of choice for larger furuncles and all abscesses, but systemic antibiotic treatment may be indicated if the patient is febrile, immunocompromised, diabetic, or at risk for MRSA or if there is a surrounding cellulitis. Cultures can distinguish MRSA from methicillin-susceptible *S. aureus* (MSSA) and can guide treatment. Elimination of *S. aureus* nasal carriage using intranasal mupirocin and elimination of *S. aureus* from body surfaces using a topical antiseptic wash may decrease relapses.

Impetigo is a superficial infection of the skin (epidermis) characterized by a group of yellowish, crusted pustules (Plate 6). Impetigo is caused by staphylococci or streptococci. Predisposing factors include poor hygiene, neglected minor trauma, and eczema. Limited disease usually can be treated effectively with topical mupirocin or bacitracin; more extensive disease can be treated with a cephalosporin, penicillinase-resistant penicillin, or β-lactam/β-lactamase inhibitor.

Ecthyma is an ulcerative infection usually caused by streptococci or staphylococci. The classic findings are superficial, saucer-shaped ulcers with overlying crusts, typically on the legs or feet (Plate 7). Effective treatment consists of cleansing with an antibacterial wash followed by topical mupirocin plus oral dicloxacillin or a first-generation cephalosporin.

Fungal Infections

Dermatophytoses (tinea) are superficial infections caused by fungi that thrive only in nonviable tissue of the skin, hair, and nails, and often cause itchy rashes but not invasive systemic infections. Predisposing factors include immunosuppression, hyperhidrosis, diabetes, corticosteroids, direct contact (e.g., towels), and hot, humid, occlusive environments. An expanding, ringlike (annular) lesion with a slightly scaly, erythematous, advancing edge and central clearing suggests a fungal infection; however, the presence of fungus should be confirmed by microscopic KOH examination of the scales before initiating treatment. *Tinea corporis* can occur on any part of the body, including the trunk and extremities. *Tinea pedis*, the most common dermatophyte infection, often presents as silvery scale and dull erythema of the soles and sides of the feet (moccasin-type; Plate 8) and/or may be characterized by interdigital scale and maceration. *Tinea cruris* typically presents as erythematous, arciform or polycyclic plaques with sharp margins and central clearing; the lesions may be located on the thighs, perineum, perianal region, buttocks, and intergluteal cleft (Plate 9). In contrast to candidiasis, tinea cruris typically spares the scrotum in males. Topical antifungal creams (clotrimazole, terbinafine) usually are effective in treating dermatophyte infections. Combination antifungal and corticosteroid products should be avoided. Oral antifungal therapy (ketoconazole, terbinafine) is needed to treat widespread or severe tinea infection. It is essential to treat tinea pedis in patients with diabetes, as tinea can create a portal of entry for bacteria and resultant cellulitis.

Tinea versicolor is caused by the yeast, *Malassezia furfur*. Lesions typically are round or oval, nonpruritic, light brown or hypopigmented macules located on the trunk and proximal upper extremities (Plate 10). The diagnosis is confirmed by the classic microscopic appearance of both spores and hyphae in a "spaghetti and meatball" pattern. Treatment consists of topical selenium sulfide solution or oral ketoconazole (a single dose is effective).

Candidiasis is an inflammatory reaction to *Candida albicans* infection. Predisposing factors include immunosuppression, diabetes, moisture, and antibiotic-induced reduction of competing flora. Candidiasis usually occurs in moist areas (skinfolds, inframammary and perianal regions, axillae) and causes itching and burning. Infected areas appear erythematous, with scattered satellite papules and pustules (Plate 11). Treatment consists of topical nystatin or imidazole cream combined with efforts to keep affected areas dry. Candidiasis often is confused with intertrigo, a skinfold dermatitis caused by moisture and rubbing, which is especially prominent in obese patients. Intertrigo usually lacks the same degree of redness and satellite lesions found in candidiasis, and KOH microscopic examination is negative.

Onychomycosis is an infection of the nail caused by dermatophytes, yeasts, or molds and characterized by a thickened, yellow or white nail with scaling under the elevated distal free edge of the nail plate (Plate 12). Nail infections can be diagnosed with KOH examination or culture (nail debris or clippings). Most patients with toenail onychomycosis are asymptomatic and do not require treatment. However, treatment with oral terbinafine, itraconazole, or fluconazole is indicated in patients with symptomatic toenail infection and in patients with peripheral arterial disease or diabetes who are at risk for complications from onychomycosis (cellulitis). The efficacy of treatment usually is <75%, and recurrence rates can approach 40%. Topical antifungal lacquers generally are not effective.

Viral Infections

Herpes zoster (shingles) results from reactivation of latent varicella-zoster virus (VZV), which resides in the nerve ganglia after an initial varicella (chickenpox) infection; it typically affects persons aged >60 years and patients who are immunosuppressed. Recurrent herpes zoster should trigger testing for possible associated HIV infection. Pain, tingling, or itching may precede the rash by 1 to 5 days. The classic morphology is grouped vesicles on an erythematous base; the vesicles occur in multiple plaques along one or several contiguous unilateral dermatomes, classically stopping at the midline (Plate 13). In patients with HIV infection or in those undergoing chemotherapy, the lesions may occur in multiple, widely separated dermatomes or may be disseminated. The vesicles become pustular and then crust with healing. Antiviral therapy with valacyclovir or famciclovir (or acyclovir, if cost is a consideration), given within 48 to 72 hours of the onset of the rash, may speed healing, decrease acute pain, and reduce the incidence and intensity of postherpetic neuralgia (PHN), a painful sequela of herpes zoster. PHN may be treated with gabapentin, pregabalin, a lidocaine patch, topical capsaicin, a tricyclic antidepressant, or an opioid analgesic. The addition of corticosteroids to antiviral therapy reduces the duration but not the incidence of PHN. Involvement of the eye, periorbital skin, or tip of the nose (trigeminal nerve) mandates urgent ophthalmologic consultation due to the risk of ocular complications. Vaccination (VZV vaccine) of immunocompetent adults aged >60 years decreases the incidence and severity of herpes zoster and PHN.

Common Rashes

Atopic dermatitis is common in persons with a personal or family history of other atopic conditions, such as asthma or allergic rhinitis. The rash characteristically involves the antecubital and popliteal fossae and flexural wrists and, when acute, results in pruritic, erythematous, poorly demarcated, eczematous, crusted, papulovesicular plaques and excoriations. The skin becomes lichenified and hyperpigmented in chronic atopic dermatitis (Plate 14). Atopic dermatitis is diagnosed clinically. Treatment consists of topical corticosteroids, antihistamines, and emollients. A potential complication of atopic dermatitis is staphylococcal superinfection.

Contact dermatitis can be caused by an irritant or allergen. Irritant contact dermatitis is a nonimmunologic, toxic reaction that results from exposure to harsh conditions or chemicals. Allergic contact dermatitis (ACD) is a delayed hypersensitivity reaction that requires initial sensitization. Common allergens include plants (e.g., poison ivy), neomycin, preservatives, and metals (e.g., nickel). In ACD, the skin is itchy, red, edematous, weepy, and crusted, and there may be vesicles or bullae (Plate 15). The skin becomes lichenified, scaly, and hyperpigmented as the dermatitis becomes chronic. Exposure history and pattern of the rash may provide clues as to the causal allergen. Patch testing is the gold standard for diagnosis. Treatment of acute and chronic ACD usually consists of mid to high potency topical corticosteroids; tapered systemic corticosteroids are used for severe or extensive

reactions. Avoidance of exposure to the offending allergen, if determined, is a key therapeutic principle.

Venous stasis dermatitis affects the skin on the lower legs, particularly around the medial malleolus, and results from venous hypertension, edema, chronic inflammation, and microangiopathy. Distinguishing stasis dermatitis from bacterial cellulitis can be difficult, but bilateral involvement, absence of fever or leukocytosis, and minimal pain suggest stasis dermatitis. The diagnosis of stasis dermatitis is clinical; edema, hyperpigmented skin due to hemosiderin deposition (most prominent at the medial ankle), and varicose veins suggest the diagnosis (Plate 16). Ulceration is a potential complication. Stasis dermatitis is treated with topical corticosteroids (if erythema and inflammation are present), leg elevation, and knee level compression stockings; topical antibiotics are not recommended.

Seborrheic dermatitis affects areas of the body that are rich in sebaceous glands; the condition may be secondary to colonization with the yeast, M. furfur. Lesions are erythematous, with dry or greasy scale and crusts, and may be pruritic (Plate 17). Common areas of involvement include the scalp (dandruff), nasolabial folds, cheeks, eyebrows, eyelids, and external auditory canals. Frequent remissions and exacerbations are common. Severe seborrheic dermatitis is common in persons with HIV infection. Treatment consists of low-potency corticosteroids (face), ketoconazole cream (face), and/or medicated shampoos that contain tar, ketoconazole, or selenium sulfide (scalp).

Psoriasis is a chronic, relapsing immune-mediated skin disorder and is one of the most common skin diseases. Exacerbating factors include stress, infection, injury to the skin, and certain medications (lithium, β-blockers). Psoriasis vulgaris can be limited or widespread. It is characterized by sharply marginated, erythematous, scaly papules and plaques covered by a silvery white scale on the extensor surfaces of the extremities, presacral skin, and/or scalp (Plate 18). Guttate psoriasis is characterized by small, droplike, scaly plaques. Palmoplantar psoriasis, although localized, may be difficult to manage and may interfere with activities of daily living. Generalized pustular psoriasis can be life threatening and frequently occurs following withdrawal of systemic corticosteroids. Nail changes (pitting, onycholysis) often occur in patients with psoriasis and correlate with a greater risk of accompanying psoriatic arthritis (Plate 19). The diagnosis of psoriasis is clinical and based on the appearance and distribution of the rash. Moderate to severe and/or recalcitrant disease is treated with topical agents (corticosteroids, calcipotriene, tazarotene, anthralin), phototherapy, and/or systemic therapy (methotrexate, acitretin, cyclosporine, biologic agents). Topical corticosteroids should be discontinued slowly to avoid rebound of psoriasis. Systemic corticosteroids have no role in the treatment of psoriasis.

Erythema multiforme (EM) is an acute, often recurrent mucocutaneous eruption characterized by circular erythematous plaques with a raised, darker central circle ("target lesions"). EM usually follows an acute infection, most often recurrent herpes simplex virus (HSV) infection; it also may be drug related or idiopathic. Lesions generally are located on the extremities, palms, and soles (Plate 20). Painful oral mucosal erosions and bullae are common. The diagnosis is clinical. Treatment of EM is primarily symptomatic. Systemic corticosteroids may provide symptomatic improvement. Antiviral therapy does not shorten the EM outbreak in HSV-associated cases.

Cutaneous drug reactions are common in both hospitalized patients and outpatients; most of these eruptions are self-limited and not severe. The most common causes are antibiotics (penicillins, β-lactams, sulfonamides), anticonvulsants, NSAIDs, thiazide diuretics, and allopurinol. Drug-induced cutaneous eruptions can mimic many different kinds of rashes and should be in the differential diagnosis in the sudden appearance of a symmetrical eruption. Pruritus may be mild, severe, or absent. The most common reaction patterns include morbilliform (Plate 21), urticaria, fixed drug eruption, photosensitivity, and EM-like reaction. Because drug reactions can occur within days or up to 2 months after exposure to the causative medication, a detailed history is essential to determine the cause. Treatment consists of stopping the offending drug, antihistamines, and systemic corticosteroids if the reaction is severe or widespread.

Pityriasis rosea is a common papulosquamous eruption that has been linked to reactivation of human herpesvirus 6 or 7. The rash typically begins with a single thin, pink, oval, 2- to 4-cm plaque (herald patch) with a thin collarette of scale at the periphery (Plate 22). Similar but smaller plaques subsequently erupt within days to weeks, usually on the torso along skin cleavage lines, in a Christmas tree–like distribution. The lesions can be asymptomatic or mildly pruritic. The eruption is self-limited and usually lasts 4 to 10 weeks. No treatment is needed, but topical corticosteroids and/or oral antihistamines may be used for pruritus.

Common Oral Lesions

Leukoplakia is a common premalignant white patch or plaque adherent to the oral mucosa. Patients should be referred for biopsy and excision.

Aphthous ulcers (aphthae, canker sores) are recurring, painful, round or oval oral ulcers with inflammatory halos; the causative factors are unknown. The diagnosis is clinical. Treatment typically consists of topical analgesics and topical corticosteroids. Severe oral ulcers may be associated with inflammatory bowel disease, celiac disease, HIV infection, and Behçet syndrome, which is characterized by aphthous ulcers plus urogenital ulcerations and iridocyclitis.

HSV type 1 infection typically causes herpes labialis. Primary infection is asymptomatic in most patients but may present as acute, painful gingivostomatitis. Recurrent episodes result from reactivation of dormant virus in the neural ganglia. Recurrences often are characterized by a prodrome of burning, stinging, or pain approximately 24 hours before the onset of lesions, which typically occur on the lips ("cold sores"). The lesions consist of grouped vesicles on an erythematous, edematous base; the lesions rupture and leave behind clustered erosions that involute (Plate 23). The diagnosis usually is made clinically, but laboratory confirmation of infection with viral culture or by direct fluorescent antibody testing may be helpful. Treatment with an oral antiviral agent (valacyclovir), given at the onset of the prodromal symptoms and prior to the outbreak of vesicles, decreases the duration of the rash by 1 to 2 days. Topical antiviral agents are not efficacious.

Acneiform Lesions

Acne vulgaris usually begins at puberty and results from 1 or more principal mechanisms: hyperkeratinization of follicles, increased sebum production secondary to increased androgenic hormone levels, proliferation of *Propionibacterium acnes*, and resulting inflammation. Topical and systemic corticosteroid therapy, hormone therapy, use of anabolic steroids, hyperandrogenism, and polycystic ovary syndrome may contribute to acneiform eruptions. Acne-prone sites include the face, neck, chest, upper back, and shoulders. In most cases, the history and physical examination are sufficient to diagnose acne. Acne is classified as either noninflammatory or inflammatory and by degree of severity. Noninflammatory acne involves open and closed comedones; inflammatory acne consists of erythematous papules, pustules, and, occasionally, nodules. Topical retinoids and benzoyl peroxide are effective treatments for noninflammatory acne. Treatment of inflammatory acne requires an antibacterial agent (topical clindamycin or erythromycin) in addition to a comedolytic or keratolytic agent. Moderate to severe inflammatory acne often requires both topical treatment and an oral antibiotic (doxycycline, minocycline, erythromycin). Treatment with oral contraceptives and spironolactone, in addition to topical acne therapy, is effective for female patients with androgen excess. Isotretinoin (an oral retinoid) is used in patients with severe nodular acne that is unresponsive to oral antibiotic therapy and may result in prolonged remissions; however, because of teratogenicity, isotretinoin should be administered only by physicians who are trained in its use and registered with the FDA.

Acne rosacea (rosacea) is a chronic inflammatory skin disorder affecting the face, typically the cheeks and nose. The cause is unknown. Rosacea is characterized by erythema with telangiectasia, pustules, and papules; comedones are absent (Plate 24). Rosacea can be differentiated from seborrheic dermatitis by the presence of pustules. In early stages, rosacea can present as only facial erythema and resemble the butterfly rash of systemic lupus erythematosus (SLE); however, the rash of SLE typically spares the nasolabial folds and areas under the nose and lower lip. Rhinophyma (large, irregular hyperplastic nose) can develop in some patients with rosacea. Treatment may consist of topical agents (metronidazole gel, benzoyl peroxide, tretinoin) or oral antibiotics (tetracycline, erythromycin).

Perioral dermatitis is characterized by discrete papules and pustules on an erythematous base, centered around the mouth (Plate 25). The eruption often follows the use of topical or inhaled corticosteroids. Treatment consists of discontinuing the corticosteroid or protecting the skin from the inhaled product. Initial treatment includes topical antibiotics and sulfur preparations.

Urticaria

Urticaria (hives) appears as raised, pruritic, erythematous wheals with sharp borders (Plate 26). The lesions can last from minutes to hours and usually involve the trunk and extremities, sparing the palms and soles. Lesions that persist >24 hours, burn, or resolve with purpura are suspicious for urticarial vasculitis and should be biopsied. Episodes of urticaria lasting <6 weeks are classified as acute and often are caused by acute infection, medication, food, or pollen. Episodes lasting >6 weeks are classified as chronic. Many patients with chronic urticaria have an IgG antibody to the IgE receptor; others are reacting to a chronic infection or ingestant. Approximately 50% of cases of chronic urticaria have no identifiable cause. Angioedema is a severe, life-threatening form of urticaria characterized by localized edema of the skin or mucosa, usually involving the lips, face, hands, feet, penis, or scrotum (Plate 27). Concurrent angioedema occurs in 40% of patients with urticaria. Urticaria is a clinical diagnosis; careful history and physical examination are essential to determine possible causes. First-line therapy is avoidance of triggers and administration of antihistamines (H_1-receptor blockers). Patients with severe acute urticaria that is unresponsive to antihistamines should be treated with a tapered dose of prednisone. Corticosteroids are not used in the management of chronic urticaria.

Pruritus

Generalized pruritus without rash can be due to local or systemic causes. Dry skin (xerosis), exacerbated by poor hydration and dry winter weather, is the most common cause of pruritus in elderly patients. Treatment consists of the use of a humidifier, moisturizers, and occlusives. Persistent generalized pruritus in the absence of skin lesions suggests a possible systemic cause and should prompt evaluation for conditions such as cholestasis, chronic kidney disease, thyroid disease, infection (HIV), hematologic disease (polycythemia vera), and malignancy.

Infestations

Scabies is a skin infestation caused by the mite, *Sarcoptes scabiei*, an obligate human parasite preferentially affecting impoverished, immobilized, or immunodeficient persons. Spread is through direct personal contact, especially sexual contact. Acquisition from bedding or clothes is rare. Scabies infestation causes intense pruritus, often worse at night, and a papular or vesicular rash; the papules often are tipped with blood crusts. Burrows are visible as short wavy lines (Plate 28). The distribution of scabies often involves the interdigital webs, flexure surface of the wrists, penis, axillae, nipples, umbilicus, scrotum, and buttocks. Treatment is with permethrin or ivermectin.

Pediculosis (lice infestation) typically presents as pruritus, possibly with excoriation. The identification of crawling lice in the scalp or hair establishes the diagnosis. Lice egg cases are called *nits* and are found sticking to the hair shaft in patients with lice. Treatment is with permethrin.

Benign Growths

Seborrheic keratoses are common benign, painless neoplasms that present as brown to black, well-demarcated papules with a waxy surface and a "stuck on" appearance (Plate 29). Seborrheic keratoses are more common in older patients. Treatment is not indicated unless the growths are inflamed, irritated, or pruritic.

Verruca vulgaris (common wart) is caused by infection with a human papillomavirus. Common warts generally appear as 5- to 10-mm, rough-surfaced, skin-colored papules. Diagnosis is based on the typical verrucous appearance of a papule or plaque noted on the hands or feet. Spontaneous involution occurs in most patients within 3 years; thus, not treating cutaneous warts often is a reasonable option. Topical salicylic acid is first-line therapy. Cryotherapy is used for warts that do not respond to initial topical management; cryotherapy should be avoided with subungual and periungual warts.

Dermatofibromas are firm, dermal nodules approximately 6 mm in diameter; the surface often is hyperpigmented (Plate 30). Dermatofibromas are most commonly seen on the legs of adult women but also occur on the trunk in both males and females. Excision is indicated only if the lesion is symptomatic, has changed, or bleeds.

Cutaneous Manifestations of Internal Disease

Up to 50% of patients infected with hepatitis C virus (HCV) develop mixed cryoglobulinemia. Mixed cryoglobulinemia consists of circulating immune complexes that deposit in postcapillary venules, causing inflammation and vessel damage, which present clinically as palpable purpura (Plate 31); the purpura may be accompanied by arthralgia, peripheral neuropathy, and glomerulonephritis. The diagnosis is confirmed by elevated serum cryoglobulin levels; a skin biopsy will demonstrate leukocytoclastic vasculitis. Treatment is directed at the underlying HCV infection.

Porphyria cutanea tarda (PCT) is a hereditary or acquired blistering disease caused by excess circulating porphyrins resulting from deficiency or reduced activity of the enzyme, uroporphyrinogen decarboxylase. Iron overload, as seen with hemochromatosis, leads to decreased activity of this enzyme. Up to 50% of patients with sporadic PCT have HCV infection. Clinically, patients present with vesicles and bullae on sun-exposed skin surfaces, most commonly on the face, dorsal hands, and scalp (Plate 32). The diagnosis can be confirmed by elevated urine uroporphyrin levels. Treatment consists of phlebotomy, low-dose antimalarial agents, and erythropoietin for patients with chronic kidney disease. Treatment of underlying HCV infection is indicated.

Erythema nodosum is characterized by the sudden onset of deep, tender, palpable erythematous nodules, typically on the anterior lower legs (Plate 2); fever and joint pain also may be present. The condition usually is acute and self-limited. Erythema nodosum is the result of a hypersensitivity immune reaction to infection or systemic inflammation or may be secondary to drugs. Common causes include sarcoidosis, tuberculosis, inflammatory bowel disease, and streptococcal pharyngitis; at least 50% of cases are idiopathic. Management consists of treating the underlying disease. NSAIDs provide symptomatic relief; systemic corticosteroids can be used if an infectious cause is ruled out.

Dermatomyositis is a condition with characteristic cutaneous manifestations combined with proximal inflammatory myopathy/muscle weakness; skin disease sometimes may be the only manifestation (see Chapter 96). The distinctive cutaneous features are heliotrope rash (a violaceous to dusky erythematous periorbital rash) and Gottron papules (slightly elevated, scaly, violaceous papules and plaques that arise over bony prominences, particularly the small joints of the hands).

SLE is a multisystem disorder whose clinical spectrum ranges from a relatively benign cutaneous eruption to a severe, potentially fatal systemic multiorgan disease. Skin lesions are categorized as chronic (usually associated with scarring and/or atrophy), subacute, and acute; this classification helps predict systemic manifestations of the disease. Acute cutaneous lupus erythematosus is characterized by a confluent malar erythema or generalized red papular or urticarial lesions on sun-exposed skin surfaces and usually is associated with systemic disease (Plate 33). Chronic cutaneous (discoid) lupus erythematosus consists of slowly progressive, scaly, infiltrative papules and atrophic red plaques on sun-exposed skin surfaces and is not associated with systemic disease (Plate 34). Patients with subacute cutaneous lupus erythematosus have bright red annular or papulosquamous (psoriasis-like) lesions that may be associated with the more benign manifestations of SLE, such as arthralgia, photosensitivity, and serositis (Plate 35). The diagnosis of cutaneous lupus erythematosus is based on the clinical lesions and findings on skin biopsy. Initial management includes sun protection, topical corticosteroids, and antimalarial agents.

Pyoderma gangrenosum is a neutrophilic, ulcerative skin condition typically associated with an underlying systemic condition, such as inflammatory bowel disease, rheumatoid arthritis, seronegative spondyloarthropathy, or a hematologic disease or malignancy (most commonly acute myelogenous leukemia). Lesions often are multiple and tend to appear on the lower extremities. They begin as tender papules, pustules, or vesicles that spontaneously ulcerate and progress to painful ulcers with a purulent base and undermined, ragged, violaceous borders (Plate 3). Treatment usually requires topical or systemic corticosteroids.

Book Enhancement

Go to www.acponline.org/essentials/general-internal-medicine-section.html. In *MKSAP for Students 5*, assess your knowledge with items 55-64 in the **General Internal Medicine** section.

Acknowledgment

We would like to thank Dr. Hanah Polotsky, who contributed to an earlier version of this chapter.

Bibliography

Bershad SV. In the clinic. Acne. Ann Intern Med. 2008;149:ITC1-1-ITC1-16. [PMID: 18591631]

Stevens DL, Eron LL. Cellulitis and soft-tissue infections. Ann Intern Med. 2009;150:ITC11. [PMID:19124814].

Tyring SK. Management of herpes zoster and postherpetic neuralgia. J Am Acad Dermatol. 2007;57(6 Suppl):S136-142. [PMID:18021865].

Williams HC. Clinical practice. Atopic dermatitis. N Engl J Med. 2005;352:2314-2324. [PMID:15930422].

Chapter 39

Approach to Lymphadenopathy

Heather Harrell, MD

ymphadenopathy, an enlargement of one or more lymph nodes, is a common condition that affects patients of all ages and backgrounds. Lymphadenopathy may be discovered incidentally as part of a physical examination or may be detected in an evaluation for a patient-reported mass or "swollen gland." The causes of lymphadenopathy are numerous, ranging from malignancy to a self-limited immunologic reaction, infection, or inflammation. This chapter reviews the evaluation of lymphadenopathy, with an emphasis on identifying findings that are more likely to be associated with underlying pathologic conditions requiring further evaluation. An overview of lymphoid malignancies also is presented.

Evaluation

The history and physical examination are critical in determining which patients need further evaluation for lymphadenopathy. The patient's age is one of the most helpful pieces of information; age >40 years is associated with a 20 times greater risk of malignancy or granulomatous disease compared with younger age. The setting in which the lymphadenopathy occurs also is important; acute onset following an infection suggests an infectious or reactive lymphadenopathy, whereas subacute onset in a person who smokes cigarettes suggests malignancy. Timing is another helpful clue, as most benign immunologic reactions resolve in 2 to 4 weeks, whereas more serious conditions are associated with persistent or progressive lymphadenopathy. Finally, the presence of systemic symptoms suggests a more serious underlying illness. For example, B symptoms (fever, night sweats, weight loss) sometimes are present in Hodgkin lymphoma, whereas rash often is associated with specific infectious or inflammatory diseases (secondary syphilis, drug hypersensitivity reaction, systemic lupus erythematosus [SLE]).

When evaluating a patient with lymphadenopathy, all lymph node regions should be carefully examined. Determine the location, size, consistency (e.g., soft, rubbery, fluctuant, firm, hard), and mobility of any involved nodes; if multiple nodes are involved, also determine whether the nodes are discrete or matted. Features concerning for malignancy include size >2 cm, hard consistency, and fixed and/or matted nodes. The location and number of involved lymph nodes provide particularly helpful clues regarding cause. For example, supraclavicular lymphadenopathy usually is a sign of a serious underlying condition, whereas inguinal lymphadenopathy is very common and often benign. Characterizing whether the lymphadenopathy is localized (limited to one anatomic region) or generalized (involving more than two anatomic regions) may suggest which diagnoses are more likely; a single supraclavicular node suggests metastatic cancer, whereas generalized lymphadenopathy suggests a systemic inflammatory or infectious disease, such as syphilis or HIV infection. In the case of localized lymphadenopathy, the anatomic region that drains into the affected lymph node system should be examined for signs of infection or malignancy. For example, if an evaluation reveals axillary adenopathy suspicious for malignancy, a thorough breast examination and mammography should be performed. Signs of inflammation (warmth, redness, tenderness, fluctuance) suggest an infectious cause. The presence of splenomegaly can be a helpful clue to the diagnosis of infectious mononucleosis, lymphoma, or leukemia. Table 1 highlights signs and symptoms that help differentiate benign and pathologic causes of lymphadenopathy.

As many as two thirds of patients with lymphadenopathy have an obvious self-limited cause that does not require further evaluation, such as a recent upper respiratory tract infection. However, there are many other, more diagnostically challenging causes of

Table 1. ALL STAGES Mnemonic for Lymphadenopathy Features Suggesting a Benign or Pathologic Cause

Feature	Greater Likelihood of Benign Cause	Greater Likelihood of Pathologic Cause
Age	<40 y	>40 y
Location	Cervical, axillary, inguinal	Supraclavicular, mediastinal, abdominal
Length of time present	<2 wk	>4 wk
Size	<2 cm	>2 cm
Texture	Soft, rubbery	Hard, matted
Associated signs	Tender, mobile	Nontender (unless massive), fixed
Generalized vs localized	Not helpful predictor	Not helpful predictor
Extranodal associations	Localized infection (e.g., cellulitis, pharyngitis)	Splenomegaly, weight loss, arthritis, persistent fever
Setting	Recent illness or injury	Risk factors for malignancy

lymphadenopathy. Table 2 presents a mnemonic, CHICAGO, useful in creating a differential diagnosis for lymphadenopathy. Given the many potential causes, the clinician must rely heavily on the history and physical examination to focus the subsequent laboratory or imaging evaluation on the most likely diagnoses. A complete blood count (CBC) with differential is a useful initial test, as it can provide clues regarding a possible infection (e.g., atypical monocytosis in the case of Epstein-Barr virus infection), connective tissue disease (e.g., anemia, thrombocytopenia, and leukopenia in the case of SLE), or malignancy (e.g., blast cells in the case of leukemia). Blood cultures and serologic studies for the presence of specific antigens or antibodies are helpful when an infectious cause is suspected but should be done only when clinical factors make a specific infection likely. Chest radiographs are performed when lymphoma, lung cancer, or granulomatous disease is in the differential diagnosis. CT and MRI may be useful when assessing for the presence of intrathoracic or intraabdominal lymphadenopathy. An empiric trial of antibiotics or corticosteroids has no role in the evaluation of lymphadenopathy.

The evaluation of lymphadenopathy often centers on whether a lymph node biopsy is needed. Generally, the more high-risk criteria that are present (see Table 1), the more urgent the biopsy. Even in the absence of multiple risk factors, persistent (>4 weeks) unexplained lymphadenopathy usually requires biopsy. Biopsies can be excisional (entire node) or core (pieces of the node). Excisional biopsy is required to fully evaluate lymphoma (demonstrate lymph node architecture and provide specimens for flow cytometry), whereas needle biopsy is sufficient for suspected squamous cell carcinoma secondary to head and neck cancers. However, many such lymph node biopsies show only nonspecific reactive changes, and a directed biopsy of the suspected primary tumor may be required. Lymph node needle aspirates also may be cultured to diagnose an infection.

Lymphoma

Malignancy is the underlying cause of lymphadenopathy in <1% of patients seen in a primary care setting, but lymphoid malignancies often are curable when diagnosed at an early stage, so it is important to diagnose these cancers without delay. Lymphoma is classified as either Hodgkin lymphoma or non-Hodgkin lymphoma (NHL). Hodgkin lymphoma is derived from B cells, whereas NHL is further classified by ontogeny (B cell, T cell, NK cell) and stage of differentiation. Approximately 80% to 85% of NHLs in adults are of B-cell origin, with the remainder derived from T cells. All B-cell–derived NHLs are CD19 and CD20. Characteristic cytogenetic markers may be found in patients with some forms of NHL, and the differential diagnosis of NHL can be narrowed by using a panel of monoclonal antibodies and genetic markers.

Hodgkin lymphoma has a bimodal age distribution, with the initial peak at age 15 to 34 years and a second peak at age 55 to 70 years. There is a suggested link between Hodgkin lymphoma and delayed exposure to common childhood infections, because patients with this disease tend to have grown up in smaller families with a higher socioeconomic status. Later onset of Hodgkin lymphoma may be a consequence of latent virus reactivation with age-related decline in immunity. Generally, the incidence of NHL increases with age. Autoimmune disease and immunodeficiency states have a known association with NHL. NHL may also be caused by viruses.

Hodgkin lymphoma has the best prognosis, with cure rates in excess of 90% for patients with early-stage disease and 60% to 70% for patients with advanced-stage disease, although rates vary by disease subtype. NHL is far more complicated and generally is classified as low, intermediate, and high grade for the purposes of treatment. Low-grade NLH often is observed without therapy and nearly always responds to chemoimmunotherapy, although it is considered incurable by most experts. The average survival for patients with low-grade NHL is >10 years. Intermediate- and high-grade NHLs are curable with chemoimmunotherapy, with cure rates varying depending on the underlying biology of the disease as well as prognostic factors, such as the patient's age and overall health status, tumor stage, and serum lactate dehydrogenase level.

Book Enhancement

Go to www.acponline.org/essentials/general-internal-medicine-section.html. In *MKSAP for Students 5*, assess your knowledge with items 65-66 in the **General Internal Medicine** section.

Bibliography

Pangalis GA, Vassilakopoulos TP, Boussiotis VA, Fessas P. Clinical approach to lymphadenopathy. Semin Oncol. 1993;20:570-582. [PMID: 8296196]

Table 2. Selected Differential Diagnosis of Lymphadenopathy: CHICAGO Mnemonic

Diagnostic Category	Example(s)
Cancer	Lymphoma, leukemia, metastatic cancer (numerous primary sites)
Hypersensitivity	Drug reaction, vaccine reaction, serum sickness
Infection	Viral (EBV, CMV, or HIV infection), bacterial (cat scratch fever, staphylococcal or streptococcal infection, syphilis, chlamydia), mycobacterial (tuberculosis, nontuberculous mycobacterial infection), parasitic (toxoplasmosis), fungal (histoplasmosis, coccidioidomycosis), rickettsial (typhus)
Connective tissue disease	Systemic lupus erythematosus, rheumatoid arthritis, Sjögren syndrome
Atypical lymphoproliferative disorder	Castleman disease (giant lymph node hyperplasia)
Granulomatous disease	Sarcoidosis, silicosis, berylliosis
Other unusual cause	Kikuchi disease (histiocytic necrotizing lymphadenitis)

CMV = cytomegalovirus; EBV = Epstein-Barr virus.

Chapter 40

Comprehensive Geriatric Assessment

Anne Eacker, MD
Jenny Wright, MD

The evaluation of an adult patient should be expanded for a geriatric patient to include a comprehensive geriatric assessment (CGA). In addition to updating the basic medical database, it is important to assess functional status and cognitive function and to evaluate for common conditions associated with aging, including hearing and vision loss, urinary incontinence, and falls. Benefits of the CGA and subsequent interventions include improved functional status and quality of life in frail elderly patients and, possibly, reduced mortality. Barriers to completion of the CGA include the time required to complete it and lack of support from a multidisciplinary team to act on the findings.

Medical Database

Geriatric patients often have multiple medical problems, take many prescription and nonprescription medications, and have several providers writing their prescriptions. In addition, many medications are poorly tolerated in the geriatric population. Reducing the number of medications patients take significantly reduces the risk of drug interactions and falls; some studies show that mortality rates also are reduced. For these reasons, it is important to regularly review all prescription and nonprescription medications to check for possible drug interactions and to eliminate any unnecessary or unsafe medications. The Beers criteria are useful for identifying medications to avoid in the elderly (http://archinte.ama-assn.org/cgi/content/full/163/22/2716/TABLEIOI20821T1).

Important aspects of the social history include asking about family and community support and the frequency of social contact, obtaining the names and contact information for persons in the patient's support network, and screening for elder abuse by asking if the patient feels safe at home. If abuse is suspected in an adult who is disabled or aged >65 years, a report must be made to Adult Protective Services. The cost of medical care may be a burden to a patient; ask about this issue, and if present, consult with a medical social worker.

Undernutrition and dietary deficiencies, such as vitamin B_{12} deficiency, are more common in the elderly. Several factors can contribute to undernutrition, including decreased enjoyment of eating due to impaired sense of taste and smell, decreased access to food as a result of social isolation, and difficulty chewing due to poor dentition and age- or drug-related dry mouth.

Assessment of Functional Ability

A patient's ability to perform *basic* and *instrumental* activities of daily living (ADLs) offers insight into the patient's functional status (Table 1). Basic ADLs such as bathing, dressing, and feeding are required for self-care. A patient who is unable to perform these functions is unlikely to be able to safely live independently. Instrumental ADLs, including taking medications and grocery shopping, are activities that further enable a patient to function independently. Generally, it is not necessary to do structured ADL assessments in all older patients, particularly if a patient is well known from previous contact or it is possible to quickly determine the patient's abilities during an office visit. However, a structured assessment is useful if a change in function is noted, such as difficulty taking medications as prescribed, missing several appointments, or appearing poorly groomed. If a patient does have declining ability to perform ADLs, it is important to establish the cause and to intervene before the patient develops significant disability.

End-of-Life Wishes

Discussions about end-of-life issues that take place when a patient is medically stable and cognitively intact offer guidance for caregivers in the event of advanced or acute illness. Ask the patient who should make decisions if the patient is unable to do so, and ask about the patient's end-of-life wishes. A living will outlines wishes regarding measures for prolonging life, such as intubation and cardiac resuscitation. A health care proxy, also referred to as a durable power of attorney for health care, makes decisions for the patient if the patient is incapacitated. If a health care proxy has not been appointed, the legal next of kin is empowered to make these decisions.

Cognitive Function

The most frequently used and extensively studied screening test for assessing mental status is the Mini–Mental State Examination (MMSE). Scores <24 correlate highly with cognitive dysfunction. Many other screening instruments can be used to identify cognitive dysfunction. The Mini-Cog is a quick test that has similar accuracy to the MMSE but takes less time. Patients are asked to recall three unrelated words after drawing a clock; if they are unable to recall any of the words or can recall one or two of the words but have an abnormal clock drawing, significant cognitive dysfunction is likely (www.hospitalmedicine.org/geriresource/toolbox/mini_cog.htm; see Chapter 66).

When cognitive dysfunction is identified, further evaluation should be performed to look for causes, particularly reversible conditions. Common reversible causes of cognitive dysfunction in the elderly include thyroid disorders, vitamin B_{12} deficiency, and hyponatremia (particularly in elderly women who are taking thiazide diuretics). Early identification of patients with dementia,

Table 1. Tools to Assess Basic and Instrumental Activities of Daily Living

Tool	Functional Activities Assessed
Katz Index of Independence in Activities of Daily Living[a]	Bathing
	Dressing
	Toileting
	Transferring
	Continence
	Feeding
Lawton and Brody Instrumental Activities of Daily Living Scale[b]	Ability to use a telephone
	Shopping
	Food preparation
	Housekeeping
	Laundry
	Mode of transportation
	Responsibility for own medications
	Ability to handle finances

[a]The Katz index is scored by assigning a score of 1 to each activity if it can be completed independently, which is defined as having no supervision, direction, or personal assistance; scores are then added for a range of 0 to 6.
[b]The Lawton and Brody scale results in a score of 0 to 8, with a score of 8 representing independence and 0 representing total dependence for activities of daily living.

particularly Alzheimer disease, is important, as treatment and palliative interventions are available (see Chapter 68).

Depression

Depression increases the risk of death in elderly patients with coronary artery disease and other chronic diseases. Elderly patients also are at higher risk for suicide than younger patients. Treatment of depression can have a positive impact on the quality of life of older patients as well as their caregivers. Diagnosis may be difficult, as geriatric patients may present with somatic complaints rather than alteration in mood. In addition, symptoms may be inappropriately attributed to comorbid conditions or medication side effects. A simple screening tool for depression consists of two questions: "Over the past 2 weeks, have you felt down, depressed, or hopeless?" and "Over the past 2 weeks, have you felt little interest or pleasure in doing things?" A positive response to both questions is highly sensitive for the diagnosis of depression.

Treatment options for depression include psychotherapy and pharmacotherapy; both are efficacious in elderly patients. Selective serotonin reuptake inhibitors are considered first-line pharmacotherapy. Tricyclic antidepressants usually are avoided due to side effects, including orthostatic hypotension, urinary retention, and cognitive impairment. Antidepressant medications are started at a lower dose in elderly patients, although the ultimate therapeutic dose is unchanged (see Chapter 30).

Sensory Impairment

Vision impairment is a common problem among the elderly. As many as one third of geriatric patients have unrecognized severe vision loss, and up to 25% are wearing improper corrective lenses. The most common causes of vision impairment in older adults are presbyopia (diminished ability of the lens to accommodate), cataracts, primary open-angle glaucoma, age-related macular degeneration, and diabetic retinopathy, all of which are potentially treatable. Because vision impairment is common in the elderly, periodic Snellen visual acuity testing is reasonable. There is consensus that accurate detection of the intraocular changes of age-related macular degeneration and glaucoma is difficult in a primary care setting; therefore, periodic examination by an eye care professional is prudent for patients aged >65 years, especially patients with risk factors for these disorders.

Hearing loss affects one third of adults aged >60 years and half of those aged >85 years. Untreated hearing loss is associated with depression and decreased quality of life. The most common cause of hearing loss in the elderly is presbycusis, a sensorineural hearing loss that initially affects high-frequency hearing. The best strategy for determining a need for formal audiometric testing is a combination of self-reported hearing loss (a positive answer to the question, "Do you have trouble hearing?") and the whispered voice test, performed in sequence. The whispered voice test assesses the patient's ability to hear the whispered voice of the examiner as he or she stands behind the patient, occluding and simultaneously rubbing the patient's external auditory canal. A handheld audioscope has diagnostic accuracy characteristics similar to the whispered voice test and is an acceptable alternative screening test. Admission of hearing difficulties or the inability to repeat back most of the numbers and letters accurately during the whispered voice test is an indication for referral for audiometry.

Falls

Falls are a major medical problem in the elderly. Assessing fall risk is an essential component of the CGA (Figure 1). All geriatric patients should be screened for fall risk by asking about a history

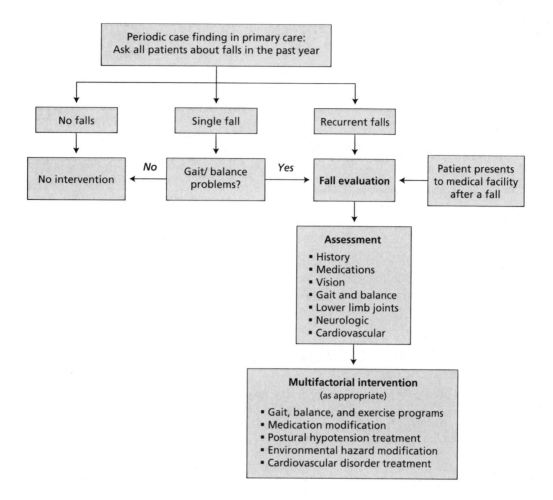

Figure 1. Assessment and management of falls. Reprinted with permission from Guideline for the prevention of falls in older persons. American Geriatrics Society, British Geriatrics Society, and American Academy of Orthopaedic Surgeons Panel on Falls Prevention. J Am Geriatr Soc. 2001;49:664-672. [PMID: 11380764] Copyright 2001 American Geriatrics Society.

of falls in the past year (a single fall is a positive test) or difficulty with gait or balance. The "Get Up and Go" test is the recommended screening test for balance and gait difficulties. Patients are timed in their ability to rise from a chair without use of their arms, walk 10 feet, turn, and then return to the chair. Most adults can complete this task in 10 seconds; most frail elderly persons take 11 to 20 seconds to complete the test. Those requiring >20 seconds need a comprehensive fall evaluation. A strong association exists between performance on this test and functional independence in ADLs.

Patients at high risk for falls should undergo a comprehensive fall evaluation, including assessment of visual acuity, medication use, basic and instrumental ADLs, and cognition; evaluation for orthostatic hypotension and gait abnormalities; and home hazard assessment. A multidisciplinary, multifactorial intervention program tailored to the patient's needs is most likely to be beneficial in preventing falls in elderly persons living in the community, reducing the relative risk of falls by as much as 20%. This type of program has multiple interventions targeting identified risk factors, including gait training by physical therapists; prescription of assistive devices and instruction in their use by occupational therapists; exercise programs, including balance training; review and

modification of medications (especially psychotropic agents); modification of home hazards; and treatment of cardiac problems, including postural hypotension. Single interventions that may be beneficial include vitamin D supplementation, muscle strengthening and balance training at home by a trained professional, home hazard assessment and modification directed by a trained professional, withdrawal of psychotropic medication, cardiac pacing for patients with carotid sinus hypersensitivity, and tai chi group exercises.

Urinary Incontinence

The incidence of urinary incontinence increases with age in both men and women. Urinary incontinence is a cause of caregiver burnout and can lead to social isolation for the patient. Patients often hesitate to report symptoms, making it important to periodically ask about them.

If incontinence is an issue, evaluation should begin by ruling out reversible causes. These are summarized by the mnemonic DIAPPERS (Delirium, Infection of the urinary tract, Atrophic urethritis/vaginitis, Pharmaceuticals, Psychological disorders [especially depression], Excessive urine output [associated with

Table 2. Types of Urinary Incontinence

Type	Notes
Urge incontinence, overactive bladder	Characteristics: daytime frequency, nocturia, bothersome urgency. Pathophysiology: involuntary contraction of the bladder, decreased control of the detrusor muscle, decreased competence of the urethral sphincter (in men). Therapy: biofeedback, bladder training, anticholinergic agents (oxybutynin, tolterodine).
Stress incontinence	Characteristics: involuntary release of urine secondary to effort or exertion (sneezing, coughing, physical exertion). Pathophysiology: pelvic muscle laxity, nerve injury (e.g., urologic surgery), poor intrinsic sphincter function. Therapy: pelvic floor muscle training (Kegel), biofeedback, electrical stimulation, open retropubic colposuspension, suburethral sling procedure.
Overflow incontinence	Characteristics: associated with overdistention of the bladder. Pathophysiology: underactive detrusor muscle or outlet obstruction. Therapy: pelvic floor muscle training with biofeedback in early postprostatectomy period, external penile clamp.
Functional incontinence	Characteristics: inability to get to the toilet in time due to impaired mobility or cognition. Therapy: regular voiding assistance, management of mobility impairment, bedside commode.

heart failure or hyperglycemia], Restricted mobility, and Stool impaction). Evaluation for reversible causes includes pelvic examination in women and prostate examination in men, in addition to urinalysis and blood chemistries.

Stress, urge, and mixed (stress plus urge) urinary incontinence are most common in women. In men, urge incontinence and incontinence as a result of prostate disease or surgery is common (Table 2). Of note, behavioral therapies, such as Kegel exercises and timed voiding, are effective for treatment of incontinence and are good initial options in frail elderly patients. The medications used to treat urge incontinence (oxybutynin, tolterodine) have anticholinergic side effects (dry mouth, constipation, confusion) that limit their utility in older patients.

Driving

All patients who drive should routinely be asked about recent accidents or moving violations. Any reported incident involving an elderly driver should trigger an assessment of the person's driving capacity. Patients with known cognitive losses, limitations in movement of the neck or extremities, cardiac arrhythmias, or a history of falls should be considered high-risk and require closer evaluation. Patients with Alzheimer dementia who continue to drive, when compared with similarly aged persons without Alzheimer dementia, have two to eight times the number of collisions.

Patients with driving concerns can be referred for a driving evaluation, either through a private group (rarely covered by insurance) or the state Department of Motor Vehicles (DMV). The American Academy of Neurology advises that patients with mild or worse dementia should be advised to stop driving. States vary in their requirements to report patients with Alzheimer disease to the DMV.

Pressure Ulcers

Risk factors for the development of pressure ulcers include increased age, limited mobility, sensory impairment, chronic illness, incontinence, vascular disease, and malnutrition. Older patients often have a combination of these risk factors. The Braden Scale for Predicting Pressure Sore Risk (www.bradenscale.com/images/bradenscale.pdf) is a tool to assess risk for pressure ulcers. Prevention requires identification of risk factors and interventions to avoid continuous pressure, friction, and shear forces on the skin, all of which lead to ulcer formation. Pressure ulcers are described by stage (Table 3), which is useful for documenting the examination findings and planning treatment. Treatment of pressure ulcers is best managed with an interdisciplinary team approach, with a care plan directed toward addressing the factors that predisposed to ulcer development. Dressings should be chosen to maintain a moist wound environment and manage exudates. When present, infec-

Table 3. Classification of Pressure Ulcers

Pressure Ulcer Stage	Description
Suspected deep tissue injury	Purple or maroon localized area of discolored, intact skin or blood-filled blister due to damage of underlying soft tissue from pressure and/or shear. May be difficult to detect in persons with dark skin tones.
Stage I	Intact skin with nonblanchable redness of a localized area, usually over a bony prominence. Darkly pigmented skin may not have visible blanching; its color may differ from the surrounding area.
Stage II	Partial-thickness loss of dermis presenting as a shallow open ulcer with a red-pink wound bed, without slough. May also present as an intact or open/ruptured serum-filled blister.
Stage III	Full-thickness tissue loss. Subcutaneous fat may be visible, but bone, tendon, or muscle is not exposed. Slough may be present but does not obscure the depth of tissue loss. May include undermining and tunneling. Depth varies by anatomic location and may be extremely deep in areas of significant adiposity.
Stage IV	Full-thickness tissue loss with exposed bone, tendon, or muscle. Slough or eschar may be present on some parts of the wound bed. Often includes undermining and tunneling.
Unstageable	Full-thickness tissue loss in which the base of the ulcer is covered by slough (yellow, tan, gray, green, or brown) and/or eschar (tan, brown, or black) in the wound bed.

Adapted with permission from National Pressure Ulcer Advisory Panel. Pressure ulcer stages revised by NPUAP. http://npuap.org/pr2.htm. Published February 2007. Accessed March 30, 2011.

tion should be controlled with topical therapies and, when cellulitis is present, systemic antibiotics. The possibility of underlying osteomyelitis should be considered. Surgical or nonsurgical debridement of eschars and nonviable tissue may be needed. Protective creams or solid barrier dressings should be used to protect the skin surrounding the wound. Air-fluidized beds are likely to improve healing compared with other pressure-relief devices, although they make it harder for patients to get into and out of bed independently.

Book Enhancement

Go to www.acponline.org/essentials/general-internal-medicine-section.html. In *MKSAP for Students 5*, assess your knowledge with items 67-72 in the **General Internal Medicine** section.

Acknowledgment

We would like to thank Dr. Ivonne Z. Jiménez-Velázquez, who contributed to an earlier version of this chapter.

Bibliography

Palmer RM. Geriatric assessment. Med Clin North Am. 1999;83:1503-1523, vii-viii. [PMID: 10584605]

Chapter 41

Hypertension

Thomas M. DeFer, MD

Hypertension is extremely common, is often asymptomatic for many years, and may result in serious and sometimes mortal complications. Less than one third of patients with hypertension in the U.S. have adequately controlled blood pressure. In >90% of cases, hypertension has no specific underlying cause (referred to as *essential, primary,* or *idiopathic hypertension*) and arises from diverse factors, such as environmental influences, salt sensitivity, disorders of renin, cell membrane defects, insulin resistance, and genetic effects. *Secondary hypertension* refers to hypertension that results from an identifiable structural, biochemical, or genetic defect (Table 1).

Prevention

Lifestyle modifications should be instituted in all patients at risk for hypertension or with prehypertension (Table 2). Therapeutic lifestyle changes include weight reduction to achieve a body weight that is <20% greater than ideal, dietary sodium intake ≤2400 mg (100 mmol) per day, regular exercise, and alcohol intake ≤2 oz (60 mL) per day. Dietary recommendations include fresh fruits and vegetables, low/non-fat dairy products, low saturated/ total fat, cholesterol, and sodium.

Table 1. Causes of Secondary Hypertension

Cause	Notes
Drug-induced hypertension	Possible causes include NSAIDs, amphetamines, cocaine, sympathomimetic agents (e.g., decongestants, dietary supplements), oral contraceptives, and corticosteroids.
Chronic kidney disease (see Chapter 62)	Late manifestations of kidney failure include elevated BUN, creatinine, potassium, and phosphate levels; low calcium level; and anemia. Most patients present at an earlier stage, with minimal signs and symptoms.
Renovascular disease (atherosclerotic and fibromuscular)	Characterized by onset of hypertension at a young age, especially in women (fibromuscular). Atherosclerotic disease often is associated with cigarette smoking, flash pulmonary edema, coronary artery disease, flank bruits, advanced retinopathy, elevated creatinine level (usually with bilateral renovascular disease), and an increase in creatinine level after treatment with an ACE inhibitor or ARB (ACE inhibitors or ARBs are preferred agents, if tolerated). Digital subtraction angiography is the diagnostic gold standard. Renal revascularization is indicated for most patients with fibromuscular dysplasia, but benefit is less clear with atherosclerotic stenosis.
Aortic coarctation	Characterized by headache, cold feet, leg pain, reduced or absent femoral pulse, delay in femoral compared with radial pulse, murmur (continuous systolic and diastolic) heard between the scapulae, and three sign on chest radiography.
Hypercalcemia (see Chapter 65)	Primary hyperparathyroidism is the most common cause of hypercalcemia in outpatients; 20% of patients have inappropriately normal PTH levels.
Thyroid disease (see Chapter 12)	Hyperthyroidism is characterized by sweating, tachycardia, weight loss, tremor, and hyperreflexia. Hypothyroidism is characterized by cold intolerance, weight gain, goiter, and slowed reflexes.
Primary hyperaldosteronism (see Chapter 13)	Characterized by muscle cramping, nocturia, thirst, and hypokalemia. Physical examination is normal.
Cushing syndrome (see Chapter 13)	Characterized by weight gain, menstrual irregularity, hirsutism, truncal obesity, abdominal striae, hypokalemia, metabolic alkalosis, and elevated urine or blood cortisol levels.
Pheochromocytoma (see Chapter 13)	Characterized by sweating, heart racing, pounding headache, pallor, tachycardia, and elevated urine or plasma levels of catecholamines or metanephrine. Hypertension may be worsened during secretion or episodic, with intervals of normal blood pressure.
Obstructive sleep apnea (see Chapter 85)	Characterized by daytime sleepiness, snoring, nonrestorative sleep, gasping or choking at night, witnessed apnea, morning headaches, obesity, large neck circumference, and crowded oropharyngeal airway. Diagnosis is established with polysomnography. Treatment with positive airway pressure may decrease blood pressure modestly in some patients.

ARB = angiotensin receptor blocker; BUN = blood urea nitrogen; PTH = parathyroid hormone.

Table 2. Classification of Blood Pressure in Adults

Classification	SBP (mm Hg)		DBP (mm Hg)
Normal	<120	*and*	<80
Prehypertension	120-139	*or*	80-89
Stage 1 hypertension	140-159	*or*	90-99
Stage 2 hypertension	≥160	*or*	≥100

DBP = diastolic blood pressure; SBP = systolic blood pressure.

Screening

Early detection of hypertension is essential in reducing the risk of stroke, coronary artery disease (CAD), peripheral vascular disease, chronic kidney disease, and retinopathy. Screen all patients at every office visit by performing office sphygmomanometry using an appropriately sized cuff and proper technique.

Diagnosis

The diagnosis of hypertension is established by a documented systolic blood pressure ≥140 mm Hg and/or diastolic blood pressure ≥90 mm Hg, based on the average of two or more readings obtained on each of two or more office visits. Hypertension also can be diagnosed on the basis of an elevated systolic blood pressure and a normal diastolic blood pressure (referred to as *isolated systolic hypertension*).

Ambulatory blood pressure monitoring should be performed if the diagnosis is uncertain or if white coat hypertension (elevated blood pressure only in the office) is suspected, self-recorded measurements are not sufficiently valid for making treatment decisions. Conversely, patients who are normotensive by in-office readings may meet criteria for hypertension by ambulatory monitoring—a phenomenon referred to as *masked hypertension*. Data suggest that masked hypertension is associated with increased cardiovascular risk; however, reasonable screening strategies for masked hypertension have not been defined.

Cardiovascular risk correlates directly with blood pressure level and, beginning at 115/75 mm Hg, doubles with each increment of 20/10 mm Hg. In persons aged >50 years, systolic blood pressure ≥140 mm Hg is a much more important cardiovascular risk factor than elevated diastolic blood pressure. The risk from hypertension is compounded by each additional risk factor for cardiovascular disease. All patients should be assessed for cardiovascular risk factors, which include smoking, obesity, physical inactivity, dyslipidemia, diabetes mellitus, microalbuminuria or estimated glomerular filtration rate (GFR) <60 mL/min/1.73 m^2, increased age, and family history of premature cardiovascular disease.

The history and physical examination can help to determine the likelihood of secondary hypertension (Table 1) and to assess for evidence of target organ damage. A history of myocardial infarction, angina, heart failure, stroke, transient ischemic attack, kidney disease, or claudication. Relevant physical findings include retinopathy; cardiac signs consistent with ischemia, infarction, or heart failure; bruits; neurologic signs consistent with stroke; and diminished or absent peripheral pulses.

Obtain the following studies in all patients: hematocrit, glucose, creatinine, electrolytes, urinalysis, fasting lipid profile, and electrocardiography. The presence of blood or protein in the urine may indicate kidney damage or suggest secondary hypertension. The urine albumin-creatinine ratio also can be used to guide treatment. An electrocardiogram showing left ventricular hypertrophy and/or signs of previous infarction is evidence of cardiovascular damage. Although echocardiography is more sensitive in diagnosing ventricular hypertrophy, it is not recommended in all patients. Specific laboratory tests usually are needed to confirm the presence of secondary hypertension suspected from the history or physical examination.

Some patients present with severely elevated blood pressure. *Hypertensive emergency* is defined as markedly elevated blood pressure (≥180/120 mm Hg) combined with symptoms or signs of end organ damage, such as encephalopathy, papilledema, retinal hemorrhages or exudates, stroke, myocardial ischemia or infarction, aortic dissection, pulmonary edema, or acute kidney injury. *Hypertensive urgency* is a severe elevation in blood pressure without acute end organ damage.

Hypertension is relatively common in pregnancy. *Gestational hypertension* is defined as ≥140/90 mm Hg on two occasions at least 6 hours apart in a previously normotensive woman presenting at >20 weeks' gestation. Hypertension arising at <20 weeks' gestation is considered evidence of previously undiagnosed chronic hypertension. The addition of proteinuria defines preeclampsia; therefore, the urine protein-creatinine ratio should be measured in all hypertensive pregnant women. Elevated blood pressure that persists beyond 12 weeks postpartum should be considered chronic hypertension. Severe gestational hypertension (blood pressure ≥160/100 mm Hg) and preeclampsia are associated with increased perinatal and maternal morbidity and mortality.

Therapy

Therapeutic lifestyle changes should be instituted in all patients with hypertension and prehypertension and should be continued even if drug therapy becomes necessary. Institute lifestyle interventions for 6 to 12 months as the sole therapy for patients with stage 1 hypertension without target organ damage or evidence of cardiovascular disease. Drug therapy is appropriate for stage 1 hypertension when therapeutic lifestyle changes have failed and is initiated immediately in conjunction with lifestyle changes for stage 2 hypertension. Modifiable risk factors should be treated. Although relieving stress may lower blood pressure, no controlled trials have shown persistent effects.

Initial drug therapy is dictated by the degree of hypertension, level of cardiovascular risk, specific patient factors, and compelling indications. The treatment goal for most patients is a blood pressure <140/90 mm Hg; for patients with diabetes or nondiabetic proteinuric (protein excretion ≥1 g/day) chronic kidney disease, the goal is <130/80 mm Hg. Hypertension, including isolated systolic hypertension, in the elderly is treated according to the usual guidelines. Older patients experience greater stroke benefit from antihypertensive drug therapy.

Thiazide diuretics, ACE inhibitors, angiotensin receptor blockers (ARBs), and calcium channel blockers all may be considered for initial treatment of hypertension, and all reduce the complications of hypertension. Thiazide diuretics are the drugs of first choice for most patients but particularly for black patients and elderly patients, as these two groups have a greater tendency to be sodium sensitive. Chlorthalidone is preferred over hydrochlorothiazide, because its use has been associated with improved cardiovascular outcomes in major clinical trials. Calcium channel blockers also are relatively more effective in these patient groups. Diuretics equalize the response of black patients to ACE inhibitors and ARBs. Loop diuretics are preferred for patients with chronic kidney disease and a serum creatinine level >1.5 mg/dL (132.6 μmol/L) or GFR <30-50 mL/min/1.73 m². Short-acting loop diuretics (e.g., furosemide) must be given more than once daily. Thiazide diuretics are much more likely than loop diuretics to cause significant hyponatremia, particularly in elderly women. ACE inhibitors and ARBs are similarly efficacious, but ARBs are less likely to cause cough.

Without compelling indications (discussed later), β-blockers are no longer considered first-line treatment, particularly in older patients, due to the lack of data supporting an independent effect on morbidity and mortality. The vasodilating β-blockers (e.g., carvedilol, nebivolol) may be preferable to more conventional β-blockers (e.g., propranolol, atenolol), which have been associated with an increased rate of stroke and risk of developing diabetes. Vasodilating β-blockers appear to have more favorable hemodynamic and endothelial effects, less deleterious metabolic effects, and better tolerability and adherence. α-Blockers are not as effective as diuretics and should not be used as monotherapy for hypertension. Direct renin inhibitors (e.g., aliskiren) are new agents that effectively lower blood pressure but lack outcome data. Aliskiren should not be used as first-line therapy, but it may be tried in patients who do not respond to or are intolerant of clearly evidence-based therapies.

Two or three antihypertensive agents often are needed to reach target blood pressure levels. Typically, a single agent decreases systolic blood pressure by 12 to 15 mm Hg and diastolic blood pressure by 8 to 10 mm Hg. Therefore, in patients with untreated stage 2 hypertension, drug therapy should be initiated with a combination of antihypertensive medications. Combined therapy with ACE inhibitors and ARBs is associated with increased adverse effects and no improvement in outcome and is not recommended.

Compelling indications for certain antihypertensive agents include CAD, heart failure, stroke, diabetes, and chronic kidney disease, particularly with proteinuria (Table 3). In these instances, the preferred agents are used first and continued regardless of whether additional agents are needed to control blood pressure.

In patients with hypertension and CAD, β-blockers are the drugs of choice, because they decrease cardiovascular mortality. Vasodilating β-blockers improve survival in patients with heart failure. The presence of asthma or chronic bronchitis may limit the use of β-blockers. ACE inhibitors are preferred for asymptomatic ventricular dysfunction and symptomatic heart failure, because they decrease cardiovascular mortality. Compared with β-blockers, ARBs may be specifically beneficial in patients with left ventricular hypertrophy. ARBs also may reduce the risk of developing diabetes in patients with impaired glucose tolerance and cardiovascular risk factors or established cardiovascular disease. Combination ACE inhibitor and thiazide diuretic therapy reduces recurrent stroke rates. ACE inhibitors and ARBs reduce albuminuria and the progression of chronic kidney disease, including diabetic nephropathy. ACE inhibitors produce greater reductions in cardiac morbidity and mortality compared with calcium channel blockers. An increase of up to 33% in serum creatinine is acceptable and not a reason to discontinue ACE inhibitor therapy; however, hyperkalemia may limit use of ACE inhibitors.

Hypertensive emergencies are treated in the hospital setting with parenteral medications and intensive care unit monitoring. Nitroprusside is the agent of choice for most patients but can cause cyanide toxicity at high doses or with prolonged use (>24-48 hours). Other potentially useful intravenous drugs are nitroglycerine, labetalol, nicardipine, and fenoldopam. Overly aggressive blood pressure lowering (i.e., to a diastolic pressure <100-110 mm Hg within 2-6 hours) is undesirable and may result in ischemic injury due to autoregulatory changes. Caution in this regard is particularly advisable during the first 24 hours after a stroke, unless thrombolytic therapy is being considered. There are exceptions as well, including aortic dissection, for which aggressive blood pressure lowering (i.e., to a systolic pressure <100-120 mm Hg) is indicated.

Parenteral drugs are avoided in hypertensive urgency, unless symptoms or progressive target organ damage is present. Initial treatment is with one or more rapid-onset oral antihypertensive drugs (e.g., clonidine or a long-acting calcium channel blocker), followed by a longer-acting formulation once blood pressure is <180/110 mm Hg. Blood pressure is rechecked within 48 hours. Avoid short-acting calcium channel blockers in patients with ischemic heart disease, because reflex adrenergic stimulation and tachycardia may lead to myocardial ischemia.

Mild gestational hypertension often is managed expectantly with frequent antepartum visits. Typical lifestyle modifications (weight loss, sodium restriction) are inappropriate. The efficacy of bed rest is unclear. Severe gestational hypertension typically is treated with antihypertensive agents. Methyldopa, labetalol, and sustained-release nifedipine generally are recommended in pregnancy. The use of thiazide diuretics is controversial, because the resultant volume depletion is undesirable. ACE inhibitors, ARBs, and direct renin inhibitors are contraindicated. Patients must be monitored frequently for progression to preeclampsia. Patients with preeclampsia, particularly if severe, are best referred to a high-risk obstetrician. When urgent blood pressure lowering is required, intravenous labetalol, hydralazine, and nicardipine can be used. Nitroprusside generally is contraindicated in pregnancy. The cure for gestational hypertension is delivery.

Table 3. Antihypertensive Drugs: Compelling Indications, Contraindications, and Side Effects

Drug Class	Compelling Indications	Contraindications	Side Effects
Diuretics	Heart failure, advanced age, systolic hypertension	Gout	Hypokalemia, hyperuricemia, glucose intolerance, hypercalcemia, hyperlipidemia, hyponatremia, impotence
β-Blockers	Angina, heart failure, post-MI, tachyarrhythmia, migraine	Asthma, COPD, heart block	Bronchospasm, bradycardia, heart failure, impaired peripheral circulation, insomnia, fatigue, decreased exercise tolerance, hypertriglyceridemia
ACE inhibitors	Heart failure, left ventricular dysfunction, post-MI, diabetic nephropathy, proteinuria	Pregnancy, bilateral renal artery stenosis, hyperkalemia	Cough, angioedema, hyperkalemia, rash, loss of taste, leukopenia
Angiotensin receptor blockers	ACE inhibitor cough, diabetic nephropathy, heart failure	Pregnancy, bilateral renal artery stenosis, hyperkalemia	Angioedema (rare), hyperkalemia
Calcium channel blockers	Advanced age, systolic hypertension, cyclosporine-induced hypertension, angina, coronary heart disease	Heart block (verapamil, diltiazem)	Headache, flushing, gingival hyperplasia, edema, constipation
α-Blockers	Prostatic hypertrophy	Orthostatic hypotension	Headache, drowsiness, fatigue, weakness, postural hypotension

MI = myocardial infarction.

Follow-Up

Follow-up should be individualized. Uncontrolled hypertension requires more vigilant follow-up, at least monthly, until control is achieved. Consider regular home blood pressure monitoring in select patients. Patients should be questioned about medication side effects. At follow-up, if there has been a partial response to a submaximal dose of the initial agent, the dose should be maximized. A second drug from a different class may be added if there is a partial response to an otherwise well-tolerated initial agent. If not used first, a thiazide diuretic should be used as the second agent, because it provides augmentation to almost any other antihypertensive agent used as monotherapy. If a diuretic was the first agent, an ACE inhibitor, an ARB, or a calcium channel blocker should be added. A third or fourth agent can be added if the target blood pressure has not been reached. β-Blockers are reasonable to add as a third or fourth agent when maximal doses of more preferred drugs are insufficient.

Resistant hypertension is blood pressure that is not at target level despite maximal doses of three antihypertensive agents, one being a diuretic. Important causes include medication nonadherence, inadequate therapy, excessive alcohol consumption, and other drugs (e.g., NSAIDs, sympathomimetic agents). White coat hypertension also may contribute to the apparent occurrence of refractory hypertension; ambulatory blood pressure monitoring is useful if this is suspected. Treatment strategies include addressing potential reasons for resistance. If a typical β-blocker is being used, changing to a vasodilating β-blocker may be helpful. Aldosterone antagonists (spironolactone, eplerenone) are potentially effective additions for resistant hypertension, even in the absence of hyperaldosteronism. The addition of hydralazine or clonidine may be necessary in a few patients. Evaluation for secondary hypertension is indicated when the clinical situation is suggestive or a patient is adherent to a four-drug regimen without adequate control.

Only half of patients who start therapy remain on therapy after 1 year. Using once daily therapy, maintaining close contact with patients, encouraging home blood pressure monitoring, and using drugs with fewer adverse effects and lower cost may improve adherence. A simple question to assess adherence in a nonthreatening and nonjudgmental manner is, "Most people have trouble remembering to take their medicine. Do you have trouble remembering to take yours?"

Book Enhancement

Go to www.acponline.org/essentials/general-internal-medicine-section.html. In *MKSAP for Students 5*, assess your knowledge with items 73-78 in the **General Internal Medicine** section.

Bibliography

ALLHAT Officers and Coordinators for the ALLHAT Collaborative Research Group. The Antihypertensive and Lipid-Lowering Treatment to Prevent Heart Attack Trial. Major outcomes in high-risk hypertensive patients randomized to angiotensin-converting enzyme inhibitor or calcium channel blocker vs diuretic: The Antihypertensive and Lipid-Lowering Treatment to Prevent Heart Attack Trial (ALLHAT) [published errata appear in JAMA. 2003;289:178 and 2004;291:2196]. JAMA. 2002;288:2981-2997. [PMID: 12479763]

Chapter 42

Anemia

Reed E. Drews, MD

Anemia is commonly encountered in clinical practice. Often identified incidentally in asymptomatic patients, anemia can be benign or related to serious underlying disease. The differential diagnosis is wide and includes congenital and acquired disorders. A structured approach is used to distinguish among the many causes of anemia and to determine management. This approach considers red cell morphology alongside other clinical and laboratory findings.

Because the life span of normal erythrocytes approaches 120 days, nearly 1% of circulating erythrocytes must be replenished daily to maintain a normal hematocrit. Normal hematopoiesis, as well as heightened production during bleeding or hemolysis, requires a healthy bone marrow microenvironment, healthy hematopoietic stem cells, ample endogenous growth factors (e.g., erythropoietin, thyroid hormone, and testosterone in the case of males), and ample and usable body stores of iron, folate, and cobalamin.

Defining Anemia

Anemia is defined as a reduction below normal in the number of erythrocytes in the circulation. Men have higher mean hematocrit and hemoglobin values than women, largely due to testosterone production in men and borderline iron stores in menstruating women. Hematocrit and hemoglobin levels have wide normal ranges, and changes in plasma volume can influence these measurements considerably, either by hemodilution or hemoconcentration. For example, in pregnant women, red blood cell mass rises; however, plasma volume increases to a greater extent. Pregnant women therefore develop lower hematocrit and hemoglobin levels (physiologic anemia). The World Health Organization defines anemia as a hemoglobin level <13 g/dL (130 g/L) in men and <12 g/dL (120 g/L) in women.

Measuring Anemia

Automated multichannel analyzers directly assess the erythrocyte count, mean corpuscular volume (MCV), red cell distribution width (the degree of variation in erythrocyte size), and hemoglobin level (the concentration of hemoglobin in whole blood after lysing erythrocytes) while calculating hematocrit, mean corpuscular hemoglobin, and mean corpuscular hemoglobin concentration (MCHC) from these measurements. Automated analyzers may

Table 1. Peripheral Blood Smear Findings and Associated Conditions

Finding	Association
Acanthocytes (erythrocytes with a small number of spicules of variable size and distribution on the cell surface)	Liver disease
Bite cells (erythrocytes with a nonstaining, clear zone)	Oxidative hemolysis, which may be due to unstable hemoglobins or potent oxidants (with or without G6PD or pyruvate kinase deficiency)
Echinocytes (erythrocytes with a small number of spicules of uniform size and distribution on the cell surface)	End-stage kidney disease
Hypochromia (increase in central pallor of erythrocytes), anisocytosis, poikilocytosis	Iron deficiency anemia
Intraerythrocytic parasites (e.g., *Plasmodium*, *Babesia*)	Hemolytic anemia
Rouleaux formation ("stacked-coins" appearance of erythrocytes)	Monoclonal protein, cold agglutinin, or increased fibrinogen (as in acute phase reaction)
Schistocytes (irregularly shaped, jagged fragments of erythrocytes)	Fragmentation hemolysis, as in micro- or macroangiopathic hemolytic anemia (e.g., DIC, TTP, malfunctioning native or prosthetic heart valve)
Sickle cells (spindle- or crescent-shaped erythrocytes)	Sickle cell anemia
Small target cells (erythrocytes with area of central density surrounded by pallor and then a rim of density), teardrop cells (cells with round main body part and an elongated end), and basophilic stippling (cells with blue granules in the cytoplasm)	Thalassemia
Spherocytes (small, round erythrocytes that are uniformly dense)	Membrane loss (as in hereditary spherocytosis, immune hemolytic anemia) without central pallor
Teardrop cells, nucleated erythrocytes, and immature myeloid forms	Myelophthisic anemia (also known as leukoerythroblastosis)

DIC = disseminated intravascular coagulation; G6PD = glucose-6-phosphate dehydrogenase; TTP = thrombotic thrombocytopenic purpura.

yield spurious findings in certain clinical circumstances (e.g., high leukocyte counts, lipemia, precipitating monoclonal proteins, cold agglutinins, hyperglycemia), and this should be suspected when measured hemoglobin levels do not approximate one third of the calculated hematocrit value.

Clinicians should evaluate erythrocyte measurements alongside leukocyte counts, platelet counts, and leukocyte differential counts. Abnormalities in these other blood cell lines may suggest a disorder of trilineage hematopoiesis. Reticulocyte counts suggest whether or not the bone marrow responses to anemia are adequate. Appropriately increased reticulocyte counts (i.e., >100,000/μL [100×10^9/L]) almost always reflect either erythrocyte loss (e.g., bleeding, hemolysis) or response to appropriate therapy (e.g., iron, folate, vitamin B_{12}). A lower than expected reticulocyte count indicates erythrocyte underproduction, including anemia due to deficient erythropoietin, nutritional deficiencies (e.g., iron, folate, vitamin B_{12}), inflammatory block, or a primary hematopoietic disorder (e.g., red blood cell aplasia, myelodysplasia). Examination of the peripheral blood smear for morphologic features of erythrocytes, leukocytes, and platelets may provide important clues to the cause of anemia (Table 1). Results of various blood chemistry tests (Table 2) help to refine or confirm diagnostic considerations suggested by the complete blood count (CBC), reticulocyte count, and peripheral blood smear.

Reticulocyte counts are determined using the same automated multichannel technologies used to obtain CBCs. By microscopic examination of Wright-Giemsa–stained peripheral blood smears, reticulocytes appear larger than more senescent erythrocytes and somewhat purple (polychromatophilic) due to increased ribonucleoprotein and nucleic acid content from the extruded erythrocyte nucleus. Reticulocyte counts are expressed as percentages; methods for interpreting reticulocyte counts are summarized in Table 3. The author prefers assessing absolute reticulocyte counts, because patients with anemia who have healthy bone marrow microenvironments, healthy hematopoietic stem cells, ample endogenous growth factors, and ample and usable body stores of iron and vitamins should have appropriately increased absolute reticulocyte counts (i.e., >100,000/μL [100×10^9/L]).

Diagnosis

Anemia due to erythrocyte underproduction generally develops and progresses slowly over weeks to months. In contrast, anemia due to bleeding or hemolysis generally occurs rapidly over days to weeks. Because anemia may be hereditary rather than acquired, knowledge of a family history of anemia is useful when considering congenital and acquired causes of anemia as well as acquired contributors to worsened congenital anemia (e.g., thalassemia).

Although symptoms and signs can offer important clues to the cause of anemia, physical examination often is normal or nonspecific. The history and physical examination are supplemented by a consideration of anemia categorized by erythrocyte size (i.e., microcytic [MCV <80 fL], normocytic [MCV 80-100 fL], or macrocytic [MCV >100 fL]) and other morphologic abnormalities. When routine laboratory test results, history, and physical examination fail to adequately explain the cause of anemia, bone marrow aspiration and biopsy help to evaluate disorders of marrow microenvironment (e.g., infiltrative myelopathies from fibrosis, cancer metastasis, or infection), disorders of myeloid maturation (e.g., leukemias, myelodysplastic syndromes), or aplasia.

Table 2. Laboratory Tests in Anemia Evaluation

Test(s)	Notes
Absolute reticulocyte count[a]	Values >100,000/μL (100×10^9/L) signify increased erythropoiesis and a shift in reticulocyte pool from bone marrow to peripheral blood; compatible with bleeding, hemolysis, or response to treatment.
Serum folate and vitamin B_{12} levels	Used to assess possible folate or vitamin B_{12} deficiency.
Serum iron, total iron-binding capacity (TIBC), and ferritin	Low serum iron and high TIBC (iron/TIBC <10%-15%) characterize iron deficiency without inflammation (low ferritin). Low serum iron and low TIBC characterize anemia of inflammation (normal to high ferritin). Caveat: 20% of patients with "anemia of inflammation" have iron/TIBC <10%.
Serum transferrin receptor concentration	Elevated in the setting of increased erythropoiesis or iron deficiency. If hemolysis or ineffective erythropoiesis is excluded, an elevated serum transferrin receptor concentration suggests iron deficiency.
ESR, CRP fibrinogen and haptoglobin	Increased levels indicate acute phase reaction due to inflammatory cytokines, which decrease erythropoietin production, decrease responsiveness to erythropoietin, and block iron transport.
Serum creatinine	High levels signify underproduction of erythropoietin, which is manufactured primarily by the kidneys.
Erythropoietin	Should rise logarithmically above normal levels in relation to decreasing hematocrit. Levels >500 mU/mL (500 U/L) predict poor response to recombinant erythropoietin administration.
Thyroid-stimulating hormone	Used to assess possible hypothyroidism, which may cause anemia.
Serum testosterone	Used to assess possible hypotestosteronism in men, which may cause anemia.
Serum lactate dehydrogenase (LDH), bilirubin, and haptoglobin	Haptoglobin levels <20 mg/dL (200 mg/L) indicate hemolysis, supported by elevated LDH and total bilirubin levels.
Urine hemosiderin and hemoglobin	Presence supports intravascular hemolysis.
SPEP, UPEP, and quantitative immunoglobulins	Hypogammaglobulinemia, positive serum monoclonal proteins, and urine free kappa or lambda light chains suggest possible plasma cell myeloma or lymphoma.

ESR = erythrocyte sedimentation rate; CRP = C-reactive protein; SPEP = serum protein electrophoresis; UPEP = urine protein electrophoresis.
[a]Absolute reticulocyte count = (erythrocyte count × reticulocyte count)/100, where erythrocyte count is expressed as n × 10^6/μL.

Table 3. Interpreting the Reticulocyte Count

Method of Interpretation	Calculation	Notes
Corrected reticulocyte count	reticulocyte percentage × (observed HCT/expected HCT)	Corrects for degree of anemia.
Reticulocyte production index (RPI)	reticulocyte percentage/correction factor	Corrects for shortened reticulocyte maturation time as anemia worsens.
		• HCT = 40-45; correction factor = 1.0
		• HCT = 35-39; correction factor = 1.5
		• HCT = 25-34; correction factor = 2.0
		• HCT = 15-24; correction factor = 2.5
		• HCT <15; correction factor = 3.0
		• RPI value <2 implies inadequate bone marrow response.
Absolute reticulocyte count	(erythrocyte count × reticulocyte count)/100 where erythrocyte count is expressed as n × 10^6/μL.	In steady state conditions, absolute reticulocyte count is 25,000-75,000/μL (25-75 × 10^9/L). Values >75,000-100,000/μL (75-100 × 10^9/L) imply stress erythropoiesis.

HCT = hematocrit.

Microcytic Anemia

Factors to consider in the differential diagnosis of microcytic anemia include a reduction in iron availability, globin chain production, and/or heme synthesis (Table 4); deficiency in one or more of these will result in hypochromic, often microcytic, anemia. Severe iron deficiency and inflammation reduce iron availability. Reduced globin production characterizes the thalassemias and other hemoglobinopathies. Certain toxins (e.g., alcohol, lead) and drugs (e.g., chloramphenicol, isoniazid) reduce heme synthesis. Decreased heme synthesis also is a characteristic of the congenital and acquired idiopathic sideroblastic anemias.

Iron Deficiency

The most common cause of microcytic anemia is iron deficiency, usually related to menstrual or gastrointestinal blood loss or mal-

absorption syndromes. Hypochromia (decreased MCHC) is the first morphologic sign of iron deficiency, followed by microcytosis (decreased MCV). As hemoglobin levels decline, erythrocytes become heterogeneous in size and shape (anisocytosis, poikilocytosis; Plate 36). Pica (a craving for ice or other unusual substances, such as clay or cornstarch) is a symptom of iron deficiency and quickly disappears with iron replacement. In men and postmenopausal women with iron deficiency, evaluation of the gastrointestinal tract for a source of blood loss is mandatory. In premenopausal women, evaluation also includes gynecologic examination. Chronic intravascular hemolysis with loss of iron in the urine is an uncommon cause of iron deficiency. Partial or total gastrectomy leads to decreased production of hydrochloric acid and diminished iron absorption. Celiac disease results in malabsorption of iron by the duodenum.

Table 4. Differential Diagnosis of Microcytic Anemia

Disorder	Notes
Iron deficiency anemia	Anemia with hypochromia, microcytosis, and increased RDW. Usually due to menstrual or GI blood loss; less commonly due to celiac disease or chronic intravascular hemolysis. Serum ferritin concentration and transferrin saturation usually are low; soluble transferrin receptor concentration usually is increased. Search for a source of chronic blood loss.
α-Thalassemia trait	Mild anemia with normal RDW due to homozygous single α-globin gene deletion or heterozygous double α-globin gene deletion. Seen in persons of African, Mediterranean, Middle Eastern, or Southeast Asian ancestry. Serum ferritin concentration and transferrin saturation are normal. Hemoglobin electrophoresis shows a normal percentage of hemoglobin A_2 and hemoglobin F. Usually a diagnosis of exclusion.
β-Thalassemia trait	Mild anemia with normal RDW due to reduced expression of β-globin gene. Seen in persons of African, Mediterranean, Middle Eastern, or Southeast Asian ancestry. Serum ferritin concentration and transferrin saturation are normal. Hemoglobin electrophoresis shows an increased percentage of hemoglobin A_2 (3.6%-8%) and a normal to slightly increased percentage of hemoglobin F (1%-3%).
β-Thalassemia intermedia	Hemoglobin levels are 7-10 g/dL (70-100 g/L) due to reduced but not absent expression of both β-globin genes. Typically, there is evidence of ineffective erythropoiesis, with a low serum haptoglobin and increased levels of indirect bilirubin and LDH in the setting of a normal reticulocyte count and increased iron stores. Serum ferritin concentration and transferrin saturation are increased. Hemoglobin electrophoresis shows an increased percentage of hemoglobin A_2 (5.4%-10%) and hemoglobin F (20%-80%).
Sickle cell–β-thalassemia	Seen in persons of African, Middle Eastern, Mediterranean, or Indian ancestry. Serum ferritin and transferrin saturation usually are normal. Hemoglobin electrophoresis shows predominantly hemoglobin S but also variable amounts of hemoglobin A (5%-30%), an increased percentage of hemoglobin A_2 (>3.5%), and a normal to variably increased percentage of hemoglobin F (2%-10%).

GI = gastrointestinal; LDH = lactate dehydrogenase; RDW = red cell distribution width.

Serum ferritin levels are the most useful test in the diagnosis of iron deficiency. However, because ferritin is an acute phase reactant, it has less diagnostic value in patients with an infection or inflammatory disorder. Virtually all patients with serum ferritin levels <10-15 ng/mL (10-15 µg/L) are iron deficient. However, 25% of menstruating women with absent stainable bone marrow iron have ferritin levels >15 ng/mL (15 µg/L). Assuming absence of inflammation, higher ferritin cutoff limits of 30-41 ng/mL (30-41 µg/L) improve diagnostic efficiency. In the presence of inflammation, the serum concentration of soluble transferrin receptor (sTfR)—a truncated fragment of the membrane receptor that is increased in iron deficiency when availability of iron for erythropoiesis is low—is not significantly different from normal. Therefore, the ratio of sTfR to log ferritin may be used to distinguish anemia of inflammation (ratio <1) from iron deficiency anemia either alone or in combination with anemia of inflammation (ratio >2).

The treatment of choice for iron deficiency almost always is an oral iron preparation. Iron salts (e.g., ferrous sulfate) are preferred over iron polysaccharide complexes. Ascorbic acid enhances absorption of iron, whereas certain dietary substances, calcium, and inhibitors of gastric acid secretion decrease iron absorption. Treatment should be continued for 6 months to 1 year until hemoglobin levels and iron stores return to normal. Indications for parenteral iron therapy include (1) inability to tolerate oral iron compounds, (2) inability to absorb oral iron, (3) repeated failure to adhere to a regular schedule of oral iron administration, (4) circumstances when iron (blood) loss exceeds oral iron replacement and/or when oral iron exacerbates symptoms of the underlying disease (e.g., inflammatory bowel disease), (5) autologous blood donation, and (6) hemodialysis.

Anemia of Inflammation

Inflammatory cytokines block iron utilization, yielding low serum iron and total iron-binding capacity levels and high serum ferritin levels. Cytokines increase serum ferritin levels by as much as threefold. Hence, serum ferritin levels <100 ng/mL (100 µg/L) may reflect iron deficiency in patients with inflammatory states. Reticulocyte counts are inappropriately low for the degree of anemia. Bone marrow biopsies generally are not indicated unless competing causes of anemia are suspected (e.g., pure red cell aplasia, sideroblastic anemia, other myelodysplastic syndromes).

The management of anemia of inflammation is treatment of the underlying inflammatory condition. When symptomatic anemia persists despite treatment of the chronic condition (e.g., rheumatoid arthritis), administration of recombinant human erythropoietin can improve anemia and diminish the need for erythrocyte transfusion.

Thalassemia

Thalassemias are congenital disorders involving imbalanced globin chain production or abnormal globin chain synthesis. Microcytic hypochromic erythrocytes in thalassemic states are accompanied by target cells (Plate 37), teardrop cells, and basophilic stippling. In contrast to patients with iron deficiency, who have low erythrocyte counts and mildly to moderately decreased MCV values, patients with thalassemia often have normal to high-normal erythrocyte counts with strikingly low MCV values. Although patients with thalassemia trait can develop iron deficiency, this is less likely among patients with severe thalassemia, where iron overload is a concern, particularly in patients who have had frequent blood transfusions.

Folic acid supplementation is a supportive therapy in all patients with thalassemia. However, other treatments vary according to the severity of the thalassemia. Patients with thalassemia trait do not require specific therapy. Patients with more severe thalassemia often require blood transfusions to maintain growth, manage symptomatic anemia, and prevent complications of extramedullary hematopoiesis. Iron chelation therapy prevents and manages iron overload. Hydroxyurea may benefit patients with β-thalassemia intermedia. Hematopoietic stem cell transplantation is an established treatment for severe β-thalassemia.

Macrocytic Anemia

First assess the reticulocyte count and rule out stress erythropoiesis (e.g., from bleeding or hemolysis). Reticulocytes are larger than senescent erythrocytes; consequently, increased reticulocyte numbers elevate the MCV, but generally not to levels >110-115 fL. Macrocytic anemia may be megaloblastic or nonmegaloblastic (Table 5).

Table 5. Differential Diagnosis of Megaloblastic Anemia (Macrocytosis, Hypersegmented Neutrophils, Macro-ovalocytes)

Disorder	Notes
Folate deficiency	Morphologically indistinguishable from vitamin B_{12} deficiency and drug-induced megaloblastosis. Inquire about excessive alcohol use, quality of diet, and history of small-bowel disease. Obtain a serum antibody test for celiac disease (anti–tissue transglutaminase).
Vitamin B_{12} deficiency	Morphologically indistinguishable from folate deficiency. Loss of vibration or position sense favors vitamin B_{12} deficiency. However, neurologic disease due to vitamin B_{12} deficiency may occur without anemia or macrocytosis.
Drug-induced changes in erythrocytes[a]	Numerous drugs prescribed for cancer, HIV infection, psoriasis, SLE, rheumatoid arthritis, and posttransplantation immunosuppression cause macrocytic and sometimes megaloblastic changes in erythrocytes. History should be revealing.
Erythroleukemia	Erythroleukemia is a morphologic diagnosis based on bone marrow evaluation. The disorder is characterized by a normal or high serum vitamin B_{12} level. Cytogenetic abnormalities are present in about half of cases.

SLE = systemic lupus erythematosus.

[a]Go to www.acponline.org/essentials/hematology-section.html to see a list of drugs that commonly cause macrocytosis.

Hemolysis

When laboratory tests suggest hemolysis (Table 2), consider the possible causes of anemia by type (spherocytic or nonspherocytic), site (intramedullary or extramedullary, intravascular or extravascular), and mechanism (immune-mediated or non–immune-mediated, intrinsic versus extrinsic to the erythrocyte). For example, spherocytic hemolytic anemia implicates a membrane defect, either acquired (e.g., warm autoimmune hemolytic anemia) or congenital (e.g., hereditary spherocytosis). Nonspherocytic hemolytic anemias include "bite cell" hemolysis (e.g., oxidant stress) and fragmentation hemolysis (e.g., thrombotic microangiopathy). Intramedullary hemolysis is seen in various disorders associated with ineffective erythropoiesis, including thalassemia. Extramedullary hemolysis may be extravascular (e.g., hemolysis mediated by the spleen) or intravascular (e.g., hemolysis associated with cold agglutinin disease or thrombotic microangiopathy). Immune-mediated hemolysis is distinguished by the Coombs test. Hemolytic disorders "intrinsic" to the erythrocyte include membrane defects, enzymopathies, and hemoglobinopathies. Table 6 summarizes various causes of hemolytic anemia. In all cases, examining the peripheral blood smear is central to identifying erythrocyte morphologies that implicate certain mechanisms of hemolysis (Table 1).

In oxidant hemolysis, a by-product is methemoglobin, which contains ferric ions. Methemoglobin has altered spectrophotometric properties from hemoglobin, which contains ferrous ions. As a consequence, patients with methemoglobinemia have arterial PO_2 values (reflecting the total concentration of oxygen in blood) that appear higher than expected in relation to the percent oxygen saturation (which specifically reflects the percent of oxygen bound to hemoglobin).

Megaloblastic Macrocytosis

Macro-ovalocytes suggest megaloblastic maturation of erythrocytes; hypersegmented neutrophils also may be present (Plate 38). Causes (Table 5) include folate and/or vitamin B_{12} deficiency, drugs affecting folate metabolism and/or DNA synthesis, and acquired idiopathic causes of megaloblastic maturation (e.g., myelodysplastic syndromes). An MCV >115 fL almost always is due to a megaloblastic cause. Because megaloblastic causes of anemia

Table 6. Differential Diagnosis of Hemolytic Anemia

Disorder	Notes
Membrane defect (hereditary spherocytosis, hereditary elliptocytosis)	Suspect in patients with a positive family history, splenomegaly, and spherocytes or elliptocytes on blood smear. Diagnosis is confirmed by osmotic fragility and negative direct Coombs test.
Enzymopathy (G6PD deficiency, pyruvate kinase deficiency)	Common forms of G6PD deficiency usually cause only episodic moderate hemolysis, precipitated by oxidant drugs or infection. Variable blood smear findings include bite cells, spherocytes, fragments (rarely), and minimal abnormalities of erythrocytes other than polychromasia (from reticulocytosis). Common drugs and chemicals that are unsafe for use in patients with G6PD deficiency include dapsone, methylene blue, nitrofurantoin, phenazopyridine, phenylhydrazine, primaquine, sulfamethoxazole, and sulfapyridine.[a] Pyruvate kinase deficiency is rare and causes moderately severe anemia; blood smear shows acanthocytes.
Hemoglobinopathy (hemoglobin S, hemoglobin C, thalassemia, hereditary unstable hemoglobins; see Chapter 44)	Chronic or episodic hemolysis. Hemoglobin A_2 level is increased with β-thalassemia; hemoglobin F also may be increased. No structural hemoglobin abnormality is detectable with α-thalassemia; diagnosis is based on hematocrit, MCV, blood smear, and family study. Abnormal hemoglobins (e.g., E and D) are uncommon in the United States. Blood smear changes suggest certain hemoglobinopathies; hemoglobin electrophoresis reveals the abnormal hemoglobin.
Autoimmune hemolytic anemia	Spherocytes on blood smear; erythrocyte agglutination is seen with cold agglutinin disease. Diagnosis is confirmed by direct and indirect Coombs tests and cold agglutinin titer; direct Coombs test is positive for C3 in cold agglutinin disease. Most cases of warm antibody disease are drug-induced or associated with an underlying disorder (e.g., SLE, lymphoproliferative disorder). Cold agglutinin disease also is frequently associated with underlying disorders (e.g., *Mycoplasma pneumoniae* infection, SLE).
Erythrocyte fragmentation (TTP, HUS, DIC; see Chapter 45)	TTP usually presents as neurologic symptoms and severe fragmentation anemia and thrombocytopenia. With HUS (children), kidney abnormalities predominate, and anemia and thrombocytopenia are milder. In other causes of microangiopathic anemia (DIC, malignant hypertension, scleroderma renal crisis), the anemia and thrombocytopenia usually are mild to moderate; these disorders are diagnosed by peripheral blood smear in the proper clinical context.
Infection (malaria, babesiosis)	Symptoms of infection, particularly fever, usually dominate. Splenomegaly is the rule with malaria; babesiosis usually produces a milder malaria-like illness, unless patients are asplenic. Finding intraerythrocytic parasites on blood smear is diagnostic.
Hypersplenism (see Chapter 25)	Splenomegaly (any cause) can cause hemolysis; hypersplenism also may decrease the number of leukocytes, platelets, or any combination of cell lines. Hypersplenism produces no erythrocyte morphologic changes in erythrocytes, but the blood smear may show changes related to the underlying cause (e.g., target cells with liver disease).

DIC = disseminated intravascular coagulation; G6PD = glucose-6-phosphate dehydrogenase; HUS = hemolytic uremic syndrome; MCV = mean corpuscular volume; SLE = systemic lupus erythematosus; TTP = thrombotic thrombocytopenic purpura.
[a]A more complete listing of unsafe and low-risk drugs can be found at www.g6pd.org/favism/english/index.mvc.

impact trilineage hematopoiesis, leukopenia and thrombocytopenia may accompany anemia. The myelodysplastic syndromes are stem cell clonal disorders characterized by ineffective hematopoiesis and various peripheral cytopenias. When a myelodysplastic syndrome is suspected, bone marrow aspiration and biopsy assess myeloid maturation and karyotypic abnormalities by metaphase analysis and interphase fluorescence in situ hybridization (FISH). FISH uses a panel of molecular probes that detect chromosomal abnormalities seen in subsets of patients with myelodysplastic syndrome (e.g., 5q deletion, 7q deletion, 20q deletion, trisomy 8).

Patients with macrocytic anemia or specific neurologic symptoms should be screened for vitamin B_{12} deficiency. However, the MCV should not be used as the only indication to exclude vitamin B_{12} deficiency, which can be present despite a normal MCV or may be present in combination with microcytic causes of anemia (e.g., iron deficiency, thalassemia), thereby yielding a normal MCV. Concomitant iron and vitamin B_{12} deficiencies can arise due to various causes, including celiac disease. Elevated serum levels of methylmalonic acid and homocysteine support vitamin B_{12} deficiency in patients with slightly low or borderline serum vitamin B_{12} levels (200-300 pg/mL [147.6-221.4 pmol/L]). Daily oral vitamin B_{12} can be used to treat most vitamin B_{12}–deficient patients. Timed-release formulations may not reliably release their vitamin B_{12} content and should be avoided.

Nonmegaloblastic Macrocytosis

Large target cells (MCV = 105-110 fL) and echinocytes (erythrocytes with a small number of spicules of uniform size and distribution on the cell surface) signify membrane changes associated with liver disease. Diminished spleen function (hyposplenism, asplenia) yields large target cells, acanthocytes (erythyrocytes with a small number of spicules of variable size and distribution on the cell surface), Howell-Jolly bodies, and variable numbers of nucleated erythyrocytes.

Normochromic Normocytic Anemia

When the MCV is normal (80-100 fL), assessing whether it is declining or rising over time may provide clues to an evolving microcytic or macrocytic pathology. Other causes of normocytic anemia (Table 7) include underproduction of erythropoietin (e.g., kidney failure), deficiency of other growth factors (e.g., thyroid hormone, testosterone), inflammation, and marrow infiltrative myelopathies, which yield teardrop cells, nucleated erythyrocytes, and immature leukocytes. With the exception of acute blood loss, the most common cause is the anemia of inflammation. Aplastic anemia, a rare cause of normocytic normochromic anemia, usually is accompanied by severe granulocytopenia and thrombocytopenia due to deficient hematopoietic stem cells.

Table 7. Differential Diagnosis of Normocytic Anemia

Disorder	Notes
Acute blood loss	Anemia with variation in erythrocyte size (increased RDW) if iron deficiency is present. Reticulocyte count usually is increased; leukocyte count and platelet count may be slightly increased, depending on the rapidity of bleeding.
Chronic kidney disease (see Chapter 62)	Anemia with a low reticulocyte count due to impaired erythropoietin production. Renal endocrine function does not correlate with renal exocrine function.
Pure red cell aplasia	Anemia with severe reticulocytopenia. Diagnosis is made by examination of a bone marrow aspirate, in which erythroblasts will be absent or severely diminished. Red cell aplasia can be idiopathic or secondary to a thymoma, solid tumor, hematologic malignancy, collagen vascular disease, viral infection (particularly human parvovirus B19 infection, which is common in immunosuppressed patients), or drug (e.g., phenytoin, azathioprine, isoniazid, chloramphenicol, mycophenolate mofetil). Red cell aplasia also may occur in patients with hemolytic anemia from any cause.
Malignancy (solid tumor, lymphoma, myelofibrosis)	Anemia with a low reticulocyte count. With bone marrow involvement by tumor, leukoerythroblastosis and extramedullary hematopoiesis occur, and nucleated erythrocytes and myelocytes are seen in the peripheral blood. Peripheral blood smear may show rouleaux formation (if a plasma cell dyscrasia is present) or teardrop-shaped erythrocytes (if splenomegaly is present).
Alcoholic liver disease	Anemia with a low reticulocyte count. Target cells and acanthocytes also may be present. Leukocyte and platelet counts will be reduced if there is portal hypertension with splenomegaly, although thrombocytopenia in liver disease is chiefly due to underproduction of thrombopoietin by the liver.
Anemia of inflammation (chronic disease)	A normocytic (but sometimes microcytic) anemia that occurs in association with another disease. The underlying disorder usually is infectious, inflammatory, or neoplastic and is characterized by distinct abnormalities of iron metabolism: low serum iron and transferrin with reduced transferrin saturation, normal or elevated serum ferritin, and normal or increased bone marrow iron stores.
Hemolytic anemia	Anemia with an elevated reticulocyte count and spherocytes, sickle cells, bite cells, or fragmented erythrocytes. There may be hemoglobinuria. If the reticulocyte count is sufficiently elevated, the MCV may be high. The serum haptoglobin level will be low whether the hemolysis is intravascular or extravascular, and if the hemolysis is antibody-mediated, the direct Coombs test result will be positive. The essential laboratory test is the peripheral blood smear, which can distinguish between the different types of hemolysis: spherocytic hemolytic anemia, erythrocyte enzyme defect, erythrocyte fragmentation, cold agglutinin disease, hemoglobinopathy, heavy metal intoxication, and paroxysmal nocturnal hemoglobinuria. Urine hemoglobin and urine hemosiderin measurements are useful for detecting intravascular hemolysis.

ESR = erythrocyte sedimentation rate; MCV = mean corpuscular volume; RDW = red cell distribution width.

Therapy of Anemia

Appropriate treatment is dictated by the underlying cause or causes of anemia. In view of the diverse causes of anemia, each dictating specific strategies for optimal management, an in-depth review of anemia treatments is not possible here. However, a few overarching principles apply.

Always ensure intact nutritional, mineral, and vitamin stores. When anemia is due to bleeding, eliminate the source of bleeding as best as possible. When anemia relates to hemolysis, identify the cause. If hemolysis is due to a congenital hemoglobinopathy, manage accordingly (e.g., supplemental folic acid, hydroxyurea for sickle cell disease). If hemolysis is acquired, identify the cause and manage accordingly (e.g., immunosuppression for autoimmune hemolytic anemia, plasmapheresis for thrombotic thrombocytopenic purpura, elimination of drugs causing oxidant stress, treatment of malaria or babesiosis, treatment of the underlying cause of disseminated intravascular coagulation, replacement of a deteriorating native or mechanical heart valve).

When anemia relates to underproduction erythropoietin (e.g., in chronic or end-stage kidney disease), consider treatment with recombinant human erythropoietin. In patients with primary hematopoietic disorders impacting normal bone marrow hematopoiesis (e.g., aplastic anemia, myelodysplastic syndrome, leukemia, plasma cell myeloma, lymphoma, myelofibrosis), proceed with the most appropriate management of the underlying primary hematopoietic disorder. For management of anemia-associated symptoms (e.g., fatigue, lethargy, exertional dyspnea), consider supportive blood transfusions versus pharmacologic doses of recombinant human erythropoietin. In some instances, allogeneic hematopoietic stem cell transplantation may be indicated.

Book Enhancement

Go to www.acponline.org/essentials/hematology-section.html. In *MKSAP for Students 5*, assess your knowledge with items 1-9 in the **Hematology** section.

Bibliography

Bain BJ. Diagnosis from the blood smear. N Engl J Med. 2005;353:498-507. [PMID: 16079373]

Chapter 43

Bleeding Disorders

Joel Appel, DO

Bleeding disorders are characterized by defects in primary and secondary hemostasis. Primary hemostasis involves the formation of a platelet plug at the site of vascular disruption, a process that begins with adhesion of platelets to exposed subendothelial matrix. Adhesion is mediated through interactions of specific platelet receptors, such as the collagen receptor and the glycoprotein Ib-IX-V complex, which binds von Willebrand factor with the subepithelial matrix. Adhesion induces platelet activation, with attendant change in platelet shape, secretion of alpha granules and dense bodies, and exposure of fibrinogen receptors that mediate platelet aggregation through binding of the dimeric fibrinogen molecule to adjacent platelets. Platelet activation also leads to rearrangement of membrane phospholipid, with increased expression of anionic phospholipid on the platelet surface and the release of platelet microparticles. Anionic phospholipid provides a surface that supports secondary hemostasis. Secondary hemostasis is initiated by the exposure of tissue factor at the site of vascular damage; tissue factor binds activated factor VII and activates factor X and factor IX. Activated factor IX, in turn, activates additional factor X, leading to the generation of thrombin and cleavage of fibrinogen to form fibrin (Figure 1).

Approach to the Patient

Obtain a detailed bleeding history, including duration, frequency, timing, and sites of bleeding. Blood transfusion history, family history, medications (e.g., aspirin, clopidogrel, NSAIDs, warfarin, antibiotics), and medical history (e.g., liver disease, uremia, poor nutrition) provide clues to possible causes and help to estimate bleeding risk.

A mucocutaneous bleeding pattern is the hallmark of disorders of primary hemostasis. Epistaxis, gingival bleeding, easy bruising, and menorrhagia are characteristic. Persistent oozing after an injury

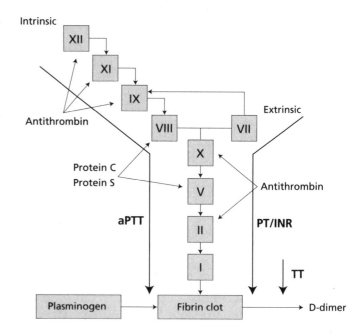

Figure 1. The coagulation cascade, showing the pathways assessed by the prothrombin time (PT)/INR, activated partial thromboplastin time (aPTT), and thrombin time (TT). The D-dimer results from the breakdown of fibrin by plasma.

is common, because the initial platelet plug is not formed. Disorders of secondary hemostasis are characterized by bleeding into muscles and joints. Delayed bleeding is common, because the platelet plug gradually succumbs to the pressures of blood flow without reinforcement from a strong fibrin mesh. Excessive bleeding after childbirth, surgery, or trauma can occur with disorders of primary or secondary hemostasis.

Table 1. Causes of Prolonged Prothrombin Time, Partial Thromboplastin Time, Thrombin Time, and Bleeding Time

Prolonged Laboratory Test	Causes
Prothrombin time (PT)	Warfarin, factor VII deficiency or inhibitor, vitamin K deficiency (nutritional or antibiotic-related), liver disease
Partial thromboplastin time (PTT)	Heparin; lupus anticoagulant (predisposes to thrombosis); von Willebrand disease; factor VIII, IX, XI, or XII deficiency or inhibitor
Combined PT and PTT	Supratherapeutic dose of heparin or warfarin; DIC (PT prolonged first); liver disease; factor V or X, prothrombin, or fibrinogen deficiency or inhibitor; direct thrombin inhibitor
Thrombin time	Heparin, direct thrombin inhibitor, factor Xa inhibitor, fibrin degradation product, low or high fibrinogen level
Bleeding time	Thrombocytopenia (<100,000/μL [100 × 10^9/L]), platelet dysfunction, von Willebrand disease

DIC = disseminated intravascular coagulation.

Table 2. Coagulation and Platelet Function Test Results Found in Various Coagulation and Platelet Disorders

Coagulation or Platelet Disorder	PT/INR	aPTT	Mixing Study[a]	TT	Fibrin-ogen	D-dimer	Platelet Count	Bleeding Time	Platelet Aggre-gation	Blood Smear[b]	Notes
Liver disease	↑	↑	Corrects	↑	↓	↑	↓	↑ or →	NI	Target cells	Findings often are variable and most prominent in advanced liver disease with cirrhosis.
Vitamin K deficiency	↑	↑	Corrects	→	→	→	→	→	→	Normal	The PT/INR rises before the aPTT because of the short half-life of factor VII.
Disseminated intravascular coagulation	↑	↑	Corrects	↑	↓	↑	↓	↑	NI	Schisto-cytes	Results vary depending on severity; some tests may be normal.
Thrombo-cytopenia	→	→	NI	→	→	→	↓	↑	Abnormal	Large platelets	Bleeding time and platelet size depend on the cause of thrombocytopenia.
Qualitative platelet defect	→	→	NI	→	→	→	→	↑	Abnormal	Normal	Platelet aggregation patterns vary depending on the defect.
Von Willebrand disease	→	↑ or →	Corrects	→	→	→	→	↑	Normal	Normal	The aPTT is dependent on factor VIII activity. Platelet aggregation does not detect abnormal adhesion; vWF level and ristocetin cofactor are abnormal. Ristocetin cofactor is a platelet aggregation study measuring the function of vWF. The structure of vWF can be determined by a vWF multimer assay.

aPTT = activated partial thromboplastin time; NI = not indicated; PT = prothombin time; TT = thrombin time; vWF = von Willebrand factor; ↑ = increased; ↓ = decreased; → = normal.
[a]A mixing study is performed on the PT or aPTT, depending on which is prolonged.
[b]Findings on blood smear are variable, depending on the severity of the disorder, and may not be present.

The prothrombin time (PT) and the activated partial thromboplastin time (aPTT) are screening assays designed to detect clotting factor deficiencies as well as inhibitors that interfere with effective fibrin clot formation (Table 1). Clotting factor levels <35% are needed to prolong the PT and aPTT, and reliance on these tests alone underestimates bleeding risk. A mixing study differentiates factor deficiency from presence of a factor inhibitor by mixing patient plasma with normal plasma; factor deficiencies correct with mixing. Bleeding time is an in vivo method of identifying disorders of platelets and vessel wall integrity. Platelet function screening is a more specific method for assessing the effects of drugs or disorders (e.g., von Willebrand disease) on platelet activity. This method uses specific platelet activators (e.g., collagen, epinephrine, ristocetin) to measure platelet aggregation in vitro. Thrombin time tests the conversion of fibrinogen to fibrin. Levels of fibrinogen, fibrinogen degradation products, and D-dimer are used to identify excessive fibrinolysis.

Disorders of Primary Hemostasis

Disorders of primary hemostasis include abnormalities of platelets or the vascular endothelium. Thrombocytopenia affects bleeding time when the platelet count is $<100,000/\mu L$ ($100 \times 10^9/L$), but spontaneous bleeding does not occur until the platelet count is $<10,000-20,000/\mu L$ ($10-20 \times 10^9/L$). Dysfunction of platelet adhesion occurs in von Willebrand disease and Bernard-Soulier syndrome. Platelet activation can be limited due to drugs such as aspirin, clopidogrel, and NSAIDs or in uremia (i.e., kidney disease). Ehlers-Danlos syndrome, Marfan syndrome, and hereditary hemorrhagic telangiectasia are associated with blood vessel abnormalities that affect hemostasis.

Von Willebrand Disease

The most common inherited bleeding disorder is von Willebrand disease (vWD), an autosomal dominant disorder that occurs in an estimated 1 in 100 to 400 people. Clinically, patients have mild to moderate bleeding evidenced by nosebleeds, heavy menstrual flow, gingival bleeding, easy bruising, and bleeding associated with surgery or trauma.

Von Willebrand factor (vWF) plays a critical role in platelet adhesion to injured vessels. It also functions as a carrier for factor VIII. Disorders of secondary hemostasis can occur due to low factor VIII levels in vWD; this distinction is important for treatment purposes. Diagnostic testing includes bleeding time, vWF antigen level, vWF activity assay, factor VIII level, and a multimer study used to diagnose subtypes of vWD (Table 2). Desmopressin releases stored vWF from endothelial cells and is first-line therapy for most subtypes of vWD; in vitro documentation of a response to desmopressin with platelet function testing or vWF assay is performed prior to administration. Intermediate-purity factor VIII concentrates, which contain vWF, also can be given. Cryoprecipitate is rich in vWF but carries the risk of transfusion-transmitted infection.

Disorders of Secondary Hemostasis

Disorders of secondary hemostasis are characterized by defects or deficiencies of coagulation factors and include inherited hemophilias, liver disease, vitamin K deficiency, acquired inhibitors of coagulation (antibodies), and consumptive processes (e.g., disseminated intravascular coagulation). Medications such as warfarin, heparin, low-molecular-weight heparin, factor Xa inhibitors (e.g., fondaparinux), and direct thrombin inhibitors (e.g., argatroban, lepirudin) also interfere with secondary hemostasis (Table 2).

Hemophilia

Factor VIII deficiency (hemophilia A) and factor IX deficiency (hemophilia B) are X-linked disorders with clinical manifestations seen almost exclusively in males. Hemophilia A affects about 1 in 10,000 people; hemophilia B occurs less frequently. All daughters of patients with hemophilia are obligate carriers, whereas all sons are normal. Sons of carrier mothers have a 50% chance of having hemophilia, and daughters have a 50% chance of being carriers. The spontaneous mutation rate is 3%. Fibrinogen deficiency and factor II, V, VII, X, and XI deficiencies usually are autosomal recessive disorders and are rare in comparison.

Both types of hemophilia are classified as mild, moderate, or severe according to baseline levels of clotting factors. Patients present in childhood with muscle hematomas, hemarthrosis, and persistent delayed bleeding after trauma or surgery. Mild hemophilia can be missed until adulthood. Assessing factor VIII and IX levels is indicated in any male who presents with a prolonged aPTT that corrects with a mixing study (Table 1).

Factor VIII and IX deficiencies are treated with factor replacement (recombinant or purified). Fresh frozen plasma is a diluted source of clotting factors with limited efficacy for high-level replacement.

Liver Disease

The liver synthesizes almost all proteins involved in hemostasis, with exceptions being vWF and tissue plasminogen activator. The PT is a sensitive indicator of hepatic synthetic function due to the short half-life of factor VII (6 hours), which the failing liver cannot maintain. The PT and aPTT both are prolonged with more severe hepatic synthetic dysfunction. Fresh frozen plasma transiently replaces all coagulation factors but is short-lived.

Vitamin K Deficiency

Clotting factors II, VII, IX, and X as well as protein C and protein S require vitamin K–dependent gamma-carboxylation for full activity. Dietary vitamin K is obtained primarily from the intake of dark green vegetables and is modified by gut flora to the active form. Interruption of bile flow prevents absorption of vitamin K. Antibiotic-related elimination of enteric bacteria limits intestinal sources of vitamin K, whereas warfarin directly antagonizes vitamin K activity.

The PT is first to prolong, but the aPTT will also lengthen with further factor deficiencies. In adults with normal hepatic function, oral or subcutaneous vitamin K usually corrects the clotting times within 24 hours; the risk of anaphylaxis is increased with intravenous vitamin K. Fresh frozen plasma is used when urgent correction is required.

Antibodies to Blood Clotting Factors

Antibodies directed against clotting factors are rare but potentially lethal acquired bleeding disorders. Most of these disorders are considered idiopathic, but antibodies to clotting factors may develop in response to drugs (penicillin, sulfonamides, phenytoin, quinolones) or as part of an underlying illness, such as a malignancy (lymphoproliferative disorder, some solid tumors) or an autoimmune disorder (systemic lupus erythematosus, rheumatoid arthritis). Patients may present with excessive bleeding following surgery, spontaneous mucosal bleeding (nasal, gastrointestinal, urinary, uterine), large ecchymoses, and large soft-tissue hematomas; hemarthrosis is unusual. Diagnosis is made by a protracted clotting time that does not correct with a mixing study. Most commonly, antibody is directed against factor VIII. Quantifying the inhibitor by obtaining an inhibitor titer helps determine treatment options. Therapy for these disorders includes factor VIII replacement (when appropriate), nonspecific immunosuppression with corticosteroids, targeted immune suppression (e.g., rituximab [monoclonal antibody against CD20]), immune globulin administration, and removal of inhibitors through plasma exchange.

Disseminated Intravascular Coagulation

Disseminated intravascular coagulation (DIC) involves widespread activation of coagulation that leads to formation of fibrin clots. Some patients have a thrombotic disorder characterized by deep venous thrombosis or pulmonary embolism. Arterial thrombi and infarction also may occur rarely. In most patients, secondary fibrinolysis dissolves the fibrin clot, and consumption of platelets and coagulation factors causes thrombocytopenia, clotting factor deficiencies, bleeding, and vascular injuries. Erythrocyte consumption manifests as a microangiopathic hemolytic anemia, with fragmented erythrocytes seen on peripheral blood smear.

DIC most commonly occurs in patients with infection, cancer (typically mucin-producing adenocarcinoma), and obstetric complications. Gram-negative sepsis is the most common infection associated with DIC, although infection due to gram-positive organisms and viruses, including HIV, also may be causative.

The diagnosis of DIC is based on the presence of a prolonged PT, aPTT, and thrombin time; a high D-dimer titer; a reduced serum fibrinogen level and platelet count; and the presence of microangiopathic hemolytic anemia. The degree of these abnormalities depends on the extent of consumption of platelets and coagulation factors and the ability of the patient to compensate for these defects.

Treatment of DIC is focused on correcting the underlying cause. Patients may require fresh frozen plasma to replace coagulation factors or transfusion of platelets or erythrocytes. Cryoprecipitate also may be given. Antithrombin III and activated protein C concentrates have been used with some effectiveness. Unfractionated heparin and low-molecular-weight heparin rarely are used today, because these formulations may increase the bleeding risk and do not improve outcomes.

Book Enhancement

Go to www.acponline.org/essentials/hematology-section.html. In *MKSAP for Students 5*, assess your knowledge with items 10-13 in the **Hematology** section.

Acknowledgment

We would like to thank Dr. Diane C. Sliwka, who contributed to an earlier version of this chapter.

Bibliography

Marks PW. Coagulation disorders in the ICU. Clin Chest Med. 2009;30: 123-129, ix. [PMID: 19186284]

Chapter 44

Sickle Cell Disease

Reed E. Drews, MD

The sickle mutation is a single base change (GAT → GTT) in the sixth codon of exon 1 of the β-globin gene, resulting in replacement of the normal glutamic acid with valine at position 6 of the β-globin polypeptide. As a consequence of this single amino acid substitution, deoxygenated hemoglobin S heterotetramers polymerize to form fibrils, causing erythrocytes to sickle and hemolyze (Plate 39). Sickle cells, forming in the relatively hypoxic regions of tissues, impede blood flow in the microvasculature and promote vaso-occlusion, resulting in profound, often disabling complications, including acute pain (crises), chronic pain, and organ dysfunction or failure (Table 1). The prevalence of sickle cell trait varies widely worldwide and may be as high as 50% in certain regions, affecting individuals of African, Hispanic, Mediterranean, Asian, and Indian descent. Among persons of African ancestry, sickle cell anemia is one of the most common genetic diseases; about 10% are carriers of the sickle gene, and 1 in 600 newborn infants have sickle cell anemia.

Screening

The goal of newborn screening is to identify infants with sickle cell anemia and to treat these patients for 5 years with prophylactic penicillin (or a macrolide, if there is an allergy to penicillin); antibiotic therapy has been shown to reduce both mortality and morbidity from pneumococcal infections in infants with sickle cell anemia and sickle cell–β-thalassemia. Abnormal hemoglobin may be identified in white people; most reports indicate that universal screening is more cost-effective than targeted screening. For possible future primary prevention, counseling the family of an affected infant should include screening of other family members, especially the parents.

Diagnosis

Sickle cell anemia is inherited in an autosomal manner. If both parents carry sickle hemoglobin or another abnormal hemoglobin, there is a 25% risk that the fetus of each pregnancy will have sickle cell anemia or another sickle cell syndrome. Prenatal diagnosis with therapeutic abortion is an option for preventing sickle cell anemia or other sickle cell syndromes. However, clinicians must offer family and genetic counseling to ensure that the parents fully understand the prenatal diagnosis, its complications, and possible outcome, including abortion.

Most patients with sickle cell anemia experience manifestations of the disease in childhood, even as early as age 6 months. Aspects of the medical history that support the possibility of sickle cell anemia or a related hemoglobinopathy include recurring episodes of acute pain, chronic pain, and symptoms and signs of anemia and its sequelae (Table 1). The average hemoglobin level in patients with sickle cell anemia is 7-8 g/dL (70-80 g/L); the anemia is normocytic normochromic, with high reticulocyte counts from stress erythropoiesis and chronic hemolysis. Microcytic hypochromic indices suggest sickle cell–β-thalassemia or coinherited α-thalassemia. High platelet and leukocyte counts relate to asplenia due to autoinfarction.

Hemoglobin electrophoresis both at alkaline pH (cellulose acetate) and acidic pH (citrate agar) distinguishes most structural variants of hemoglobin. High hemoglobin F levels are associated with less severe disease. Elevated hemoglobin A_2 levels signify the presence of β-thalassemia. Knowledge of the molecular lesion in a patient with sickle cell anemia may predict disease severity, assist with family counseling and planning, and guide use of aggressive therapeutic modalities (e.g., allogeneic bone marrow transplantation).

Additional laboratory testing documents organ dysfunction caused by sickle cell anemia. Urinalysis and serum creatinine level identify patients with proteinuria and kidney failure. In patients who have received multiple transfusions, indirect antibody testing detects alloantibodies relevant to future transfusions; liver enzymes, viral hepatitis serologies, and serum iron chemistries identify patients who have contracted viral hepatitis and/or developed iron overload. Pulmonary hypertension, correlating with older age and prior history of acute chest syndrome, is the most common abnormality on echocardiography, with electrocardiography demonstrating signs of right ventricular hypertrophy or strain (marked right axis deviation, tall R waves in lead V_1, delayed precordial transition zone with prominent S waves in leads V_5 and V_6, inverted T waves and ST-segment depression in leads V_1 to V_3, and peaked P waves in lead II due to right atrial enlargement). Physical examination findings associated with sickle cell disease are summarized in Table 2.

Therapy

Hydroxyurea augments levels of hemoglobin F, which inhibits intracellular polymerization of hemoglobin S. Hydroxyurea decreases the incidence of acute painful episodes by approximately 50% in responders; it also reduces the incidence of acute chest syndrome and the need for blood transfusion. Nine-year follow-up of adult patients taking hydroxyurea showed that hydroxyurea was associated with a 40% reduction in mortality. In addition to inducing fetal hemoglobin, other beneficial effects of hydroxyurea in sickle cell disease include improved erythrocyte hydration,

Table 1. Major Complications of Sickle Cell Disease

Complication	Notes
Acute chest syndrome (ACS) vs. pneumonia, fat embolism, venous thromboembolism (VTE)	• ACS correlates with risk of pulmonary hypertension and is the most frequent cause of death. ACS is associated with chlamydia, mycoplasma, respiratory syncytial virus, coagulase-positive *Staphylococcus aureus*, *Streptococcus pneumoniae*, *Mycoplasma hominis*, parvovirus, and rhinovirus infections (in decreasing order of frequency). • Pneumonia usually is a localized infiltration, whereas ACS usually is characterized by diffuse pulmonary infiltrates. Cultures of bronchial washings or deep sputum usually are positive in pneumonia. • Fat embolism presents as chest pain, fever, dyspnea, hypoxia, thrombocytopenia, and multiorgan failure. Fat embolism is a component of ACS and usually is associated with acute painful episodes. It is best differentiated by the presence of fat bodies in bronchial washings or in deep sputum and by multi-organ involvement (e.g., stroke, kidney failure). • The presence of lower extremity thrombophlebitis may differentiate VTE from ACS, but in some cases pulmonary arteriography may be needed. Newer contrast agents may be safer than hypertonic contrast agents, which precipitate intravascular sickling.
Avascular necrosis	Involves the hips and shoulders; may require surgery. More common in sickle cell–α-thalassemia than in other sickle cell syndromes.
Stroke	Occurs in 8%–17% of patients. Infarction is most common in children; hemorrhage is most common in adults. Brain imaging and lumbar puncture establish the diagnosis.
Cholecystitis vs. hepatic crisis	Chronic hemolysis may result in gallstones and acute cholecystitis. Fever, right upper quadrant pain, and elevated aminotransferase levels may also be due to sickle cell–related ischemic hepatic crisis. Abdominal ultrasonography can help differentiate the conditions.
Dactylitis vs. osteomyelitis	Dactylitis is associated with painful, usually symmetric swelling of the hands or feet, erythema, and low-grade fever; it is more common in children aged <5 y. Osteomyelitis usually involves one bone.
Heart failure	Related to pulmonary and systemic hypertension and ischemia.
Infection	Related to functional asplenia.
Leg ulcers	Most common in hemoglobin S disease.
Liver disease	Viral hepatitis and/or iron overload from transfusions and ischemia-induced hepatic crisis.
Sickle cell pain syndrome vs. myocardial infarction (MI), appendicitis	• Sickle cell pain crisis involving the chest may suggest acute MI. The quality of pain of MI (central pressure) is different from that of sickle cell pain (sharp, pleuritic). Serial determination of cardiac enzymes will differentiate the conditions. • Abdominal pain, fever, and leukocytosis may suggest appendicitis. Elevated serum LDH level and normal bowel sounds support sickle cell pain syndrome.
Priapism	Prolonged or repeated episodes may cause impotence.
Proteinuria and kidney failure	Prevalence of proteinuria and kidney failure is approximately 25% and 5%, respectively.
Pulmonary hypertension	Risk of development correlates with increasing age and prior history of ACS.
Retinopathy	More common in patients with compound heterozygosity for hemoglobin SC.
Sickle anemia vs. aplastic crisis, hyperhemolysis	A hemoglobin level that decreases by ≥2 g/dL (20 g/L) during a painful crisis could be due to aplastic crisis or hyperhemolysis. Aplastic crisis could be idiopathic or due to coexistent infection (e.g., parvovirus B19) or cytotoxic drugs. Hyperhemolysis could be due to infection (e.g., mycoplasma), transfusion reaction, or coexistent G6PD deficiency. Reticulocyte count is decreased with aplastic crisis and increased with hyperhemolysis. Serum bilirubin, LDH, and aminotransferase levels are elevated in hyperhemolysis.
Splenomegaly and splenic sequestration	Common in children aged <5 years who afterward manifest asplenia from splenic infarction. Patients with hemoglobin SC often have splenomegaly persisting into adulthood.

G6PD = glucose-6-phosphate dehydrogenase; LDH = lactate dehydrogenase.

macrocytosis, and lower neutrophil and reticulocyte counts with decreased adhesiveness and improved rheology of circulating neutrophils and reticulocytes. Together, these beneficial effects reduce intracellular sickling and result in reduced hemolysis and improved hemoglobin levels.

Exchange transfusions, a technique that removes the patient's blood while transfusing normal, crossmatched donor blood, should be considered to decrease and maintain hemoglobin S levels <30% as an ongoing stroke-prevention program in children who are considered at high risk for developing stroke based on transcranial Doppler studies or who have had a prior stroke. Incidence of iron overload requiring chelation therapy, which increases morbidity and mortality, is less in patients receiving exchange transfusions compared with those on simple blood transfusion. However, there is growing evidence that hydroxyurea therapy also offers multiple benefits in children. Beginning hydroxyurea in childhood or adolescence may help to prevent chronic and long-term end-organ damage, thereby supplanting the need for chronic management strategies such as exchange transfusion and chelation therapy.

Table 2. Physical Examination (PE) Findings Associated with Sickle Cell Disease

PE Component	Notes
Temperature	Acute painful episodes often are associated with low-grade fever. If temperature is >38.3°C (101.0°F), rule out infection.
Pulse	Anemia, infection, and pain often are associated with tachycardia.
Respiration rate	Respiration rate usually is 16-20/min in the steady state. A rate <10/min suggests opioid overdose.
Blood pressure	Blood pressure usually is low-normal. Hypertension increases morbidity and mortality risk.
Cardiac examination	A systolic murmur due to anemia is common. The absence of a murmur is associated with mild anemia and no cardiomegaly. Findings associated with pulmonary hypertension and right ventricular hypertrophy or strain include increased intensity of the pulmonic component of S_2, right-sided murmurs and gallops (increased intensity with inspiration), and a prominent a wave in the jugular venous pulse.
Pulmonary examination	The lungs usually are clear in the steady state. Rhonchi may be heard in patients with a history of recurrent acute chest syndrome (ACS). Decreased breath sounds and/or pulmonary crackles in a febrile patient suggest pneumonia or ACS.
Abdominal examination	With age and repeated episodes of sickling, the spleen becomes small, fibrosed, and devoid of any function (autosplenectomy). However, splenomegaly may persist into young adulthood, especially in patients with hemoglobin SC, sickle cell–β-thalassemia, or sickle cell–α-thalassemia. Hepatomegaly could be a sign of iron overload or heart failure. Tender hepatomegaly suggests hepatic crisis.
Skin examination	Leg ulcers develop in 5%-10% of patients; ulcers most often are located on the medial or lateral aspect of the ankle.
Neurologic examination	Focal findings suggestive of stroke. Not all patients with a history of stroke have residual weakness.

ACE inhibitors prevent progressive kidney disease by lowering intraglomerular pressures. Additionally, ACE inhibitors can lower protein excretion and should be used in patients with albuminuria, even in the absence of hypertension. Recombinant erythropoietin stimulates erythropoiesis to achieve hemoglobin levels similar to steady state values (i.e., 7-9 g/dL [70-90 g/L]) in patients who have kidney failure or to limit blood transfusions in patients who are alloimmunized and for whom crossmatch-compatible blood is difficult to find.

Supplemental folic acid prevents folate deficiency (arising from chronic hemolysis) and subsequent elevation of homocysteine levels, which may be a risk factor for stroke. Periodic retinal examinations are recommended for monitoring and managing (photocoagulation) progressive proliferative sickle retinopathy. Polyvalent (23-valent) pneumococcal polysaccharide vaccine, *Haemophilus influenzae* type b conjugate vaccine, and influenza vaccine prevent infections. Relaxation and biofeedback methods, cognitive coping strategies, and self-hypnosis are techniques that reduce emergency department visits, hospital admissions, hospital days, and analgesic use. Goals of these interventions are to improve quality of life by increasing activity and enhancing normal function and to decrease dependence on opioid analgesics.

Patients are hospitalized when severe acute painful episodes (crises) do not resolve at home with oral analgesics after 1 to 2 days or do not resolve or improve significantly after a minimum of 4 to 6 hours of treatment with parenteral opioids. Effective pain relief is best achieved with combined use of acetaminophen, NSAIDs, opioid analgesics, and adjuvant therapies (antihistamines, antidepressants, anticonvulsants). Meperidine is not recommended as opioid therapy, because it is less effective than morphine or hydromorphone and is associated with more side effects (e.g., seizures). NSAIDs should be avoided in patients with kidney failure.

Supplemental oxygen should be used only in the presence of demonstrated hypoxia (oxygen saturation <92% or arterial PO_2 ≤70 mm Hg [9.3 kPa]). For severe symptomatic anemia or acute organ failure, blood/exchange transfusions improve blood oxygen-carrying capacity and microvascular perfusion by diluting circulating sickled erythrocytes. To avoid increased blood viscosity, transfusions should not yield hemoglobin levels >10 g/dL (100 g/L).

Exchange transfusions should be considered to decrease hemoglobin S levels <30% in managing specific acute complications, including cerebral infarction, fat embolism, acute chest syndrome, unresponsive acute priapism, and nonhealing leg ulcers.

Allogeneic bone marrow transplantation (in patients aged <16 years with severe complications) may cure sickle cell anemia; its success depends on the availability of donors and the severity of the disease of the patient in question. Recipients of HLA-matched donor marrow have 75% to 85% event-free survival, 15% graft rejection, and 10% mortality.

Book Enhancement

Go to www.acponline.org/essentials/hematology-section.html. In *MKSAP for Students 5*, assess your knowledge with items 14-18 in the **Hematology** section.

Bibliography

Frenette PS, Atweh GF. Sickle cell disease: old discoveries, new concepts, and future promise. J Clin Invest. 2007;117:850-858. [PMID: 17404610]

Ware RE. How I use hydroxyurea to treat young patients with sickle cell anemia. Blood. 2010;115:5300-5311. [PMID: 20223921]

Chapter 45

Thrombocytopenia

Richard S. Eisenstaedt, MD

Thrombocytopenia occurs through one of two mechanisms: decreased platelet production or accelerated platelet destruction (Table 1). Most disorders that produce thrombocytopenia through inadequate bone marrow production also affect other marrow cell lines and cause additional cytopenias. Platelet production may be decreased due to bone marrow injury mediated by toxins (e.g., alcohol) or idiosyncratic drug reaction, metastatic cancer, miliary tuberculosis or other infections, deficiency of vitamin B_{12} or folic acid, or bone marrow disease (e.g., acute leukemia, myelodysplastic syndrome, aplastic anemia). Accelerated peripheral platelet destruction occurs in patients with splenomegaly and hypersplenism or disseminated intravascular coagulation. This chapter focuses on three other causes of accelerated platelet destruction: immunologic thrombocytopenic purpura (ITP), heparin-induced thrombocytopenia (HIT), and thrombotic thrombocytopenic purpura–hemolytic uremic syndrome (TTP-HUS).

Table 1. Differential Diagnosis of Thrombocytopenia

Disorder	Notes
Decreased Platelet Production	
Vitamin B_{12} or folate deficiency (see Chapter 42)	Associated with pancytopenia, macrocytosis, macro-ovalocytes, hypersegmented neutrophils, and, possibly, neurologic signs.
Bone marrow disorder (e.g., acute leukemia, aplastic anemia, myelodysplastic syndrome)	Associated with pancytopenia, abnormal blood smear (e.g., nucleated erythrocytes, teardrop cells, immature leukocytes), and abnormal bone marrow examination.
Toxin- or drug-related bone marrow injury	History of alcohol abuse, environmental or occupational exposures, or drug use. Mechanism may also include accelerated destruction. Often associated with anemia or pancytopenia.
Infection	Thrombocytopenia is seen in HIV infection, hepatitis B and C, EBV infection, rubella, disseminated tuberculosis, and other infections. Mechanism may also include accelerated destruction.
Accelerated Destruction	
Immunologic thrombocytopenic purpura (ITP)	Isolated thrombocytopenia in the absence of systemic disease, lymphadenopathy, and splenomegaly. Associated with large platelets on peripheral smear and increased megakaryocytes on bone marrow evaluation (marrow evaluation usually is not required for diagnosis in the absence of other features listed for bone marrow disorders).
Heparin-induced thrombocytopenia	History of exposure to heparin. May be associated with modest thrombocytopenia and devastating arterial and venous thrombosis.
Chronic liver disease (see Chapter 25)	Portal hypertension can lead to splenic sequestration of platelets and thrombocytopenia. Liver disease may be associated with target cells. Liver disease may be occult.
Thrombotic thrombocytopenic purpura–hemolytic uremic syndrome (TTP-HUS)	Syndromes associated with hemolytic anemia and thrombocytopenia. HUS is characterized by more severe renal involvement, TTP by more frequent neurologic symptoms. Associated with elevated serum LDH level, decreased haptoglobin concentration, and schistocytes on peripheral blood smear.
Disseminated intravascular coagulation (see Chapter 43)	Coagulopathy that typically occurs in the setting of sepsis, metastatic cancer, or obstetric catastrophe. Associated with prolonged prothrombin time and activated partial thromboplastin time, low fibrinogen level, and thrombocytopenia.
HELLP syndrome (hemolysis, elevated liver enzymes, low platelets)	Late pregnancy complication of thrombocytopenia associated with microangiopathic hemolytic anemia, and elevated liver enzymes, and hypertension.
Chronic lymphocytic leukemia (see Chapter 48)	ITP is an autoimmune complication of chronic lymphocytic leukemia.
Other	
Pseudothrombocytopenia	In vitro clumping of platelets caused by EDTA-dependent agglutinins leads to falsely decreased platelet counts. Excluded by examination of a peripheral blood smear; no therapy is needed.
Gestational thrombocytopenia	Mild, asymptomatic thrombocytopenia first noted late in pregnancy; resolves following delivery without therapy.

EBV = Epstein-Barr virus; EDTA = ethylenediaminetetraacetic acid; LDH = lactate dehydrogenase.

Immunologic Thrombocytopenic Purpura

Although ITP was formerly known as *idiopathic* thrombocytopenic purpura, *immunologic* thrombocytopenic purpura is a more appropriate term. Thrombocytopenia in ITP occurs when antibodies targeting platelet antigens mediate accelerated destruction. Antibodies arise in three distinct clinical settings: in response to a drug, in association with a disease, and when neither an offending drug nor a related underlying disease process can be identified (idiopathic).

Almost any drug can trigger platelet-targeted antibody production, but the syndrome most often is linked to quinine or quinidine. Although these drugs are used infrequently, quinine-related compounds are found in diverse naturopathic or herbal products. A careful drug history, including a review of all prescriptions, over-the-counter drugs, herbal products, and supplements, is important to identify the offending agent. Stopping the drug hastens recovery from ITP.

ITP may be part of a broader disease affecting immune regulation, such as HIV infection, systemic lupus erythematosus, and, especially in older patients, lymphoproliferative malignancy. HIV-infected patients may develop ITP before the infection has been diagnosed and immunosuppression and opportunistic infections occur. Therefore, screening for HIV infection is warranted in all patients with ITP who have any behavioral risks, including heterosexual contact. Recent reports link ITP to *Helicobacter pylori* infection, although platelet count response to antibiotic therapy is unpredictable.

ITP commonly presents as easy bruising or petechial rash. At times, asymptomatic thrombocytopenia is noted on routine blood tests. ITP is a disease of exclusion; the diagnosis is most probable in patients with isolated thrombocytopenia. The leukocyte count should be normal, and the hemoglobin concentration is normal or reduced as a result of blood loss secondary to thrombocytopenia (Table 2). Measurement of platelet-associated antibody is not helpful, because the test lacks both sensitivity and specificity. The physical examination is normal, with the exception of signs of bleeding, most often petechiae (punctuate red macular lesions that do not blanch with pressure) on the skin or mucous membranes. Patients may have ecchymoses on the skin or more overt bleeding, especially in the gastrointestinal tract. The presence of fever or hepatosplenomegaly suggests another diagnosis. The blood smear will show decreased platelets and occasional large platelets (megathrombocytes). Bone marrow aspirate, if necessary to exclude other diagnoses, will show increased numbers of megakaryocytes and normal erythroid and myeloid precursors. Hematology consultation is advised for patients with severe thrombocytopenia or an uncertain diagnosis.

Patients with ITP require treatment when thrombocytopenia is severe enough to cause clinical bleeding. Such bleeding is expected when the platelet count is $>10,000/\mu L$ $(10 \times 10^9/L)$. Both corticosteroids and intravenous gamma globulin (IVIG) are effective therapy, but thrombocytopenia often relapses when treatment is discontinued. In patients with chronic ITP, the risks of prolonged therapy with corticosteroids or IVIG must be balanced against the benefits. Some patients with tolerable bleeding are best managed without immunosuppressive therapy. Alternative immunosuppressive agents may be used for patients who do not respond to or who have intolerable toxicity from IVIG or corticosteroids. $Rh_o(D)$-positive patients with ITP may be treated with anti-$Rh_o(D)$ immunoglobulin. Another second-line immunosuppressive agent, rituximab, a chimeric monoclonal antibody directed against the CD20 surface marker on B lymphocytes, will lead to doubling of the platelet count in 40% in patients. Romiplostim, a thrombopoiesis-stimulating agent, also is effective in augmenting platelet counts in patients with ITP, but the expense of therapy, need for continued treatment to maintain response, and uncertainty about the safety profile common to any new treatment have tempered enthusiasm for this option.

Rarely, patients with significant bleeding unresponsive to immunosuppressive medication require splenectomy. Although platelet counts will improve, perioperative complications and long-term asplenia sequelae (i.e., infection with encapsulated bacteria) must be anticipated. Pneumococcal, meningococcal, and *Haemophilus influenzae* vaccines are administered before splenectomy.

Table 2. Laboratory Tests to Support the Diagnosis of Immunologic Thrombocytopenic Purpura (ITP)

Test	Notes
CBC	Low platelet count with normal hemoglobin, hematocrit, and leukocyte count is evidence for the diagnosis of ITP.
Peripheral blood smear	Exclude platelet clumping (pseudothrombocytopenia). Myeloid and erythroid morphology should be normal. Platelets should appear normal or large in size. Abnormal or immature leukocytes should be absent. The presence of schistocytes is associated with TTP, DIC, and HELLP syndrome and is evidence against ITP. The presence of polychromatophilia, poikilocytosis, and spherocytes suggests hemolytic anemia. Nucleated erythrocytes should be absent.
Bone marrow	Consider bone marrow aspiration and biopsy to establish the diagnosis in patients with atypical or nondiagnostic findings, especially with additional cytopenias or immature leukocytes or with additional abnormalities on peripheral blood smear. ITP will show normal or increased numbers of megakaryocytes, normal myeloid and erythroid morphology, and no malignant cells.
HIV antibodies	Indicated in patients with any risk factors for HIV infection, including heterosexual contact.
PT/PTT	Coagulation testing is not recommended for routine diagnosis; however, an abnormal PT or PTT is evidence against ITP.
ANA and other serologic tests	ANA is not recommended for routine diagnosis; however, consider ANA and other serologic tests (e.g., rheumatoid factor, complement levels, anti-DNA) in patients with rash, synovitis, arthralgia, or other signs of rheumatologic disease.

ANA = antinuclear antibody; CBC = complete blood count; DIC = disseminated intravascular coagulation; HELLP = hemolytic anemia, elevated liver enzymes, low platelets; PT = prothrombin time; PTT = partial thromboplastin time; TTP = thrombotic thrombocytopenic purpura.

Heparin-Induced Thrombocytopenia

HIT is a unique, drug-triggered platelet disorder that develops in 1% to 2% of patients receiving unfractionated heparin. The incidence of HIT is reported to be lower in patients receiving low-molecular-weight heparin, but that benefit has not been demonstrated in randomized controlled studies and may be related to differing patient populations treated with one form of heparin versus the other. For example, patients undergoing open-heart surgery have a higher incidence of HIT than do patients receiving heparin products for thromboembolism prophylaxis. Most patients develop clinical signs of HIT, including a decrease of approximately 50% in platelet count from baseline levels, 5 to 10 days after initiating heparin therapy. A small subset of patients, perhaps 5%, will have a delayed onset a mean of 14 days after heparin exposure, and those patients may have the first clinical signs of HIT noted after the heparin has been discontinued. Onset of HIT may be detected as early as 10 hours after heparin exposure in patients with a history of heparin exposure in the prior 1 to 3 months. Thrombocytopenia nadir in HIT is modest; mean platelet counts are approximately 60,000/µL (60 × 10^9/L), and patients typically do not bleed excessively. To the contrary, patients with HIT have a dramatic risk of thromboembolic complications, including deep venous thrombosis and pulmonary embolism, as well as unusual clotting problems such as portal vein thrombosis or acute arterial occlusion.

The early stages of HIT are asymptomatic; all patients receiving heparin should have periodic screening platelet counts. In patients on heparin who develop thrombocytopenia, laboratory tests will reveal antibodies that cause heparin-induced serotonin release or platelet aggregation, although the clinical circumstances may suggest the diagnosis before confirmatory laboratory data are available.

Heparin must be discontinued and an alternative rapidly acting anticoagulant must be used instead. Warfarin is not a suitable alternative agent. Direct thrombin inhibitors (e.g., lepirudin, argatroban) should be administered, often under a hematologist's guidance.

Thrombotic Thrombocytopenic Purpura–Hemolytic Uremic Syndrome

Patients with TTP-HUS develop consumptive thrombocytopenia and microangiopathic hemolysis from platelet thrombi that form throughout the microvasculature. The multisystem nature of this syndrome is unpredictable. Fever, acute kidney injury, and fluctuating neurologic abnormalities are components of the syndrome, but all are seldom present during earlier phases of the illness. Patients with little to no kidney involvement and prominent neurologic symptoms fall more into the TTP category, whereas those with acute kidney injury and fewer neurologic manifestations (often seen in children with significant diarrhea) fit better with HUS. Clinical features often overlap, and a precise distinction between TTP and HUS may be difficult to make. TTP-HUS is a syndrome with diverse triggers and pathophysiology, including abnormal von Willebrand factor metabolism and very high molecular weight polymers that predispose to platelet microthrombi. Most patients with TTP have an autoantibody that inhibits a metalloproteinase (ADAMTS13) that normally cleaves unusually large von Willebrand factor multimers into smaller fragments. Pregnant women, HIV-infected patients, and patients receiving cancer chemotherapy or immunosuppressive agents following organ transplantation are at increased risk. Children develop HUS with prominent gastrointestinal symptoms from Shiga toxin–producing enteric bacteria (e.g., *Escherichia coli* O157:H7).

Laboratory findings suggestive of TTP-HUS syndrome include microangiopathic hemolysis with prominent schistocytes on peripheral blood smear (Plate 40), decreased haptoglobin, elevated serum lactate dehydrogenase, and thrombocytopenia. Assays for ADAMTS13 activity may help to confirm the diagnosis, but the test is neither uniformly standardized nor easily available, and therapy should not be withheld while awaiting test results. Malignant hypertension, disseminated intravascular coagulation, and prosthetic heart valves can be associated with microangiopathic hemolysis, although the additional presence of thrombocytopenia and fever, kidney, and neurologic findings strongly supports the diagnosis of TTP-HUS.

Some patients with TTP-HUS respond to plasma infusion, whereas others require the removal of plasma (plasmapheresis). As it is impossible to predict which option will be effective, all patients are managed with plasma exchange therapy. Automated equipment and large-bore, secure intravenous access are needed for plasma exchange; plasma infusion therapy may be initiated in the interim. Corticosteroids also are recommended. Patients with more severe disease, especially with prominent neurologic manifestations, or those with delayed response to plasma exchange and corticosteroids may be treated with alternative immunosuppressive agents (e.g., rituximab). Platelet transfusions in patients with untreated TTP-HUS are associated with acute kidney injury, stroke, and sudden death.

Book Enhancement

Go to www.acponline.org/essentials/hematology-section.html. In *MKSAP for Students 5*, assess your knowledge with items 19-22 in the **Hematology** section.

Bibliography

George JN. Clinical practice. Thrombotic thrombocytopenic purpura. N Engl J Med. 2006;354:1927-1935. [PMID: 16672704]

Chapter 46

Thrombophilia

Patrick C. Alguire, MD

Thrombosis can represent a normal response to blood vessel injury or an unwanted response to an inciting factor. Thrombosis may be limited by rapid blood flow and dilution of activated coagulation factors, a nonthrombogenic endothelium, inhibitors to coagulation factors, and a fibrinolytic system that degrades fibrin clots. Conversely, venous stasis limits blood flow and allows activated factors to accumulate, vascular injury disrupts the endothelium and exposes surfaces that aggregate platelets and activate coagulation factors, and a defect or deficiency of inhibitors or lytic factors allows coagulation activation to go unchecked.

Thrombophilia refers to an increased tendency for thrombosis. Thrombophilia risk factors can be congenital or acquired as well as permanent or transient. Risk factors act by disrupting the blood flow, the blood vessel, or the procoagulant/anticoagulant regulatory pathways. In the normally functioning anticoagulant pathway, thrombin bound to thrombomodulin on the endothelial cell surface activates protein C, which binds to cofactor protein S on the platelet surface, resulting in the degradation of factors V and VII. Antithrombin is another major regulatory protein of the coagulation cascade. It irreversibly binds and neutralizes activated factors II, IX, and X. Genetic amino acid defects or vitamin B_{12}, vitamin B_6, or folate deficiency may result in an elevated homocysteine concentration, which in turn may result in thrombotic and atherosclerotic reactions.

The evaluation of thrombophilia begins by establishing which risk factors are present (Table 1). A family history is a particularly strong indicator of risk and prompts consideration of congenital disorders. Of the inherited thrombophilic conditions, factor V Leiden is the most common. A single mutation in the factor V gene results in an amino acid substitution (Arg to Gln at position 506), rendering factor V more resistant to cleavage by activated protein C. This mutation can be detected by genetic analysis or by the activated protein C resistance assay (a coagulation assay); results for the latter test may also be abnormal because of other circumstances. In the United States, the factor V Leiden mutation occurs in approximately 6% of the white population and less frequently in other ethnic populations. This mutation is found in approximately 20% of all individuals with a deep venous thrombosis (DVT) and occurs much more frequently in those with idiopathic DVT; it also is associated with DVT in women who take oral contraceptives.

Another common genetic thrombophilia is a $G \rightarrow A$ mutation in the prothrombin gene at position 20210; individuals with this gene mutation ($PT^{G20210A}$) have increased prothrombin levels. $PT^{G20210A}$ occurs in approximately 3% of white individuals in the United States and confers a three- to fourfold increased risk for venous thromboembolism (VTE). Surprisingly, neither the heterozygote factor V Leiden nor the $PT^{G20210A}$ phenotype is associated with a significantly increased risk for recurrent VTE, possibly

Table 1. Risk Factors for Venous Thromboembolism (VTE)

Risk Factor	Notes
Immobility	Prolonged immobilization (>72 h) increases the risk for VTE. Recent stroke with paresis, MI, HF, and pulmonary disease are associated with high risk.
Inherited thrombophilia	Risk factors include family history of thrombosis or thrombophilia; personal history of VTE at age <45 y, recurrent thrombosis, or thrombosis at an unusual site; personal history of arterial thrombosis at age <50 y (MI, stroke); or personal history of pregnancy complications (fetal demise, abruption).
Malignancy	Malignancies include solid and hematologic cancers, especially myeloproliferative disorders. Ongoing treatment, palliation, or a diagnosis within the prior 6 mo all increase risk. Screen all patients with VTE for malignancy with age- and sex-appropriate screening (e.g., mammograms for women aged >50 y, Pap tests for women aged >18 y), CBC and liver tests, and chest radiographs (all smokers). The utility of screening for malignancies, with regard to morbidity and survival, is not known.
Previous thrombosis	Even in the absence of a recognized thrombophilic condition, the risk for VTE increases in any patient with a history of thrombosis.
Surgery	All but minor procedures in the prior month represent an increased risk for VTE. Hip, knee, and pelvic surgeries carry the highest risk.
Trauma	Trauma within the prior month increases risk for VTE. Risk is highest with spinal injuries and trauma of the lower limb, with or without plaster immobilization.
Erythropoiesis-stimulating agents	When administered to patients with cancer to treat chemotherapy-associated anemia, erythropoietin and darbepoietin alfa are associated with increased risk of VTE and mortality.

CBC = complete blood count; HF = heart failure; MI = myocardial infarction.

because patients with an initial episode of thrombosis or pulmonary embolism have an alternative predisposing risk.

Antithrombin (previously known as antithrombin III) deficiency is an autosomal dominant disorder, and the prevalence of the heterozygous condition is 0.02% in the general population (homozygous antithrombin deficiency generally is not compatible with life). Antithrombin deficiency is associated with a risk for VTE of approximately 1% per year. Protein C and protein S are vitamin K–dependent proteins. Protein C requires activation by thrombin-thrombomodulin complex on the endothelial surface to neutralize factors VIIIa and Va, whereas protein S is a cofactor in this reaction. Protein C deficiency is inherited as an autosomal recessive trait, with 1 in 200 to 300 individuals affected, many of whom are asymptomatic. Protein C has a half-life of approximately 6 hours, decreases to low levels soon after initiation of warfarin therapy, and is the cause of warfarin-induced skin necrosis in some patients. Concomitant treatment with heparin can prevent this adverse effect. Protein S deficiency is inherited as an autosomal dominant trait; its frequency is less than that of protein C deficiency. Protein S circulates bound to C4b-binding protein, 40% of which is free and active. Deficiencies of protein C, protein S, and antithrombin all lead to an increased risk for VTE. Arterial thrombotic events are rare.

Acquired thrombophilia usually occurs as part of a defined clinical condition (e.g., cancer, pregnancy) or following traumatic injury or a surgical procedure, particularly hip or knee replacement. Although on occasion the VTE may precede recognition of the predisposing condition, as in patients with occult cancer, no additional cancer screening is recommended beyond what would ordinarily be done based on patient age and gender.

The antiphospholipid syndrome is the most common molecular form of acquired thrombophilia; the antiphospholipid antibody is actually an antibody to a protein (β_2-glycoprotein 1) that is bound to phospholipid. Other proteins (e.g., prothrombin, protein C) may function as the epitope for binding. The antiphospholipid antibody sometimes interferes with the coagulation cascade, as measured by the activated partial thromboplastin time or the prothrombin time, causing a prolongation that is not corrected with a corresponding mix including normal plasma (i.e., a lupus anticoagulant). Although they prolong in vitro coagulation tests, these antibodies are associated with approximately a two-thirds increased risk for venous and arterial thromboembolism. There also is a strong correlation between antiphospholipid syndrome and pregnancy loss, presumably due to placental insufficiency in affected patients secondary to thrombosis. Criteria for the diagnosis of the antiphospholipid syndrome are listed in Table 2.

Screening

A family history of thrombosis in a first-degree relative has a positive predictive value of only 14% for factor V Leiden, the most common of the thrombophilias; therefore, the clinical utility of thrombophilia screening has been questioned. Nevertheless, some experts believe that the benefits of screening family members of patients with a documented hereditary thrombophilia can be clinically important to the affected family member, particularly if they are exposed to high-risk situations, such as use of oral contraceptives or hormone replacement therapy.

Diagnosis

Whether knowledge of an inherited thrombophilia provides important information in managing patients with a thromboembolic event remains controversial. In particular, it is unclear whether the intensity or duration of anticoagulation should differ in patients with a thromboembolic event based on whether or not there is an underlying genetic predisposition. If testing is to be done, it should be based on whether patients are determined to be strongly or weakly thrombophilic; testing may not be cost-effective in the latter group. Patients who are considered strongly thrombophilic will often have had their first idiopathic VTE before 50 years of age, may have a history of recurrent thrombotic episodes, and may have one or more first-degree relatives in whom a documented thromboembolism has occurred before 50 years of age. Patients with a VTE and none, or perhaps one, of these characteristics are considered weakly thrombophilic. Patients who are

Table 2. Criteria for Diagnosis of the Antiphospholipid Syndrome[a]

Clinical Criteria

1. Vascular thromboses: One or more episodes of a vascular thrombotic event.

2. Pregnancy morbidity:

    a. One or more unexplained deaths of a morphologically normal fetus beyond the 10th week of gestation.

    b. One or more premature births of a morphologically normal neonate before the 34th week of gestation because of eclampsia or severe preeclampsia or recognized features of placental insufficiency.

    c. Three or more unexplained consecutive spontaneous abortions before the 10th week of gestation.

Laboratory Criteria

1. Lupus anticoagulant: Presence of lupus anticoagulant on two or more occasions at least 12 weeks apart.

2. Anticardiolipin antibody: Presence of anticardiolipin antibody of IgG and/or IgM isotype, in medium or high titer, on two or more occasions at least 12 weeks apart.

3. Anti–β_2-glycoprotein 1 antibody: Presence of anti–β_2-glycoprotein 1 antibody of IgG and/or IgM isotype on two or more occasions at least 12 weeks apart.

[a]Diagnosis of antiphospholipid syndrome requires that at least one clinical criterion and at least one laboratory criterion are met.
Adapted with permission from Miyakis S, Lockshin MD, Atsumi T, et al. International consensus statement on an update of the classification criteria for definite antiphospholipid syndrome (APS). J Thromb Haemost. 2006;42:295-306. [PMID: 16420554]

Table 3. Laboratory and Other Studies for Thrombophilia

Condition	Test
Activated protein C resistance	Factor V Leiden gene mutation accounts for 95% of activated protein C resistance; thus, the activated protein C resistance assay is a good screen. False-positive results occur in pregnancy and with oral contraceptive use. Confirm a positive test result with testing for factor V Leiden gene mutation.
Factor V Leiden gene mutation	A direct PCR gene test and the test of choice for activated protein C resistance in patients who are pregnant or receiving estrogen or oral contraceptives.
Prothrombin gene mutation	A direct PCR gene test.
Protein C deficiency	Select both antigenic and functional assays. Active thrombosis and use of warfarin may cause false-positive results.
Protein S deficiency	Select both antigenic and functional assays. Active thrombosis, use of warfarin, and pregnancy may cause false-positive results.
Antithrombin III deficiency	Select both antigenic and functional assays. Active thrombosis and use of heparin may cause false-positive results.
Hyperhomocysteinemia	The risk for thrombosis increases as fasting plasma homocysteine levels increase >1.35 mg/L (10 µmol/L). Kidney failure and vitamin deficiencies can cause false-positive results. Pregnancy may artificially lower levels.
Lupus anticoagulant	Test with partial thromboplastin time. If prolonged, perform a mixing study; mixing with normal plasma will not correct the study if lupus anticoagulant is present.
Anticardiolipin antibodies (IgG, IgM)	An ELISA test. Levels fluctuate; thus, positive tests should be repeated several weeks apart.

ELISA = enzyme-linked immunosorbent assay; PCR = polymerase chain reaction.

strongly thrombophilic should undergo testing for activated protein C resistance, factor V Leiden, PT^{G20210A}, antiphospholipid antibody, lupus anticoagulant, antithrombin deficiency, protein C deficiency, and protein S deficiency. Those who are weakly thrombophilic should undergo either no special testing or testing only for the most common disorders: activated protein C resistance, factor V Leiden, PT^{G20210A}, antiphospholipid antibody, and lupus anticoagulant. Testing for antithrombin deficiency, protein C deficiency, and protein S deficiency is not indicated in weakly thrombophilic patients.

Testing should not be done in the setting of an acute thrombotic event but should be delayed until weeks or months afterward, after anticoagulant therapy has been discontinued, because active thrombosis may alter the level of some proteins. Avoid testing while a patient is taking anticoagulants. In particular, heparin may decrease antithrombin levels or mimic a lupus anticoagulant, and warfarin will decrease protein C and protein S levels. Finally, confirm all test results before assigning a specific diagnosis; laboratory abnormalities can be transient, and a single positive test may be unreliable (Table 3).

Therapy

Certain thrombophilias (hyperhomocysteinemia, lupus anticoagulant, anticardiolipin antibody) are associated with increased arterial vascular disease, and smoking may increase this risk. Advise all patients who smoke to stop smoking.

Patients with VTE and certain thrombophilias are at especially high risk for recurrent VTE. The benefit of long-term anticoagulation (usually with warfarin) in these high-risk patients may outweigh the risk of bleeding complications. Some experts recommend lifelong therapeutic anticoagulation for patients with VTE and any of the following thrombophilias: lupus anticoagulant, anticardiolipin antibody, homozygosity for factor V Leiden mutation, homozygosity for PT^{G20210A}, combined heterozygosity for factor V Leiden mutation and PT^{G20210A}, and antithrombin III deficiency. Patients with other documented thrombophilias are provided with temporary prophylactic anticoagulation (usually with low-molecular-weight heparin) only during high-risk situations, such as surgery, prolonged immobilization, or pregnancy.

In patients with hyperhomocysteinemia, reducing levels of homocysteine with vitamin B$_6$, vitamin B$_{12}$, or folic acid has not resulted in a subsequent reduction in the incidence of VTE.

Follow-Up

Do not obtain regular laboratory studies once the diagnosis of a thrombophilia has been established, except in patients who require monitoring of anticoagulant therapy. Do not repeat thrombophilia testing or regular routine blood testing in patients in whom a diagnosis of a thrombophilia has been established. Periodically check platelet levels in patients with anticardiolipin antibody or lupus anticoagulant, because these individuals may have thrombocytopenia as part of their clinical picture.

Book Enhancement

Go to www.acponline.org/essentials/hematology-section.html. In *MKSAP for Students 5*, assess your knowledge with items 23-25 in the **Hematology** section.

Bibliography

Whitlatch NL, Ortel TL. Thrombophilias: when should we test and how does it help? Semin Respir Crit Care Med. 2008;29:25-39. [PMID: 18302084]

Chapter 47

Multiple Myeloma

Richard S. Eisenstaedt, MD

Multiple myeloma (MM) is a malignant clonal proliferation of plasma cells. Most cases are believed to arise from an asymptomatic premalignant proliferation of monoclonal plasma cells in a condition referred to as *monoclonal gammopathy of unknown significance* (MGUS). Although most cases of MGUS remain stable for many years, approximately 1% to 2% per year transform into MM. Several chromosomal abnormalities have been implicated in the pathogenesis of MM, including translocation at a chromosome region involved in immunoglobulin synthesis, oncogene activation, and inactivation of kinase inhibitors. The net result of these abnormalities is a malignant expansion of a plasma cell clone that secretes a specific immunoglobulin (most often an intact IgG, less often IgA or IgM). In approximately 20% of cases, the malignant plasma cells secrete a monoclonal light chain (kappa or lambda). These monoclonal proteins, whether in the form of intact immunoglobulins or light chains, are termed *M proteins*. MM accounts for approximately 1% of cancer cases and typically occurs in the seventh decade. New chemotherapy options and the use of autologous stem cell transplantation have improved the outlook for what was a uniformly fatal disease. Today, approximately one third of patients aged <60 years achieve a 10-year survival.

In MM, the uncontrolled clonal proliferation of plasma cells leads to bone marrow failure, initially manifesting as a normocytic anemia and progressing to other cytopenias. The clonal expansion also results in inadequate numbers of normal plasma cells, with subsequent hypogammaglobulinemia predisposing to infection with encapsulated bacteria (e.g., *Streptococcus pneumoniae*). Neoplastic proliferation within the marrow also is associated with osteoclast activation, resulting in hypercalcemia and bone damage that produces pain and increases the risk of compression fracture of the spine and pathologic fracture of weight-bearing bones. Some patients develop plasma cell tumors (plasmacytomas), which may arise adjacent to or directly from bony structures or in extramedullary sites. Clinical features vary with location, but plasmacytomas arising from the vertebrae increase the risk of spinal

Table 1. Differential Diagnosis of Multiple Myeloma (MM)

Disorder	Notes
Monoclonal gammopathy of undetermined significance	M protein <30 g/dL; bone marrow plasma cells <10%; normal hemoglobin, serum calcium, serum creatinine, and bone survey. May be precancerous, but no therapy reduces the likelihood of malignant transformation.
Polyclonal hypergammaglobulinemia	A nonclonal increase in serum immunoglobulins. No increased risk of evolving into MM. Associated with liver disease, connective tissue disease, chronic infections (e.g., HIV), lymphoproliferative disorders, and nonhematologic malignancies.
Plasma cell leukemia	2000/µL (2000 × 10⁶) circulating plasma cells. Worse prognosis than typical MM.
POEMS syndrome	Rare variant of MM consisting of peripheral neuropathy, organomegaly, endocrinopathy, monoclonal plasma cell proliferative disorder, skin changes, sclerotic bone lesions, papilledema, fingernail clubbing, edema, effusions, and, possibly, Castleman disease.[a] Not all features required for diagnosis; minimum of peripheral neuropathy, plasma cell dyscrasia, and either sclerotic bone lesion or Castleman disease. Better overall prognosis than MM.
Primary systemic amyloidosis (AL amyloidosis)	A clonal plasma cell proliferative disorder in which fibrils of monoclonal light chains are deposited in the kidney and other tissues (liver, heart, peripheral nervous system), causing nephrotic syndrome, cardiomyopathy, orthostatic hypotension, cholestatic liver disease, peripheral neuropathy, "pinch purpura," fatigue, weight loss, peripheral edema, macroglossia, xerostomia, arthropathy, and carpal tunnel syndrome. Most patients have small serum M proteins and approximately 5% bone marrow plasma cells; 6%-15% of patients with AL amyloidosis have coexisting MM.
Waldenström macroglobulinemia	An IgM monoclonal gammopathy characterized by anemia, hyperviscosity, lymphadenopathy, and bone marrow plasmacyte infiltration. More responsive to purine nucleoside analogues and anti-CD20 immunotherapy.
Plasmacytoma	A localized collection of plasmacytes that may occur as a single lytic lesion in bone or extramedullary (upper respiratory tract, especially sinuses, nasopharynx, or larynx). Patients may or may not have M protein in the serum or urine. No increase in bone marrow plasma cells, anemia, hypercalcemia, or renal insufficiency. Treated with local therapy (excision, radiation). Patients have increased risk for developing MM.

[a]A lymphoproliferative disorder association with HIV and human herpesvirus 8.

cord compression. The M protein, when filtered through the glomerulus, can cause renal tubular injury; large M proteins (e.g., IgM or multimers of IgA) also may cause symptoms related to hyperviscosity. Symptoms of hyperviscosity include bleeding (hyperviscosity interferes with normal coagulation factor activation and platelet function), decreased vision and other neurologic symptoms, dyspnea, and heart failure.

The amyloidoses are a group of diseases that share a common feature of extracellular deposition of pathologic, insoluble fibrils in various tissues and organs. Within this group of disorders, AL amyloidosis is the most common systemic amyloidosis associated with an underlying clonal plasma cell dyscrasia. The plasma cell burden in this disorder usually is low, at 5% to 10%, although AL amyloidosis is associated with overt MM in 10% to 15% of cases. Clinical manifestations are variable but most commonly include nephrotic syndrome, cardiomyopathy, hepatosplenomegaly, gastrointestinal dysmotility, orthostatic hypotension, and peripheral neuropathy. Table 1 summarizes a differential diagnosis of MM.

Diagnosis

Suspect MM in patients with anemia, bone pain, osteopenia or osteoporosis, pathologic fracture, lytic bone lesions, hypercalcemia, recurrent infections (particularly pneumococcal infections), or kidney failure. Asymptomatic disease may be found in patients who have elevated total serum protein levels on routine laboratory screening, with subsequent electrophoresis revealing an M protein. Rarely, the uniform cationic electrical charge of monoclonal

proteins may create a seemingly narrow anion gap on the basic metabolic panel. The large numbers of monoclonal proteins also alter blood rheology and lead to erythrocytes sticking to one another (rouleaux formation on peripheral blood smear).

Evaluation of MM (Table 2) begins with serum protein electrophoresis and urine protein electrophoresis on a 24-hour urine sample. Up to 20% of patients with MM secrete lambda or kappa light chains rather than an intact immunoglobulin. The smaller molecular weight of the light chains allows them to be filtered by the glomerulus and excreted in the urine. Thus, electrophoresis of the serum will not reveal an M protein, although it may reveal hypogammaglobulinemia. A monoclonal protein in either urine or serum would be further characterized by immunoelectrophoresis. Light chains in the urine (Bence Jones proteins) are not detected in a routine urinalysis, emphasizing the need for urine protein electrophoresis and subsequent immunoelectrophoresis in patients in whom MM is suspected. Additional studies include a complete blood count (CBC); a radiographic bone survey (Figure 1); and serum creatinine, blood urea nitrogen, and serum calcium levels. Normochromic anemia is the most common CBC abnormality, whereas patients with more advanced disease may also have leukopenia and thrombocytopenia. MM may be associated with kidney disease ("myeloma kidney") caused by several mechanisms, most commonly the direct renal tubular toxicity of light chains. Associated hypercalcemia may cause acute kidney injury, and amyloidosis often is associated with nephrotic syndrome and azotemia. Although diffuse lytic bone lesions are more specific for MM, osteopenia is a more common finding. Bone

Table 2. Laboratory and Other Studies for Diagnosis of Multiple Myeloma (MM)

Test	Notes
Complete blood count	Anemia is present in about 60% of patients at diagnosis and eventually develops in all patients. Thrombocytopenia and leukopenia are possible.
Peripheral blood smear	Rouleaux formation, due to increased serum proteins.
Serum calcium (see Chapter 60)	Hypercalcemia initially is seen in 15%-20% of patients, due to cytokine-mediated destruction of bone.
Serum creatinine	At diagnosis, 20% of patients have serum creatinine levels >2 mg/dL (176.8 mmol/L). Causes include hypercalcemia, "myeloma kidney," dehydration, and hyperuricemia.
Serum protein electrophoresis	Characteristic M protein is seen in approximately 80% of patients; presence or absence does not guarantee or exclude the diagnosis. Note whether there is a spike or a diffuse increase in M protein levels. A spike in γ-globulin is more consistent with a monoclonal protein; a diffuse increase correlates with a polyclonal gammopathy. A polyclonal gammopathy almost never relates to MM.
Immunofixation of serum	At diagnosis, 93% of patients have a monoclonal protein in the serum by immunofixation.
Quantitative immunoglobulin measurement (IgA, IgG, IgM)	Confirms monoclonal gammopathy; >90% of patients also have suppression of at least one uninvolved immunoglobulin at diagnosis.
β_2-Microglobulin	Important for prognosis; measures tumor burden.
24-Hour urine protein electrophoresis with immunofixation	75% of patients have M protein in their urine by immunofixation. Because approximately 20% of patients have light chain only, the free monoclonal light chain may be missed in the serum in these patients; this test is essential, especially in this subgroup of patients.
Radiographic bone survey	75% of patients have punched-out lytic lesions, osteoporosis, or fractures on conventional radiography. Because myelomatous bone lesions are lytic, conventional radiography is superior to technetium 99m bone scanning.
Bone marrow aspirate and biopsy	Essential but not sufficient for the diagnosis of MM. Plasma cells account for ≥10% of bone marrow cells.
Bone marrow plasma cell labeling index	Specifically measures plasma cell proliferation. Prognostic for survival.
Cytogenetic and FISH studies	Obtained at diagnosis. Certain chromosomal abnormalities (e.g., deletion of the long arm of chromosome 13) are associated with shorter disease-free and overall survival.

FISH = fluorescence in situ hybridization.

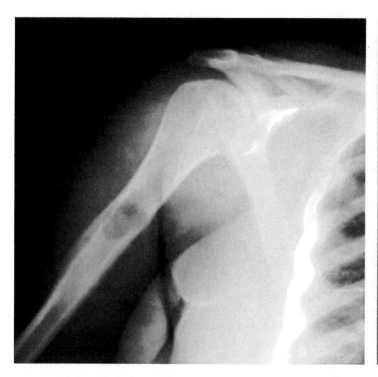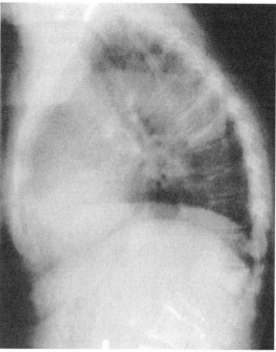

Figure 1. Lytic lesion of the right humerus (*left*) and osteoporosis and compression fracture of the thoracic spine (*right*) in a patient with multiple myeloma.

scans are not obtained, because the myeloma lesions usually are lytic and lack the associated increase in osteoblast activity that leads to positive bone scans typical of other forms of metastatic cancer. A bone marrow aspirate and biopsy are performed to document the presence of increased plasma cells. Although excessive in number, plasma cells are normal in individual appearance in most patients; however, in some patients, binucleate or other frankly dysplastic plasma cell morphologies may assist in the diagnosis. Quantitative immunoglobulin measurement will show depressed amounts of nonmonoclonal immunoglobulins, aiding in the diagnosis and providing clinically relevant information (i.e., depressed levels of normal immunoglobulins predisposes the patient to recurrent infection). Significant elevations in serum lactate dehydrogenase and β_2-microglobulin suggest a high myeloma tumor burden and are used to determine prognosis and guide therapy.

Patients found to have M proteins are stratified into three categories: MGUS (a premalignant condition that may remain stable for decades), MM, and an in-between condition termed *smoldering myeloma*. Patients with MGUS are asymptomatic. They have smaller amounts of M protein and normal amounts of the other immunoglobulins. Examination of the bone marrow reveals <10% plasma cells. These patients do not have signs of bone marrow failure, skeletal abnormalities, hypercalcemia, or kidney injury. Conversely, patients with MM have larger quantities of M protein associated with hypogammaglobulinemia. Most have anemia and/or bone pain or other radiographic signs of bone involvement. Hypercalcemia and kidney disease may be noted, and the bone marrow will show a higher percentage of plasma cells. Patients with smoldering myeloma have increased numbers of plasma cells in the bone marrow and a correspondingly larger amount of M protein, but they are otherwise asymptomatic. The differentiation of MM from MGUS is summarized in Table 3.

Therapy

MM is a heterogeneous illness, ranging from smoldering myeloma, which usually requires no therapy, to rapidly progressive disease. The first goal in determining therapy is assessing the risk for death and complications and determining the patient's eligibility

Table 3. Diagnosis of Multiple Myeloma[a] and Monoclonal Gammopathy of Undetermined Significance (MGUS)

Multiple myeloma major criteria

1. Plasmacytoma on tissue biopsy

2. Bone marrow clonal plasma cells >30%

3. High M protein (IgG >3.5 g/dL [35 g/L], IgA >2.0 g/dL [20 g/L]) or Bence Jones proteinuria >1.0 g/24 h

Multiple myeloma minor criteria

A. Bone marrow clonal plasma cells: 10%-30%

B. IgG <3.5 g/dL (35 g/L), IgA <2.0 g/dL (20 g/L)

C. Lytic bone lesions

D. Diminished levels of nonmonoclonal immunoglobulins (IgM <50 mg/dL [0.5 g/L], IgA <100 mg/dL [1 g/L], or IgG <600 mg/dL [6 g/L])

MGUS criteria

• IgG <3.5 g/dL (35 g/L), IgA <2.0 g/dL (20 g/L)

• Bence Jones proteinuria <1.0 g/24 h

• Bone marrow clonal plasma cells <10%

• No end-organ damage (no symptoms, bone lesions, or anemia; normal kidney function)

[a]Diagnosis of multiple myeloma is based on the presence of at least 1 major criterion + 1 minor criterion *or* the presence of at least 3 minor criteria that include A and B.

for autologous stem cell transplantation. Markers of poor prognosis include various cytogenetic abnormalities, such as deletion of chromosome 13 and certain chromosome translocations. Other high-risk markers include acute kidney injury, hypercalcemia, severe anemia, elevated β_2-microglobulin, hypoalbuminemia, and >50% plasma cells on bone marrow aspirate.

Patients aged <75 years with good performance status are candidates for autologous stem cell transplantation, which is now considered the best therapy for symptomatic MM. Contraindications to autologous stem cell transplantation beyond advanced age and poor performance status include unstable and progressive kidney disease, decompensated cirrhosis, and New York Heart Association class III or IV heart failure. Patients who are eligible for transplantation are treated with an induction chemotherapy regimen for 2 to 4 months to reduce the tumor burden and to demonstrate responsiveness to chemotherapy. In general, agents such as melphalan, which will be used during the transplantation, should be avoided during induction treatment. Initial treatment typically includes high-dose dexamethasone and thalidomide. Lenalidomide (which is related to thalidomide in its antineoplastic action) and bortezomib (a proteasome inhibitor) are newer agents used at some centers for induction therapy. Thalidomide and lenalidomide are potent teratogens and must be used cautiously in women of childbearing age, although most female patients are postmenopausal. Patients receiving either thalidomide or lenalidomide with dexamethasone as combination therapy have a very high risk for venous thromboembolism and require thromboprophylaxis with aspirin, low-molecular-weight heparin, or warfarin. The response to treatment is determined by monitoring serum protein electrophoresis and/or urine protein electrophoresis; the amount of immunoglobulin should decrease significantly after 3 to 4 months of treatment. If a response is achieved, the patient is referred for autologous stem cell transplantation. Patients who are not candidates for transplantation are treated with chemotherapy regimens similar to those used for induction therapy. Melphalan may also be used.

Beyond specific chemotherapy and stem cell transplantation, a number of interventions can prevent complications of MM. Although the immune response may be blunted, pneumococcal vaccine and annual influenza vaccine should be given to all patients. Some experts advise the prophylactic use of antibiotics (trimethoprim-sulfamethoxazole or a quinolone) to prevent infectious complications. Trimethoprim-sulfamethoxazole also should be administered to prevent *Pneumocystis* pneumonia in all patients receiving prolonged corticosteroids, and acyclovir prophylaxis is recommended for patients receiving bortezomib to prevent varicella-zoster virus reactivation. Bisphosphonates (pamidronate or zoledronate) are used for hypercalcemia and for patients with bone pain, lytic lesions, or osteopenia. Bisphosphonate therapy has been shown to reduce the rate of subsequent bone fractures and to decrease pain. Prior to their initiation, pay careful attention to den-

tition and have any necessary dental work completed before treatment. Monitor patients carefully for side effects, including acute kidney injury and osteonecrosis of the jaw, which may be more likely to occur if dental work is done after long-term bisphosphonate treatment. Bisphosphonate therapy is limited to 2 years.

Radiation therapy can provide effective palliation of localized bone pain. Patients with MM and back pain need prompt radiographic evaluation, often with MRI, to rule out spinal cord compression. The evaluation should be done even if there is no motor or sensory deficit or other neurologic manifestation of cord compression. Paralysis, sensory loss, or incontinence would be more worrisome, and once patients develop neurologic deficits, emergent management with corticosteroids (typically dexamethasone), radiation therapy, or neurosurgery leads to neurologic recovery in only 50% of patients. Consider radiation therapy or surgery to treat impending long bone fracture unresponsive to chemotherapy.

Maintain hydration and avoid nephrotoxic drugs and contrast dyes in patients with MM to prevent acute kidney injury. Mild hypercalcemia may resolve with hydration alone, and early acute kidney injury may improve with hydration and treatment of hypercalcemia. Patients with severe kidney injury may require dialysis. Erythropoietic stimulating agents will improve symptomatic anemia. Initiate plasmapheresis for symptomatic hyperviscosity.

Follow-Up

Patients with MGUS have a transformation rate to MM that is proportional to the size of the M protein peak in their serum or urine. For example, patients with IgG levels <15 g/dL have a low risk of transformation over the next year compared with patients with levels ≥25 g/dL. Thus, patients with MGUS and low paraprotein concentrations are checked once a year, and those with larger concentrations are checked more often. Patients with MM are followed on a monthly basis to determine their response to therapy and to assess kidney function, blood cell counts, and calcium levels.

Book Enhancement

Go to www.acponline.org/essentials/hematology-section.html. In *MKSAP for Students 5*, assess your knowledge with items 26-28 in the **Hematology** section.

Acknowledgment

We would like to thank Dr. Mark M. Udden, who contributed to an earlier version of this chapter.

Bibliography

Palumbo A, Anderson K. Multiple myeloma. N Engl J Med. 2011;364: 1046-1060. [PMID: 21410373]

Chapter 48

Common Leukemias

Richard S. Eisenstaedt, MD

Leukemias are clonal malignant proliferations of hematopoietic cells. Leukemias are classified according to their cell of origin (myeloid or lymphoid) and by the tempo of their progress (chronic or acute). Chronic lymphocytic leukemia (CLL) is characterized by an indolent clonal proliferation of mature lymphocytes and is more similar to well-differentiated or follicular lymphoma than to acute leukemia. Chronic myeloid leukemia (CML) is a myeloproliferative disease characterized by clonal proliferation of myeloid cells that are able to mature and function normally. Acute myeloid leukemia (AML) and acute lymphoid leukemia (ALL) are clonal proliferations of myeloid or lymphoid cells that are arrested at an immature, nonfunctional stage of maturation and that replicate aggressively, causing bone marrow failure and neoplastic infiltration of other organs. Although some clinical features distinguish ALL from AML, and different chemotherapy is to treat these two acute leukemias, there is considerable similarity in the presentation of ALL and AML as well as similar general principles of evaluation, risk stratification, and management. ALL, which is more frequent in childhood, will not be discussed here.

Chronic Lymphocytic Leukemia

Diagnosis

CLL is the most common leukemia encountered in adults. Patients may be asymptomatic. The disease most often is diagnosed by the incidental finding of lymphocytosis detected on complete blood count (CBC), with or without diffuse lymphadenopathy. Some patients have symptoms related to bulky lymph node enlargement, or they may have early satiety, abdominal fullness, or other symptoms related to splenomegaly. Patients also may have systemic symptoms, including fever, malaise, night sweats, and weight loss.

Look for signs of anemia (pallor, tachycardia), lymphadenopathy, and hepatosplenomegaly. The key to diagnosis is the recognition of an increased blood leukocyte count due to increased numbers of mature lymphocytes and "smudge" cells (lymphocytes that appear flattened or distorted) during the process of preparing the peripheral smear (Plate 41). Bone marrow aspirates and biopsy may be performed to evaluate thrombocytopenia or anemia but most often reveal an expansion of mature lymphocytes that reflects findings in the peripheral blood.

The diagnosis of CLL is confirmed by an absolute increase in mature lymphocytes ($>5000/\mu L$ [$5 \times 10^9/L$]) in the absence of an acute viral illness or other trigger for benign or reactive lymphocytosis. The chronicity and, at times, the magnitude of the lymphocytosis distinguish CLL from infectious or other reactive causes. Immunophenotyping by flow cytometry will show a mon-

oclonal proliferation of mature B lymphocyte phenotype with expression of CD19 and CD20, along with expression of a T lymphocyte antigen (CD5). Such immunophenotyping, in addition to distinguishing CLL from reactive lymphocytosis, will identify less common variants of CLL, including those arising from clonal T lymphocytes rather than B lymphocytes.

Staging of CLL is based on the physical examination and CT to assess lymphadenopathy and hepatosplenomegaly. Two staging schemes are used:

- The Rai staging system applies stage 0 to asymptomatic patients with lymphocytosis; these patients account for about 25% of the population and have a mean survival of >10 years. Patients with stage I CLL (lymphocytosis plus lymphadenopathy) or stage II CLL (lymphocytosis, lymphadenopathy, and hepatosplenomegaly) account for 50% of the popuation and survive 6 to 9 years. Patients with stage III CLL (anemia) or stage IV CLL (thrombocytopenia) account for the remaining 25% and have a more lethal course, with a mean survival <2 years.

- The Binet system is based on the number of lymph node sites involved. For example, bilateral cervical lymph node enlargement is counted as one site, bilateral cervical and axillary lymphadenopathy is counted as two sites, and an enlarged liver and enlarged spleen each count as one lymph node site. Stage A has fewer than three sites involved, and survival is comparable to age-matched controls without CLL. Stage B has three or more sites involved, with survival of 7 years. Stage C, defined as the additional presence of either anemia or thrombocytopenia, is associated with survival of approximately 2 years.

Patients with early-stage disease require only observation. Later-stage disease, which often is associated with symptoms, requires active treatment. Specialized testing, such as cytogenetic studies and determination of the mutational status of the immunoglobulin variable (V) gene, is becoming increasingly important in establishing risk for disease progression in CLL.

CLL-associated symptoms may arise from lymph node enlargement or hepatosplenomegaly. Malaise, fatigue, exertional dyspnea, or bleeding manifestations may be secondary to anemia or thrombocytopenia. Associated systemic symptoms (anorexia, weight loss) may become debilitating. Patients with CLL may develop various immune defects that predispose to infectious complications, the most common being infection with encapsulated organisms (e.g., *Streptococcus pneumoniae*), which arises from inadequate B cell function or hypogammaglobulinemia. Patients may also have cell-mediated immune defects that predispose to recurrent herpes simplex virus infections. Different forms of chemotherapy produce additional immunodeficiencies. Patients with CLL also are at increased risk for autoimmune disease, most commonly autoimmune thrombocytopenia; autoimmune hemolytic anemia is less common. Management of the underlying autoimmune disorder often requires concomitant treatment of CLL.

Therapy

Pneumococcal and yearly influenza vaccinations are recommended. Patients with recurrent bacterial infections and hypogammaglobulinemia may benefit from immunoglobulin infusion therapy. The small numbers of viable stem cells present in the peripheral blood may cause a graft-versus-host disease in severely immunosuppressed patients who receive transfused blood products, which is analogous to that seen following allogeneic bone marrow transplantation (BMT). The transfusion graft-versus-host syndrome is characterized by diffuse erythroderma, diarrhea, abnormal liver function, and bone marrow failure. The syndrome usually is lethal but may be prevented by irradiating all transfused blood products.

Asymptomatic patients with early-stage disease may be followed with no active treatment. Most symptomatic patients are treated with the purine analogue, fludarabine. Patients with very advanced disease sometimes are given a combination of fludarabine, cyclophosphamide, and humanized antibody against CD20 (rituximab). About 10% of patients will develop autoimmune thrombocytopenia or hemolytic anemia. These patients may respond to chemotherapy for CLL, prednisone, or anti-CD20 treatment. Radiation therapy sometimes is used to control painful or bulky lymph nodes. Very young patients are considered for BMT.

Follow-Up

Most patients with CLL are elderly, and many never require treatment for their leukemia. Follow the CBC periodically to look for a rapid increase in the lymphocyte count, anemia, or thrombocytopenia. Patients who have received fludarabine-based treatment are profoundly immunosuppressed and may develop atypical infections, such as *Pneumocystis* pneumonia. About 10% of patients experience a transformation of their chronic leukemia to a very aggressive and difficult-to-treat diffuse large B-cell lymphoma; this is known as *Richter transformation*.

Chronic Myeloid Leukemia

Diagnosis

CML is a clonal proliferation of mature granulocytes associated with a translocation between chromosomes 9 and 22, t(9;22)(q34;q11), which results in a truncated chromosome 22 (the Philadelphia chromosome). This reciprocal translocation results in the BCR-ABL fusion gene and the production of a unique tyrosine kinase protein. Although patients usually present in the chronic phase of disease and may do well for years, CML, if untreated, will invariably transform into acute leukemia (myeloid in two thirds of patients, lymphoid in one third). The transformation may be preceded by an "accelerated phase" of disease characterized by progressive leukocytosis and splenomegaly, extreme thrombocytosis or thrombocytopenia, and systemic symptoms, all of which are resistant to treatment. CML is one of four myeloproliferative disorders, all characterized by their clonal origin, disordered hematopoiesis (typically manifest by excessive proliferation of at least one cell line) associated features (e.g., hepatosplenomegaly), and an associated risk of evolving to acute leukemia. The other myeloproliferative diseases are polycythemia rubra vera, essential thrombocythemia, and myelofibrosis with myeloid metaplasia.

Patients with CML present with fatigue, lethargy, low-grade fever, and weight loss. Splenomegaly may be striking and is associated with early satiety, abdominal distention, or left upper quadrant pain. Physical examination may reveal pallor and splenomegaly, but lymphadenopathy is not common in the chronic phase.

CML is recognized by an elevated blood leukocyte count and increased number of granulocytic cells in all phases of development on the peripheral blood smear (Plate 42). The magnitude of the leukocytosis varies from $15,000/\mu L$ [15×10^9/L] to $50,000/\mu L$ [50×10^9/L]) but is still within the range that could be triggered by an infectious disease (termed a *leukemoid reaction*). In some patients, the leukocyte count will be >$100,000/\mu L$ [100×10^9/L], which is more pathognomonic of a myeloproliferative disorder. Very immature cells, such as myeloblasts and promyelocytes, may be seen in small numbers in the peripheral blood smear, but myelocytes and metamyelocytes are more predictably found. Basophils and eosinophils are increased, as they are in other myeloproliferative disorders. The platelet count often is elevated, and striking thrombocytosis (>$1,000,000/\mu L$ [1000×10^9/L]) may be seen. Patients often have anemia. The bone marrow aspirate tends to mirror findings in the peripheral blood, with marked expansion of myeloid cells and a shift toward less mature forms. When blasts represent >10% of the leukocytes, accelerated or blast phase should be considered. Increased megakaryocytes are seen, and increased collagen and reticulin fibrosis will be noted on bone marrow biopsy.

The diagnosis is confirmed by cytogenetic studies of the bone marrow aspirate showing a t(9;22) chromosomal abnormality or the presence of the novel BCR-ABL gene produced by the translocation. The BCR-ABL gene is detected and quantitated by polymerase chain reaction (PCR). Patients with abdominal pain or discomfort should undergo abdominal ultrasonography or CT to identify splenomegaly or splenic infarction.

Therapy

The treatment of CML was revolutionized by the development of therapy targeting the novel tyrosine kinase produced by the BCR-ABL gene. Inhibition of this kinase by imatinib reduces the leukocyte count, shrinks the spleen, and clears the bone marrow of Philadelphia chromosome–positive cells. Imatinib treatment often achieves molecular remissions in which no BCR-ABL transcripts can be identified in the blood or bone marrow. Imatinib must be given indefinitely; BCR-ABL–positive cells will appear 3 to 4 months after discontinuation of therapy. Dasatinib and nilotinib are newer options that may work more rapidly and cause more noticeable inhibition of tyrosine kinase. These newer agents may be used to initiate therapy or to treat patients who become resistant to imatinib.

Allogeneic BMT was the preferred treatment option for patients with CML before the discovery of tyrosine kinase inhibitors. BMT remains the most definitive option to cure the disease, albeit at the cost of significantly greater treatment toxicity (including mortality) and subsequent complications from graft-versus-host disease. There are no randomized trials to compare BMT to tyrosine kinase inhibitors, and most experts recommend beginning therapy with a tyrosine kinase inhibitor. Allogeneic BMT might be used as initial therapy in very young patients with CML but will more typically is used in patients showing signs of resistance to tyrosine kinase inhibitors. Once the disease has transformed into an accelerated phase or acute leukemia, the prognosis is poor, regardless of treatment option.

Patients may require transfusion occasionally to treat anemia and rarely for thrombocytopenia. Massive splenomegaly with splenic infarction may require splenectomy for patient comfort.

Follow-Up

Patients typically are seen every 1 to 2 weeks during the initiation of treatment with imatinib. Once stable blood counts are achieved, patients are followed every month to monitor blood counts. Peripheral blood or bone marrow samples are obtained periodically to assess the efficacy of treatment; the best results are associated with a fourfold reduction of BCR-ABL transcripts determined by quantitative PCR. Increasing leukocyte counts, basophilia, fever, and an enlarging spleen are signs of accelerated phase and blast crisis.

Acute Myeloid Leukemia

Diagnosis

AML is a malignant clonal proliferation of myeloid cells that do not fully mature. AML most commonly occurs in patients with no antecedent risk factors; its incidence is increased in patients who are exposed to radiation or benzene or following therapy with chemotherapy, especially alkylating agents. AML also occurs as a result of transformation of a myeloproliferative disorder (CML, polycythemia vera) or in patients with a preexisting myelodysplastic syndrome.

Patients with AML present with nonspecific symptoms of fatigue, pallor, and easy bleeding. Of all the leukemias, AML is most likely to cause significant thrombocytopenia, with bleeding, bruising, and petechiae; in addition, inadequate numbers of mature functioning leukocytes lead to infection. Patients have a variable degree of lymphadenopathy and hepatosplenomegaly. Leukemic cells may infiltrate extramedullary sites, such as the gingivae, skin, and meninges. When the leukocyte count is very high, patients may present with leukostasis syndrome, which is presumed to be secondary to leukemic blasts occluding the microcirculation and leading to respiratory failure and cerebral dysfunction.

The diagnosis of AML is suggested by an elevated leukocyte count, anemia, thrombocytopenia, and blasts on the peripheral blood smear (Plate 43). At times, patients may have an "aleukemic" form of AML with severe leukopenia (often pancytopenia), and a scarcity of circulating immature blast forms. The diagnosis of AML is confirmed by bone marrow aspiration and biopsy showing >20% blasts. Typical myeloblasts demonstrate

antigens found on immature cells, such as CD34 (stem cell marker) and HLA-DR, as well as antigens more specific for granulocytic maturation, such as CD33 and CD13. Cytogenetic studies are crucial, because specific genetic abnormalities are associated with either a favorable or a poor prognosis. The morphology of the bone marrow cells combined with immunophenotype and results of cytogenetic studies are used to classify AML according to the World Health Organization and French-American-British (FAB) classification systems.

Acute promyelocytic leukemia is a special subset of AML characterized by a t(15;17) translocation (which disturbs a retinoic acid receptor) and by proliferation of promyelocytes, with their characteristic primary granules. Patients with acute promyelocytic leukemia have significant bleeding at the time of their presentation due to fibrinolysis and disseminated intravascular coagulation.

Therapy

Patients require immediate hospitalization for placement of durable venous access (Hickman catheter, subcutaneous port), initiation of chemotherapy, irradiated blood and platelet transfusion support, and, if febrile and leukopenic, antibiotics for presumed infection.

The standard chemotherapy induction regimen is 3 days of an anthracycline, such as idarubicin, and 7 days of a continuous infusion of cytarabine. With the initiation of chemotherapy, some patients are at risk for abrupt necrosis of a large mass of leukemia cells and release of their intracellular contents into the circulation, or *tumor lysis syndrome*. The syndrome is characterized by hyperuricemia, hyperphosphatemia, hypocalcemia, hyperkalemia, and acute kidney injury. Tumor lysis syndrome may be prevented or attenuated with vigorous intravenous hydration, allopurinol or rasburicase (recombinant urate oxidase), and, if needed, phosphate binders and hemodialysis. After induction therapy, patients remain pancytopenic for many days, and infectious and bleeding complications are common. Patients with neutropenic fever should receive broad-spectrum antibiotics until the bone marrow recovers, regardless of whether cultures remain negative. Persistent neutropenic fever despite antibiotics warrants empiric antifungal therapy.

Younger patients and patients with favorable cytogenetic abnormalities do well, with remission rates of 60% to 70%; remission is defined as normalization of the blood count, <5% bone marrow blasts, and normalization of the karyotype. Most of these patients will remain in remission and achieve 10-year disease-free survival. Older patients with significant comorbidities and high-risk cytogenetic abnormalities have much lower remission rates as well as a higher risk of treatment mortality; these patients may be better treated palliatively rather than with induction chemotherapy. In addition to advanced age, poor performance status, and certain cytogenetic abnormalities, AML that is related to prior cancer chemotherapy or a preexisting myeloproliferative or dysmyelopoietic syndrome has a poor prognosis.

Once remission is achieved, consolidation chemotherapy is given and patients with high-risk disease are referred for allogeneic BMT. Treatment for acute promyelocytic leukemia is initiated with all-*trans*-retinoic acid, which induces maturation of the promyelocyte and ameliorates disseminated intravascular coagulation.

Follow-Up

Patients with AML who relapse tend to do so within 18 to 24 months of achieving complete remission. Patients are seen monthly during the first 2 years after remission to perform an interim history, physical examination, and blood count; bone marrow aspiration is performed only if there are abnormalities in the CBC. Patients who have undergone allogeneic BMT should be managed at centers familiar with posttransplantation complications, including opportunistic infections and graft-versus-host disease.

Book Enhancement

Go to www.acponline.org/essentials/hematology-section.html. In *MKSAP for Students 5*, assess your knowledge with items 29-31 in the **Hematology** section.

Acknowledgment

We would like to thank Dr. Mark M. Udden, who contributed to an earlier version of this chapter.

Bibliography

Betz BL, Hess JL. Acute myeloid leukemia diagnosis in the 21st century. Arch Pathol Lab Med. 2010;134:1427-1433. [PMID:20923295]

Goldman JM. Chronic myeloid leukemia: a historical perspective. Semin Hematol. 2010;47:302-311. [PMID:20875546]

Gribben JG, O'Brien S. Update on therapy of chronic lymphocytic leukemia. J Clin Oncol. 2011;29:544-550. [PMID:21220603]

Testa U. Leukemia stem cells. Ann Hematol. 2011;90:245-271. [PMID:21107841]

Chapter 49

Approach to Fever

Joseph T. Wayne, MD

Fever is a complex adaptive biologic response that alters the body's temperature set-point. Fever results from the production of cytokines, including interleukins 1 and 6, tumor necrosis factor, interferons, and prostaglandin E_2. Normal body temperature ranges from 35.6°C (96.0°F) to 38.2°C (100.8°F), with a mean of 36.8°C (98.2°F). There is a diurnal variation, with a nadir near 6 AM and a peak near 4 PM. Fever is defined as a body temperature ≥37.2°C (99.0°F) in the morning or ≥37.7°C (100.0°F) in the afternoon. Hyperthermia occurs when thermoregulatory control is overwhelmed by the combination of exogenous heat exposure and excess heat production without a change in the hypothalamic set-point or cytokine production.

Approach to the Patient

Fever can be a presenting symptom or sign in infectious and noninfectious conditions. Subjective patient reports of fever are accurate only about 50% to 75% of the time. Body temperature can be measured with digital thermometers, infrared tympanic thermometers, and liquid crystal thermometers, which measure surface temperature of the skin. Digital thermometers are the most accurate, with rectal temperature the most reproducible. Infrared tympanic thermometers and liquid crystal thermometers can vary as much as 0.5-1.5°C (0.9-2.7°F). Newer infrared thermometers measuring temporal artery temperatures are accurate and reliable. It is best to record body temperature from the same site every time (e.g., all oral).

The approach to a febrile patient varies depending on clinical setting (outpatient or inpatient) and whether the patient is immunocompromised. For all patients, first determine the duration of the fever, rapidity of fever onset (abrupt or gradual), and presence or absence of constitutional symptoms (e.g., chills, rigor, sweating). Next, look for localizing clues (e.g., cough, coryza, dyspnea, dysuria, diarrhea, localized pain, wounds, rash, unusual discharge, history of recent medical interventions or instrumentation), and focus the physical examination based on these findings. Medication history is always important. Drug reactions can cause confounding and recurrent fever, some with shaking chills. It often is possible to determine if a drug interaction is the cause of fever by eliminating the suspected drug and observing for 48 to 72 hours.

Outpatient Fever

Most cases of fever seen in the outpatient setting are due to viral illness and will resolve in <2 weeks. If a patient is seriously ill (e.g., pale, dyspneic, cool, clammy, hypotensive, tachycardic, cyanotic,

confused or with an otherwise altered mental state), bacterial infection is more likely. If there are no localizing symptoms, a detailed history and thorough physical examination, including a pelvic examination in a female patient, are necessary. In stable patients, this information can be gathered over several visits. Address recent medication use or transfusions, implanted devices or prostheses, exposure to known illnesses, animal exposures, travel history, drug use, sexual habits, dietary habits (e.g., raw seafood or undercooked meat), and family history of connective tissue disease. This process is repeated to assess any new symptoms and to monitor for changes. If fever has been of short duration and no potential source for the fever is suggested at the first visit, testing should be directed at any potentially localizing symptoms or physical findings (e.g., rapid antigen detection test for pharyngitis). A fever that persists for >3 weeks despite three or more visits and appropriate investigation is designated a fever of unknown origin.

Inpatient Fever

Fever that occurs in the inpatient setting requires assessment for localizing signs and symptoms as well as potential sources of infection or fever, including intravascular catheters (bacteremia), urinary catheters (urinary tract infection), nasogastric tubes (sinusitis), foreign bodies (infected prosthetic joint, vascular graft, or pacemaker), and blood transfusions (febrile transfusion reaction). Problems due to prolonged immobility (deep venous thrombosis, decubitus ulcers, atelectasis) also should be considered.

Investigate any localized findings, check all invasive sites for signs of infection, inspect dependent parts of the body for skin breakdown (redness, warmth, tenderness, swelling, discharge), examine the legs for swelling, and look for medications associated with hyperthermia or fever. Examinations should be repeated daily until a source is found or the fever resolves. In addition, perform standard laboratory tests, chest radiography, and additional tests as directed by the physical findings. A fever that persists without a diagnosis for >3 days in an immunocompromised inpatient or >1 week in an immunocompetent inpatient is designated a fever of unknown origin.

Fever of Unknown Origin

The most common categories of illness associated with fever of unknown origin (FUO) are infectious diseases, systemic inflammatory disorders, and malignancies. The most common infectious cause is tuberculosis; intraabdominal or pelvic abscess is another common cause. Vertebral osteomyelitis occasionally is characterized by FUO without localizing back pain or symptoms. When endocarditis causes FUO, it usually is associated with culture-negative organisms, such as *Coxiella burnetii*, *Bartonella quintana*, or the HACEK organisms (*Haemophilus* species, *Actinobacillus actinomycetemcomitans*, *Cardiobacterium hominis*, *Eikenella corrodens*, and *Kingella kingae*). Febrile illnesses often are associated with rash. The distribution of the rash (e.g., extremities [Rocky Mountain spotted fever], trunk [infectious mononucleosis, typhoid fever], or palms and soles [syphilis]), the chronicity of the rash relative to fever, and the character of the rash (e.g., vesicular [smallpox, chickenpox] or petechial [vasculitis]) are important in determining a potential cause. Some fever-associated skin lesions suggest serious underlying illnesses, such as Janeway lesions, Osler nodes, or subconjunctival petechiae, which occur in infective endocarditis. In approximately 80% of patients with HIV infection, an additional infection is the cause of fever.

One of the more common vasculitides is temporal arteritis, which can present as FUO in adults aged >50 years, even in the absence of the classic symptoms of headache, jaw claudication, or polymyalgia rheumatica. Other vasculitides (e.g., Wegener granulomatosis) and systemic inflammatory disorders (e.g., systemic lupus erythematosus, adult-onset Still disease) also should be considered.

The most common FUO-associated malignancy is non-Hodgkin lymphoma. Renal cell carcinoma, any malignancy that metastasizes to the liver, and leukemia are other common causes.

Patients with FUO require a through history, physical examination, and laboratory evaluation (Table 1). Obtain a complete blood count with differential, a peripheral blood smear, an erythrocyte sedimentation rate (ESR), a C-reactive protein (CRP) level, and urinalysis. Immature neutrophils (band forms), toxic granulations, or Döhle bodies may indicate a bacterial cause of fever. Leukopenia most often is due to viral illness but also may be seen with autoimmune or marrow infiltrative disorders. Lymphocytosis with atypical lymphocytes is associated with acute Epstein-Barr, cytomegalovirus, and HIV infections; monocytosis can be seen with typhoidal disease and tuberculosis. In stable patients, there is no need to initiate antibiotic therapy until a diagnosis is established.

If no infectious cause is identified, further evaluation is directed toward autoimmune diseases, connective tissue diseases, and granulomatous disorders (i.e., sarcoidosis). In the miscellaneous category, thyroiditis, pulmonary embolism, drug fever, and factitious fever need to be considered. If ESR and CRP level are normal at the time symptoms are present, factitious fever should be considered.

Despite an extensive workup, one third to half of patients may not receive a specific diagnosis. These patients generally have a good prognosis, with resolution of fever in several months.

Management

Fever, as a symptom, does not always require treatment. When antipyretic agents are administered, studies have shown prolonged time to crusting in varicella and increased viral shedding and suppressed neutralizing antibody production in herpes zoster and rhinovirus infections. Cooling blankets have been shown to increase oxygen consumption (by induced shivering) and to cause coronary artery vasospasm. Antipyretic agents also have adverse effects; aspirin is associated with gastrointestinal and renal adverse effects, and acetaminophen is associated with hepatic and renal adverse effects. Antipyretic therapy may be considered for patient comfort and is considered safe when appropriate dosing guidelines are followed. In stable patients without localizing signs, empiric antibiotic therapy typically is withheld. In unstable patients without localizing signs, empiric broad-spectrum antibiotics may be initiated (see Chapter 50).

Hyperthermia

Hyperthermia is a noninfectious disorder of thermoregulation that results in elevation of body temperature above the normal range. Body temperatures >40.0°C (104.0°F) are life threatening, and brain death begins at 41.0°C (105.8°F). The most important causes of severe hyperthermia are heat stroke, malignant hyperthermia, neuroleptic malignant syndrome, and the serotonin syndrome.

Nonexertional heat stroke from impaired thermoregulation occurs in various cardiovascular, neurologic, and psychiatric disorders and in patients taking diuretics and anticholinergic agents, particularly with exposure to a hot environment. Exertional heat stroke results from strenuous exercise in very hot and humid weather. The first sign of serious heat stroke is the absence of sweating and warm, dry skin. Fans, cooling blankets, ice packs, cold intravenous fluids, and oxygen are used; for severe hyperthermia, cold gastric and peritoneal lavage also is used. Benzodiazepines decrease excessive shivering during treatment.

Malignant hyperthermia is an inherited skeletal muscle disorder characterized by a hypermetabolic state precipitated by exposure to volatile inhalation anesthetics (halothane, isoflurane, enflurane, desflurane, sevoflurane) and depolarizing muscle relaxants (succinylcholine, decamethonium). Malignant hyperthermia usually occurs on exposure to the drug. Increased intracellular calcium leads to sustained muscle contractions, with resultant skeletal mus-

Table 1. Typical Laboratory Evaluation for Persistent Fever

For all patients

Complete blood cell count with differential, peripheral blood smear

Comprehensive metabolic panel

Urinalysis and microscopy

Blood and urine cultures

Antinuclear antibody and rheumatoid factor testing

HIV antibody testing

Chest radiography

For select patients

Viral serology in patients with mononucleosis-like syndrome (cytomegalovirus, heterophil)

Q fever serology (if exposure to farm animals)

Hepatitis serology (if abnormal liver enzyme levels)

cle rigidity and masseter spasm, tachycardia, hypercarbia, hypertension, hyperthermia, tachypnea, and cardiac arrhythmias. Rhabdomyolysis and acute kidney failure can develop. Malignant hyperthermia is life threatening if not treated immediately. Treatment includes discontinuing the offending drug and supportive care (hydration, oxygen, cooling measures). Dantrolene sodium, a skeletal muscle relaxant, is the treatment of choice.

The neuroleptic malignant syndrome is a life-threatening disorder caused by an idiosyncratic reaction to neuroleptic tranquilizers and some antipsychotic agents. The most common offending neuroleptic agents are haloperidol and fluphenazine. The syndrome can occur with all drugs that cause central dopamine receptor blockade and usually occurs soon after starting a new drug or with dose escalation. Most patients with the syndrome develop muscle rigidity, hyperthermia, cognitive changes, autonomic instability, diaphoresis, sialorrhea, seizures, arrhythmias, and rhabdomyolysis within 2 weeks after initiating the drug. Death may occur from respiratory or cardiac failure, disseminated intravascular coagulation, or acute kidney failure.

Drug therapy with dantrolene sodium and/or bromocriptine decreases mortality and duration of symptoms.

The serotonin syndrome presents as high fever, muscle rigidity, and cognitive changes. Unique findings include shivering, hyperreflexia, myoclonus, and ataxia. The serotonin syndrome most often is caused by the use of selective serotonin reuptake inhibitors. Stopping the offending medication(s) and supportive care are the mainstays of therapy.

Book Enhancement

Go to www.acponline.org/essentials/infectious-disease-section. html. In *MKSAP for Students 5*, assess your knowledge with items 1-3 in the **Infectious Disease Medicine** section.

Bibliography

Tolia J, Smith LG. Fever of unknown origin: historical and physical clues to making the diagnosis. Infect Dis Clin North Am. 2007;21:917-936, vii. [PMID: 18061082]

Chapter 50

Sepsis Syndrome

Isaac O. Opole, MD

Sepsis syndrome is a continuum of four clinical entities with a stepwise increase in morbidity and mortality: systemic inflammatory response syndrome (SIRS), sepsis, severe sepsis, and septic shock. Severe sepsis accounts for 20% of all admissions to intensive care units (ICUs) and is the leading cause of death in noncardiac ICUs. Approximately 750,000 cases of severe sepsis occur in the United States each year, with mortality rates of 20% to 50%. The incidence of sepsis rises exponentially after age 65 to 70 years, and age-specific mortality rates are much higher in patients with baseline comorbidities, such as diabetes mellitus or heart disease. Sepsis is most common in men, nonwhites, and the elderly, with gram-positive organisms accounting for >50% of all cases. The predicted mortality for a patient with severe sepsis increases by 15% to 20% for each sepsis-induced dysfunctional organ. Early diagnosis of sepsis syndrome and early goal-directed therapy reduce mortality.

Sepsis is a complex dysregulation of both inflammation and coagulation. Primary cell injury may result directly from infection or occur when a toxic microbial stimulus initiates a deleterious host inflammatory response. A network of inflammatory mediators are generated, including tumor necrosis factor (TNF)-α, interleukin-1 (IL-1), and other cytokines and chemokines that activate leukocytes and promote leukocyte vascular endothelial adhesion and damage. Endothelial damage leads to tissue factor expression and activation of the tissue factor–dependent clotting cascade and subsequent formation of thrombin. The result is the development of microaggregates of fibrin, platelets, neutrophils, and erythrocytes, which cause impaired capillary blood flow and decreased oxygen and nutrient delivery to tissues. Higher levels of circulating and intracellular TNF-α, IL-1, interleukin-6 (IL-6), and soluble adhesion molecules, which are markers for activated or damaged endothelium, are detected in older patients with sepsis. Even in the absence of sepsis, increased age is associated with elevated circulating levels of IL-6, D-dimer, activated coagulation factor VII, and other coagulation factors, indicating activation of inflammatory and coagulation pathways. This may explain in part the increased morbidity and mortality associated with sepsis in older patients.

Diagnosis

The diagnosis of sepsis syndrome relies on the early identification of SIRS, which is defined by four clinical criteria that lead to a high index of suspicion for infection or sepsis (Table 1). Sepsis is defined as the presence of two or more SIRS criteria plus the presence of a known or suspected infection (documented positive cultures are not required). Severe sepsis is defined as the presence of sepsis plus evidence of sepsis-induced dysfunction of at least one organ; such

Table 1. Definition of Systemic Inflammatory Response Syndrome

Presence of two or more of the following in the absence of other known causes of these:

- Temperature >38.0°C (100.4°F) or <36.0°C (96.8°F)
- Heart rate >90/min
- Respiration rate >20/min or arterial P_{CO_2} <32 mm Hg (4.3 kPa)
- Leukocyte count >12,000/μL (12×10^9/L) or < 4000/μL (4×10^9/L) with 10% bands

evidence may include hypoxemia, shock, delirium, thrombocytopenia, acute kidney injury (rising serum creatinine level), or hepatic injury (rising bilirubin or transaminase level). Septic shock occurs when there is profound sepsis-induced hypotension and hypoperfusion despite adequate fluid resuscitation. The differential diagnosis of septic shock should include other causes of shock, such as cardiogenic shock, neurogenic shock, severe hypovolemia, adrenal insufficiency, and anaphylaxis (Table 2).

The initial evaluation of the patient with sepsis includes a rapid yet thorough history and physical examination, with an emphasis on identifying a possible source of infection. Vital signs are crucial for diagnosis as well as assessment of the stability of the patient. Vital signs require continuous monitoring but are not always sensitive in older or immunosuppressed patients. For example, fever may be blunted or absent in approximately 15% of older patients with bacteremia compared with <5% of patients aged <65 years. There must be a high index for suspicion (especially in older patients) when any of the following nonspecific clinical signs or symptoms of infection are present: delirium, weakness, anorexia, malaise, urinary incontinence, or falls.

Laboratory evaluation is focused on finding evidence of end-organ dysfunction related to sepsis, such as acute kidney injury, liver dysfunction, disseminated intravascular coagulation, or mental status changes. Initial laboratory studies include a complete blood count with differential, serum electrolyte and creatinine levels, urinalysis, liver chemistry tests, and coagulation parameters. Serum lactate level should be measured, because it has been correlated with the degree of global tissue hypoxia, the severity of sepsis, and mortality risk. Blood, urine, and sputum cultures as well as cultures from other sites of potential infection should be obtained as soon as the diagnosis of sepsis is suspected. Radiography and other imaging studies should be obtained as directed by the patient's symptoms. Various biologic markers of sepsis have been studied (e.g., procalcitonin, C-reactive protein, IL-6), but none has been validated for routine clinical use.

Table 2. Differential Diagnosis of Shock

Disorder	Notes
Septic shock	Characterized by high cardiac output (early) that can become depressed (late), low systemic vascular resistance, and low filling pressures. Fever, leukocytosis, and source of infection are characteristically present.
Cardiogenic shock	Typically occurs in ACS, in valve dysfunction, or from cardiac tamponade. Characteristics include cardiogenic pulmonary edema, high filling pressures, low cardiac index, and high systemic vascular resistance. An ECG is useful in evaluating patients with suspected sepsis to exclude ACS. An echocardiogram also is useful in this regard.
Hypovolemic shock	Characterized by low cardiac output, high systemic vascular resistance, and low cardiac filling pressures. Patients may have a history of hemorrhage or volume depletion from other causes (e.g., severe diarrhea).
Anaphylactic shock	Clinical presentation includes urticaria, angioedema, or both; shortness of breath and wheezing; stridor due to laryngeal edema; pulmonary edema; and hypotension. As may be seen in severe sepsis, the systemic vascular resistance typically is low, and the cardiac output is elevated. Diagnosis is made when the typical signs and symptoms occur shortly after exposure to a suspected antigen. Treatment with epinephrine should be part of the initial management. Corticosteroids and antihistamines also are indicated.
Neurogenic shock (spinal shock)	Occurs after injury to the spinal cord or other severe CNS injury. Thought to be caused by failure of the autonomic nervous system; as a result, it is associated with low systemic vascular resistance and, typically, bradycardia. Bradycardia and hypotension in a patient with spinal cord injury should raise suspicion for neurogenic shock.
Adrenal crisis	Patients with adrenal crisis often have shock and abdominal symptoms (tenderness, nausea, vomiting) and may have fever. In addition, weakness, fatigue, lethargy, and confusion are common. Patients may have hyponatremia and hyperkalemia. If adrenal insufficiency is suspected, tests of adrenal function should be initiated without delay.
Obstructive shock	Characterized by hypotension, tachycardia, and low cardiac output; may mimic septic shock. Causes of obstructive shock include cardiac tamponade, pulmonary embolism, and tension pneumothorax. All of these diagnoses are rapidly life threatening.

ACS = acute coronary syndrome; CNS = central nervous system; ECG = electrocardiogram.

Therapy

Almost universally, patients are admitted to the hospital if they meet SIRS criteria. Patients with sepsis, severe sepsis, or septic shock are managed in the ICU. Most patients will require central venous access for fluid administration and invasive monitoring. Early goal-directed therapy aimed at restoration of hemodynamic stability should be instituted immediately on admission and during the first 6 hours of hospitalization. The initial goal of therapy is to maintain tissue perfusion, balancing oxygen delivery with oxygen demand to prevent tissue hypoxia. The Surviving Sepsis Campaign and the Institute for Healthcare Improvement have advocated the use of management "bundles" (groups of interventions that result in better outcomes when they are implemented together) in patients suspected of having severe sepsis or shock. The "severe sepsis resuscitation bundle" includes early assessment of serum lactate, aggressive fluid resuscitation, blood culture before initiation of antibiotics, early broad-spectrum antibiotic administration, and vasopressor administration (Table 3).

Early serum lactate measurement is important in assessing tissue perfusion; a lactate level >4 meq/L (4 mmol/L) is indicative of inadequate tissue perfusion. Aggressive fluid resuscitation with crystalloid or colloid should be initiated and continued until a central venous pressure (CVP) of 8 to 12 mm Hg or a mean arterial pressure (MAP) ≥65 mm Hg is attained. Adequate initial fluid resuscitation with resolution of lactic acidosis has been shown to be the most important factor in improving survival. There is no evidence supporting a benefit of one choice of fluid replacement over another. A 500- to 1000-mL bolus of fluid is given initially, and the CVP is monitored to direct subsequent fluid replacement.

Most patients need at least 4 to 6 L of fluid within the first 6 hours, and one of the biggest pitfalls of management is underestimating the intravascular volume deficit. Some protocols have suggested maintaining a superior vena cava oxygen saturation >70%. However, this practice has not yet been widely adopted.

If a fluid challenge fails to achieve an MAP ≥65 mm Hg, vasopressors are added as part of early goal-directed therapy. The most commonly used vasopressor for septic shock is norepinephrine. Norepinephrine is a potent peripheral vasoconstrictor effective in reversing the endotoxin-induced vasodilation that is the hallmark of septic shock. Dobutamine also is acceptable but is associated with more tachycardia and arrhythmia, because it acts as both an α- and a β-agonist. Vasopressin has been investigated for the treatment of severe shock resistant to other vasopressor agents and may be of some benefit. Vasopressin is avoided in patients with cardiac dysfunction, because it commonly depresses cardiac output.

Whenever possible, source control, including removal of sources of infection (e.g., indwelling catheters), drainage of abscesses, and surgical debridement of wounds, should occur promptly upon diagnosis of sepsis. Empiric antibiotic therapy should be initiated within 1 hour of recognition of sepsis and after blood has been drawn and samples from other suspected sites of infection have been taken for culture. Inadequate initial antibiotic therapy is independently associated with poor outcomes, and initial empiric therapy should include agents with activity against all probable pathogens. Because of increasing antibiotic resistance, broad and early antibiotic therapy must be balanced with de-escalation based on identified organisms and/or cessation of antibiotics once the infection has resolved. In selecting empiric antibiotics, recognize that gram-positive infections now cause most

Table 3. Severe Sepsis Resuscitation Bundle

Serum lactate measured

Blood cultures obtained prior to antibiotic administration

From the time of presentation, broad-spectrum antibiotics administered within 3 h for emergency department admissions and 1 h for intensive care unit admissions

In the event of hypotension and/or lactate >4 meq/L (4 mmol/L):

    Deliver an initial minimum of 20 mL/kg of crystalloid (or colloid equivalent)

    Apply vasopressors for hypotension not responding to initial fluid resuscitation to maintain mean arterial pressure >65 mm Hg

In the event of persistent hypotension despite fluid resuscitation (septic shock) and/or lactate >4 meq/L (4 mmol/L):

    Achieve central venous pressure >8 mm Hg

    Achieve central venous oxygen saturation >70%

Adapted with permission from Levy MM, Dellinger RP, Townsend SR, et al. The Surviving Sepsis Campaign: results of an international guideline-based performance improvement program targeting severe sepsis. Intensive Care Med. 2010;36:224. [PMID: 20069275]

cases of sepsis; however, gram-negative infections are still prevalent, and fungal infections must be considered in high-risk patients (e.g., neutropenic patients, patients receiving immunosuppression therapy).

In septic patients at high risk for death, recombinant human activated protein C (rhAPC or drotrecogin alpha) can be given. Risk is determined by a severity-of-illness scoring system, such as APACHE II (Acute Physiology and Chronic Health Evaluation II), or by the presence of septic shock requiring vasopressors, sepsis-induced acute respiratory distress syndrome requiring mechanical ventilation, or the presence of sepsis-induced dysfunction in two or more organs. In such patients, rhAPC has been shown to have a modest effect on mortality. However, bleeding complications are significantly increased in all patients taking rhAPC, with no demonstrated benefit in patients who are not at high risk; therefore, the drug should not be given to such patients. Where indicated, rhAPC is given as a continuous 96-hour infusion.

Although an early study reported improved mortality rates in patients with relative adrenal insufficiency who were treated with hydrocortisone and fludrocortisone, the landmark CORTICUS study failed to demonstrate any survival advantage for patients in septic shock with a systolic blood pressure ≥90 mm Hg. Therefore, corticosteroid therapy currently is not indicated in patients with sepsis or septic shock, except possibly for those patients with systolic blood pressure <90 mm Hg despite aggressive fluid resuscitation and vasopressors. Patients receiving corticosteroids should be monitored for hyperglycemia, immunosuppression, poor wound healing, delirium, and ICU-acquired weakness.

Hyperglycemia and insulin resistance are common in patients who are critically ill. Following initial stabilization, blood glucose levels should be controlled by continuous insulin infusion. Although blood glucose levels of 80-110 mg/dL (4.4-6.1 mmol/L) may be beneficial in patients with other forms of critical illness, tight glucose control does not have universal benefits and

Table 4. Treatment of Sepsis

Agent(s)	Notes
Crystalloid	Restores intravascular volume, which is depleted in patients with severe sepsis. Improves cardiac output, organ perfusion, and mortality in severe sepsis. Commonly given as repeated, rapid bolus infusions as long as the patient remains in shock or on vasopressor agents and continues to show a beneficial response without major adverse effects. Patients may require 4-6 L during initial stabilization.
Antibiotics (fourth-generation cephalosporin, extended-spectrum [antipseudomonal] penicillin, carbapenem)	Early appropriate antibiotic therapy is associated with improved outcomes. Appropriate empiric therapy should be initiated rapidly, even if the source of infection is unknown. A more appropriate, source-directed antibiotic selection should be initiated if the source is known or becomes known. For example, add vancomycin if MRSA is suspected, add double coverage with an intravenous fluoroquinolone or aminoglycoside if a highly resistant gram-negative pathogen is suspected, or add clindamycin if toxic shock syndrome is suspected; consider additional agents (e.g., fluoroquinolones, macrolides, tetracyclines, antifungal agents, antiviral agents) depending on the clinical presentation.
Norepinephrine	Improves blood pressure and cardiac output. Associated with less tachycardia than other vasopressor agents with β-effects. More effective than dopamine in refractory septic shock. Currently considered by many to be the first-choice vasopressor for patients with septic shock.
Dobutamine	Improves cardiac output. May be used in combination with a vasopressor to increase cardiac output if it is inappropriately low.
Vasopressin	Improves blood pressure in patients with septic shock. Because vasopressin works on receptors other than adrenergic receptors, it may be useful in refractory septic shock treated with high-dose adrenergic vasopressors. No randomized controlled trials exist to show a mortality benefit in this setting.
Drotrecogin alfa	Replaces activated protein C, which is depleted in severe sepsis. Activated protein C has antithrombotic, profibrinolytic, anti-inflammatory, and anti-apoptotic properties. Improves survival in patients with severe sepsis at high risk for death. Associated with a mild increase in the incidence of serious bleeding.

MRSA = methicillin-resistant *Staphylococcus aureus*.

in some cases may increase mortality. A glucose target of <180 mg/dL (1.0 mmol/L) results in lower mortality, and in septic patients, a modest goal of 140-180 mg/dL (7.8-8.3 mmol/L) is commonly recommended.

Low-dose unfractionated heparin or low-molecular-weight heparin is given for deep venous thrombosis prophylaxis. Mechanical compression devices are an alternative if anticoagulation is contraindicated. Proton pump inhibitors or H_2-receptor antagonists are given for stress ulcer prophylaxis. Erythrocyte transfusions should be considered conservatively. A large randomized trial showed that a target hemoglobin concentration of 7-9 g/dL (70-90 g/L) resulted in no additional mortality compared with the traditional target of 10 g/dL (100 g/L). Except in select cases, such as elderly patients with myocardial infarction, hemoglobin target concentrations of 7 g/dL (70 g/L) should be considered adequate. In mechanically ventilated patients, a lung-protective strategy of ventilation is recommended (tidal volume of 6 mL/kg predicted weight and an end-inspiratory passive recoil [plateau] pressure <30 cm H_2O), and the head of the bed should be raised to 45 degrees to reduce the risk of ventilator-associated pneumonia. Table 4 summarizes the various interventions used to treat sepsis.

Book Enhancement

Go to www.acponline.org/essentials/infectious-disease-section.html. In *MKSAP for Students 5*, assess your knowledge with items 4-8 in the **Infectious Disease Medicine** section.

Acknowledgment

We would like to thank Dr. Charin L. Hanlon, who contributed to an earlier version of this chapter.

Bibliography

Levy MM, Dellinger RP, Townsend SR, et al. The Surviving Sepsis Campaign: results of an international guideline-based performance improvement program targeting severe sepsis. Intensive Care Med. 2010;36:222-231. [PMID: 20069275]

Chapter 51

Common Upper Respiratory Problems

Jennifer Bierman, MD

This chapter addresses four common upper respiratory problems: upper respiratory infection, pharyngitis, sinusitis, and otitis media.

Upper Respiratory Infection

Upper respiratory infection (URI) is an undifferentiated, usually viral syndrome that is benign and self-limited, lasting 3 to 10 days. Viruses (rhinovirus, coronavirus, respiratory syncytial virus, meta pneumovirus) cause infection by gaining entrance to epithelial cells of the upper respiratory tract, leading to vasodilation and increased vascular permeability, cholinergic stimulation, and host inflammatory responses.

Prevention

Contact with secretions is the most likely principal mode of transmission. Frequent hand washing has been proved to prevent transmission. The use of vitamin C or *Echinacea* is not supported by strong evidence.

Diagnosis

Viral URIs have an incubation period of 24 to 72 hours and cause a combination of sore throat, cough, rhinorrhea, fever (body temperature ≤39°C [102°F]) lasting <72 hours, and/or laryngitis. Influenza is differentiated from a viral URI by a typically sudden onset of high fever (body temperature >39°C [102°F]), severe myalgia, and headache. Physical examination of the patient with a viral URI may reveal a red nose, glassy-appearing nasal mucosa, nasal discharge, and mild oropharyngeal erythema. Laboratory testing and imaging studies are unnecessary for diagnosis. A small percentage of patients will develop secondary acute bacterial sinusitis. Upper respiratory viruses can cause lower respiratory tract infections in patients with underlying cardiopulmonary disease or immunosuppression. Viral URIs also can heighten symptoms of asthma and COPD. Table 1 summarizes the differential diagnosis of URI.

Therapy

Inhaling heated vapor, such as steam from a hot shower, may decrease nasal symptoms. Other symptomatic measures include increasing fluid intake, gargling with salt water or using saline nasal spray, sucking on throat lozenges, and getting adequate rest. Although these measures lack good evidence of effectiveness, they are safe and inexpensive. For relief of nasal congestion, oral decongestants (pseudoephedrine) or short-term (<3 days) use of topical nasal decongestants (phenylephrine) is beneficial. In patients with rhinorrhea and sneezing, a short course of a first-generation antihistamine or intranasal ipratropium may be considered. In patients with a productive cough and wheezing, an inhaled β-agonist may reduce the duration of cough. Naproxen, ibuprofen, or acetaminophen may be used for headache, myalgia, and malaise. Codeine and over-the-counter antitussive agents have not proved to be effective for acute cough in URIs. Antibiotics are not indicated for uncomplicated URIs, even when purulent sputum or nasal discharge is present. In the United States, antibiotics are overprescribed for URIs, leading to increased antibiotic resistance. Patients should be instructed to follow up if they develop persistent cough, shortness of breath, hemoptysis, chest pain, wheezing, dysphagia, trismus (inability to open the mouth), severe headache, persistent nasal discharge, or ear pain.

Pharyngitis

Pharyngitis is a common condition encountered in the ambulatory setting. Although viruses (e.g., rhinovirus) are the most frequent cause of pharyngitis, infection caused by group A β-hemolytic streptococcus (GABHS) is a concern. GABHS is the major treatable pathogen but causes only about 5% to 15% of cases of acute pharyngitis in adults. Sequelae of GABHS pharyngitis include toxic shock syndrome, suppurative complications (peritonsillar abscess, pneumonia, sepsis), and nonsuppurative postinfectious complications (rheumatic fever, glomerulonephritis, reactive arthritis). *Chlamydophila pneumoniae* and *Mycoplasma pneumoniae* are other bacterial causes of pharyngitis, but treatment has not proved to be beneficial. Much less common causes include Epstein-Barr virus infection and acute HIV infection. *Fusobacterium necrophorum* is an emerging cause of nonstreptococcal pharyngitis in adolescents and young adults, accounting for up to 10% of cases in some series. *F. necrophorum* is a gram-negative anaerobe that can cause suppurative complications; it also is the pathogenic agent of Lemierre syndrome (septic thrombophlebitis of the internal jugular vein). Lemierre syndrome has a mortality rate of approximately 4.4%.

Prevention

In the general population, proper diagnosis and treatment of patients who present with symptomatic group A streptococcal pharyngitis usually are sufficient to control the transmission and rapid spread of virulent GABHS strains. Do not use prophylactic antibiotics in asymptomatic individuals to prevent the spread of infection.

Table 1. Differential Diagnosis of Upper Respiratory Infection

Disorder	Notes
Streptococcal pharyngitis	Fever, tonsillar exudates, and tender anterior cervical adenopathy; cough is absent. Trismus, unilateral tonsillar swelling, and deviation of the uvula suggest peritonsillar abscess.
Sinusitis	Purulent nasal discharge, unilateral sinus pain or tenderness, maxillary toothache, poor response to decongestants, and worsening illness after initial improvement. Recurrent sinusitis is an indication for ENT consultation.
Acute cough illness (bronchitis, pneumonia)	Chest pain, wheezing, dyspnea, and fever. Obtain chest radiographs to exclude pneumonia if the pulse is >100/min, respiration rate is >24/min, or temperature is >38.0°C (100.4°F).
Epiglottitis	Severe sore throat with a benign-appearing oropharynx. Adults may have dyspnea, drooling, and stridor. Obtain urgent ENT consultation, and do not attempt to examine the throat. A lateral neck film may show an enlarged epiglottis ("thumb sign").
Mononucleosis (EBV infection)	A 1- to 2-wk prodrome of fatigue, malaise, and myalgia followed by adenopathy (particularly of posterior cervical nodes), sore throat, fever, splenomegaly, hepatomegaly, and lymphocytosis (atypical lymphocytes).
Allergic rhinitis	Seasonal nasal symptoms, including clear rhinorrhea and watery, itchy eyes. Patients may have a history of asthma.
Asthma	Wheezing, dyspnea, and persistent dry cough. Symptoms may worsen at night and be triggered by cold air, exercise, or strong odors.
Influenza	Coryza, fever up to 41.0°C (105.8°F), myalgia, headache, and sore throat. Severity of symptoms associated with high fever and myalgia suggest influenza.
Otitis media	Ear pain, fever, decreased hearing acuity, and a tympanic membrane that is red, opaque, bulging, or retracted. Otitis media is more common in children than in adults.
Meningococcal disease	Patients with meningococcal disease may present with sore throat, rhinorrhea, cough, headache, and conjunctivitis before developing invasive disease.

EBV = Epstein-Barr virus; ENT = ear, nose, and throat.

Diagnosis

When diagnosing GABHS pharyngitis, it is important to consider the prevalence of GABHS in the community. GABHS is more common in the autumn and winter and is associated with crowded living conditions and recent close contact with a person with GABHS infection. Characteristic symptoms include sudden-onset sore throat, pain on swallowing, headache, fever, and malaise. Coryza, cough, and hoarseness typically are not present. Look for tonsillopharyngeal erythema with or without exudates, and examine for tender and enlarged anterior cervical lymph nodes. Non-GABHS pharyngitis is indistinguishable from GABHS pharyngitis, and the use of a clinical prediction tool, such as the Centor score (Table 2), is recommended. In the diagnosis of GABHS pharyngitis, the rapid antigen detection test (RADT) has comparable sensitivity (80%-90%) and specificity (95%) to throat culture and is supplanting culture in many settings. The throat swab for either culture or RADT should be obtained from both tonsils or tonsillar fossae and the posterior pharyngeal wall.

Therapy

Antimicrobial therapy should be used only when GABHS pharyngitis is highly likely. Patients fulfilling all Centor criteria should be treated with antibiotics without testing. A 10-day course of oral penicillin is the treatment of choice; erythromycin is an alternative treatment for patients who are allergic to penicillin. Consider giving a single injection of intramuscular penicillin G benzathine to patients who are unlikely to complete a full 10-day course of oral therapy. Macrolides should be avoided in adolescents and young adults, as they do not cover *F. necrophorum*. Advise patients to return if they do not respond to appropriate therapy within 12 to 24 hours or if they develop severe throat pain, dysphagia, drooling (epiglottitis), or unilateral neck swelling (Lemierre syndrome).

Sinusitis

Sinusitis, also referred to as rhinosinusitis, is an inflammation of the paranasal sinuses and, often, nasal mucosa. Rhinitis is a common symptom with a differential diagnosis that includes allergic, irritant, vasomotor, and infectious causes. Most sinus infections are viral in origin, with only 0.5% to 2% having a bacterial cause. Typical organisms include *Streptococcus pneumoniae, Haemophilus influenzae*, and, occasionally, *Moraxella catarrhalis*. Dental disease or instrumentation can cause anaerobic infections, whereas immunodeficiency may give rise to fungal infections. Symptoms may be classified as acute (<4 weeks), subacute (4-12 weeks), or chronic (>12 weeks). Complications include local spread (osteitis of the sinus bones, orbital cellulitis) or metastasis to the central nervous system (meningitis, brain abscess, infection of the intracranial venous sinuses).

Diagnosis

Ask about allergies, systemic diseases, and exposure to irritants. The symptoms of acute sinusitis include nasal congestion, rhinorrhea, and facial pain; more severe infections may be associated with fever and malaise. Examine for rhinorrhea, purulent secretions in the nasal cavity, and local pain. When present, abnormal nasal sinus transillumination may help to confirm the diagnosis. The probability of bacterial sinusitis is low (<25%) if only one of the following three diagnostic criteria is present: symptoms lasting >7 days, facial pain, and purulent nasal discharge. Diagnostic probability is

Table 2. Testing and Treatment Guidelines for Adult Pharyngitis

Centor Score[a]	Recommended Testing	Treatment
0	No test	No treatment
1	No test	No treatment
2	RADT	Penicillin V if test is positive
3	No test[b] or RADT	Empiric penicillin V[b] if test is positive
4	No test	Empiric penicillin V

RADT = rapid antigen detection test.
[a]One point is given for each of fever, absence of cough, tender anterior cervical lymphadenopathy, and tonsillar exudates.
[b]Strategy endorsed by Centor RM, Allison JJ, Cohen SJ. Pharyngitis management: defining the controversy. J Gen Intern Med. 2007;22:127-130. [PMID: 17351852]

higher (50%) when two or more of criteria are present. Avoid sinus imaging in uncomplicated acute sinusitis. Sinus puncture, although the gold standard, is performed by specialists only when a precise diagnosis is needed to determine optimal therapy (e.g., in immunocompromised patients). Patients with ophthalmic or neurologic symptoms or signs may need diagnostic imaging.

Therapy

Antibiotics have been found to have little if any role in the treatment of acute sinusitis in the primary care setting. Nonetheless, some guidelines do conclude that antibiotics are reasonable if at least two of the diagnostic criteria are present; however the probability of infection is still only 50%. A review concluded that after 10 days of sinusitis symptoms, antibiotic therapy and watchful waiting are equally acceptable and efficacious. First-line antibiotics include amoxicillin, doxycycline, and trimethoprim-sulfamethoxazole. Nonmedical therapy includes saline nasal spray or sinus irrigation, which may help increase mucosal moisture and remove inflammatory debris and bacteria. Intranasal steroids may reduce inflammation, mucolytic agents (e.g., guaifenesin) may reduce viscosity of nasal secretions, and topical decongestants (e.g., xylometazoline) may reduce mucosal inflammation and improve ostial drainage. Although these therapies have not proved to be efficacious in studies, they often are prescribed.

Otitis Media

Obstruction of the eustachian tube due to allergy or URI results in accumulation of secretions in the middle ear. Secondary bacterial or viral infection of the resulting effusion causes suppuration and features of otitis media. Risk factors for otitis media include age (younger age for acute otitis media, older age for chronic otitis media), smoking, allergic rhinitis, and chronic eustachian tube dysfunction. Viruses responsible for otitis media include respiratory syncytial virus, influenza virus, rhinovirus, and adenovirus. The most common bacterial causes include *S. pneumoniae*, *H. influenzae*, and *M. catarrhalis*. Rare complications of otitis media include meningitis, epidural abscess, brain abscess, lateral sinus thrombosis, cavernous sinus thrombosis, and carotid artery thrombosis.

Diagnosis

Symptoms of otitis media include ear pain and decreased conductive hearing. Examine for fluid in the middle ear and a retracted or bulging erythematous tympanic membrane. The absence of tympanic membrane mobility on pneumatic otoscopy adds additional diagnostic information (sensitivity 89%, specificity 80%). Tenderness to palpation over the mastoid area may indicate extension of infection into the mastoid. Chronic otitis media may be suppurative or associated with formation of a cholesteatoma (a mass consisting of excess squamous epithelium), which can erode into surrounding structures and lead to otorrhea, pain, hearing loss, or neurologic symptoms.

Therapy

Management of acute otitis media begins with decongestant therapy and pain control. Reserve antibiotic therapy for patients with evidence of purulent otitis media or for patients whose symptoms (congestion, eustachian tube dysfunction) do not respond to treatment. First-line therapy includes amoxicillin or a macrolide (for patients who are allergic to penicillin). Antibiotic treatment usually is for 10 to 14 days. Follow-up is not necessary unless symptoms persist or progress. Consider referral for ventilation tube insertion in patients with recurrent otitis media and/or associated hearing loss.

Book Enhancement

Go to www.acponline.org/essentials/infectious-disease-section. html. In *MKSAP for Students 5*, assess your knowledge with items 9-13 in the **Infectious Disease Medicine** section.

Acknowledgment

We would like to thank Dr. Robert W. Nelson, Jr., who contributed to an earlier version of this chapter.

Bibliography

Centor RM. Expand the pharyngitis paradigm for adolescents and young adults. Ann Intern Med. 2009;151:812-815. [PMID: 19949147]

Chapter 52

Urinary Tract Infection

Irene Alexandraki, MD

The majority of acute uncomplicated urinary tract infections occur in women aged 18 to 24 years. Urinary tract infections are unusual in men aged <50 years. Approximately 10% of adult women will have at least one urinary tract infection (UTI) annually. UTIs may involve only the lower urinary tract or the upper and lower urinary tract. A urinary tract infection in an individual with an indwelling urinary catheter, neurogenic bladder, stones, obstruction, immunosuppression, pregnancy, renal disease, or diabetes is defined as complicated and may predispose to treatment failure or require modified approaches to management due to infection with antibiotic-resistant organisms. *Asymptomatic bacteriuria* is defined as $\geq 10^5$ colony-forming units (CFU) of bacteria per milliliter of urine in the absence of typical symptoms of UTI.

UTIs may involve only the lower urinary tract or both the upper and lower urinary tracts. Most bacteria gain access to the bladder via the urethra. Uropathogens from fecal flora can colonize the vagina and migrate to the bladder through the urethra. Pyelonephritis can develop if these organisms ascend to the kidneys via the ureters. Sexual intercourse and contraceptive use increase the risk for developing an uncomplicated UTI in women. In women with recurrent UTIs, genetic factors increase susceptibility to vaginal colonization with uropathogenic coliform bacteria that adhere to uroepithelial cells. Infection of the kidney, including abscess, can occur hematogenously in patients with staphylococcal bacteremia or endocarditis. Bladder outlet obstruction due to benign prostatic hyperplasia may be associated with urinary stasis and an increased risk of UTI in older men. Complications may range from acute prostatitis and cystitis to more complex infections, including pyelonephritis and urosepsis.

Escherichia coli causes 80% of all UTIs. *Staphylococcus saprophyticus* accounts for 10% to 15% of acute symptomatic UTIs in young females. Typical causes of complicated UTIs include *Staphylococcus aureus*, enterococci, and gram-negative bacilli, including *Proteus, Klebsiella, Serratia,* and *Pseudomonas* species. Isolation of *S. aureus* should raise suspicion of hematogenously acquired infection, which most often occurs in debilitated patients.

Prevention

Asymptomatic bacteriuria is treated only in the following circumstances: during pregnancy, in a patient with urinary tract obstruction or neutropenia, following removal of an indwelling urinary catheter, or prior to an invasive urologic procedure. Chronic prophylactic antibiotic therapy is beneficial in pregnant women with recurrent asymptomatic bacteriuria; if untreated, 20% to 40% of these cases will progress to symptomatic UTI, including pyelonephritis, which is associated with low birth weight and prematurity. Postcoital antibiotic prophylaxis is considered in women with two or more episodes of postcoital UTI per year. Cranberry juice may decrease the incidence of acute cystitis in women, particularly those with recurrent UTIs.

Screening

Screening for asymptomatic bacteriuria is recommended before transurethral resection of the prostate, urinary tract instrumentation involving biopsy, or other tissue trauma resulting in mucosal bleeding. Screening is not recommended for simple catheter placement or cystoscopy without biopsy. Pregnant women should be screened for asymptomatic bacteriuria.

Diagnosis

Table 1 summarizes the differential diagnosis of UTI. Symptomatic cystitis is associated with dysuria, urinary frequency and urgency, and suprapubic pain. An abrupt onset of symptoms is more consistent with a UTI, whereas a gradual onset and vaginal symptoms suggest a sexually transmitted disease. The combination of dysuria and urinary frequency without vaginal discharge or irritation raises the probability of cystitis to >90%. A history of urologic abnormalities, underlying medical conditions (e.g., diabetes), and modifying host factors (e.g., advanced age) can predict infection with resistant organisms, delayed or incomplete response to therapy, relapse, and infectious complications (e.g., kidney abscess, emphysematous pyelonephritis, perinephric abscess, sepsis).

Pyelonephritis is associated with an abrupt onset of fever, chills, sweats, nausea, vomiting, diarrhea, myalgia, and flank or abdominal pain; hypotension and septic shock may occur in severe cases (see Table 1). Urinary frequency and dysuria may precede pyelonephritis. Search for complicating conditions, such as recent instrumentation of the urethra and bladder, diabetes, pregnancy, or prior UTIs. Infection at distant sites suggests the possibility of hematogenous pyelonephritis.

Acute prostatitis presents as a rapid onset of fever, chills, low back and perineal pain, urinary frequency and urgency, nocturia, dysuria, and generalized malaise. Physical examination may reveal a tender and boggy prostate.

The physical examination in cystitis generally reveals only tenderness of the urethra or suprapubic area. Pyelonephritis may be associated with fever and tachycardia. Physical examination usually reveals marked costovertebral angle tenderness; unilateral abdominal tenderness may be present. Pelvic examination may be

Table 1. Differential Diagnosis of Urinary Tract Infection

Disease	Notes
Vaginitis, cervicitis, or genital herpes (see Chapter 53)	*History*: Vaginal discharge, no urinary frequency or urgency, possibly new sex partner or unprotected sexual activity; history of previous STDs, recurrent genital HSV, or vaginitis; gradual onset of symptoms (*Chlamydia*). Dysuria can result from urine coming into contact with inflamed and irritated vulvar epithelial surfaces in the absence of bacterial UTI. Women may be able to differentiate between "internal" (UTI-associated) and "external" (vulvovaginal) dysuria, which helps to guide the evaluation. *Pelvic exam*: Vulvovaginal or cervical erythema, exudate, or ulcers; cervical discharge; adnexal tenderness or mass; cervical motion tenderness. *Laboratory*: Abnormal vaginal fluid findings; viral test from vulvovaginal ulcers positive for HSV; cervical swab with PMN leukocytes (± gram-negative diplococci) on Gram stain (if done), and positive by culture (or other test) for *Chlamydia* and/or *N. gonorrhoeae* (if indicated); urinalysis with PMNs but no bacteria; urine culture negative or with low counts of non-pathogens.
Sexually transmitted urethritis (see Chapter 53)	*History*: New sex partner, unprotected sexual activity, gradual onset of symptoms (*Chlamydia*); history of previous STDs or recurrent genital HSV, ± vaginal discharge; ± urinary frequency or urgency. Inflammation of the urethra from sexually transmitted pathogens can mimic bacterial cystitis quite closely. Sexual history can suggest the diagnosis. Specific tests are needed for confirmation, in conjunction with the negative routine urine culture. *Pelvic exam*: Possible normal, or evidence of coexistent vulvovaginitis or cervicitis/salpingitis. *Laboratory*: Urinalysis with PMNs but no bacteriuria; urine culture negative or low counts of non-pathogens; urine or urethral swab positive (by culture or other specific test) for *Chlamydia* or *HSV* (or *M. genitalium* or *U. urealyticum*).
Pyelonephritis	*History*: Fever, malaise, sweats, headache; anorexia, nausea, vomiting, abdominal pain; back, flank or loin pain; ± voiding symptoms. *Exam*: Fever, tachycardia; costovertebral angle tenderness; possibly abdominal tenderness. *Laboratory*: Elevated leukocyte count, ESR, and/or C-reactive protein; urinalysis with PMNs and bacteria (as in cystitis), ± leukocyte casts; urine culture with >10^4 colony-forming units/mL of a typical uropathogen (*E. coli, Proteus*). Imaging studies (not routinely indicated for uncomplicated pyelonephritis): ultrasound, intravenous pyelogram, enhanced CT (looking for obstruction, stone).
Acute prostatitis	*History*: Spiking fever, chills, dysuria, pelvic or perineal pain, and cloudy urine; possible obstructive symptoms (dribbling, hesitancy, and anuria). *Exam*: Edematous and tender prostate. *Laboratory*: Pyuria, positive urine culture.
Chronic prostatitis	*History*: Dysuria and frequency in the absence of the signs of acute prostatitis; recurrent urinary tract infections. *Exam*: Prostate tenderness and edema, but is frequently normal. *Laboratory*: Cultures of urine or expressed prostatic secretions are almost always positive.
Painful bladder syndrome/interstitial cystitis	*History*: Chronic bladder pain associated with bladder filling and/or emptying; urinary frequency, urgency, and nocturia. *Exam*: Diffuse tenderness in lower abdomen and pelvis. Diagnosis based upon characteristic symptoms and exclusion of other conditions.

CT = computed tomography; ESR = erythrocyte sedimentation rate; GI = gastrointestinal; HSV = herpes simplex virus; PMN = polymorphonuclear; STD = sexually transmitted disease; UTI = urinary tract infection.

indicated if the history suggests sexually transmitted disease. Suspect UTI if there is evidence of bladder distention on physical examination, pericatheter leakage of urine (in catheterized patients), or decreased or absent urine output despite a sensation of bladder fullness.

Urinalysis can be omitted for healthy women with acute cystitis if there are no complicating factors. However, obtain a urine culture for women with suspected cystitis if the patient is pregnant, the diagnosis is not clear from the history and physical examination, an unusual or antimicrobial-resistant organism is suspected, therapeutic options are limited because of a history of medication intolerance, the episode represents a suspected relapse or treatment failure after recent treatment for UTI, or underlying complicating conditions are identified.

The presence of pyuria and ≥10^5 CFU/mL of bacteria on quantitative urine culture confirm the diagnosis of UTI. If pyuria is absent, the diagnosis of UTI should be reconsidered. When the diagnosis is not clear, a urine dipstick test for leukocyte esterase and/or nitrite is an acceptable screening tool but may be less sensitive than microscopic urinalysis with low-count bacteriuria. Gram stain of the urine sediment increases specificity, suggests the type of microorganism, and is particularly useful in complicated UTI.

Proper urine specimen collection and handling is crucial. High concentrations of gram-negative bacilli (>10^3 CFU/mL) may be significant in symptomatic women; high bacterial concentrations in asymptomatic women usually are irrelevant, regardless of the degree of pyuria. In complicated UTI, almost any organism can be causative and must be considered seriously if the patient is symptomatic.

Bacteriuria and pyuria are the gold standard for the diagnosis of pyelonephritis if they are associated with a suggestive history and physical findings; urine culture usually shows bacterial concentrations ≥10^4 CFU/mL. Obtain blood cultures in clinically ill patients; blood cultures are positive in 25% of patients with pyelonephritis. Obtain a complete blood count, urinalysis, and urine culture in patients with acute prostatitis; blood cultures generally are indicated only in immunosuppressed patients.

Use imaging studies only if an alternative diagnosis or a urologic complication is suspected. Obtain kidney and bladder ultrasonography as the initial imaging study. Transrectal ultrasonography (TRUS) may be useful in the diagnosis of complicated prostatitis. Consider CT and MRI for patients with ultrasound findings suggesting an anatomic abnormality and for persistent or relapsing pyelonephritis despite normal findings on ultrasonography. CT may be useful in the diagnosis and drainage of a prostatic abscess and in ruling out other pelvic pathology mimicking prostatitis.

Therapy

Treat nonpregnant women with uncomplicated cystitis empirically with trimethoprim-sulfamethoxazole (TMP-SMZ) for 3 days. Fluoroquinolones also are effective but are less preferred as initial therapy because of their additional cost and resistance concerns. If there is a high prevalence of resistance to TMP-SMZ or intolerance to the drug, substitute nitrofurantoin, a β-lactam, or a fluoroquinolone for 3 days. Patients with underlying complicating conditions are more likely to have a drug-resistant infection, to exhibit a poor response to antimicrobial therapy even when the organism is susceptible, and to develop complications if initial therapy is suboptimal. For these patients, obtain a urine culture and treat empirically for 7 to 14 days with a fluoroquinolone or, if the organism is known to be susceptible, with TMP-SMZ. Acute cystitis in an elderly woman is not automatically considered complicated unless the patient has multiple comorbidities, was recently treated with antibiotics, or is a nursing home resident. Obtain a urine culture and susceptibility testing for pregnant women with cystitis and treat for 3 to 7 days with an oral antimicrobial agent that is safe in pregnancy, such as amoxicillin or nitrofurantoin.

For women with recurrent uncomplicated UTIs, consider daily prophylaxis with nitrofurantoin or TMP-SMZ or self-treatment with 3 days of TMP-SMZ or a fluoroquinolone beginning at the onset of symptoms. Recommend alternative contraception to women with recurrent UTIs who use spermicide-based contraception. Consider prophylaxis with single-dose TMP-SMX, nitrofurantoin, or ciprofloxacin after sexual intercourse for women with two or more episodes of postcoital UTI per year. Daily topical application of intravaginal estrogen cream reduces the frequency of symptomatic UTIs in postmenopausal women. Young men with UTIs should be treated with short-course antibiotic regimens approved for women with cystitis. Consider evaluating these patients further to rule out urinary obstruction or other anatomic abnormalities.

Consider outpatient management for patients with pyelonephritis who are medically stable and able to take oral medication. Use fluoroquinolones as first-line empiric oral therapy (except in pregnancy) because of the higher urine drug concentrations achieved compared with TMP-SMX. Ampicillin, TMP-SMX, and first-generation cephalosporins are no longer used for empiric therapy because of unacceptably high rates of resistance.

Patients with pyelonephritis who are acutely ill, hypotensive, nauseated, or vomiting are admitted to the hospital for intravenous fluids and parenteral antibiotics. If obstruction is present, catheter drainage of the bladder (or other drainage procedures) and replacement of an existing catheter are indicated in conjunction with antimicrobial therapy. Begin empiric therapy with a fluoroquinolone, an extended-spectrum cephalosporin or penicillin, or an aminoglycoside, and treat for 7 to 14 days; cephalosporins or aminoglycosides alone are insufficient for treating enterococci. Persistent fever and unilateral flank pain despite adequate treatment suggest perinephric or intrarenal abscess and the need for kidney CT.

Consider an intravenous fluoroquinolone or an extended-spectrum cephalosporin (with or without an aminoglycoside) for patients with acute prostatitis who are too ill for oral therapy. Patients who fail to respond within 72 hours should have a urologic consultation and TRUS or CT to rule out a prostatic abscess. Treat acute prostatitis for 4 to 6 weeks. In all cases of UTI, change from parenteral to oral therapy once the patient can tolerate oral intake.

Follow-Up

Following treatment of acute cystitis in pregnant women, obtain a urine culture to confirm eradication of bacteriuria, and repeat urinalyses or urine cultures at intervals through the time of delivery to confirm sterility of the urine. Following treatment of complicated cystitis in nonpregnant women, obtain a urine culture and confirm the resolution of symptoms.

Confirm eradication of bacteriuria in patients treated for acute pyelonephritis or prostatitis by repeating a urinalysis and urine culture. Treat recurrences with antimicrobial drugs based on susceptibility tests. Consider urologic consultation for patients with complicated kidney infections, stones, prostatic abscess, or urinary tract obstruction.

Book Enhancement

Go to www.acponline.org/essentials/infectious-disease-section. html. In *MKSAP for Students 5*, assess your knowledge with items 14-18 in the **Infectious Disease Medicine** section.

Bibliography

Neal DE Jr. Complicated urinary tract infections. Urol Clin North Am. 2008;35:13-22, v. [PMID: 18061020]

Nicolle LE. Uncomplicated urinary tract infection in adults including uncomplicated pyelonephritis. Urol Clin North Am. 2008;35:1-12, v. [PMID: 18061019]

Ramakrishnan K, Salinas RC. Prostatitis: acute and chronic. Prim Care. 2010;37:547-563, viii-ix. [PMID: 20705198]

Chapter 53

Sexually Transmitted Diseases

Sara B. Fazio, MD

Sexually transmitted diseases (STDs) are common problems in both the inpatient and the outpatient setting. Diseases characterized by urethritis and cervicitis include gonorrhea and chlamydia, while herpes simplex, primary syphilis and chancroid are the most common infectious diseases characterized by genital ulceration. Human papilloma virus (HPV) causes genital warts as well as cervical dysplasia. Human immunodeficiency virus (HIV) infection is discussed in Chapter 54.

Prevention

Key to the prevention of STDs is patient education about safe sexual practices. All patients should be encouraged to use a latex condom for vaginal or anal intercourse and fellatio. Variables associated with STD acquisition include young age (<25 years), lower socioeconomic status, substance abuse, lack of or inconsistent use of a barrier method of protection, use of an intrauterine device, and douching. Additionally, new or multiple sexual partners and a history of an STD increases the risk of disease transmission. Consistent and correct use of condoms reduces transmission of all STDs as well as pelvic inflammatory disease (PID) and its sequelae (ie, chronic pelvic pain, infertility). Many STDs are spread asymptomatically. The presence of an ulcerative genital lesion greatly increases the risk of HIV transmission, making prevention that much more critical. Partner treatment of patients diagnosed with an STD is an essential public health approach to prevention. HPV vaccination should be offered to all females between the ages of 9 and 26 years to prevent HPV infection and cervical dysplasia.

Screening

Any person who engages in high-risk sexual behavior should be screened for gonorrhea, chlamydia, syphilis, and HIV infection. All sexually active women aged <25 years should be screened routinely for chlamydia, based on evidence that screening reduces the incidence of PID by >50%. Men who have sex with men should be screened for STDs on an annual basis or more frequently based on risk behavior. Pregnant women should be offered screening for HIV infection, syphilis, and chlamydia at the first prenatal visit, as well as screening for gonorrhea in areas of high prevalence. A repeat test for gonorrhea should be offered in the third trimester to women at continued risk to prevent neonatal conjunctivitis (ophthalmia neonatorum). Prophylactic cesarean section is indicated in a woman with active herpes simplex virus (HSV; human herpesvirus 3) lesions at the time of delivery to prevent infection in the newborn. The presence of one STD requires screening for other STDs. Pap testing to

screen for HPV infection and cervical dysplasia is discussed in Chapter 77. Although some experts recommend anal Pap smears for HIV-infected homosexual men, the current Centers for Disease Control and Prevention STD treatment guidelines do not recommend routine screening given the limited data available on the natural history of anal squamous intraepithelial lesions and treatment efficacy.

Diagnosis

Genital herpes is suggested by the presence of multiple painful vesicular or ulcerative lesions (Plate 44) and is the most common cause of genital ulcers. The first episode of genital herpes is more severe than recurrent episodes and often involves systemic symptoms. Primary genital herpes outbreaks are characterized by fever, headache, and numerous painful, ulcerated, vesicular lesions. Grouped vesicles on an erythematous base are the classic clinical presentation. Recurrences often are unilateral and may be preceded by a neuropathic prodrome about 24 hours before lesions develop. Diagnosis is primarily with culture; direct fluorescent antibody testing and polymerase chain reaction (PCR) testing are useful when the diagnosis is unclear. A positive HSV type 2 antibody test indicates only previous infection and is not a clinically useful diagnostic test. Culture becomes less sensitive as genital lesions begin to heal. Reliance on the Tzanck test (showing multinucleated giant cells) is not recommended due to lack of sensitivity.

In primary syphilis, patients present with a painless ulcer (chancre) with a clean base and raised indurated edges (Plate 45) as well as painless regional lymphadenopathy. Secondary syphilis typically occurs weeks to months after the onset of primary disease and is characterized by a generalized mucocutaneous rash that involves the palms and soles (Plate 46), generalized lymphadenopathy, and constitutional symptoms. Inflammation may develop in other organs, resulting in hepatitis, glomerulonephritis, aseptic meningitis, patchy alopecia, and mucous patches (Plate 47). Diagnosis of primary and secondary-stage mucocutaneous lesions can be established by darkfield microscopy visualization of motile *T. pallidum* in exudative fluid from the lesions. In a patient with suggestive clinical findings, a presumptive diagnosis can be based on reactive syphilis serology, which entails the use of a nontreponemal serologic test (rapid plasma reagin [RGR] or VDRL test) followed by a more specific treponemal serologic test (fluorescent treponemal antibody absorption [FTA-ABS] test or *T. pallidum* particle agglutination assay [TP-PA]). Tertiary syphilis, which occurs years to decades after the initial infection, is characterized by neurologic findings (meningitis, tabes dorsalis, Argyll Robertson pupil, mental status changes), cardiac abnormalities (thoracic aortic aneurysm), or gummatous disease. Latent syphilis is characterized by positive serology without symptoms. Neurosyphilis requires cerebrospinal fluid examination for diagnosis. Treponemal serologies typically remain positive for life, whereas nontreponemal serology titers regress after appropriate treatment and are used to assess disease activity.

Chancroid (*Haemophilus ducreyi* infection) presents as one or more painful genital ulcers, often with unilateral suppurative inguinal lymphadenopathy. Diagnosis can be made by culture. However, because chancroid is relatively rare in the United States, culture medium often is not readily available, and the diagnosis is often one of exclusion (Table 1).

Gonorrhea should be suspected in a man with purulent or mucopurulent urethral discharge or in a woman with mucopurulent cervicitis. *Neisseria gonorrhoeae* and *Chlamydia trachomatis* both cause cervicitis, urethritis, and proctitis (in persons who engage in anal receptive intercourse), but gonorrhea is characterized by a more exudative polymorphonuclear immune response and, consequently, a more visibly purulent discharge. However, diagnosis cannot reliably be based on clinical findings. *N. gonorrhoeae* and *C. trachomatis* also are common causes of epididymitis in sexually active men aged <35 years; epididymitis typically presents as testicular pain with or without dysuria. Infection at any site may be asymptomatic, most notably infection of the pharynx (causing pharyngitis) and rectum (causing proctitis), allowing for unrecognized sexual transmission. Most endocervical gonococcal or chlamydial infections are asymptomatic; thus, a high index of suspicion is necessary. Untreated gonococcal infection of mucosal sites can result in bacteremia and disseminated gonococcal infection, characterized by fever and the triad of dermatitis (papular and pustular skin lesions that are typically few in number; Plate 48), tenosynovitis (tendon sheath inflammation, usually involving the distal extremities), and mono- or oligoarthritis. Perihepatitis (Fitz-Hugh–Curtis syndrome) and peritonitis also may occur with intraperitoneal extension of untreated pelvic infection in women. In the newborn, unrecognized perinatal acquisition of gonococcal infection may result in ophthalmia neonatorum. Chlamydial infection is the most commonly diagnosed sexually transmitted bacterial infection in the United States, with the highest prevalence among sexually active teenagers and adults aged <25 years. Women with chlamydia frequently are asymptomatic, and untreated infections can cause severe sequelae, including PID, infertility, ectopic pregnancy, and chronic pelvic pain. Men with chlamydia may have urethral discharge or may be asymptomatic. *C. trachomatis* also can cause conjunctivitis, which is most common in impoverished nations and is a leading cause of blindness worldwide.

Gonorrhea and chlamydia are best diagnosed by culture or PCR testing (greater sensitivity). PCR testing in men may be performed with a urine specimen; in women, a urine sample is suitable to test for chlamydia, but an endocervical specimen is needed for gonorrhea testing. In men with gonococcal urethritis, Gram stain reveals gram-negative intracellular diplococci in 95% of cases (Plate 49), allowing for a rapid, specific diagnosis. However, Gram stain of endocervical specimens is less sensitive

Table 1. Differential Diagnosis of Genital Ulcers

Disease	Characteristics
Syphilis (*Treponema pallidum*)	*Incubation*: 9-90 d. *Primary lesion*: papule. *Number of lesions*: usually one. *Pain*: none. *Size of lesion*: 5-15 mm. *Edges*: indurated. *Base*: clean. *Depth*: moderate. *Lymph nodes*: enlarged, nontender. *U.S. epidemiology*: Southeast, urban areas. The characteristics described are those seen in the classic presentation of infection. Atypical chancres may be small, nonindurated, or painful or have unusual shapes.
Herpes (herpes simplex virus types 1 and 2)	*Incubation*: days to years. *Primary lesion*: vesicle. *Number of lesions*: multiple. *Pain*: yes. *Size of lesion*: 1-2 mm. *Edges*: flat, red. *Base*: red, exudate. *Depth*: superficial. *Lymph nodes*: enlarged, tender. *U.S. epidemiology*: most common cause of genital ulcers. Herpes ulcers differ from primary syphilis in that they are much shallower, often appear in crops, begin as a vesicle, and are painful.
Chancroid (*Haemophilus ducreyi*)	*Incubation*: 1-14 d. *Primary lesion*: pustule. *Number of lesions*: one or many. *Pain*: exquisite. *Size of lesion*: 5-25 mm. *Edges*: ragged, undermined. *Base*: friable, purulent exudate. *Depth*: deep, excavated. *Lymph nodes*: tender, may suppurate/form buboes. *U.S. epidemiology*: rare, occasionally seen in warmer climates (many of these cases are imported from Mexico or the Caribbean). Chancroid differs from primary syphilis in that the ulceration usually is deeper and more destructive, the edges are ragged rather than punched out, and there is significant associated pain and tenderness as well as significant lymphadenopathy, which also is painful and tender.
Behçet disease	Behçet disease is a systemic disease with genital ulcers as one component; the ulcers often are painful. Other features include recurrent oral aphthous ulcers, uveitis, pathergy, arthritis, gastrointestinal manifestations, and central nervous system disease. In Behçet disease, serologic tests for syphilis will be negative.
Lymphogranuloma venereum (LGV; *Chlamydia trachomatis* serovars L1, L2, and L3)	LGV is extremely rare in the United States. The infection can begin as a small papule, erosion, or ulcer in the genital or perineal region; the lesion usually is asymptomatic and heals quickly without scarring. Patients with LGV rarely, if ever, present in this early ulcerative stage. Subsequently, patients develop the painful lymphadenopathy and buboes. During this stage, patients may have fever and other constitutional symptoms and develop draining fistulae. The early ulcerative lesions of LGV differ from those of primary syphilis in that they are smaller and less destructive and heal promptly.
Donovanosis[a]	Donovanosis is extremely rare in the United States. Ulcers most commonly are large, nontender, and beefy red and bleed easily when touched. The lesions differ from the syphilitic chancre in that they are larger, may be multiple in number, and usually have a very beefy red base. The ulcers do not heal spontaneously and can be present chronically.

[a]Also known as granuloma inguinale (*Calymmatobacterium granulomatis*).

and thus should not be used to diagnose infection in women. Nongonococcal urethritis is defined by two criteria: the presence of urethritis (dysuria or a thin mucoid discharge) and leukocytosis on Gram stain of the discharge. The failure of urethritis to respond to antibiotic treatment for gonorrhea and chlamydia suggests a less common cause, such as *Trichomonas vaginalis* or HSV. HSV also causes cervicitis and proctitis.

PID is a polymicrobial infection of the endometrium, fallopian tubes, and ovaries. The diagnosis is suggested by the presence of abdominal discomfort, uterine or adnexal tenderness, or cervical motion tenderness. Other criteria include body temperature >38.3°C (101.0°F), cervical or vaginal mucopurulent discharge, leukocytes in vaginal secretions, and documentation of gonorrhea or chlamydia. PID is most likely to occur within 7 days of the onset of menses. Although *N. gonorrhoeae* and *C. trachomatis* are the primary causes of PID, more recent studies have implicated organisms of bacterial vaginosis. All women with suspected PID should be tested for gonorrhea and chlamydia and have a pregnancy test

to rule out normal or ectopic implantation. In severe cases, imaging should be performed to rule out a tubo-ovarian abscess.

Most HPV infection is asymptomatic. Transmission of HPV can occur with skin-to-mucosa or skin-to-skin contact. HPV serotypes 6 and 11 are most often responsible for genital warts (condylomata acuminata), whereas high-risk HPV serotypes (16, 18, 31, 33, and 35) are associated with cervical dysplasia and cervical cancer. Genital warts may be flat or pedunculated and are typically diagnosed by appearance alone, although biopsy can be used if necessary.

Therapy

Counsel all patients with active symptoms to abstain from sexual contact until at least 1 week of treatment has been completed. Because HSV persists in a dormant state, patients must be educated that treatment does not eradicate the virus and that asymptomatic shedding and transmission can occur, particularly during

Table 2. Recommended Treatment of Common Sexually Transmitted Infections

Clinical Situation	Recommended Regimen
Syphilis	
Primary, secondary, or early latent (<1 y) syphilis	Penicillin G benzathine 2.4 MU IM, given in a single dose
Late latent (>1 y) syphilis or latent syphilis of unknown duration	Penicillin G benzathine 7.2 MU total, given as three doses of 2.4 MU IM at 1-wk intervals
Neurosyphilis	Aqueous crystalline penicillin G 18-24 MU/d, given as 3-4 MU IV every 4 h or continuous infusion, for 10-14 d
HIV infection	For primary, secondary, and early latent syphilis, treat as previously described; some specialists recommend three doses. For late latent syphilis or latent syphilis of unknown duration, perform CSF examination before treatment.
Pregnancy	Penicillin is the only recommended treatment for syphilis during pregnancy. Women who report allergy should be desensitized and then treated with penicillin.
Gonococcal Infections[a]	
Infection of cervix, urethra, or rectum	Ceftriaxone 125 mg IM, given in a single dose, *or*
	Cefixime 400 mg orally, given in a single dose
Chlamydial Infections	
Adults and adolescents	Azithromycin 1 g orally, given in a single dose *or*
	Doxycycline 100 mg orally twice daily for 7 d
Pregnancy	Azithromycin 1 g orally, given in a single dose *or*
	Amoxicillin 500 mg orally three times daily for 7 d
Nongonococcal urethritis	Azithromycin 1 g orally, given in a single dose *or*
	Doxycycline 100 mg orally twice daily for 7 d
Pelvic inflammatory disease (outpatient management)	Ceftriaxone 250 mg IM, single dose, plus doxycycline 100 mg orally twice daily for 14 d
Pelvic inflammatory disease (inpatient management)	Cefoxitin 2 g IV, every 6 hours plus doxycycline 100 mg orally twice
Genital Herpes	
First clinical episode of genital herpes	Acyclovir 400 mg orally three times daily for 7-10 d *or*
	Acyclovir 200 mg orally 5 times daily for 7-10 d *or*
	Famciclovir 250 mg orally three times daily for 7-10 d *or*
	Valacyclovir 1 g orally twice daily for 7-10 d

CSF = cerebrospinal fluid; IM = intramuscularly; IV = intravenously; MU = million units.
[a]Treat also for chlamydial infection if not ruled out by a sensitive test (nucleic acid amplification test).

the first year of infection. Syphilis, gonorrhea, and chlamydia are reportable infectious diseases in every state. Table 2 summarizes the recommended treatments for common STDs.

Treat primary HSV infection for 7 to 10 days and recurrent disease for 3 to 5 days. Treatment decreases the duration of symptoms and reduces viral shedding. Suppressive therapy may be necessary to decrease the frequency of recurrences. Topical therapy is ineffective.

Chancroid is treated with a single dose of azithromycin or ceftriaxone, 3 days of ciprofloxacin, or 7 days of erythromycin base.

Primary or secondary syphilis is treated with one dose of intramuscular (IM) penicillin G benzathine. Late latent syphilis or tertiary non-neurosyphilis is treated with three weekly doses of IM penicillin G benzathine. Doxycycline and tetracycline are alternative choices for penicillin-allergic nonpregnant patients. Failure of nontreponemal serologic titers to decline fourfold in the 6 to 12 months after treatment indicates treatment failure or reinfection. Neurosyphilis requires intravenous penicillin or ceftriaxone; in penicillin-allergic patients, desensitization is required. The Jarisch-Herxheimer reaction is an acute febrile illness occurring within 24 hours of treatment for any stage of syphilis and probably represents an immune response to cell wall proteins released by dying spirochetes.

Patients with documented or suspected gonorrhea, including men aged <35 years with presumed epididymitis, are treated for both gonorrhea and chlamydia, given the high frequency of coinfection. Fluoroquinolones are no longer recommended in the treatment of gonorrhea due to the emergence of resistance.

Chlamydia is effectively treated with a single dose of azithromycin, 7 days of doxycycline, or a fluoroquinolone.

In patients with suspected PID, the choice of antibiotic should cover gonorrhea, chlamydia, gram-negative rods, and anaerobic bacteria. The duration of treatment is 14 days. PID often can be treated on an outpatient basis. Hospitalization should be considered if there is no clinical improvement after 48 to 72 hours of antibiotic therapy, inability to tolerate oral antibiotics, severe illness (nausea, vomiting, or high fever), suspected intra-abdominal abscess, pregnancy, or nonadherence with outpatient therapy.

Treatment of genital warts involves removal either by patient-applied regimens (podofilox, imiquimod), provider-administered regimens (cryotherapy, podophyllin resin, trichloracetic or bichloracetic acid), or surgery. Treatment may reduce, but does not eliminate, HPV.

Follow-up of patients with STDs is important to resolve infection and to ensure adequate partner management (Table 3).

Book Enhancement

Go to www.acponline.org/essentials/infectious-disease-section.html. In *MKSAP for Students 5*, assess your knowledge with items 19-23 in the **Infectious Disease Medicine** section.

Bibliography

Wilson JF. In the clinic. Vaginitis and cervicitis. Ann Intern Med. 2009; 151:ITC3-1-ITC3-15; Quiz ITC3-16. [PMID: 19721016]

Table 3. Follow-Up for Patients with Sexually Transmitted Disease (STD)

Clinical Situation	Recommended Follow-Up
Primary HSV infection	Counsel patient regarding the natural history of herpes recurrence and use of barrier contraception.
Primary syphilis	Perform follow-up quantitative nontreponemal serologies at 6, 12, and 24 mo.
Tertiary syphilis, HIV-infected person with late latent syphilis, treatment failure	Perform lumbar puncture and cerebrospinal fluid analysis for neurosyphilis.
Sexual partner of patient with syphilis	Perform serologic testing if >90 d after sexual contact. Treat empirically if <90 d after sexual contact.
Gonorrhea or chlamydia	Repeat diagnostic testing if symptoms persist 3-4 d after treatment.
Sexual partner of patient with gonorrhea or chlamydia	Treat all sexual contacts of the last 60 d.
Pelvic inflammatory disease	Reevaluate within 48-72 h of initiation of therapy and again at the end of antibiotic treatment. Patients not responding to therapy may require parenteral therapy or broader antibiotic coverage, additional diagnostic tests, drainage of an abscess or fluid collection, or surgical intervention.
Any patient with an STD diagnosis	Test for other STDs, including HIV and HBV infection.

HBV = hepatitis B virus; HSV = herpes simplex virus.

Chapter 54

Human Immunodeficiency Virus Infection

Peter Gliatto, MD

HIV, the cause of AIDS, slowly destroys the immune system and can lead to deadly opportunistic infections. Combination antiretroviral therapy has changed the face of HIV/AIDS illness, offering many affected persons the chance to live for decades. Despite these advances, it is sobering to remember that of the roughly 1 million persons infected with HIV in the United States, one quarter to one third do not know they are infected. The greatest proportion of newly diagnosed cases of HIV/AIDS is made up of men who have sex with men, followed by adolescents and adults infected through heterosexual contact. The effects of HIV/AIDS illness on the developing world are devastating. In Sub-Saharan Africa, the prevalence of HIV/AIDS is 12.5%. All physicians must have a basic understanding of how HIV infection is acquired, diagnosed, and treated.

HIV is a retrovirus that enters the bloodstream via mucosal contact. The virus enters cells through use of an external glycoprotein (gp120), which binds to the CD4 receptor on helper T cells. After fusion with the cell, facilitated by binding to a coreceptor (CCR5 or CXCR4), the virus inserts its core, and viral RNA is reverse transcribed into DNA and incorporated into host cell DNA. The reverse transcriptase has a high error rate, contributing to a high viral mutation rate, which influences the virulence of the virus and its response to host defenses and drug therapy. New virions leave the cell via endocytosis to infect other cells. Infected T cells or virions enter the bloodstream and then multiply in the gastrointestinal tract, spleen, and bone marrow. With this amplification, symptoms of acute HIV infection can result within 2 to 6 weeks of infection. Host defenses to contain the spread of virus include CD8 responses, which reduce the viremia to a stable level. The virus causes destruction of CD4 cells over a period of years. As the CD4 cell count declines, the risk for opportunistic infections increases.

Prevention

Counsel all patients about the routes of HIV transmission and risk-reduction strategies. Teach patients that all forms of sexual contact involving mucosal exposure to genital secretions or blood, including oral sex, involve risk of HIV transmission. Screening for other sexually transmitted infections, particularly genital ulcer diseases, is essential, because open lesions increase the likelihood of HIV transmission. Routinely offer HIV testing to pregnant patients; antiretroviral treatment administered to an HIV-infected woman during pregnancy can significantly reduce maternal-fetal transmission. Counsel patients who use injection drugs about risk-reduction behaviors (not sharing needles). HIV transmission to health care workers can be prevented by educating those at risk for occupa-

tional exposures to HIV-infected blood or bodily fluids about safety precautions (not capping used needles) and offering postexposure treatment in appropriate circumstances (immediately after a high-risk needle-stick injury). A vaccine is still in development and will not be available for use in the immediate future.

Screening

Early recognition of HIV infection facilitates effective counseling about antiretroviral therapy, monitoring of disease progression, and prevention and treatment of opportunistic infections and other complications; it also reduces the risk of HIV transmission to others. The 2006 Centers for Disease Control and Prevention (CDC) guidelines recommend screening all persons aged 13 to 64 years for HIV infection. In an attempt to increase the number of persons tested, the CDC does not recommend separate written consent for HIV screening.

Diagnosis

The presentation of HIV/AIDS can be protean and nonspecific. It is essential to maintain a high index of suspicion based on exposures, risk factors, symptoms, and findings on physical examination and diagnostic testing.

Certain diagnoses warrant HIV testing. These include severe or treatment-refractory herpes simplex virus infection, esophageal candidiasis, *Pneumocystis jirovecii* pneumonitis, cryptococcal meningitis, disseminated mycobacterial infection, cytomegalovirus retinitis or gastrointestinal disease, and toxoplasmosis.

HIV testing is indicated in any patient with signs or symptoms of immunologic dysfunction, weight loss, generalized lymphadenopathy, fever and night sweats of >2 weeks' duration, oral thrush, severe aphthous ulcers, severe seborrheic dermatitis, or oral hairy leukoplakia. Herpes zoster in a younger person, recurrent pneumonia, chronic diarrhea, or unexplained hematologic abnormalities (anemia, leukopenia, thrombocytopenia, polyclonal gammopathy) also should prompt consideration of HIV infection. Suspect primary (acute) HIV infection as the cause of a febrile illness occurring within several weeks of a potential exposure. Obtain a detailed sexual history and ask about other risk factors when evaluating a patient for unexplained acute febrile illness, especially if fatigue, adenopathy, pharyngitis, rash, or headache also is present.

HIV testing involves a two-step approach. The first step is a highly sensitive enzyme-linked immunosorbent assay (which may include any one of the approved tests involving blood, oral secretions, or urine) or a rapid test (which may give results within 1

Table 1. Complications of HIV Infection

Condition	Associated CD4 Count (cells/μL or cells × 10⁶/L)	Key Characteristics
Candidiasis	<100	Involves the oropharynx, esophagus, trachea, bronchi, or lungs
Cryptococcosis	<100	Causes subacute meningitis; often associated with cryptococcemia
Cryptosporidiosis	Any, but <100 with more severe disease	Persistent watery diarrhea
Cytomegalovirus	<50	Retinitis, esophagitis, colitis
Kaposi sarcoma	Any	Raised discrete red lesions, often on the lower extremities; primarily in homosexual men coinfected with human herpesvirus 8
Lymphoma	Any	Burkitt, immunoblastic, or primary CNS lymphoma
Mycobacterium tuberculosis	Any	Pulmonary or extrapulmonary infection
M. avium complex	<50	Disseminated infection, often with liver and bone marrow involvement and diffuse adenopathy
Pneumocystis pneumonia	<200	Dyspnea on exertion, hypoxia; diffuse infiltrates on chest radiograph
Progressive multifocal leukoencephalopathy	<100	Caused by JC virus (a human polyomavirus); white matter lesions seen on imaging; presents with focal neurologic defects including altered mental status
Toxoplasmosis	<100	Fever, headache, focal neurologic deficits; multiple ring-enhancing lesions on CNS imaging; positive *Toxoplasma* serology

CNS = central nervous system.

hour). All positive results require a confirmatory test, the Western blot, which is highly specific. Seroconversion typically occurs within 6 weeks after infection. During this window, patients have extremely high levels of circulating virus, detectable either by assays for viral nucleic acid (viral load) or viral antigen (p24 antigen). Use these tests if acute HIV infection is suspected.

In HIV-positive patients, assessing the viral load and CD4 cell count offers important prognostic information as well as baseline values to monitor response to therapy. The viral load is the most reliable marker for predicting prognosis and rate of decline of CD4 cells. The CD4 cell count is the most reliable marker for the current risk of opportunistic complications of HIV infection. Immunosuppression due to HIV infection can lead to several characteristic infectious and neoplastic conditions (Table 1).

Suspect *P. jirovecii* pneumonia in patients with HIV/AIDS who have a CD4 cell count <200/μL (200 × 10⁶/L) and who develop fever, dry cough, and dyspnea over days to weeks. Chest radiographs typically show diffuse interstitial infiltrates, but radiologic findings vary widely. Diagnosis is made by silver stain examination of sputum (induced or obtained by bronchoscopy). Suspect toxoplasmic encephalitis in patients who have a CD4 count <100/μL (100 × 10⁶/L), fever, and neurologic findings. Brain MRI or head CT will show ring-enhancing lesions. Failure of the lesions to shrink after a trial of therapy for toxoplasmosis raises concern for primary central nervous system (CNS) lymphoma. Primary CNS lymphoma tends to be periventricular in location and also may involve single or multiple ring-enhancing lesions; toxoplasmosis typically presents as multiple lesions.

Therapy

Caution HIV-infected persons about using alcohol or other substances that may be toxic to the liver. Many persons with

HIV/AIDs are coinfected with hepatitis B or C virus, and drugs to treat HIV infection or its complications can also affect the liver and drug metabolism.

Suppressing the viral load slows the progression of disease, partially reconstitutes immune deficits, improves quality of life, and prolongs survival of many HIV-infected patients. Highly active antiretroviral therapy (HAART) is a drug regimen of three or more active compounds that inhibit HIV. Timing for the initiation of therapy is controversial, but guidelines currently support treatment in patients with a history of an AIDS-defining illness and/or a CD4 count <350/μL (350 x 10⁶/L). Additionally, patients who are pregnant or have hepatitis B or HIV nephropathy should be treated regardless of CD4 count.

Six classes of antiretroviral agents currently are available. Initial combination therapy for treatment-naïve patients usually involves a "base" that consists of a nonnucleoside reverse transcriptase inhibitor (typically efavirenz) or one or two protease inhibitors (the second protease inhibitor is ritonavir, which boosts the levels of the first by inhibiting the cytochrome P-450 system), combined with a "backbone" that consists of two nucleoside/nucleotide reverse transcriptase inhibitors. (The fixed combination of emtricitabine/tenofovir often is a first choice.) Regimens that use protease inhibitors are of concern because of long-term side effects. Select a combination regimen based on drug characteristics, side effect profile, patient comorbidities, and testing for virus resistance.

Drug selection for patients who have been on antiviral therapy and need to switch medications because of virologic failure or intolerable side effects should be based on treatment history and pattern on testing for virus resistance. Use at least two drugs that are new to the patient when changing a regimen.

Combination therapy maximizes treatment efficacy by reducing the chance of resistance, but it increases the chance of drug interactions. Certain antiretroviral drugs are associated with rare but potentially fatal hepatic steatosis, pancreatitis, myopathy, and lactic acidosis (Table 2). Protease inhibitors are associated with a cluster of metabolic effects, including hyperlipidemia, body fat redistribution, and insulin resistance. In a small subset of patients, initiation of antiretroviral therapy can lead to an inflammatory response as the immune system recovers and mounts a response to pathogens that may be present. This is called the immune reconstitution inflammatory syndrome. Treatment usually is supportive.

Provide prophylaxis against certain opportunistic infections based on the level of immunosuppression and other clinical factors (Table 3). Vaccinate HIV-infected patients against influenza, pneumococcal pneumonia, and, if not already immune, hepatitis A and B. Vaccination is likely more effective in patients with higher CD4 counts. Treat patients with *P. jirovecii* pneumonia with trimethoprim-sulfamethoxazole, and add corticosteroids for patients with hypoxia (arterial Po_2 <70 mm Hg [9.3 kPa] or alveolar arterial gradient >35 mm Hg [4.7 kPa]).

Follow-Up

The broad goal of antiretroviral therapy is to achieve the lowest possible viral load while minimizing the adverse effects of treatment. Assess the viral load and CD4 count 4 weeks after starting or changing antiretroviral therapy and every 3 to 4 months thereafter. Available evidence indicates that suppression of the viral load to <50 copies/mL is associated with improved outcomes and prolonged survival. Generally, an effective antiretroviral regimen should decrease the viral load by 90% to 99% within 2 weeks and to <50 copies/mL at 4 to 6 months. Failure to meet these criteria suggests poor adherence, poor absorption, or viral resistance. Significant ongoing viral replication in the face of ongoing therapy may contribute to the selection of multidrug resistance. Suspected viral resistance should prompt a complete change in the antiretroviral regimen, usually based on resistance testing and consultation with an infectious disease expert.

Table 2. Antiviral Agents and Common Side Effects

Drug Category and Examples	Common Side Effects
Nucleoside/Nucleotide Reverse Transcriptase Inhibitors	
Abacavir	Hypersensitivity reaction
Didanosine	GI upset, peripheral neuropathy, pancreatitis
Emtricitabine	Lactic acidosis, fat redistribution, hepatotoxicity
Stavudine	Neuropathy, lactic acidosis, superficial fat atrophy, pancreatitis
Tenofovir	Generally well tolerated
Zalcitabine	Neuropathy, rash, stomatitis, pancreatitis, fever
Zidovudine	Anemia, neutropenia, myopathy, hepatopathy
Nonnucleoside Reverse Transcriptase Inhibitors	
Delavirdine	Occasional rash
Efavirenz	Sleep disturbance, psychiatric alterations, vivid dreams or hallucinations
Etraverine	Rash (including Stevens-Johnson syndrome)
Nevirapine	Rash (including Stevens-Johnson syndrome), fever, drug-induced hepatitis
Protease Inhibitors	
Atazanavir	GI upset, jaundice
Darunavir	GI upset, hyperlipidemia, pancreatitis, fat redistribution, insulin resistance
Fosamprenvir	GI upset, hyperglycemia, skin rash
Indinavir	GI upset, kidney stones, jaundice, hyperlipidemia, fat redistribution, insulin resistance
Lopinavir/ritonavir	GI upset, hyperlipidemia, pancreatitis, fat redistribution, insulin resistance
Ritonavir	GI upset, paresthesias, insulin resistance, fat redistribution, hyperlipidemia, hepatopathy
Saquinavir	GI upset, hyperlipidemia, pancreatitis, fat redistribution, insulin resistance
Tipranavir	GI upset, hyperlipidemia, insulin resistance, fat redistribution, hepatotoxicity
Fusion Inhibitors	
Enfuvirtide	Injection site reactions, severe reactions (sometimes with eosinophilia and signs of allergy)
Coreceptor Antagonists	
Maraviroc	Cough, fever, upper respiratory infections, rash, musculoskeletal symptoms
Integrase Inhibitors	
Raltegravir	Generally well tolerated

GI = gastrointestinal.

Table 3. Prophylaxis for Opportunistic Infections

Condition	Prophylaxis
Toxoplasmosis	*When*: CD4 count <100/µL (100 × 10^6/L) and toxoplasma seropositive
	What: Daily trimethoprim-sulfamethoxazole
	Discontinue: CD4 count >200/µL (200 × 10^6/L) for >3 mo
Mycobacterium avium complex	*When*: CD4 count <50/µL (50 × 10^6/L)
	What: Weekly azithromycin
	Discontinue: CD4 count >100/µL (100 × 10^6/L) for >3 mo
Pneumocystis	*When*: CD4 count <200/µL (200 × 10^6/L)
	What: Daily trimethoprim-sulfamethoxazole
	Discontinue: CD4 count >200/µL (200 × 10^6/L) for >3 mo
Mycobacterium tuberculosis	*When*: Induration of ≥5 mm on purified protein derivative skin test
	What: Isoniazid and pyridoxine
	Discontinue: After 9 mo of therapy
Candidiasis	Not recommended
Cryptococcosis	Not recommended
Cryptosporidiosis	Not recommended
Cytomegalovirus	Not recommended

Regular physical examinations and laboratory testing can help detect drug toxicities, opportunistic infections, and treatment failure due to resistance or nonadherence. Depending on the drug regimen, obtain a complete blood count, a chemistry profile, an amylase or a lipase value, and cholesterol and triglyceride levels every 3 to 4 months to monitor for possible drug toxicities. The physical examination also should assess for potential drug toxicities, including rash, fat redistribution, hepatic enlargement or tenderness, muscle tenderness, and/or peripheral neuropathy. Patients infected with HIV should be tested for hepatitis B and C viruses. Tuberculin skin testing using purified protein derivative should be performed annually. A tuberculin skin test resulting in induration of ≥5 mm is considered positive and should prompt prophylactic therapy in the absence of evidence of active tuberculosis. It is also critical for women to have regular gynecologic evaluations, including Pap testing; women with HIV infection have a much higher rate of cervical cancer than women who are not infected with HIV.

Book Enhancement

Go to www.acponline.org/essentials/infectious-disease-section. html. In *MKSAP for Students 5*, assess your knowledge with items 24-28 in the **Infectious Disease Medicine** section.

Bibliography

Thompson MA, Aberg JA, Cahn P, et al; International AIDS Society-USA. Antiretroviral treatment of adult HIV infection: 2010 recommendations of the International AIDS Society-USA panel. JAMA. 2010;304:321-333. [PMID: 20639566]

Chapter 55

Health Care–Associated Infections

Gonzalo Bearman, MD

A health care–associated infection is a systemic or localized infection that was not present or incubating at the time of hospital admission and that occurs ≥48 hours after admission or within 48 to 72 hours of discharge. The most common health care–associated infections in medical patients are urinary tract infections (UTIs), pneumonia (including ventilator-associated pneumonia), and bloodstream infections. In addition, antibiotic-associated (*Clostridium difficile*) diarrhea is on the rise in hospitals, long-term care facilities, and the community.

More than 2.1 million health care–associated infections occur annually, significantly increasing the morbidity, mortality, and costs associated with health care. Many of these infections can be prevented. Even with a growing body of literature on risk-reduction practices, the single most important way to prevent health care–associated infections is by diligent hand hygiene with medicated soap and water or with an alcohol-based hand rub. The most important risk factor for a health care–associated infection is the presence of an invasive device (urinary or vascular catheter, endotracheal tube) in an acutely ill patient. Infection prevention programs perform surveillance of health care–associated and device-associated infections in high-risk patients and intensive care units to track their incidence and prevalence. Infection prevention programs also guide health care workers in implementing risk-reduction practices across the health care setting. Patients with communicable diseases or drug-resistant pathogens should be isolated appropriately and quickly to minimize transmission of pathogens to other patients, hospital visitors, and health care workers (Table 1).

Catheter-Associated Urinary Tract Infections

The most common health care–associated infections are UTIs, most of which are caused by indwelling urinary catheters. Bacteriuria occurs in 3% to 10% of catheterized patients daily, with the incidence directly related to the duration of catheterization. An estimated 5% of patients will become colonized for each day of catheterization beyond 2 days, and 10% to 25% of these patients will develop symptomatic UTIs. Urinary catheters pose a significant UTI risk for several reasons, including (1) bacteria can be inoculated directly into the bladder during insertion, (2) catheters are conduits to the bladder, (3) the glycocalyx that forms on the catheter surface protects bacteria from antibiotics and host defenses, and (4) residual urine serves as a reservoir for bacterial growth. Other risk factors for catheter-associated urinary tract infection (CAUTI) include advanced age, female sex, diabetes, malnutrition, kidney dysfunction, and improper catheter care.

The most effective way to prevent CAUTIs is to decrease catheter use. Devices should be used for specific indications, not for convenience, and should be removed as soon as possible. If a urinary catheter is needed, measures should be taken to decrease the risk of colonization and infection. These include hand washing, using an aseptic catheter placement technique and sterile equipment for catheter insertion and care, securing the catheter properly, maintaining unobstructed urine flow with closed sterile drainage, and using antibiotic-coated catheters (Table 2). Manipulation and irrigation should be minimized. Urine specimens should be

Table 1. Infection Control Precautions for Health Care Institutions

Transmission Mode	Precautions	Patients
Airborne	Patient is isolated in a private room with negative air pressure, the door remains closed, and all entering persons wear masks with a filtering capacity of 95%. Transported patients must wear masks.	For patients with known or suspected illnesses transmitted by airborne droplet nuclei, such as tuberculosis, measles, varicella, or disseminated varicella-zoster virus infection.
Droplet	Patient is isolated in a private room, and hospital personnel wear masks when within 3 ft of the patient.	For patients with known or suspected illnesses transmitted by large-particle droplets, such as *Neisseria meningitidis* infections and influenza.
Contact	Patient is isolated in a private room or with patients who have the same active infection. Nonsterile gloves and gowns are required for direct contact with the patient or any infective material; gowns and/or gloves are removed before exiting isolation rooms.	For patients with known or suspected illnesses transmitted by direct contact, including infections due to vancomycin-resistant enterococci and methicillin-resistant *Staphylococcus aureus*.

Table 2. Best Practices to Prevent Health Care–Associated Infections

Practice	Notes
Hand hygiene	• Cleanse hands with soap and water or waterless alcohol product before and after contact with patients or contaminated surfaces. • Install alcohol-based waterless cleaning products inside and outside all patient rooms and in other locations where clinical care will be provided. • Do not allow clinical staff to wear artificial nails.
Prevention of catheter-related bloodstream infections	• Remove unnecessary vascular lines. • Use recommended hand hygiene before insertion or manipulation of vascular lines. • Use maximal barrier precautions (gowns, gloves, masks, head covers) for insertion of vascular lines. • Apply appropriate skin antiseptics (chlorhexidine is the agent of choice) for insertion of vascular lines, dressing changes, and reinsertion. • Use the subclavian site whenever possible, because this site is associated with the lowest risk for infection. • Maintain clean and dry dressings. • Do not use prophylactic antibiotics for insertion of vascular lines.
Prevention of urinary tract infections	• Remove all unnecessary catheters. • Use sterile technique for insertion of catheters. • Do not remove urine samples from lines or open systems. • Do not use antibiotics prophylactically.
Prevention of ventilator-associated pneumonia	• Sterilize and maintain respiratory equipment appropriately. • Raise the head of the bed to a 45-degree angle (use the semi-recumbent position). • Use noninvasive ventilation techniques when possible. • Use oscillation or rotate the patient. • Use good oral care. • Use endotracheal tubes that allow for subglottic suctioning in high-risk patients.

collected using the drainage bag valve. Antibiotics should not be used as prophylaxis for CAUTIs.

Patients with CAUTIs often do not present with typical signs of a UTI. If a patient develops cloudy urine, fever, or other systemic manifestations compatible with infection, blood and urine cultures should be obtained. If a CAUTI is suspected, management includes removal of the catheter, with catheter replacement only if necessary. A urine culture should be obtained prior to administration of antibiotics. Common pathogens include *Escherichia coli*, *Klebsiella*, *Proteus*, *Enterococcus*, *Pseudomonas*, and *Staphylococcus*; fungi (*Candida*) are prevalent in patients with diabetes or chronic indwelling catheters. A third-generation cephalosporin (cefotaxime, ceftriaxone) or fluoroquinolone (ciprofloxacin, levofloxacin) is used for a suspected gram-negative bacterial infection, and vancomycin is used for a suspected staphylococcal or enterococcal infection. Antibiotics often are modified by pathogen susceptibility data obtained from the urine culture. Complications from CAUTIs include pyelonephritis and prostatitis. Secondary bacteremia occurs in about 3% of patients with CAUTIs.

Catheter-Related Intravascular Infections

Primary bloodstream infections (BSIs) occur without a recognizable focus of infection at another anatomic site. The increased use of intravascular catheters is believed to have contributed to the large increase in BSIs over the years. Approximately 250,000 central line–associated BSIs (CLABSIs) occur in the United States annually. Reported case fatality rates have ranged from 14% to 40%.

Use of intravenous catheters should be reserved for patients with proven need, with catheters removed as soon as clinically possible. Use of sterile technique and maximal sterile barriers minimizes risk. Specifically, full body sterile drape, gown, mask, and gloves should be used for central catheter insertion. Chlorhexidine is the most effective agent for skin decontamination before catheter insertion and is the antiseptic of choice over povidone-iodine or alcohol alone (see Table 2). The risk for infection is highest with femoral placement and lowest with subclavian placement.

Mechanisms of CLABSI include contamination from skin flora, intraluminal or hub contamination, and secondary seeding from other sources. Microorganisms from the patient's skin or from health care workers migrate along the catheter and cause contamination. Thrombosis, contaminated infusion products, and flushing can cause contamination.

Antibiotic-coated catheters may decrease the risk of early CLABSI and should be considered. Because hub contamination is an important source of CLABSI, using sterile technique when accessing the catheter and limiting the number of access events help prevent CLABSI. Although routine replacement of peripheral catheters may prevent infection, the same is not recommended for central venous catheters. In addition, routine changes of dressings for catheters do not seem to prevent CLABSI.

In any patient with fever and a central venous catheter, CLABSI is a diagnostic consideration. Purulence and cellulitis around the catheter site often are absent at the time of diagnosis. Clinical factors predicting CLABSI include difficult or emergent insertion of a central venous catheter, placement of a multiple lumen catheter, central venous catheterization for >4 days, catheter thrombosis, a high number of manipulations per day, prior positive blood cultures, respiratory infection, and immunocompromise.

As clinical features are poor predictors, diagnosis typically relies on culture data. A CLABSI is defined as bacteremia or fungemia in a patient who has an intravascular device, at least one positive blood culture result obtained from a peripheral vein, clinical manifestations of infection (fever, chills, and/or hypotension), and no apparent source for BSI with the exception of the catheter. The organism isolated on the peripheral blood culture should be the same as the organism isolated on a culture of blood drawn from the central catheter or a culture of the catheter tip. In the absence of clinical features, positive catheter cultures often represent colonization or contamination. Persistent bacteremia strongly suggests endovascular infection. Endocarditis must be excluded in the setting of BSI and a heart murmur or previous valvular heart disease.

In most cases, the central venous catheter must be removed as part of management. In cases of coagulase-negative staphylococcal CLABSI, the catheter may be retained if the infection is uncomplicated (defined as resolution of fever in 72 hours and absence of endovascular hardware, such as a prosthetic heart valve) and if there is no evidence of endocarditis. Begin empiric treatment with broad-spectrum antibiotics and then narrow the regimen once culture data are available. Coagulase-negative staphylococci, enterococci, *Staphylococcus aureus*, and gram-negative rods (*E. coli, Klebsiella, Pseudomonas*) are common pathogens. Use vancomycin for empiric coverage, given its activity against coagulase-negative staphylococci and *S. aureus*. In severely ill or immunocompromised patients, additional empiric coverage with a third-generation cephalosporin (ceftriaxone, ceftazidime) or fourth-generation cephalosporin (cefepime) may be needed for enteric gram-negative bacilli and *Pseudomonas aeruginosa*. Systemic antifungal agents such as an echinocandin (caspofungin, micafungin) or an azole (fluconazole) must be prescribed when fungemia is suspected, as in patients with sepsis and risk factors for candidiasis (total parenteral nutrition, prolonged use of broad-spectrum antibiotics, hematologic malignancy, bone marrow or solid organ transplantation). Uncomplicated infections are treated for 10 to 14 days (most pathogens); coagulase-negative staphylococci may be treated for 5 to 7 days if the infected catheter is removed.

Complications of CLABSIs include septic thrombosis, endocarditis, osteomyelitis, meningitis, and abscess. Patients with complicated infection require ≥6 weeks of antibiotic therapy.

Hospital-Acquired and Ventilator-Associated Pneumonia

Hospital-acquired pneumonia (HAP) is defined as pneumonia that develops ≥48 hours after hospitalization and includes ventilator-associated pneumonia (VAP), non–ventilator-associated pneumonia, and postoperative pneumonia. Pneumonia is the leading cause of death from hospital-acquired infection.

The most common cause of HAP is microaspiration of bacteria that colonize the oropharynx and upper airways in seriously ill patients. Although gram-negative bacilli and *S. aureus* are the most common pathogens, the number of drug-resistant organisms continues to escalate. Endotracheal intubation with mechanical ventilation poses the greatest overall risk for HAP, with 85% of all cases of HAP occurring in ventilated patients. Endotracheal intubation breaches airway defenses, impairs cough and mucociliary clearance, and facilitates microaspiration of bacteria-laden secretions that pool above the inflated endotracheal tube cuff. Major risk factors for postoperative pneumonia are age >70 years, abdominal or thoracic surgery, malnutrition, increased gastric pH, and reintubation.

Removing an endotracheal tube as quickly as possible will reduce the risk for VAP. Minimizing manipulation of an endotracheal tube and ventilator tubing and performing meticulous hand hygiene before and after any contact with the system can prevent infection. Following weaning protocols can facilitate timely extubation and reduce the risk of infection. Patients should have daily "sedation vacations" and be assessed for extubation readiness. While intubated, patients should be in a semi-upright or upright position, as this decreases aspiration of upper airway secretions. Mouth care also may reduce the risk of infection. Although ventilator circuits do not need to be changed regularly, any accumulating condensate should be drained carefully into a patient-specific drainage container (see Table 2). Continuous aspiration of subglottic secretions using a specially designed endotracheal tube attached to a suction device may reduce the risk for aspiration, but data for this procedure are inconclusive. Selective decontamination of the oropharynx (using topical gentamicin, colistin, or vancomycin) or of the entire gastrointestinal tract is controversial and not uniformly recommended.

The diagnosis of VAP is based on clinical presentation, leukocytosis, and new or changing findings on chest radiographs. Suspect VAP if a patient has a radiographic infiltrate that is new or progressive, along with clinical findings suggesting infection (fever, purulent sputum, leukocytosis) and a decline in oxygenation. The presence of neutrophils or an organism on Gram stain can refine the diagnostic accuracy for VAP.

Do not delay initiating empiric antibiotic therapy to perform diagnostic studies. Antibiotic selection is based on risk for multidrug-resistant pathogens, with risk factors including prolonged duration of hospitalization (≥5 days), admission from a health care–related facility, and recent prolonged antibiotic therapy. Antibiotic selection is based on local antimicrobial susceptibility and anticipated side effects and takes into consideration antibiotics that were recently administered. Common pathogens include *Enterobacter, Pseudomonas, Klebsiella, E. coli, Streptococcus,* and *S. aureus* (including methicillin-resistant *S. aureus*). In patients with no risk factors, use ceftriaxone or levofloxacin. Patients with risk factors should be treated with an antipseudomonal agent and vancomycin. For suspected pseudomonal infections, therapy includes a β-lactam plus either an antipseudomonal quinolone or an aminoglycoside.

Antibiotic-Associated Diarrhea

C. difficile diarrhea occurs in about 20% of hospitalized patients taking antibiotics. The combination of health care–associated exposure to *C. difficile* and loss of normal protective colonic bacteria leads to *C. difficile* colonization. The colitis is produced by two enterotoxins (A and B), which have different mechanisms of action but both cause cytotoxicity at extremely low concentrations. Risk factors for *C. difficile* diarrhea include use of antibiotics, enemas, intestinal stimulants, and chemotherapeutic agents that alter the colonic flora.

Limiting unnecessary antibiotic exposure is a key factor in preventing *C. difficile* infection. Routine infection-control measures to prevent the spread of *C. difficile* include adherence to strict hand hygiene procedures and use of universal precautions (see

Table 2). Alcohol-based hand rubs are not sporicidal. Although there is a theoretical potential for alcohol-based hand hygiene products to increase the incidence of *C. difficile* infection because of their relative ineffectiveness at eliminating spores from the hands, there has not been any clinical evidence to support this thus far. Patients with known or suspected illness should be placed under contact isolation.

Consider *C. difficile* infection in patients with diarrhea who have received antibiotic therapy in the previous 2 months or have been recently hospitalized. Patients may complain of abdominal pain, fever, anorexia, malaise, or vomiting. Physical examination may demonstrate signs of volume depletion, abdominal tenderness, and, in severe cases, abdominal rigidity and rebound tenderness. Obtain an enzyme-linked immunosorbent assay of the stool for both endotoxins; sensitivity is improved by serial testing. Cytotoxin assay is the gold standard for diagnosis but is not widely available. In select patients, colonoscopy may help establish the diagnosis by demonstrating typical pseudomembranes. In severe cases, complications include toxic megacolon, perforated colon, severe ileus, ascites, and death.

For a mild to moderately severe initial episode of *C. difficile* infection, oral or intravenous metronidazole is the first-line agent. For a severe initial episode in a patient exhibiting a leukocyte count ≥15,000/µL (15×10^9/L) or a serum creatinine level 1.5 times greater than baseline, oral vancomycin is the drug of choice. Treat a first relapse with a second course of the initial antibiotic used for first-line therapy. For a second relapse, vancomycin in a tapered and/or pulsed regimen is preferred.

New therapies are needed to manage the increasing incidence, severity, and high rate of recurrence of *C. difficile* infection. A recent randomized placebo-controlled study found that a single infusion of monoclonal antibodies to both *C. difficile* endotoxins, along with standard-of-care antibiotic management, significantly reduced the recurrence of *C. difficile* infection.

Book Enhancement

Go to www.acponline.org/essentials/infectious-disease-section.html. In *MKSAP for Students 5*, assess your knowledge with items 29-33 in the **Infectious Disease Medicine** section.

Acknowledgment

We would like to thank Dr. Brijen Shah, who contributed to an earlier version of this chapter.

Bibliography

Klompas M. Does this patient have ventilator-associated pneumonia? JAMA. 2007;297:1583-1593. [PMID: 17426278]

Mermel LA, Allon M, Bouza E, et al. Clinical practice guidelines for the diagnosis and management of intravascular catheter-related infection: 2009 Update by the Infectious Diseases Society of America [published errata appear in Clin Infect Dis. 2010;50:457 and 2010;50:1079]. Clin Infect Dis. 2009;49:1-45. [PMID: 19489710]

Yokoe DS, Mermel LA, Anderson DJ, et al. A compendium of strategies to prevent healthcare-associated infections in acute care hospitals. Infect Control Hosp Epidemiol. 2008;29 Suppl 1:S12-S21. [PMID: 18840084]

Chapter 56

Tuberculosis

Arlina Ahluwalia, MD

Tuberculosis is a common infectious disease worldwide, with mortality rates up to 80% in untreated persons. Infection by *Mycobacterium tuberculosis* primarily involves the lungs but has the potential to affect nearly any organ. Inhalation of infected airborne droplets initiates a cell-mediated immunologic response. Macrophages initially engulf the inhaled bacilli but cannot arrest mycobacterial multiplication, and a granuloma forms. As immunity develops, the patient becomes reactive to the tuberculin skin test (TST). If the infection is contained, a state of latent tuberculosis infection (LTBI) without systemic manifestations may ensue; however, the risk for reactivation of dormant bacilli and resultant active infection remains for years. Treatment of LTBI, the most prevalent form of tuberculosis in the United States, decreases rates of reactivation tuberculosis by up to 90%. Reactivation tuberculosis usually is localized to the lungs.

In the case of an initial inadequate immune response, infection may spread to nearly every organ hematogenously or via lymphatics. HIV/AIDS is a major risk factor for both primary progression and reactivation of quiescent tuberculosis, but malnutrition and other immunosuppressed states also increase risk.

Recent challenges to tuberculosis control in the United States include the association with HIV infection, risks of reactivation (especially in settings of decreased cell-mediated immunity), spread of new disease (occasionally in epidemic form), and emergence of multidrug-resistant strains. Multidrug resistance complicates efforts to eradicate tuberculosis and constitutes a major factor in mandating lengthy drug regimens monitored by a health care worker or public health program. Aggressive screening programs and a high index of suspicion form the cornerstone of control of active tuberculosis infection.

Prevention

Implement primary prevention of tuberculosis by isolating infected patients, and promote secondary prevention by treating patients with evidence of LTBI; the risk of reactivation tuberculosis is greatest in the first 1 to 2 years following initial infection. Hospitalized patients with suspected or confirmed active tuberculosis should be isolated in a private room with negative air pressure, the door should remain closed, all entering persons should wear masks with a filtering capacity of 95% (different from regular surgical masks), and the hospital infection control department should be notified. All cases of active tuberculosis must be reported to the public health department.

Offer LTBI treatment to all high-risk persons with a positive TST (or other diagnostic test) regardless of age, unless prior treatment is documented or is medically contraindicated. Bacille Calmette-Guérin (BCG) vaccination has no role in prevention of tuberculosis in the United States.

Screening

Screen individuals at high risk for exposure to or contraction of tuberculosis using purified protein derivative (PPD) with the Mantoux TST method or interferon gamma release assay. High-risk populations include (1) anyone who has close contact with a person with known or suspected active tuberculosis, (2) persons who were born in areas with high rates of tuberculosis (Asia, Africa, Latin America, Eastern Europe, Russia), (3) persons who reside or are employed in high-risk congregate settings, (4) persons who provide health care to high-risk persons, (5) medically underserved or low-income populations, (6) populations with increased prevalence of tuberculosis (Asian and Pacific Islanders, Hispanics, blacks, American Indians, migrant farm workers, homeless persons), (7) persons who use illicit injection drugs, and (8) patients who are beginning chronic immunosuppressive therapy (e.g., prednisone, TNF-α inhibitors, transplant recipients). A positive TST is defined by the diameter of the indurated area, not the size of the erythema; taking into account a person's risk profile increases the specificity of a TST test (Table 1). Educational outreach to health care workers improves the case detection rate of tuberculosis.

Skin tests do not always convert after BCG vaccination, and history of vaccination alters neither testing nor consideration of treatment in most adults. Because the skin test result may not become positive for up to 12 weeks after exposure to active tuberculosis, consider retesting or treating empirically, especially in high-risk persons (e.g., those with HIV infection). Patients exposed to tuberculosis in the more distant past initially may have a negative skin test; a second skin test 7 to 21 days after the first may be helpful in reducing the false-negative response rate. Such two-step testing often "boosts" a negative test to positive as the immune system recalls its previous exposure, thus uncovering a true-positive result. Two-step testing may be particularly helpful for regular testing programs (e.g., nursing home resident/employee or hospital employee programs) to distinguish new from old exposure. A newer screening option is the interferon-gamma release assay (IGRA), which assesses the T-cell response to specific *M. tuberculosis* antigens. IGRA shows excellent specificity, especially with BCG-vaccinated persons, and may be preferred for patients unlikely to return for TST reading results, although the optimal role of this newer method has yet to be established. Chest radiography, in addition to a history and physical examination, is mandatory to rule out active disease in all patients with a positive skin test being considered for LTBI treatment.

Table 1. Criteria for Tuberculin Positivity by Risk Group

Induration ≥5 mm	Induration ≥10 mm	Induration ≥15 mm
Person with HIV infection	Person who recently (<5 y) arrived from a country with high TB prevalence	All others with no risk factors for TB
Person with recent contact with case of active TB	Injection drug user	
Person with fibrotic changes on chest radiograph consistent with old TB	Resident or employee of high-risk congregate setting (prison, jail, nursing home or other long-term facility for the elderly, hospital or other health care facility, residential facility for patients with AIDS, homeless shelter)	
Person with an organ transplant or other immunosuppressive condition (e.g., receiving equivalent of ≥15 mg/d of prednisone for >4 wk)	Health care worker	
	Employee of mycobacteriology laboratory	
	Person with a clinical condition associated with high risk for active TB	
	Children age <4 years or exposed to adults in high-risk categories	

TB = tuberculosis.

Diagnosis

Patients with pulmonary tuberculosis often are asymptomatic. However, constitutional symptoms (anorexia, fatigue, weight loss, chills, fever, night sweats) as well as local symptoms (cough) may develop. Hemoptysis and chest pain from pleural involvement indicate advanced disease. The pulmonary examination often is minimally abnormal. HIV-infected or otherwise immunocompromised patients have a greater likelihood of disseminated or extrapulmonary infection, but classic signs or symptoms of tuberculosis often are absent, and chest radiographs may be normal. Maintain a high level of suspicion for active tuberculosis to enable rapid diagnosis. Gather information about active tuberculosis exposures, previous tuberculosis, and previous skin testing. Table 2 summarizes the differential diagnosis of tuberculosis.

Bacteriologic confirmation and susceptibility testing form the cornerstone of management. Obtain acid-fast bacilli smears and cultures (pulmonary and any suspected site of infection), chest radiographs, and skin tests in patients suspected of having active tuberculosis (Table 3). In patients with infection, the TST usually is positive within 48 to 72 hours. A false-negative skin test may occur in anergic patients and in up to 25% of those with active tuberculosis. On 3 separate days, send early-morning induced sputum (or early-morning gastric washings if voluntary sputum is unattainable) for rapid nucleic acid amplification testing, culture, and staining (Ziehl-Neelsen or Kinyoun). Nucleic acid amplification tests of sputum may be used to exclude tuberculosis in patients with false-positive sputum (nontuberculous mycobacteria) or to confirm the disease in some patients with false-negative smears. Patients with active disease may have only a single positive culture. For patients suspected of having pleural tuberculosis, consider thoracentesis to obtain fluid for testing (adenosine deaminase, microbiology, and cell count) or pleural biopsies. In persons with unknown HIV status, test for HIV infection.

Table 2. Differential Diagnosis of Tuberculosis (TB)

Disorder	Notes
Nontuberculous mycobacterial infection	Signs and symptoms may be the same as for TB; patients usually have less fever and weight loss than patients with TB. Presence of multiple nodules with bronchiectasis on lung CT is highly specific for *Mycobacterium avium* complex.
Sarcoidosis (see Chapter 86)	Patients have dyspnea and cough. Chest radiography shows diffuse infiltrative lung disease with bilateral hilar adenopathy. Biopsy reveals noncaseating granulomas. Diagnosis is made after exclusion of other possibilities.
Aspiration pneumonia	May have an indolent course. Radiologic infiltrates are more common in dependent areas. Patients may have decreased mental status or evidence of reduced gag reflex.
Lung abscess	Frequently involves the posterior upper segments of the upper lobes; may be acute or indolent. Patients usually have foul-smelling sputum.
Histoplasmosis or coccidioidomycosis	Patients may have fever, cough, and night sweats. These diseases usually are geographically specific (histoplasmosis, Midwest; coccidioidomycosis, Southwest). Chest radiography may show a miliary (histoplasmosis) or cavitary lesion.
Wegener granulomatosis (see Chapter 97)	Necrotizing granulomas in the lung and necrotizing glomerulonephritis. Patients have fever and cough. Chest radiography shows a cavitary lesion in up to 70% of cases.
Actinomycosis	Characterized by cough, hemoptysis, and (eventually) draining sinuses. Has an indolent course; patients may have respiratory symptoms for up to 5 months before diagnosis. Sulphur granules are seen in stained specimens from draining sinuses.
Lung cancer (see Chapter 75)	Symptoms may be the same as occur in TB (weight loss, cough). Cytology or biopsy to rule out. Patients may have both a lung cancer and TB.

Table 3. Laboratory and Other Studies for Tuberculosis (TB)

Test	Notes
Complete blood count	Anemia is present in 10% of patients with TB, particularly if infection is disseminated. Leukocytosis is present in 10% of patients with TB.
Electrolytes	Hyponatremia is present in up to 11% of patients with TB.
Chest radiography	The classic appearance of reactivation TB is lesions in the apical posterior segments of the upper lung and superior segments of the lower lobe. Chest radiographs may be normal in patients with endobronchial disease or peribronchial node with fistula or in symptomatic HIV-infected patients with active TB. In disseminated disease, 50%-90% have a miliary pattern on chest x-ray.
Tuberculin skin test (TST)	TST has a sensitivity of 59%-100% and specificity of 44%-100%. Sensitivity and specificity change with specific patient risk factors and cutoff point (see Table 1). A positive test may indicate latent TB. False-positive results can occur with exposure to nontuberculous mycobacteria. False-negative results occur in anergic patients and in up to 25% of patients with active TB.
Interferon-gamma release assay (IGRA)	IGRA is more specific than TST in the setting of previous BCG vaccination and may be more sensitive in cases of immune deficiency. IGRA cannot distinguish between LTBI and active infection.
Sputum smear for acid-fast bacilli	Sputum smear has a sensitivity of 50%-80%; with multiple specimens, the sensitivity increases to up to 96%. At least 5000 to 10,000 organisms should be present for a smear to be positive. The more acid-fast bacilli seen, the more infectious is the patient. Induced sputum or gastric washings may be obtained if a patient does not have a productive cough. Nontuberculous mycobacteria may produce positive smears. *Nocardia* is acid fast on the modified acid-fast stain.
Sputum culture for acid-fast bacilli	Sputum culture has a sensitivity of 67%-82% and specificity of 99%-100%. Solid media cultures in conjunction with liquid media often are the gold standard used for diagnosis. The only false-positive results that occur are as a result of laboratory error or contamination of the specimen. False-negative results do occur and often are due to nontuberculous mycobacterial overgrowth and antibiotic treatment.
Nucleic acid amplification of smear-positive sputum	Nucleic acid amplification has a sensitivity of 95% and specificity of 98%. Results are available in a few hours. False-positive results occur only with laboratory contamination, although the test does not indicate if bacteria are alive or dead (i.e., may remain positive for some time after treatment).

BCG = Bacille Calmette-Guérin; LTBI = latent tuberculosis infection.

Radiologic abnormalities of reactivation tuberculosis classically include lesions in the apical posterior segments of the upper lung and superior segments of the lower lobe. Primary progressive tuberculosis may manifest as hilar adenopathy or infiltrates in any part of the lung, similar to bacterial pneumonia. Atypical or absent radiologic findings are common in immunocompromised patients but may also be the case for immunocompetent patients. Bronchoscopy may aid in the diagnosis in certain circumstances.

Therapy

The standard treatment for suspected or confirmed active tuberculosis is at least 6 months of a 3- to 4-drug regimen usually consisting of isoniazid, rifampin, pyrazinamide, and ethambutol. Base all treatment on resistance patterns in the area where the patient was likely exposed to tuberculosis. Directly observed therapy programs are ideal. A repeat sputum smear and culture after the initial 2-month phase of therapy may aid in determining whether the continuation phase of treatment requires 4 or 7 months of drugs, especially in cavitary disease. These approaches decrease the incidence of acquired drug resistance, relapse, reactivation, and transmission. Consider the possibility of potential drug interactions (e.g., concurrent HIV drug therapy). Multidrug-resistant (MDR) tuberculosis is resistant to isoniazid and rifampin and possibly to other chemotherapeutic agents. Extensively drug-resistant (XDR) tuberculosis is resistant to isoniazid; rifampin; fluoroquinolones; and aminoglycosides, capreomycin, or both. Treatment of MDR or XDR tuberculosis requires an individualized regimen based on comprehensive drug susceptibility testing and consultation with an expert.

LTBI is treated with isoniazid for 9 months or, alternatively, with rifampin for 4 months, although therapy must be individualized. Before treatment is initiated, exclude active tuberculosis by history, physical examination, and chest radiography. Discuss with the patient the risks and benefits of drug therapy as well as the patient's perceptions of LTBI treatment to optimize adherence to treatment. Before starting therapy, obtain baseline blood tests specific to potential drug toxicities to detect abnormalities that might complicate treatment (e.g., hepatic dysfunction complicated by isoniazid, pyrazinamide, or rifampin). Baseline or follow-up audiometry (streptomycin toxicity) or visual acuity testing (ethambutol toxicity) also may be required.

Isolation is paramount to limit spread of disease. Hospitalization is especially appropriate in cases of respiratory distress, marked hemoptysis, or other indicators of systemic disease requiring hospital support or to remove the index case from an unstable housing situation or other high-risk setting (e.g., nursing home). Consider maintenance of isolation in MDR tuberculosis until sputum cultures are negative. Surgical resection of diseased tissue rarely is required but may be considered in certain circumstances (e.g., bronchopleural fistula, lack of response in MDR or XDR tuberculosis).

Follow-Up

Ensure careful monitoring for treatment adherence in patients with active tuberculosis or LTBI, and provide written patient information (including explanation of methods to limit spread of infection and factors that increase risk of liver damage) to improve adherence and avoid complications. Instruct patients to stop medications immediately in the event of adverse drug reactions and to report these events promptly. Consider monthly sputum cultures to monitor treatment response, and adjust the drug regimen based on susceptibilities and length of therapy. A tuberculosis expert should be consulted if the sputum culture remains positive or if the patient has not improved clinically after 3 months of therapy. Perform periodic (at least monthly) assessments for adverse reactions in patients on treatment, including evaluating for hepatitis, anemia, thrombocytopenia, visual changes, and gout. Assessment should focus on signs and symptoms surveillance rather than scheduled laboratory testing. Periodic laboratory monitoring is reasonable, however, in patients at higher risk for hepatitis (elderly patients, patients with a history of alcohol abuse, patients with viral hepatitis or HIV infection). Ensure that household members and other close contacts of patients with tuberculosis are tested for LTBI.

Book Enhancement

Go to www.acponline.org/essentials/infectious-disease-section. html. In *MKSAP for Students 5*, assess your knowledge with items 34-38 in the **Infectious Disease Medicine** section.

Bibliography

Escalante P. In the clinic. Tuberculosis [published erratum appears in Ann Intern Med. 2009;151:292]. Ann Intern Med. 2009;150:ITC61-614; quiz ITV616. [PMID: 19487708]

Chapter 57

Community-Acquired Pneumonia

Irene Alexandraki, MD

Community-acquired pneumonia (CAP) affects 4 million adults per year in the United States, 20% of whom will require hospitalization. CAP is the leading cause of death from infectious disease in the United States and the sixth-leading cause of death overall.

Host defense mechanisms keep the lower airways sterile. Pneumonia develops when there is a defect in host defenses, exposure to a particularly virulent organism, or an overwhelming inoculum. The pathogens descend from the oropharynx to the lower respiratory tract (90% of cases) or are acquired through inhalation (viruses), hematogenously (*Staphylococcus*), or directly from a contiguous infected site. Alterations in anatomic barriers and impairment of humoral or cell-mediated immunity or phagocytic function are risk factors for pneumonia.

Streptococcus pneumoniae is the most common pathogen isolated from patients with CAP; drug-resistant *S. pneumoniae* accounts for up to 40% of isolates. Other common bacterial pathogens include *Haemophilus influenzae* and atypical pathogens, such as *Mycoplasma pneumoniae, Chlamydophila pneumoniae,* and *Legionella*. Gram-negative bacteria may be a cause in patients with comorbidities (chronic cardiopulmonary disease, chronic kidney or liver disease, diabetes mellitus, active malignancy, recent antibiotic therapy) and in nursing home residents. *Klebsiella pneumoniae* causes severe pneumonia in patients with alcoholism. *Pseudomonas aeruginosa* is more common in patients with structural lung disease (bronchiectasis) and after recent antibiotic therapy or hospitalization. When aspiration is a possibility, enteric gram-negative and anaerobic organisms should be considered. Viral pathogens (influenza virus, parainfluenza virus, adenovirus, respiratory syncytial virus) also cause CAP. Influenza increases the susceptibility of previously healthy persons to invasive pneumococcal or methicillin-resistant *Staphylococcus aureus* (MRSA) pneumonia, resulting in increased morbidity and mortality during influenza epidemics and pandemics.

Prevention

Influenza vaccine prevents or attenuates illness due to influenza and reduces pneumonia-related mortality during influenza season by 27% to 50%. In 2010, the U.S. Advisory Committee on Immunization Practices recommended influenza vaccination for all persons aged ≥6 months. The vaccine should be administered as soon as it becomes available, usually in September. Consider empiric use of oseltamivir or zanamivir in unvaccinated high-risk persons during an influenza epidemic.

Administer pneumococcal vaccine to all adults aged ≥65 years and to all adults aged <65 years who live in long-term care facilities or who have coronary artery disease, heart failure, COPD, diabetes, alcoholism, cirrhosis, cerebrospinal fluid leaks, or anatomic or functional asplenia, including sickle cell disease. Also immunize adults aged <65 years who are immunocompromised due to HIV infection, an immune disorder or malignancy, multiple myeloma, leukemia, lymphoma, Hodgkin disease, chronic kidney disease, nephrotic syndrome, or immunosuppressive therapy (including long-term corticosteroids).

Review the vaccination status and risk factors in all persons aged >50 years. Among those aged >65 years, revaccinate once after 5 years anyone who was initially vaccinated before age 65. Revaccinate immunocompromised patients once, 5 years after the initial vaccination. Consider giving the vaccine to any hospitalized patient before discharge. The current pneumococcal vaccine contains purified, capsular polysaccharide from 23 serotypes that cause 85% to 90% of invasive pneumonia in adults and children and is effective in preventing pneumococcal bacteremia and meningitis in healthy, immunocompetent adults.

Diagnosis

Consider pneumonia in a patient with cough, sputum, fever, chills, or dyspnea. Ask about the duration of symptoms and about pleuritic chest pain, night sweats, and weight loss. Symptoms may develop abruptly or may gradually worsen over days. Patients with chronic illness may present with nonrespiratory symptoms or deterioration of their illness. Elderly patients may have confusion, weakness, lethargy, poor oral intake, or complaints of falling; older patients may be afebrile and remain undiagnosed until late in the course of illness.

Ask about chronic heart and lung disease (pneumococci, enteric gram-negative bacteria, *H. influenzae*); travel to the southwestern United States (*Coccidioides*) or Southeast Asia (*Mycobacterium tuberculosis*); alcohol abuse (anaerobes, *K. pneumoniae*); injection drug use (MRSA, anaerobes, *M. tuberculosis*); and exposure to farm animals (*Coxiella burnetii*), birds (*Chlamydophila psittaci, Cryptococcus, Histoplasma*), and bats (*Histoplasma*). Assess risk for aspiration, such as history of stroke, seizures, alcoholism, or poor dentition (anaerobes). Information about residence and recent antibiotic therapy also may help predict likely pathogens.

Look for tachypnea, fever, crackles, bronchial breath sounds, and signs of pleural effusion, such as egophony and dullness to percussion with reduced breath sounds. Consider using the CURB-65 criteria (Confusion, blood Urea nitrogen >19.6 mg/dL [7.0 mmol/L], Respiration rate ≥30/min, systolic Blood pressure <90 mm Hg or diastolic blood pressure <60 mm Hg, and age ≥65 years) to identify high-risk patients and to predict a complicated course. Patients who meet at least two criteria usually are admitted to the hospital, and those with at least three criteria are considered for intensive care unit (ICU) admission. Another prognostic model, the Pneumonia Severity Index, may be used to predict mortality risk based on patient age, comorbidities, physical examination findings, and laboratory data. Admit patients who have failed outpatient therapy, have decompensated comorbid illness, have complex social needs, or require intravenous antibiotics or oxygen. Although there is a need to reduce unnecessary hospitalizations for CAP, the decision for admission is complex, and no single rule can replace clinical evaluation.

Obtain a chest radiograph in patients with clinical features suggesting CAP. Chest radiography documents the presence of pneumonia and complications, such as pleural effusion, lung abscess, cavitation, and multilobar illness. Limit laboratory testing in uncomplicated outpatient cases to chest radiography and pulse oximetry to assess oxygenation. The presence of cavities with airfluid levels suggests abscess formation, whereas the presence of cavities without air-fluid levels suggests tuberculosis or fungal infection. If there is evidence of volume loss, bronchial obstruction must be excluded. Enlargement of mediastinal or hilar lymph nodes suggests fungal or mycobacterial infection. If a pleural effusion is present, obtain a decubitus film or chest CT scan. The presence of pleural fluid may indicate empyema possibly requiring thoracentesis.

For hospitalized patients, order chest radiography, two sets of blood cultures, a routine metabolic panel, pulse oximetry, and a complete blood count. Obtain arterial blood gas when carbon dioxide retention is suspected (e.g., patients with COPD). Obtain a sputum culture for any patient at risk for infection with drug-resistant or unusual pathogens and to correlate with sputum Gram stain results. Use rapid antigen tests for influenza A and B during the appropriate season and during epidemics. Consider testing concentrated urine for pneumococcal and Legionella antigens. Suspect Legionella in patients with risk factors (age ≥50 years, smoking history, immunocompromising condition) who present with severe pneumonia and extrapulmonary symptoms (headache, confusion, diarrhea, kidney failure). Hyponatremia occurs more often in Legionnaire disease than in other causes of pneumonia. The urine antigen test detects only Legionella serogroup 1.

Consider unusual pathogens (M. tuberculosis, fungi, viruses, Pneumocystis) in patients who do not respond to empiric therapy within 48 to 72 hours. Also consider empyema, lung abscess, metastatic infectious complications (e.g., endocarditis), and noninfectious processes (Table 1). In such circumstances, order additional diagnostic tests (chest CT, pulmonary angiography, bronchoscopy) and obtain an infectious disease or a pulmonary consultation.

Therapy

In the outpatient setting, treat patients without cardiopulmonary disease or other comorbidities with a macrolide (azithromycin, clarithromycin) or doxycycline. For patients with cardiopulmonary disease or modifying factors (Table 2), use an antipneumococcal quinolone (levofloxacin, gatifloxacin, moxifloxacin) or a combination of a β-lactam or β-lactam/β-lactamase inhibitor (cefuroxime, cefpodoxime, amoxicillin-clavulanate) and a macrolide or doxycycline. Macrolides, quinolones, and doxycycline will provide coverage of atypical organisms. Because Chlamydophila and Legionella species are intracellular organisms and Mycoplasma has no cell wall, β-lactam antibiotics are not effective against these atypical organisms.

Table 1. Differential Diagnosis of Community-Acquired Pneumonia

Disorder	Notes
Bronchiolitis obliterans with organizing pneumonia	Subacute illness (4-6 wk) with fever and alveolar infiltrates (often peripheral). Diagnosis is based on biopsy (transbronchial or open lung) or characteristic clinical picture and response to corticosteroids.
Lung cancer (see Chapter 75)	May cause postobstructive pneumonia. Suspect in patients who smoke, especially if there is hemoptysis and radiographic evidence of volume loss or a mass effect.
Eosinophilic pneumonia (see Chapter 86)	Presents as an acute illness with the radiographic "photo negative" of pulmonary edema, usually with peripheral eosinophilia. Biopsy may not be needed with a classic presentation.
Hypersensitivity pneumonitis (see Chapter 86)	Recurrent episodes of fever and dyspnea, with rapid resolution of infiltrates; chronic infiltrates after multiple episodes. Diagnose with precipitating antibodies to the antigen (molds etc.), characteristic history, or open lung biopsy.
Interstitial pneumonia (see Chapter 86)	A nonspecific radiographic pattern resulting from infection (viral, atypical pathogen), inflammation (usual interstitial pneumonia), or drug toxicity (amiodarone). A careful exposure history and duration of illness can help distinguish between several diagnostic possibilities, but open lung biopsy may be required.
Pulmonary embolism (see Chapter 87)	If infarction is present, there may be fever, lung infiltrate, dyspnea, and hemoptysis. Suspect in patients with appropriate risk factors (immobilization, heart failure, recent surgery). The infiltrate of infarction may "melt away" rapidly.
Sarcoidosis (see Chapter 86)	May present as lung infiltrate of any type, with or without mediastinal adenopathy. Suspect if the radiographic abnormalities in the lung parenchyma are extensive and the patient is not as ill as suggested by the radiographic pattern. An elevated ACE level enhances suspicion. Diagnosis can be made by transbronchial lung biopsy.
Wegener granulomatosis (see Chapter 97)	Associated with characteristic nodular and cavitary infiltrates, hemoptysis, and otitis media. May be limited to the lung or involve the kidneys (rapidly progressive glomerulonephritis). In general, diagnosis is based on the characteristic clinical picture, presence of c-ANCA, and absence of p-ANCA. If uncertain, perform open lung biopsy to document vasculitis.

c-ANCA = cytoplasmic antineutrophil cytoplasmic antibody; p-ANCA = perinuclear antineutrophil cytoplasmic antibody.

Table 2. Modifying Factors that Increase the Risk of Infection with Specific Pathogens

Modifying Factor	Pathogen
Age >65 y, β-lactam therapy (in previous 3 mo), alcoholism, immunosuppression (illness, corticosteroids), multiple medical comorbidities, exposure to a child in a day care center	Penicillin-resistant and drug-resistant pneumococci
Residence in a nursing home, underlying cardiopulmonary disease, multiple medical comorbidities, recent antibiotic therapy	Enteric gram-negative bacteria
Structural lung disease (bronchiectasis), corticosteroid therapy, broad-spectrum antibiotic therapy for >7 d; malnutrition	*Pseudomonas aeruginosa*
Endobronchial obstruction (tumor)	Anaerobes, *Streptococcus pneumoniae, Haemophilus influenzae, Staphylococcus aureus*
Intravenous drug use	Anaerobes, *S. aureus, Mycobacterium tuberculosis, S. pneumoniae*
Influenza epidemic in the community	Influenza virus, *S. pneumoniae, S. aureus, H. influenzae*
COPD, smoking history	*S. pneumoniae, H. influenzae, Moraxella catarrhalis, P. aeruginosa, Legionella* species, *Chlamydophila pneumoniae*
Poor dental hygiene, aspiration, lung abscess	Oral anaerobes
Animal exposure	*Coxiella burnetii* (farm animals); *Chlamydophila psittaci, Cryptococcus* (birds); *Histoplasma* (birds, bats)

For hospitalized patients, administer oxygen, titrating to an oxygen saturation level of ≥90%. Do not delay antibiotic therapy while awaiting sputum sampling for culture. Give intravenous antibiotics within 6 hours of the patient's arrival to the hospital, after rapid assessment of oxygenation and routine blood work and culture. Monitor oxygen therapy carefully in patients with COPD, who may further retain carbon dioxide. Provide intravenous hydration to patients with signs of dehydration and chest physiotherapy to patients with large volumes of respiratory secretions.

Give intravenous azithromycin to hospitalized patients without cardiopulmonary disease or modifying factors (see Table 2). Treat patients with cardiopulmonary disease or modifying factors with an oral or intravenous quinolone (levofloxacin, moxifloxacin) or the combination of a β-lactam or β-lactam/β-lactamase inhibitor (cefotaxime, ceftriaxone, ampicillin-sulbactam) and a macrolide or doxycycline. Use clindamycin or a β-lactam/β-lactamase inhibitor (ampicillin-sulbactam, piperacillin-tazobactam) when aspiration is suspected. Treat a lung abscess secondary to aspiration with clindamycin, and consider surgery if there is inadequate response to medical therapy or concern for a noninfectious cause and a need for tissue diagnosis.

ICU admission is required for patients at increased risk for death. Admit patients to the ICU who meet at least three of the following criteria: respiration rate ≥30/min, arterial PO_2/FiO_2 <250 mm Hg, multilobar infiltrates, confusion or disorientation, blood urea nitrogen ≥20 mg/dL (7.1 mmol/L), leukocyte count <4000/μL (4×10^9/L), platelet count <100,000/μL (100×10^9/L), body temperature <36.0°C (96.8°F), and hypotension requiring aggressive fluid resuscitation. Patients with respiratory failure requiring mechanical ventilation or with septic shock require ICU admission. Respiratory failure is defined as the inability to maintain an oxygen saturation level of >90% on maximal mask oxygen, or the presence of hypercarbia. Intubation may be required for patients with an inability to clear secretions or for airway protection. Alert and cooperative patients with isolated hypoxemia or hypercarbia might be candidates for non-invasive positive pressure ventilation.

Treat patients in the ICU who do not have risk factors for *P. aeruginosa* infection with intravenous ceftriaxone or cefotaxime plus azithromycin or an antipneumococcal quinolone (levofloxacin, moxifloxacin). If *Pseudomonas* infection is a possibility, select either an antipseudomonal β-lactam (piperacillin-tazobactam, cefepime, imipenem, meropenem) plus an intravenous quinolone effective against *Pseudomonas* (ciprofloxacin, high-dose levofloxacin). Alternatively, treat with an antipseudomonal β-lactam combined with an aminoglycoside (amikacin, gentamicin, tobramycin) plus intravenous azithromycin or an antipneumococcal quinolone. If community-acquired MRSA infection is a consideration, add linezolid or vancomycin in combination with clindamycin. In the ICU, it is important for empiric therapy to be active against *Legionella*; observational evidence suggests quinolones may be more effective than macrolides.

Treat patients with mild-to-moderate CAP for ≤7 days if there is a good clinical response, no fever for 48 to 72 hours, and no sign of extrapulmonary infection. Treat patients with *Legionella* infection for 5 to 10 days when a quinolone is used. Treat patients with severe illness, empyema, lung abscess, meningitis, or documented infection with pathogens such as *P. aeruginosa* or *S. aureus* for ≥10 days. Patients with bacteremic *S. aureus* pneumonia need 4 to 6 weeks of therapy and testing to rule out endocarditis, whereas patients with uncomplicated bacteremic pneumococcal pneumonia may need only a 7- to 10-day course of therapy if they have a good clinical response.

Switch patients to oral antibiotic therapy once symptoms improve and patients have no fever on two occasions 8 hours apart and are able to take medications by mouth. Discharge patients once the switch to oral therapy is made.

Follow-Up

Follow-up is necessary to ensure that the pneumonia has resolved, to exclude other pulmonary disease, and to focus on prevention of future episodes. If the patient has clinical response to therapy, obtain chest radiographs 4 to 6 weeks after initial therapy.

Radiographic resolution lags behind clinical resolution, taking as long as 6 to 8 weeks. Lung cancer, inflammatory disease, or infection with unusual or resistant pathogens may be present if the x-ray fails to resolve. Administer pneumococcal and influenza vaccines if they have not previously been given, and advise patients who smoke cigarettes to stop smoking.

Book Enhancement

Go to www.acponline.org/essentials/infectious-disease-section.html. In *MKSAP for Students 5*, assess your knowledge with items 39-43 in the **Infectious Disease Medicine** section.

Bibliography

Niederman M. In the clinic. Community-acquired pneumonia [published erratum appears in Ann Intern Med. 2009;151:827]. Ann Intern Med. 2009;151:ITC4-2-ITC4-14; quiz ITC4-16. [PMID: 19805767]

Chapter 58

Infective Endocarditis

Fred A. Lopez, MD

Most patients with infective endocarditis have an underlying cardiac lesion. Endothelial damage created by turbulent blood flow in this setting is the inciting event for formation of nonbacterial thrombotic endocarditis (NBTE), which consists of fibrin, platelets, and other coagulation-associated proteins. Bacteria with adherence properties colonize NBTE lesions during episodes of transient bacteremia, forming infective vegetations. Bacteremia results from disruption of a mucosal surface during daily activities such as flossing and brushing the teeth and certain dental procedures. The ability of bacteria to avoid host-associated immune defenses by enveloping themselves within the vegetation contributes to the propagation and persistence of infection.

Staphylococci (*Staphylococcus aureus,* coagulase-negative staphylococci), streptococci (particularly *Streptococcus viridans*), and enterococci are the most common organisms causing native valve infective endocarditis. Prosthetic valve infective endocarditis is categorized according to its temporal relationship to surgery. Infections within the first 2 months are most frequently due to coagulase-negative staphylococci; afterward, the microbiology is similar to native valve infective endocarditis. Due to virulence factors that facilitate adherence, colonization, persistence, tissue invasion, abscess formation, and dissemination, *S. aureus* can cause infective endocarditis in normal cardiac valves. *S. aureus* also is the most common cause of infective endocarditis in injection drug users (usually involving the tricuspid valve) and in patients on hemodialysis. Nosocomial infective endocarditis usually is caused by staphylococci or enterococci and often is associated with vascular catheters or invasive procedures.

Suspect endocarditis when blood culture results are positive in a patient with valvular disease or in a patient with an unexplained febrile or chronic illness. The mortality rate is approximately 10% for streptococcal endocarditis, 35% for staphylococcal endocarditis, and 25% to 50% for prosthetic valve endocarditis.

Prevention

Do not recommend antibiotic prophylaxis to patients with low- or moderate-risk cardiac conditions undergoing any type of procedure, and do not offer antibiotic prophylaxis to patients undergoing low-risk procedures, regardless of the patient's cardiac condition. Low-risk procedures include genitourinary and gastrointestinal procedures, cardiac catheterization, and incision of clean skin. Offer antibiotic prophylaxis to patients with both an increased risk of infection and an increased risk of adverse outcomes should infective endocarditis develop (Table 1). The goal is to achieve sufficiently high serum antibiotic concentrations to prevent attachment and growth of bacteria on predisposed cardiac structures. The choice of antibiotics is based on the predicted type of bacteremia. Because certain dental or respiratory tract procedures result in viridans group streptococcal bacteremia, a single dose of oral amoxicillin is given 30 to 60 minutes before the procedure. Clindamycin or azithromycin is used in patients with a history of anaphylaxis, angioedema, or urticaria with penicillins or ampicillin. Dental procedures for which prophylaxis is indicated include those in which there is perforation of the oral mucosa or manipulation of the periapical region of the teeth or gingival tissue. Respiratory tract procedures for which prophylaxis is reasonable include those in which there is perforation of the respiratory mucosa (tonsillectomy, adenoidectomy). Specific recommendations for prevention of infective endocarditis are available in guidelines published by the American Heart Association.

Diagnosis

The diagnosis of infective endocarditis is established on the basis of specific clinical criteria or definitive histopathologic confirmation from involved valves. Risk factors for infective endocarditis include injection drug use, recent procedures associated with risk of transient bacteremia, presence of a prosthetic valve, and certain cardiac abnormalities (see Table 1).

Fever, malaise, and fatigue are sensitive but nonspecific symptoms associated with infective endocarditis. Symptoms suggestive of septic emboli in patients with tricuspid valve endocarditis include shortness of breath, chest pain, and cough. Blindness, focal weakness, localized back or flank pain, hematuria, and gangrenous skin lesions may be embolic manifestations of left-sided infective endo-

Table 1. Indications for Bacterial Endocarditis Antibiotic Prophylaxis

Prosthetic heart valve

Previous endocarditis

Heart transplant recipient with valvulopathy

Uncorrected complex cyanotic congenital heart disease

Corrected complex congenital heart disease (receive prophylaxis for 6 mo following correction)

carditis. Physical examination findings suggestive of infective endocarditis include a new cardiac murmur, new-onset heart failure, focal neurologic signs, splenomegaly, and cutaneous manifestations (petechiae, splinter hemorrhages). The presence of Osler nodes (violaceous, circumscribed, painful nodules found in the pulp of the fingers and toes) or Janeway lesions (painless, erythematous, macular lesions found on the soles and palms) is highly suggestive of infective endocarditis.

Nonspecific laboratory abnormalities associated with infective endocarditis include leukocytosis, normocytic normochromic anemia, electrocardiographic conduction defects (atrioventricular block from extension of infection into the conduction system), hematuria, and low serum complement levels (glomerulonephritis). Radiologic findings suggesting heart failure or septic emboli from right-sided endocarditis (multiple bilateral small nodules on chest radiograph) raise suspicion for infective encarditis.

Obtain an echocardiogram to detect valvular abnormalities, particularly in bacteremic patients with underlying valvular disease, a history of infective endocarditis or injection drug use, or an unrecognized source of bacteremia. Transthoracic echocardiography is noninvasive and the initial diagnostic test of choice, but it has a sensitivity of only 50% to 80% for detection of valvular vegetations; use of transesophageal echocardiography increases both the sensitivity and specificity to approximately 95%. Transesophageal echocardiography is particularly useful to better delineate the anatomy of a native valve and is essential to more accurately identify paravalvular abscesses and evaluate prosthetic valves.

Obtain blood cultures to identify the microbiologic cause of infective endocarditis. Additional serologic tests for *Coxiella burnetii* (Q fever) and for *Bartonella, Legionella, Brucella,* *Mycoplasma*, and *Chlamydophila* species can be obtained when there is a high clinical suspicion of infective endocarditis but blood cultures are negative in the absence of antibiotic therapy. Additional causes of culture-negative endocarditis include a group of gram-negative pathogens constituting the HACEK group (*Haemophilus, Actinobacillus, Cardiobacterium, Eikenella,* and *Kingella* species), nutritionally variant streptococci (*Abiotrophia* species, *Trophermyma whippelii*), and fungi (*Aspergillus* species, *Histoplasma capsulatum*).

Local extension of infection can result in paravalvular abscesses, heart failure due to valvular damage, pericarditis, and myocardial infarction from vegetation-associated emboli. Suspect a paravalvular abscess in patients with persistent fever despite appropriately targeted antibiotics and with electrocardiographic manifestations of atrioventricular block. Neurologic complications include stroke (embolic or hemorrhagic), brain abscess, and meningitis. Emboli can result in renal and splenic infarction and abscesses and vertebral osteomyelitis. Mycotic aneurysm (infection-induced dilatation of an artery) can occur anywhere in the vascular system. Right-sided infective endocarditis can result in pulmonary artery occlusion or multiple bilateral pulmonary abscesses. Immunologically mediated glomerulonephritis should be suspected in patients with low complement levels and hematuria, erythrocyte cell casts, or proteinuria.

The Duke criteria are validated clinical and laboratory criteria for the diagnosis of infective endocarditis, with a sensitivity >80% (Table 2). Consider other medical conditions that can mimic the syndrome of infective endocarditis, especially when patients with negative blood cultures do not respond to empiric antibiotic therapy or when transesophageal echocardiography is unrevealing (Table 3).

Table 2. Modified Duke Criteria for the Diagnosis of Infective Endocarditis

Major criteria

1. Microbiologic (any of the following):

    Typical microorganisms (including *Staphylococcus aureus*) grown from 2 blood cultures

    A microorganism grown from persistently positive blood cultures

    Positive serologic test or single positive blood culture for *Coxiella burnetii*

2. Evidence of endocardial involvement (either of the following):

    Echocardiogram: oscillating intracardiac mass, abscess, or new partial dehiscence of a prosthetic valve

    Physical examination: new valve regurgitation (change in preexisting murmur is not sufficient)

Minor criteria

1. Predisposing heart condition or injection drug use

2. Fever >38.0°C (100.4°F)

3. Vascular phenomena: major arterial emboli, septic pulmonary infarcts, mycotic aneurysm, intracranial hemorrhage, conjunctival hemorrhage, or Janeway lesions

4. Immunologic phenomena: glomerulonephritis, Osler nodes, Roth spots, positive rheumatoid factor

5. Microbiologic: serologic evidence of infection or positive blood cultures not meeting the major criteria (a single blood culture for coagulase-negative staphylococci is not sufficient)

Diagnosis

Definite endocarditis = 2 major criteria *or* 1 major + 3 minor criteria *or* 5 minor criteria

Possible endocarditis = 1 major + 1 minor criterion *or* 3 minor criteria

Adapted from Li JS, Sexton DJ, Mick N, et al. Proposed modifications to the Duke criteria for the diagnosis of infective endocarditis. Clin Infect Dis. 2000;30:633-638. [PMID: 10770721]

Table 3. Differential Diagnosis of Infective Endocarditis

Disorder	Notes
Pulmonary embolism (see Chapter 87)	Low-grade fever with pulmonary symptoms. Diagnosis is based on clinical algorithms using radiologic or nuclear medicine studies.
Bacteremic infections	Disseminated infection from a focal source. Transesophageal echocardiography is negative.
Acute leukemia (see Chapter 48)	Fever, systemic symptoms, and splenomegaly. CBC and bone marrow examination are diagnostic.
Malignancy with metastases	Low-grade fever and systemic symptoms associated with known primary neoplasm. Imaging studies and biopsy are diagnostic.
Collagen vascular disease with angiitis (see Chapter 97)	Low-grade fever, systemic symptoms, and positive rheumatoid factor (RF). Similar symptoms and a false-positive RF may be seen in infective endocarditis. Specific immunologic tests help with the diagnosis.
Atrial myxoma	Low-grade fever, embolic phenomena, and specific imaging characteristics on echocardiogram. Blood cultures are negative.
Nonbacterial thrombotic endocarditis (see Chapter 95)	Fever and emboli. Blood cultures are negative.
Stroke (see Chapter 71)	Acute loss of motor function, speech or mental status changes. Patients are afebrile, echocardiogram is normal; blood cultures are negative.

CBC = complete blood count.

Therapy

Begin empiric antibiotic therapy in patients with proven or suspected infective endocarditis after at least three sets of blood cultures are obtained from separate sites. Empiric therapy for community-acquired native valve infective endocarditis includes vancomycin and gentamicin for streptococci (especially *S. viridans* and *Streptococcus bovis*), staphylococci (particularly in injection drug users and those with indwelling vascular catheters), and enterococci. Empiric therapy for early prosthetic valve infective endocarditis includes vancomycin, gentamicin, and rifampin for multidrug-resistant bacteria, particularly coagulase-negative staphylococci. Pathogen-directed therapy is instituted once the microbiologic cause has been identified; recommended regimens are published in a scientific statement developed by the American Heart Association (http://circ.ahajournals.org/cgi/content/full/111/23/e394). Although vancomycin is used to treat methicillin-resistant *Staphylococcus aureus*, it should not be used to treat methicillin-sensitive *S. aureus* (for which a β-lactam agent such as nafcillin or oxacillin is preferred) or penicillin-sensitive streptococci (for which penicillin or ceftriaxone is preferred), unless the patient is unable to tolerate a β-lactam antibiotic. Intravenous antibiotics usually are administered for at least 4 to 6 weeks. Oral antibiotics are not recommended due to unreliable absorption; oral agents are used only when patients refuse parenteral therapy or when parenteral therapy is not possible.

A distinct trend of improved outcomes has been documented with surgical resection of the infected valve in select patients with infective endocarditis. Absolute indications for surgical intervention of native valve infective endocarditis include valvular dysfunction with heart failure or infection refractory to antibiotic therapy. Relative indications include onset of atrioventricular block, extension of infection into perivalvular tissue, fungal endocarditis, relapse after prolonged antibiotic therapy, recurrent emboli despite antibiotic therapy, or persistent fever during empiric antibiotic therapy for culture-negative infective endocarditis. In prosthetic valve endocarditis, relapse after prolonged therapy and the presence of *S. aureus* are indications for surgery.

Follow-Up

Most patients with infective endocarditis will be cured. With the exception of infection with *S. aureus*, fever resolves after 3 to 5 days of antimicrobial therapy. Outpatient treatment can be considered if vital signs are stable, symptoms are improving, and therapy is tolerated. Monitoring for refractory infection, development of heart failure, and antibiotic toxicity is important. An echocardiogram is obtained at the completion of therapy to establish a new baseline, because there is an increased risk for recurrent infective endocarditis. Valve replacement may be required months or years after successful medical therapy. All patients will require antibiotic prophylaxis for certain bacteremia-associated procedures (see Prevention).

Book Enhancement

Go to www.acponline.org/essentials/infectious-disease-section.html. In *MKSAP for Students 5*, assess your knowledge with items 44-48 in the **Infectious Disease Medicine** section.

Bibliography

Murdoch DR, Corey GR, Hoen B, et al. Clinical presentation, etiology, and outcome of infective endocarditis in the 21st century: the International Collaboration on Endocarditis-Prospective Cohort Study. Arch Intern Med. 2009;169:463-473. [PMID: 19273776]

Wilson W, Taubert KA, Gewitz M, et al. Prevention of infective endocarditis. guidelines from the American Heart Association: a guideline from the American Heart Association Rheumatic Fever, Endocarditis, and Kawasaki Disease Committee, Council on Cardiovascular Disease in the Young, and the Council on Clinical Cardiology, Council on Cardiovascular Surgery and Anesthesia, and the Quality of Care and Outcomes Research Interdisciplinary Working Group [published erratum appears in Circulation. 2007;116:e376-e377]. Circulation. 2007;116:1736-54. [PMID: 17446442]

Chapter 59

Osteomyelitis

David C. Tompkins, MD

O steomyelitis is an infection of bone caused by various bacteria and, less commonly, mycobacteria and fungi. Normal bone is highly resistant to infection, and the development of osteomyelitis often requires trauma, the presence of a foreign body, or inoculation with particular pathogens. *Staphylococcus aureus*, for example, expresses several receptors for bone components (fibronectin, laminin, collagen) that allow adherence to bone and the establishment of infection.

Osteomyelitis can be characterized by the duration of illness (acute or chronic), mechanism of infection (hematogenous spread, extension from a contiguous focus, direct contamination), affected bone, physiologic status of the host, and presence of orthopedic hardware. The clinical presentation and treatment vary depending on the type of osteomyelitis.

Hematogenous spread is responsible for <20% of cases of osteomyelitis in adults and occurs in patients at risk for bloodstream infections (including those on hemodialysis with tunneled intravascular catheters and those with long-term intravascular catheters) and in patients with high-grade bacteremia, endocarditis, or sickle cell disease. The intervertebral disk space and two adjacent vertebrae are the most common sites of hematogenous osteomyelitis in adults. Typically, only one microorganism is isolated in patients with hematogenous osteomyelitis; 40% to 60% of cases are caused by *S. aureus.*

Osteomyelitis from contiguous spread of infection is much more common in adults, particularly in persons aged >50 years who have diabetes mellitus or peripheral vascular disease. Patients with osteomyelitis from contiguous spread usually have a polymicrobial infection. Direct contamination of bone exposed by an open fracture or by surgery may lead to osteomyelitis, depending on the degree of contamination and associated soft tissue injury. Table 1 summarizes clinical risk factors and associated pathogens for osteomyelitis.

Prevention

Patients with diabetes or peripheral vascular disease are at increased risk for osteomyelitis, particularly involving the small bones of the feet. These patients should be educated about the importance of meticulous attention to foot care and proper management of minor foot injuries. In addition, patients with diabetes should have a yearly foot examination by a health care provider and custom-made footwear to accommodate foot deformities.

Hematogenous seeding of orthopedic implants can occur following dental and other invasive procedures. The administration of antimicrobial agents before an invasive procedure can reduce the risk of transient bacteremia and seeding of an orthopedic implant. Consider antimicrobial prophylaxis prior to high-risk dental procedures in high-risk patients, such as those who have undergone joint replacement within the previous 2 years or who have a history of prosthetic joint infection. A single dose of antibiotic with activity against streptococci (amoxicillin, cephalexin, cephradine) within 60 minutes of the procedure is recommended for such patients.

Diagnosis

Patients should be assessed for predisposing conditions (diabetes, previous surgery, rheumatoid arthritis, peripheral vascular disease) and risk factors for bacteremia (recent infections, illicit injection

Table 1. Clinical Risk Factors and Associated Bacterial Agents Causing Osteomyelitis

Risk Factor	Possible Organisms
Contiguous infection (e.g., diabetic foot, wound)	Polymicrobial infection; most commonly *S. aureus* and coagulase-negative staphylococci. May also include streptococci, enterococci, gram-negative bacilli (e.g., *Pseudomonas* sp., *Enterobacter* sp., *E. coli, Serratia* sp.) and anaerobes (e.g., *Peptostreptococcus, Clostridium* sp., *Bacteroids fragilis*)
Contaminated open fracture	*Staphylococcus* sp., aerobic gram-negative bacilli (e.g., *Pseudomonas* sp., *Enterobacter* sp., *E. coli, Serratia* sp.)
Dog bite, cat bite	*Pasteurella multocida*
Foot puncture wound (wearing sneakers)	*Pseudomonas aeruginosa*
Hematogenous (e.g., bacteremia)	*Staphylococcus aureus*
Illicit intravenous drug use	Varies in different communities but typically includes *S. aureus* and gram-negative bacilli.
Sickle cell disease	*Salmonella* sp.
Hemodialysis	*Staphylococcus* sp., *P. aeruginosa*

Table 2. Differential Diagnosis of Osteomyelitis

Disorder	Notes
Soft tissue infection	Imaging studies show sparing of the bone. Probe to bone test is negative.
Infectious arthritis (see Chapter 90)	Severe functional limitation and joint swelling often are present. Bone is not infected early in the disease course.
Metastatic malignancy to the bone	Usually associated with a primary lesion (breast, prostate, lung). Metastasis usually is multifocal and tends to remain isolated to one vertebral body, whereas osteomyelitis often crosses the end plate.
Neuropathic arthropathy in diabetes	Radiologic features should be suggestive. Systemic signs and symptoms of infection are absent. May be difficult to distinguish from infection.
Osteoarthritis	Radiologic features should be suggestive. Systemic signs and symptoms of infection are absent. CRP level, ESR, and leukocyte count are normal.

CRP = C-reactive protein; ESR = erythrocyte sedimentation rate.

drug use, long-term intravenous catheters). The clinical hallmarks of osteomyelitis are local pain and fever, particularly in patients with acute hematogenous osteomyelitis; however, these findings may be absent in chronic or contiguous osteomyelitis. Vertebral osteomyelitis often presents as an insidious onset of progressively more severe, dull back pain. The infection can trigger paravertebral muscle spasm, with an associated decrease in mobility of the spine. On examination, there often is tenderness to percussion over the involved vertebral bodies. The presence of a sinus tract (fistula to the skin, draining pus from a deep tissue infection) overlying a bone and the palpation of bone when using a sterile, blunt, stainless steel probe in the depth of a foot ulcer almost always are associated with osteomyelitis. In patients with diabetic foot infections, the presence of visible bone, an ulcer persisting for >2 weeks, and an ulcer >2 cm are correlated with the presence of osteomyelitis. Table 2 summarizes the differential diagnosis of osteomyelitis.

Prosthetic joint infection should be suspected in patients who have had joint pain since surgery. Prosthetic loosening in the first 2 years after arthroplasty should raise suspicion for a prosthetic joint infection.

Various bone imaging techniques can help to establish a diagnosis of osteomyelitis (Table 3). A plain radiograph has a low overall sensitivity but may reveal surrounding soft tissue swelling within the first days to first week of infection. Bone changes such as periosteal elevation, cortical erosion, and reactive sclerosis take several weeks to months to develop. MRI has largely supplanted the technetium 99m bone scan as an aid in the diagnosis of osteomyelitis. The inflammatory process associated with osteomyelitis results in bone marrow edema that can be demonstrated on MRI, often within 1 week of the onset of infection. The absence of bone marrow edema in a patient with symptoms present for longer than 1 to 2 weeks has a high negative predictive value in ruling out osteomyelitis.

Laboratory values typically include a normal leukocyte count. Markers of inflammation, such as elevated erythrocyte sedimentation rate (ESR) and C-reactive protein (CRP) level, can be helpful in supporting the diagnosis and monitoring the response to therapy. The ESR can be normal early in the disease process, becomes markedly elevated in established infections, and takes several months after therapy to normalize. The CRP level often rises

Table 3. Laboratory and Other Studies for Osteomyelitis

Test	Notes
Leukocyte count	Absence of leukocytosis cannot be used as evidence against the diagnosis of infection (sensitivity 26%).
Erythrocyte sedimentation rate and C-reactive protein level	Most sensitive in acute hematogenous osteomyelitis but often normal in early disease (sensitivity 50%-90%).
Sinus tract culture	Correlation is best for Staphylococcus aureus (sensitivity 80%). The association is poor for other microorganisms (sensitivity <40%).
Blood culture	Obtain in patients with fever or systemic signs of sepsis. Less sensitive in chronic osteomyelitis and orthopedic implant–associated osteomyelitis (sensitivity <20%).
Plain bone radiography	Obtain in all patients. Soft tissue swelling and subperiosteal elevation are the earliest abnormalities but may not be seen for several weeks (sensitivity 62%).
Technetium 99m methylene diphosphonate scan	Usefulness is limited by a lack of specificity (sensitivity 70%-100%, specificity 38%-82%).
MRI	MRI is excellent in distinguishing soft tissue infection from osteomyelitis. MRI is more sensitive than plain radiography and allows better identification of optimal areas for needle aspiration or biopsy (sensitivity 91%-95%).
Fluorodeoxyglucose positron emission tomography (PET) scan	PET has the highest diagnostic accuracy of all imaging tests for confirming or excluding the diagnosis of chronic osteomyelitis (sensitivity 69%-100%).
Percutaneous bone biopsy	Not as invasive as an open biopsy. Mainly used in disk space infection or diabetic foot infection (sensitivity 87%).
Surgical bone biopsy	The gold standard for diagnosing osteomyelitis (sensitivity 100%, specificity 100%).

and falls more quickly with the onset of infection and in response to effective therapy.

The choice of antimicrobial therapy is ideally based on identification of the infecting organism(s) and in vitro sensitivities. Blood cultures are obtained when signs and symptoms of infection are present. Superficial cultures obtained from drainage sites often are contaminated with skin flora and correlate poorly with deep cultures. If possible, obtain a bone biopsy (percutaneous or open) for cultures prior to the initiation of antibiotics. Open biopsy facilitates procurement of a larger piece of bone than that obtained through percutaneous biopsy, thereby increasing the diagnostic yield and facilitating debridement of the bone and surrounding tissues, if necessary. Biopsy material should be incubated in anaerobic and aerobic media. Bone biopsy may not be needed for patients with suspected osteomyelitis and a supportive imaging study in the setting of positive blood cultures. Table 3 summarizes laboratory and other studies useful in the diagnosis of osteomyelitis.

Therapy

Surgical debridement usually is warranted in cases of chronic osteomyelitis, contiguous osteomyelitis, and orthopedic implant–associated osteomyelitis. Complete drainage and debridement of all necrotic soft tissue and resection of dead and infected bone is required. Failure to remove an infected orthopedic implant allows the offending microorganisms to form a biofilm and, therefore, escape the effect of antimicrobial agents. In patients with peripheral vascular disease, revascularization is extremely important to allow adequate oxygenation of soft tissues, promote bone healing, and allow access of antibiotics and the host humoral response to the infected area.

Antibiotic treatment typically is begun immediately after appropriate cultures are obtained. Initial intravenous antimicrobial therapy is directed against the most common bacteria responsible for hematogenous osteomyelitis, including S. aureus. Nafcillin, cefazolin, or vancomycin is a reasonable empiric antibiotic. Patients with sickle cell disease have an increased risk for salmonella as well as streptococcal infection; illicit injection drug users are at increased risk for gram-negative infections. For both of these groups, levofloxacin plus nafcillin (or oxacillin) or vancomycin is a reasonable choice for empiric coverage. Surgical intervention should be considered in patients with acute hematogenous osteomyelitis and (1) femoral head involvement, (2) failure to make a specific microbiologic diagnosis with noninvasive techniques, (3) neurologic complications, (4) fragments of dead bone (sequestra), or (4) failure to improve while on appropriate antimicrobial therapy.

Osteomyelitis that complicates diabetic foot infections usually is polymicrobial in nature; initial antimicrobial therapy should target S. aureus, streptococci, enterococci, Enterobacteriaceae organisms, Pseudomonas, and anaerobes. Appropriate empiric antibiotic therapy includes a β-lactam/β-lactamase inhibitor (piperacillin-tazobactam, ampicillin-sulbactam), a carbapenem (imipenem, meropenem), or metronidazole with cefepime, ciprofloxacin, or aztreonam. In patients with diabetes, because of recurrent infections and repeated use of antibiotics, there is an increased risk of methicillin-resistant S. aureus infection, and vancomycin often is included in the initial antibiotic combination pending culture results.

The optimal duration of antibiotic therapy in osteomyelitis is not clear; however, animal models and clinical experience have demonstrated a higher failure rate with a shorter duration of therapy (<4 weeks). Adult patients with uncomplicated acute hematogenous vertebral osteomyelitis are treated with 4 to 6 weeks of antimicrobial therapy.

In patients with chronic osteomyelitis without acute soft tissue infection or sepsis syndrome, withhold antimicrobial therapy until deep bone cultures have been obtained. Patients with chronic or contiguous osteomyelitis usually require a combination of surgical debridement and extended antimicrobial therapy based on culture results. Antimicrobial agents should be administered for 4 to 6 weeks to allow the debrided bone to be covered by vascularized soft tissue and to reduce the high relapse rate.

The duration of antimicrobial therapy in orthopedic implant–associated osteomyelitis is adjusted according to the surgical therapeutic modality. Following removal of all hardware and infected bone, administer 4 to 6 weeks of antimicrobial therapy. Antibiotic-impregnated polymethylmethacrylate can deliver high local levels of antimicrobial agents and sometimes is used at the time of surgical debridement. If removal of a foreign body is not possible (mechanical instability or contraindications to surgery), initial parenteral therapy is followed by prolonged suppression using an oral antimicrobial agent.

Follow-Up

Patients receiving treatment for osteomyelitis require regular follow-up to monitor for drug-related toxicity, vascular access complications, and disease recurrence. A persistently elevated ESR or CRP level despite appropriate antibiotic therapy may reflect the presence of a persistent focus of infection. Interpretation of imaging studies often is difficult, particularly following surgical therapy for osteomyelitis; therefore, follow-up images are not routinely obtained.

Book Enhancement

Go to www.acponline.org/essentials/infectious-disease-section. html. In MKSAP for Students 5, assess your knowledge with items 49-52 in the **Infectious Disease Medicine** section.

Bibliography

Butalia S, Palda VA, Sargeant RJ, Detsky AS, Mourad O. Does this patient with diabetes have osteomyelitis of the lower extremity? JAMA. 2008;299:806-813. [PMID: 18285592]

Chapter 60

Approach to Kidney Disease

John A. Walker, MD

Acute kidney injury (AKI) is defined as an absolute increase in the serum creatinine level of ≥0.3 mg/dL (26.5 μmol/L) over 48 hours, an increase in the serum creatinine level of ≥50%, or urine output <0.5 mL/kg/h for >6 hours. Chronic kidney disease (CKD) is defined by an estimated glomerular filtration rate <60 mL/min/1.73 m² or kidney damage (abnormal findings on urinalysis, kidney imaging, or kidney biopsy) of at least 3 months' duration. The two key components of the laboratory assessment of kidney function are a determination of the glomerular filtration rate (GFR) and a quantitative and qualitative analysis of the urine.

Determination of Glomerular Filtration Rate

The GFR may be estimated (eGFR) by the serum concentration of certain endogenous solutes or measured (mGFR) by the clearance of endogenous or exogenous filtration markers.

Azotemia is defined as an increased concentration of blood urea nitrogen (BUN) and is an important indicator of a reduced GFR. BUN often is measured simultaneously with serum creatinine. The normal BUN-creatinine ratio ranges from 10:1 to 15:1. BUN is a relatively poor indicator of eGFR. Although urea is freely filtered at the glomerulus, it also undergoes tubular reabsorption. Urea reabsorption is increased in states of decreased kidney perfusion. Therefore, prerenal conditions (e.g., dehydration, heart failure) are associated with a disproportionate increase in the BUN-creatinine ratio, typically to 20:1 or higher; other causes of an elevated BUN include a high-protein diet, catabolic states, and gastrointestinal bleeding. Causes of a reduced BUN include liver failure and malnutrition.

Creatinine is generated by muscle at a relatively constant rate in proportion to muscle mass and is excreted by the kidneys. Because serum creatinine level increases as GFR falls, creatinine level is used to evaluate kidney function. However, serum creatinine level is not an ideal marker for GFR for several reasons. A large change in GFR initially is required to raise serum creatinine levels significantly; in CKD, GFR may decrease as much as 50% before the serum creatinine level rises above the upper limit of normal. A reduction in muscle mass may cause a low serum creatinine level, which may result in an overestimation of GFR. Although freely filtered, creatinine also is excreted via tubular secretion; in CKD, tubular secretion of creatinine may account for as much as 50% of total creatinine excretion and, thus, lead to an overestimation of the true GFR.

Two estimating equations may provide more accurate quantitative information about kidney function. The Cockcroft-Gault equation predicts creatinine clearance as:

$$C_{Cr} = \frac{(140 - age\,[y]) \times (weight\,[kg])}{S_{Cr} \times 72} \, (\times 0.85 \text{ if female})$$

The Modification of Diet in Renal Disease (MDRD) equation provides the most reliable estimation of GFR in patients with moderate to severe CKD. The MDRD equation requires input of a patient's serum creatinine measurement, age, gender, and race (African-American versus all others). Although the equation is operationally complex, it is available for online calculation (www.kidney.org/professionals/kdoqi/gfr_calculator.cfm). Many laboratories provide an MDRD-derived eGFR when reporting serum creatinine concentration. The Cockcroft-Gault and MDRD equations are valid only when the serum creatinine concentration is at steady state; the equations should not be used in patients with AKI, as the serum creatinine concentration changes rapidly in AKI. The MDRD equation underestimates GFR when the true GFR is ≥60 mL/min/1.73 m², so its use should be restricted to those patients with stage 3 or higher CKD.

A more accurate estimate of GFR (eGFR) may be obtained by a urinary clearance study or by various radionuclide scanning techniques. Creatinine is the endogenous solute most commonly measured in urinary clearance studies, but tubular secretion of creatinine may yield clearance values that exceed the true GFR. Moreover, urinary clearance studies require an accurate, timed urine collection (usually of 24 hours' duration); over- or under-collection of the urine sample will result in an inaccurate clearance calculation. Radionuclide kidney clearance scanning is the gold standard for the estimation of GFR in healthy persons and in those with AKI.

Urinalysis by Multi-reagent Dipstick

Urine pH may range between 4.5 and 8.0. Measurement of urine pH is useful when evaluating patients with suspected renal tubular disorders, where renal acid excretion may be impaired and the urine pH may be inappropriately high in the face of a systemic acidosis (e.g., renal tubular acidosis).

Specific gravity quantifies the density of a solution. Urine specific gravity ranges between 1.003 and 1.035. Excretion of urine with a persistently low specific gravity (<1.007) is called *hyposthenuria* and may indicate a loss of concentrating ability (e.g., diabetes insipidus). High urine specific gravity may reflect an appropriate response to water loss/dehydration or may indicate a pathologic state of fluid retention (e.g., heart failure). Excretion of urine with a specific gravity fixed at about 1.010 regardless of the state of hydration is known as *isosthenuria* and usually accompanies severe kidney damage involving disruption of both concentrating and diluting abilities.

Glycosuria occurs when the filtered load of glucose exceeds the reabsorptive capacity of sodium-glucose cotransporters in the proximal tubule. Glycosuria usually is detected by dipstick when blood glucose levels exceed approximately 200 mg/dL (11.1 mmol/L) and is seen most often in diabetes mellitus. Glycosuria without hyperglycemia usually is associated with proximal renal tubular dysfunction (e.g., Fanconi syndrome, multiple myeloma).

Albumin is the only protein reliably detected by dipstick. The detection of proteinuria implies an albumin excretion rate of ≥300 mg/24 h. However, the detection of microalbuminuria (albumin excretion rate of 30-300 mg/24 h) requires other quantitative methods. The dipstick protein indicator is insensitive to tubular proteins and immunoglobulins; identification of the latter (e.g., Bence-Jones proteins secondary to multiple myeloma) is best accomplished by a 24-hour urine collection for total protein with protein electrophoresis and immunofixation.

The dipstick indicator is sensitive to intact erythrocytes but will also yield a positive reaction in the setting of hemoglobinuria or myoglobinuria. If fewer than 3 erythrocytes per high-power field are reported for a urine sample that tests positive for blood, evidence for hemolysis or rhabdomyolysis should be sought.

Lysed neutrophils and macrophages release indoxyl esterase, which can be detected by multi-reagent dipstick technology (leukocyte esterase–positive). A positive reaction for urine nitrite may indicate the presence of bacteria that reduce nitrate, most commonly gram-negative pathogens. A positive result for both urine leukocyte esterase and urine nitrites is 68% to 88% sensitive for urinary tract infection, whereas a negative result for both assays has a high negative predictive value for urinary tract infection.

Microscopic Examination of the Urine Sediment

A freshly voided sample should be viewed, as urine elements begin to lyse within 2 to 4 hours of urine collection. Among the most useful findings are casts; these cylindrical structures are composed of a Tamm-Horsfall glycoprotein matrix, within which cells (erythrocytes, leukocytes, epithelial cells) may be trapped. Casts are formed only within the tubules. Thus, any cell contained within a cast is of renal parenchymal origin.

Microscopic hematuria is defined as the presence of ≥3 erythrocytes per high-power field. In patients with microscopic hematuria, the location of bleeding (glomerular or nonglomerular) should be identified to guide further diagnostic studies. Erythrocyte casts are specific for glomerular bleeding, but the sensitivity for glomerular pathology is poor (Plate 50). Glomerular hematuria also is characterized by the presence of dysmorphic erythrocytes (often recognized as erythrocyte blebs or budding), resulting in erythrocytes of variable shape and size. Transient glomerular bleeding has been noted in normal individuals after vigorous physical activity. However, the combination of microscopic hematuria and proteinuria signifies glomerular disease. Nonglomerular bleeding is suggested by the presence of isomorphic, normal-appearing erythrocytes and the absence of proteinuria. Figure 1 outlines a suggested approach to evaluation of a patient with microscopic hematuria.

Up to 3 leukocytes per high-power field may be seen in normal urine. Greater numbers define pyuria, most often caused by a urinary tract infection. Pyuria in the face of a negative urine culture may reflect a viral or mycobacterial infection. However, sterile pyuria also may indicate interstitial nephritis, where the presence of leukocyte casts establishes the renal parenchymal disease and usually is associated with non-nephrotic proteinuria (Plate 51). Eosinophils may be seen in the urine of patients with AKI due to drug-induced interstitial nephritis and in a variety of other conditions, including rapidly progressive glomerulonephritis, prostatitis, renal atheroemboli, and small-vessel vasculitis.

Renal tubular epithelial cell casts may be produced by desquamation of epithelial cells associated with acute tubular necrosis, proliferative glomerulonephritis, or interstitial nephritis. The broad, muddy brown casts associated with acute tubular necrosis are diagnostically helpful (Plate 52). Hyaline casts are composed of Tamm-Horsfall glycoprotein secreted by the epithelial cells of the thick ascending limb of Henle. Hyaline casts normally may be seen in increased numbers in concentrated urine specimens. Granular casts are hyaline casts containing aggregated filtered proteins and may be seen in patients with albuminuria and nephritic-range proteinuria. Degenerated cellular casts may appear granular and upon further degeneration are described as *waxy casts*.

Lipiduria is associated with various glomerular diseases and usually is accompanied by heavy proteinuria. Lipids may be seen within tubular epithelial cells or macrophages. Lipids embedded within hyaline casts form fatty casts. When viewed under polarized light, lipid particles in the urine display a Maltese cross pattern.

Measurement of Urine Albumin and Total Protein Excretion

An increase in urine albumin excretion often is the earliest sign of glomerular injury. Screening for microalbuminuria is recommended for individuals with risk factors for kidney disease (e.g., diabetes, hypertension). Microalbuminuria may be identified and quantified via a urine albumin-creatinine ratio on a single voided specimen or a timed 24-hour urine collection. Microalbuminuria is defined as a urine albumin excretion rate of 30-300 mg/24 h (30-300 mg/g on a spot urine albumin-creatinine ratio). The urine total protein-creatinine ratio is preferable to a 24-hour urine collection because of the inconvenience and difficulties in properly collecting a 24-hour urine specimen. A urine protein-creatinine ratio >0.2 mg/mg and <2 mg/mg is associated with chronic tubulointerstitial, renovascular, and glomerular disease; a ratio >3.5 mg/mg is classified as nephritic-range proteinuria.

Electrophoresis can identify the types and relative quantities of urine proteins and may assist in distinguishing glomerular from tubulointerstitial disease. In proteinuria of glomerular origin, albumin constitutes 60% to 90% of the total urine protein. In tubular proteinuria, low-molecular-weight proteins typically predominate, and this may indicate either impaired tubular uptake or overpro-

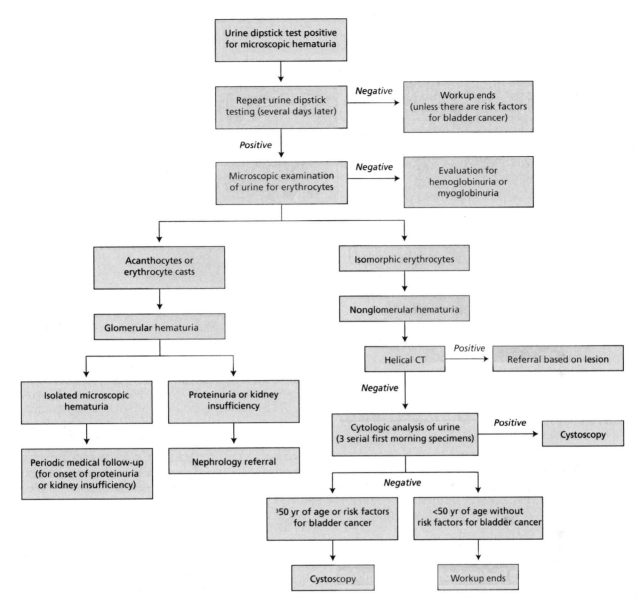

Figure 1. Evaluation of microscopic hematuria. If hematuria is determined to be nonglomerular in origin and a kidney stone is suspected, CT should be performed without contrast or first without and then with contrast. Ultrasonography should be performed instead of CT in pregnant patients and in patients with hypersensitivity to contrast. Risk factors for bladder cancer include cigarette smoking, occupational exposure to chemicals used in certain industries (e.g., leather, dye, rubber, and tire manufacturing), heavy phenacetin use, past treatment with high-dose cyclophosphamide, and ingestion of aristolochic acid found in some herbal weight-loss preparations. Modified with permission from Cohen RA, Brown RS. Clinical practice. Microscopic hematuria. N Engl J Med. 2003;348:2330-2338. [PMID: 12788998] Copyright © 2003, Massachusetts Medical Society.

duction and filtration of low-molecular-weight proteins (e.g., multiple myeloma).

Proteinuria does not always indicate significant kidney disease. Isolated or transient proteinuria (usually <1 g/24 h) may be associated with febrile illness or heavy exercise. This condition typically is benign and does not warrant further evaluation.

Orthostatic proteinuria refers to protein excretion that increases during the day but decreases to a normal value (<50 mg/8 h) during recumbency. The diagnosis is established by comparing the urine protein excretion rate during the day with that from a separate urine collection obtained during the night.

Nephrotic and Nephritic Syndromes

Glomerular disease can produce clinical patterns of kidney disease classified as either the nephrotic syndrome or the nephritic syndrome. Recognition of these syndromes can be helpful in the creation of a differential diagnosis for patients with kidney disease. Some patients have characteristics of both syndromes.

The nephrotic syndrome is characterized by heavy proteinuria (>2+ protein by dipstick, urine protein-creatinine ratio >3.5 mg/mg) and a relatively bland urine sediment, which may contain hyaline or hyaline-granular casts, lipids, and none to moderate numbers of per erythrocytes. The nephrotic syndrome may manifest as a primary kidney disease or occur secondary to a systemic disease. Primary nephrotic syndrome usually is diagnosed when a secondary cause for the nephrotic syndrome has not been identified. Common causes of primary nephrotic syndrome include minimal change disease, membranous glomerulopathy, and focal segmental glomerulosclerosis. Diabetes is the most common cause of secondary nephrotic syndrome (diabetic nephropathy). Other causes include dysproteinemia (glomerulopathy due to amyloidosis and multiple myeloma), HIV infection (focal segmental glomerulosclerosis), and hepatitis B (membranous glomerulopathy).

The nephritic syndrome is characterized by varying degrees of proteinuria and an active urine sediment, which may contain granular casts, moderate to large numbers of dysmorphic erythrocytes, and erythrocyte casts. Some patients with the nephritic syndrome have dermal inflammation that manifests as palpable purpura, necrosis, ulcers, or nodules. These patients may have renal-dermal syndromes, such as systemic lupus erythematosus, Henoch-Schönlein purpura, antineutrophil cytoplasmic antibody (ANCA)-associated vasculitis, and cryoglobulinemia. Pulmonary-renal syndrome also may develop in patients with the nephritic syndrome. Assays for anti–glomerular basement membrane antibody, ANCA, and markers for immune complex diseases (e.g., antinuclear antibodies, anti–double-stranded DNA antibodies, cryoglobulins, antibodies to hepatitis B or C virus, complement levels) may further refine the diagnosis; low complement levels suggest lupus nephritis, postinfectious and membranoproliferative glomerulonephritis, and mixed cryoglobulinemia. Rapidly progressive glomerulonephritis is a clinical syndrome characterized by swift loss of kidney function, hematuria, proteinuria, and glomerular crescent formation. The syndrome may be idiopathic or caused by many primary or secondary glomerular diseases, including those previously listed.

Imaging Studies

Assessment of kidney function often requires imaging of the urinary tract (Table 1). Because kidney ultrasonography is noninvasive and does not require the administration of contrast agents or radiation exposure, it is the imaging modality of choice in the initial diagnostic evaluation of most patients with kidney disease. Ultrasonography can identify simple and complex cysts, solid masses, and kidney stones; it also provides a reasonably reproducible estimate of kidney size and will reveal the uncommon patient with a solitary kidney. Ultrasonography detects hydronephrosis with high sensitivity.

Kidney function should be evaluated prior to determining the most appropriate radiographic study. This evaluation is particularly important before performing studies that require use of radiocontrast agents, to avoid contrast-induced nephropathy. Patients with AKI or with CKD (eGFR <60 mL/min/1.73 m^2) are at increased risk for contrast toxicity. Recently, the incidence of

Table 1. Use of Radiographic Imaging Studies in the Assessment of Kidney Function and Kidney Disease

Imaging Study	Indications
Kidney ultrasonography	Urinary tract obstruction, nephrolithiasis, cyst, mass lesion, location for kidney biopsy
Duplex ultrasonography, angiography	Renal artery stenosis
Abdominal CT	Urinary tract obstruction, nephrolithiasis, mass lesion
CT angiography	Renal artery stenosis, renal vascular lesion
MRI	Cyst, mass lesion, renal artery stenosis
Radionuclide kidney clearance scanning (GFR scanning)	GFR estimation, urinary tract obstruction, kidney infarction

GFR = glomerular filtration rate.

nephrogenic systemic fibrosis (formerly known as nephrogenic fibrosing dermopathy) has increased in patients with reduced kidney function who are exposed to intravenous gadolinium contrast agents during MRI. Although several measures (e.g., isotonic intravenous hydration, use of low-osmolality or iso-osmolality contrast) appear to have value in preventing iodinated radiocontrast-related kidney injury, no proven regimen currently exists for preventing or treating gadolinium-related nephrogenic systemic fibrosis; therefore, patients with CKD should avoid MRI procedures with gadolinium. Optimal selection of additional imaging modalities often is best informed by consultation with an experienced diagnostic or interventional radiologist.

Kidney Biopsy

Kidney biopsy is performed when histologic confirmation is needed to help diagnose kidney disease, implement medical therapy, or change medical treatment. Kidney biopsy is used predominantly to diagnose and categorize glomerular disease. The most common indications for kidney biopsy include the nephrotic syndrome, acute glomerulonephritis, AKI of uncertain etiology, and kidney transplant dysfunction.

Book Enhancement

Go to www.acponline.org/essentials/nephrology-section.html. In *MKSAP for Students 5*, assess your knowledge with items 1-4 in the **Nephrology** section.

Bibliography

Fogazzi GB, Verdesca S, Garigali G. Urinalysis: core curriculum 2008. Am J Kidney Dis. 2008;51:1052-1067. [PMID: 18501787]

Rosner MH, Bolton WK. Renal function testing. Am J Kidney Dis. 2006;47:174-183. [PMID: 16377400]

Chapter 61

Acute Kidney Injury

Harold M. Szerlip, MD

To better reflect the range of structural and functional changes that occur during acute injury to the kidney, the term *acute kidney injury* (AKI) is preferred over the older term *acute renal failure*. AKI is defined as an abrupt increase in the serum creatinine concentration or decrease in urine output. AKI can be divided into three stages (Table 1). AKI may occur secondary to decreased perfusion from prerenal causes; intrarenal injury due to ischemia, toxins, tubular obstruction, immunologic events, or allergic reactions; or postrenal obstruction of urine outflow (Figure 1). Because renal hypoperfusion and urinary outflow obstruction both can lead to renal parenchymal injury, it is paramount to promptly diagnose and correct these disorders.

Blood perfusing the corticomedullary portion of the kidney has a low oxygen content. As a result, those parts of the nephron that reside within this area (i.e., the straight segment of the proximal tubule and the ascending loop of Henle) function under near-hypoxic conditions. In addition, these tubular segments use large amounts of energy-reabsorbing sodium. Insults that result in decreased renal perfusion or toxins that interfere with tubular cell energetics will cause oxygen demand to exceed oxygen delivery. The resultant ischemia and subsequent reperfusion activate cellular processes that cause tubular cell apoptosis and necrosis. The loss of polarity of the tubular epithelial cells interferes with the vectorial transport of electrolytes out of the lumen back into the renal interstitium. The sloughing of these cells into the tubular lumen causes obstruction.

Prevention

An increase in serum creatinine concentration of as little as 0.3 mg/dL (26.5 μmol/L) is associated with an increase in morbidity and mortality; therefore, it is important to prevent AKI from developing. This is best accomplished by identifying patients who are at risk. AKI is most likely to occur in patients who already have decreased renal function or whose intravascular volume is depleted. Patients with hypertension or diabetes mellitus and elderly patients are especially at risk. The use of NSAIDs, which can compromise renal hemodynamics, also places patients at risk. Routinely estimate glomerular filtration rate (GFR) in patients at risk for AKI. Serum creatinine concentration alone is a poor indicator of renal function. Validated equations for estimating GFR are available and are easy to use (see Chapter 61). These equations are more precise and more convenient than 24-hour urine collections. A GFR <60 mL/min/1.73 m² represents significant renal dysfunction.

In at-risk individuals, if possible, avoid the use of nephrotoxins (e.g., iodinated contrast, aminoglycoside antibiotics) and stop NSAIDs. In high-risk patients requiring imaging with contrast, use the smallest possible dose of a low-osmolality or iso-osmolality contrast agent and treat with isotonic saline or bicarbonate prior to and immediately after the procedure. The use of *N*-acetylcysteine also may be beneficial. All patients at high risk for AKI and any patient requiring a nephrotoxic drug should have an estimated GFR calculated. When prescribing aminoglycosides, consider once-daily dosing, or follow peak and trough levels and discontinue the medications as early as possible. Avoid overdiuresis in patients with heart failure, the nephrotic syndrome, or cirrhosis. Patients who rely on an activated renin-angiotensin axis to maintain glomerular filtration are especially prone to develop AKI when ACE inhibitors or angiotensin II receptor blockers (ARBs) are added. This includes patients who are volume depleted from overdiuresis; patients with decompensated heart failure, hepatic dysfunction, chronic kidney disease, or renal artery stenosis; and patients who are using NSAIDs. In high-risk patients with poor oral intake or excessive fluid loss (e.g., diarrhea, vomiting, burns), maintain intravascular volume using intravenous fluids.

Diagnosis

The diagnosis of AKI is made when there is an abrupt increase in serum creatinine concentration or decrease in urine volume (Table 1). After establishing the presence of AKI, it is essential to determine the cause. Intrinsic AKI is divided into oliguric (≤400 mL/24 h) and nonoliguric (>400 mL/24 h) forms; the lower the urine output, the worse is the prognosis. Prerenal and postrenal causes of AKI often are rapidly reversible and, thus, must be distinguished from intrinsic renal parenchymal disease (Table 2).

Table 1. Stages of Acute Kidney Injury (AKI)

Stage	Serum Creatinine Criteria	Urine Output Criteria
1 (risk)	Increase of ≥150%-200%	<0.5 mL/kg/h for >6 h
2 (injury)	Increase of ≥200%-300%	<0.5 mL/kg/h for >12 h
3 (failure)	Increase of >300% or >4 mg/dL (353.6 μmol/L) with acute increase ≥0.3 mg/dL (26.5 μmol/L)	<0.5 mL/kg/h for >24 h or anuria for 12 h

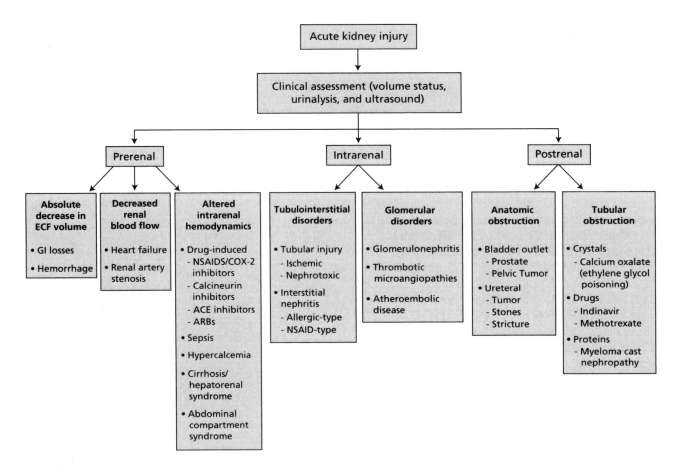

Figure 1. Approach to acute kidney injury. ARBs = angiotensin receptor blockers; COX-2 = cyclooxygenase-2; ECF = extracellular fluid; GI = gastrointestinal.

Prerenal

Important historical clues to prerenal causes of AKI include a history of volume loss (e.g., vomiting, diarrhea), the presence of orthostatic symptoms, decreased urine volume, or urine that appears more concentrated. After abdominal surgery, patients may sequester large amounts of fluid within tissues and have reduced effective circulating volume. Look for a history of heart failure, liver disease, and the nephrotic syndrome, which are other conditions associated with decreased effective circulating volume. For hospitalized patients, review blood pressure records for evidence of prolonged hypotension, particularly in surgical patients. Obtain a complete list of all medications that can alter effective circulating volume, such as NSAIDs, ACE inhibitors, ARBs, diuretics, and vasodilators. An extreme form of prerenal failure is hepatorenal syndrome. This syndrome is seen in patients with acute liver failure or decompensated liver disease. Renal vasoconstriction is severe and cannot be reversed by intravascular volume repletion.

On physical examination, look for signs of hypovolemia, such as tachycardia, a postural pulse rate increase of >30/min, dry axillae, flat neck veins, and dry oral mucosa. Decreased renal perfusion due to decreased effective circulating volume is associated with heart failure; look for elevated jugular venous pressure, an S₃ gallop, and pulmonary crackles on lung examination. Spider

telangiectasia, jaundice, and ascites support a diagnosis of liver disease. Increases in intra-abdominal pressure from massive ascites or edematous bowel can lead to abdominal compartment syndrome, which limits both renal arterial perfusion and renal venous outflow. A distended tense abdomen supports a diagnosis of abdominal compartment syndrome, which can be confirmed by placing a pressure transducer into the bladder.

Postrenal

Postrenal causes of AKI are most common in elderly men with prostatic hypertrophy, children with a history of congenital urinary tract abnormalities, and patients with a history of pelvic malignancy. Other causes include renal stone disease, particularly in patients with a solitary kidney, and neuropathic conditions affecting bladder emptying (e.g., diabetic neuropathy). Historical clues may include difficulty passing urine, lower abdominal or flank pain, dysuria, or hematuria. Prostatic enlargement, suprapubic fullness, or an abdominal or pelvic mass suggests urinary obstruction.

Renal Parenchymal

Renal parenchymal disease is divided into processes that affect the tubules (acute tubular necrosis [ATN]), the interstitium (intersti-

Table 2. Differential Diagnosis of Acute Kidney Injury (AKI)

Disorder	Notes
Prerenal	Characterized by BUN-creatinine ratio >15:1, urine sodium <10 meq/L (10 mmol/L) or FENa <1%, bland urine sediment, and urine specific gravity >1.018. Consider volume depletion, cirrhosis (including HRS), heart failure, sepsis, or impaired renal autoregulation.
Renal parenchymal	
Atheroembolic and thromboembolic disease	Atheroembolic disease characterized by urinary eosinophils; associated with recent manipulation of the aorta. May be associated with livedo reticularis or blue toe syndrome. Atrial fibrillation or recent myocardial infarction may be associated with thromboembolic disease.
Intrarenal vascular disease	Characterized by hematuria with erythrocyte or granular casts, mild proteinuria, and leukocytes. Consider vasculitis (i.e., PAN), malignant hypertension, or TTP-HUS.
Acute glomerulonephritis	Characterized by hematuria with erythrocyte casts, mild or nephritic-range proteinuria, and FENa >1%. Consider SLE, IgA nephropathy, postinfectious glomerulonephritis, anti-GBM antibody disease, or Wegener granulomatosis.
Acute tubular necrosis (ATN)	Characterized by muddy brown casts, tubular epithelial cell casts, and FENa >1%. Consider radiocontrast agents, drugs (aminoglycosides, amphotericin B), and episodes of hypotension. Aside from prerenal AKI, ATN is the most common cause of AKI in the hospital setting.
Acute interstitial nephritis	Characterized by pyuria, leukocyte casts, urine eosinophils, and nephritic-range proteinuria (in the case of drug- or NSAID-induced minimal change disease). Associated with medication use (methicillin, NSAIDs, but can include nearly any drug) and rash. Discontinue any unnecessary or suspicious medications.
Intrarenal tubular obstruction	Characterized by coarse tubular casts (including muddy brown granular casts), crystalluria, and urinary light chains. Consider rhabdomyolysis, tumor lysis syndrome, or multiple myeloma.
Renal vein obstruction	Characterized by hematuria and nephritic-range proteinuria. Consider nephrotic syndrome (membranous nephropathy), clotting disorder, malignancy, trauma, or compression.
Postrenal (urinary tract obstruction)	Characterized by micro- or macroscopic hematuria, bacteriuria, pyuria, and crystal deposition; urinalysis also may be normal. Consider nephrolithiasis, malignancy, granuloma, pregnancy, hematoma, radiation, neurogenic bladder, benign prostatic hypertrophy, or retroperitoneal fibrosis.

BUN = blood urea nitrogen; FENa = fractional excretion of sodium; GBM = glomerular basement membrane; HRS = hepatorenal syndrome; PAN = polyarteritis nodosa; SLE = systemic lupus erythematosus; TTP-HUS = thrombotic thrombocytopenic purpura–hemolytic uremic syndrome.

tial nephritis), the glomeruli (glomerulonephritis), or the vasculature (vasculitis, microangiopathic hemolytic anemia). The most common cause of ATN is sepsis. Also look for possible renal toxins (e.g., aminoglycosides, amphotericin B, cisplatin, intravenous contrast), and review all medications including over-the-counter preparations, herbal remedies, and illicit drugs for potential renal toxicities. Patients who are using cocaine or who are found comatose from drug ingestion may develop rhabdomyolysis, which results in release of myoglobin, a renal tubular toxin.

Renal tubular obstruction and AKI can occur in patients with lymphoma or leukemia who develop tumor lysis following chemotherapy; these patients will have significantly elevated serum and urine uric acid concentrations. In patients with multiple myeloma, immunoglobulin light chains can precipitate within the renal tubules. The antiviral drugs acyclovir and indinavir and sulfonamide antibiotics also can precipitate within the renal tubules and cause obstruction.

Inquire about recent invasive vascular procedures that may result in atheroembolic kidney disease (e.g., angiography, aortic stenting, aneurysm repair). Clues to vasculitis include palpable purpura (Plate 31), petechiae, joint swelling, and skin rashes. The presence of a fine, reticular (net-like) red to purple rash (livedo reticularis) or blue toes ("blue toe syndrome") suggests atheroembolic disease (Plate 53). Underlying collagen vascular disease or chronic infection (e.g., hepatitis B) may be associated with glomerular disease; ask about fever, joint pain, fatigue, rashes, or jaundice.

Diagnostic Studies

Examine the urine for casts, cells, and crystals (Table 3). Muddy brown granular casts (Plate 52) are consistent with renal injury secondary to tubular necrosis; erythrocyte casts (Plate 50) and proteinuria of >3 g/day are pathognomonic for glomerular disease; and leukocytes, leukocyte casts, and, rarely, eosinophils are associated with acute interstitial nephritis (Plate 51). Prerenal disease is associated with a normal urinalysis. Blood on urine dipstick analysis without erythrocytes detected on microscopic examination suggests the presence of myoglobin and supports a diagnosis of rhabdomyolysis; obtain a serum creatine phosphokinase concentration to confirm the diagnosis.

In all patients with AKI, routinely measure BUN and serum electrolyte, creatinine, calcium, phosphorous, uric acid, glucose, and albumin concentrations and obtain a complete blood count with differential. Routinely measure urine sodium and creatinine concentrations and urine osmolality. Low urine flow is associated with reabsorption of urea along the nephron, and patients with prerenal failure frequently have a BUN-creatinine ratio >20:1. Volume depletion leads to activation of hormonal systems aimed at conserving salt and water and is characterized by high urine osmolality and low urine sodium concentration (<10 meq/L [10 mmol/L]) with a fractional excretion of sodium of <1%. Acute glomerular disease can produce the same findings but is also associated with proteinuria, microscopic hematuria, and erythrocyte casts in the urine.

Table 3. Laboratory and Other Studies for Acute Kidney Injury (AKI)

Test	Notes
Urinalysis with microscopic examination	Significant proteinuria suggests glomerular disease. Dipstick hematuria without erythrocytes suggests rhabdomyolysis. Dysmorphic erythrocytes suggest acute glomerulonephritis.
BUN-creatinine ratio	BUN-creatinine ratio >20:1 suggests prerenal azotemia.
Fractional excretion of sodium (FENa)	FENa >1 suggests ATN. FENa ≤1 suggests prerenal azotemia (when oliguria is present) and AGN.
Spot urine sodium	Urine sodium <10 meq/L (10 mmol/L) suggests prerenal azotemia.
Serum phosphorus	Severe hyperphosphatemia suggests acute rhabdomyolysis or tumor lysis syndrome.
Serum calcium	Hypercalcemia can cause AKI via several mechanisms.
Serum uric acid	Serum uric acid >15 mg/dL (0.9 mmol/L) suggests rhabdomyolysis or tumor lysis syndrome.
Antinuclear antibody (ANA)	Indicated in acute nephritis or systemic disease (SLE).
Antineutrophil cytoplasmic antibody (ANCA)	c-ANCA (cytoplasmic ANCA) is more specific for Wegener granulomatosis. p-ANCA (perinuclear ANCA) is specific for microscopic polyangiitis or pauci-immune glomerulonephritis.
Anti–glomerular basement membrane antibody	Positive in 90% of patients with Goodpasture syndrome.
Complete blood count	Anemia can occur with severe AKI; decreased platelets suggest HUS-TTP.
Complement (C3) level	C3 level is decreased in 60%-70% of patients with type I or type II MPGN.
Cryoglobulins	Especially indicated for AKI in the setting of hepatitis C.
Anti–double-stranded DNA antibody	Sensitivity of 75% for SLE.
Hepatitis serology	AGN, hepatorenal syndrome.
Renal biopsy	Biopsy is indicated when there is evidence of intrinsic renal disease and results will affect management or clarify diagnosis.
Serum and urine protein electrophoresis	Obtain in the setting of AKI, anemia, or hypercalcemia, especially in patients aged >60 y or when serum anion gap is low to diagnose multiple myeloma.
Urine eosinophils	Suggest acute interstitial nephritis or atheroembolic disease.
Renal ultrasonography	Sensitivity of 93%-98% for acute obstruction.

AGN = acute glomerulonephritis; ATN = acute tubular necrosis; MPGN = mesangioproliferative glomerulonephritis; SLE = systemic lupus erythematosus; TTP-HUS = thrombotic thrombocytopenic purpura–hemolytic uremic syndrome.

If the history and physical examination suggest an underlying thrombotic or vasculitic process or the urinalysis shows erythrocytes, erythrocyte casts, or proteinuria suggesting glomerular disease, obtain assays for antinuclear antibodies, cytoplasmic and perinuclear antineutrophil cytoplasmic antibodies, anti–glomerular basement membrane antibody, hepatitis B surface antigen, hepatitis C antibodies, complement levels, and anti–double-stranded DNA antibodies. Look for schistocytes and decreased platelets on peripheral smear, which imply a thrombotic microangiopathy, such as hemolytic uremic syndrome or thrombotic thrombocytopenia purpura. If present, confirm hemolysis with serum lactate dehydrogenase and haptoglobin concentrations.

The first imaging test of choice is renal ultrasonography, which can show hydronephrosis from obstruction and demonstrate increased echogenicity or loss of size associated with chronic kidney disease. A renal biopsy will diagnose acute glomerulonephritis and should be performed in patients with normal-appearing kidneys on renal imaging who do not improve with conservative therapy.

Therapy

In patients with prerenal and postrenal causes of AKI, therapy is aimed at increasing renal perfusion and relieving obstruction.

Treat volume depletion with normal saline; if severe anemia is present, transfuse packed red blood cells. If the serum albumin level is extremely low, or if a patient has portal hypertension and ascites, albumin may be beneficial as a volume expander. Discontinue all drugs that decrease renal perfusion (e.g., NSAIDs) and stop all diuretics in volume-depleted patients. Reduce the dose of ACE inhibitors and ARBs or discontinue these mediations if the serum creatinine level increases >50%. If there is evidence of urinary obstruction, place a urinary catheter to relieve bladder outlet obstruction; if the obstruction is above the bladder, either retrograde or antegrade nephrostomy will be necessary.

For patients with suspected renal parenchymal disease, discontinue all nephrotoxins (e.g., aminoglycosides, cisplatin, amphotericin B) unless absolutely necessary. In patients with rhabdomyolysis, intravenous normal saline may prevent renal toxicity from myoglobin. Whenever possible, identify and specifically treat the underlying cause of AKI. This may include treating collagen vascular diseases, vasculitides, or pulmonary-renal syndromes (e.g., Goodpasture syndrome, Wegener granulomatosis) with cytotoxic and immunosuppressant drugs and, depending on the disease, plasmapheresis. Increases in abdominal pressure can be reduced by therapeutic paracentesis or even surgical decompression.

Most complications associated with AKI can be managed with dialysis; however, in patients who do not yet require dialysis or when dialysis is not promptly available, drug therapy is required. The treatment of metabolic acidosis is controversial, but many experts use sodium bicarbonate when the pH is <7.0. Immediately treat hyperkalemia with electrocardiographic changes (i.e., peaking of T waves, lengthening of the PR and QRS intervals) with intravenous calcium gluconate to stabilize the myocardium. Shift potassium from the extracellular to the intracellular space with intravenous regular insulin and glucose; inhaled nebulized albuterol may be added if necessary. In patients with underlying metabolic acidosis, intravenous administration of sodium bicarbonate will also shift potassium into cells. These short-term measures must be followed by removal of potassium from the body. If the patient has a normal intravascular volume and is making urine, administration of a loop diuretic will help with potassium excretion; otherwise, give a cation-exchange resin (sodium polystyrene sulfonate in sorbitol) by mouth. Initiate emergency hemodialysis if these measures are not successful in reducing the serum potassium level. In patients who develop hyperphosphatemia, begin phosphate binders, such as calcium carbonate, calcium acetate, aluminum hydroxide, lanthanum carbonate, or sevelamer hydrochloride.

Avoid overly aggressive treatment of hypertension. In patients with extremely elevated blood pressure, use intravenous nitroglycerine, labetalol, fenoldopam, nicardipine or clevidipine to lower the mean arterial blood pressure by 10% to 15%. If there is evidence of volume overload, use loop diuretics. Avoid the use of ACE inhibitors or ARBs. When initiating or switching to oral medications for blood pressure control, use short-acting β-blockers (e.g., metoprolol), calcium channel blockers, centrally acting α-blockers, or vasodilators (e.g., hydralazine).

Adjust the dose of all medications that are excreted by the kidney. In patients with a rising serum creatinine level, assume a GFR <10 mL/min; GFR cannot be measured in non–steady state conditions using any formulas. Confirm correct drug dosages by measuring drug levels if possible. Avoid drugs that have no proven benefit for the prevention or treatment of AKI, including loop diuretics, (unless clinically volume overloaded, mannitol, and dopamine).

Begin renal replacement therapy (dialysis) in all patients with uremic signs or symptoms (nausea, vomiting, change in mental status, seizures, pericarditis) as well as patients who have hyperkalemia, metabolic acidosis, or volume overload that cannot be easily managed with medication. In patients who are critically ill and oliguric as well as nonoliguric patients whose serum creatinine level continues to rise without a readily reversible cause, begin renal replacement therapy before symptoms or laboratory findings make dialysis mandatory.

Book Enhancement

Go to www.acponline.org/essentials/nephrology-section.html. In *MKSAP for Students 5*, assess your knowledge with items 5-9 in the **Nephrology** section.

Bibliography

Abuelo JG. Normotensive ischemic acute renal failure. N Engl J Med. 2007;357:797-805. [PMID: 17715412]

Chapter 62

Chronic Kidney Disease

John Jason White, MD

Chronic kidney disease (CKD) is a worldwide epidemic and is associated with significant morbidity and increased utilization of health care resources. CKD is defined as the presence of decreased kidney function (glomerular filtration rate [GFR] <60 mL/min/1.73 m^2) or kidney damage that persists ≥3 months. Irrespective of the cause of CKD, several comorbidities may develop, including accelerated cardiovascular disease, anemia, disordered bone mineral metabolism, metabolic acidosis, malnutrition, and electrolyte disturbances.

Diabetes mellitus, hypertension, and glomerular diseases account for most cases of CKD in the United States. In diabetes, hyperglycemia leads to pathologic changes in the kidney that usually follow a characteristic clinical course. Kidney disease manifests initially as microalbuminuria, then as clinical proteinuria, and ultimately as loss of kidney function. Hypertensive nephropathy is characterized by long-standing hypertension, left ventricular hypertrophy, minimal proteinuria, and progressive kidney failure. Glomerular diseases are a heterogeneous group of disorders with a variable clinical course; the disorders are generically divided into the nephritic syndrome and the nephrotic syndrome (see Chapter 60). Recognition and early diagnosis of glomerular disease is vital, as many forms progress to end-stage kidney failure. CKD that occurs following kidney transplantation may be caused by chronic rejection, drug toxicity, or recurrence of the original kidney disease.

Prevention

To prevent CKD, the underlying causes need to be aggressively managed. Treatment goals for patients with diabetes include a target hemoglobin A_{1c} (HbA_{1c}) level <7% and blood pressure <130/80 mm Hg. Target blood pressure for patients without diabetes or preexisting kidney disease is <140/90 mm Hg.

Screening

CKD often is unrecognized. Therefore, it is important to screen individuals at high risk, including the elderly, patients with diseases that cause CKD (e.g., hypertension, diabetes, systemic lupus erythematosus), and ethnic populations with increased risk (e.g., blacks, American Indians, Hispanics, Asians, Pacific Islanders). Measure blood pressure in all patients. Screen for urine protein using standard dipstick or albumin-specific dipsticks; positive results should be quantified by the protein-creatinine or albumin-creatinine ratio (normal protein-creatinine ratio is <200 mg/g). First morning urine specimens are preferred. Obtain urinalysis to look for leukocytes, erythrocytes, or casts, which may suggest underlying glomerular disease.

Screen patients with diabetes for microalbuminuria with an albumin-creatinine ratio using a spot urine sample (normal albumin-creatinine ratio is <30 mg/g). Screen patients with type 1 diabetes beginning 5 years after diagnosis, at puberty, and yearly thereafter. Screen patients with type 2 diabetes at the time of diagnosis then yearly. If kidney disease is discovered, measure the serum creatinine concentration, estimate the GFR (eGFR) using the Modification of Diet in Renal Disease (MDRD) or Cockcroft-Gault equation, and classify the stage of CKD (Table 1).

Diagnosis

Focus the history on possible causes of CKD. Ask about diabetes, hypertension, and high-risk behaviors predisposing to infectious diseases associated with CKD and proteinuria (e.g., HIV infection, hepatitis B and C, syphilis). Ask about a family history of kidney disease (e.g., polycystic kidney disease, Alport syndrome). Inquire about symptoms of urinary obstruction and urinary tract infection.

Table 1. Stages of Chronic Kidney Disease

Stage	Description	GFR[a] (mL/min/1.73 m^2)	Action
1	Kidney damage with normal GFR	≥90	Treatment of comorbid conditions, interventions to slow disease progression and reduce risk factors for cardiovascular disease
2	Kidney damage with mildly decreased GFR	60-89	Estimation of disease progression
3	Moderately decreased GFR	30-59	Evaluation and treatment of disease complications (anemia, renal osteodystrophy)
4	Severely decreased GFR	15-29	Preparation for kidney replacement therapy (dialysis, transplantation)
5	Kidney failure	<15 (or dialysis)	Kidney replacement therapy if uremia is present

GRF = glomerular filtration rate.
[a]GFR as estimated using the Modification of Diet in Renal Disease equation: GFR (mL/min/1.73 m^2) = 186 × [serum creatinine]$^{-1.154}$ × (age)$^{-0.203}$ × 0.742 (if female) × 1.21 (if black).

Table 2. Laboratory and Other Studies for Chronic Kidney Disease (CKD)

Test	Notes
Spot urine protein-creatinine ratio	The preferred quantitative measure for diagnosing proteinuria; 24-hour urine collections are inaccurate and not recommended. Urine dipsticks can be used to screen patients who are not diabetic, but positive results should be followed with a quantitative measurement. Normal ratio is <200 mg/g. First morning urine specimens are preferred, but random specimens are acceptable. Patients with two or more positive quantitative test results 1-2 wk apart are diagnosed with persistent proteinuria and must undergo further evaluation and management.
Spot urine albumin-creatinine ratio	Normal ratio is <30 mg/g; 30-300 mg/g is defined as microalbuminuria. In adults, albuminuria is a more sensitive marker than total protein for CKD due to diabetes, hypertension, or glomerular disease.
Urinalysis	Hematuria, proteinuria, casts, and leukocytes are some of the abnormalities seen in CKD. The presence of dysmorphic erythrocytes suggests active glomerular disease.
Electrolytes	Hyperkalemia and metabolic acidosis often develop in CKD; hyponatremia may occur in edematous states associated with CKD.
Serum calcium	Hypocalcemia can be seen in patients with CKD. Corrected total calcium (mg/dL) = total calcium (mg/dL) + $0.8 \times [4 -$ serum albumin (g/dL)].
Serum phosphorus	Phosphorus retention is common in CKD and leads to development of secondary hyperparathyroidism.
Serum intact parathyroid hormone (PTH)	PTH level is used to detect secondary hyperparathyroidism. Measure PTH in patients with stage 3 or higher CKD.
Albumin	Serum albumin level is a marker of nutritional status and an independent predictor of mortality in patients on dialysis.
Lipid profile	Patients with CKD are at high risk for cardiovascular disease.
Complete blood count	If the hemoglobin level is <11 g/dL (110 g/L), check erythrocyte indices, iron stores, reticulocyte count, and stool for occult blood to evaluate the need for iron replacement or an erythropoiesis-stimulating agent.
Renal ultrasonography	Hydronephrosis may be found on ultrasonography in patients with urinary tract obstruction or vesicoureteral reflux. The presence of multiple discrete macroscopic cysts suggests autosomal dominant or recessive polycystic kidney disease. Increased cortical echogenicity and small kidney size are nonspecific indicators of CKD.
Other imaging studies	IVP, CT, MRI, or nuclear medicine scanning can be used for specific situations, such as stone disease, renal artery stenosis, or obstruction.

IVP = intravenous pyelography.

Table 3. Classification of Chronic Kidney Disease (CKD)

Disease	Notes
Diabetic kidney disease (see Chapter 8)	Diabetic kidney disease is the leading cause of CKD in the United States. Kidney disease in diabetes, particularly type 1 diabetes, usually follows a characteristic course, manifesting first as microalbuminuria, followed by clinical proteinuria, hypertension, and declining GFR. Diabetic nephropathy often is accompanied by diabetic retinopathy, particularly in type 1 diabetes. In patients with type 2 diabetes, the presence of retinopathy strongly suggests coexisting diabetic nephropathy. Even in the absence of retinopathy, diabetic nephropathy is likely, but an evaluation for other causes of proteinuria is reasonable.
Glomerular disease	Patients may present with either nephritic or nephrotic syndrome. Nephritic syndrome is characterized by hematuria, variable proteinuria, and hypertension, often with other systemic manifestations. Common causes include postinfectious glomerulonephritis, IgA nephropathy, and membranoproliferative glomerulonephritis. Nephrotic syndrome is characterized by high-grade proteinuria (often >3 g/24 h), hypoalbuminemia, and edema. Common causes include minimal change disease, focal glomerulosclerosis, membranous nephropathy, and amyloidosis. SLE commonly affects the kidney and may cause nephritic or nephrotic syndrome. A kidney biopsy often is needed to make a specific diagnosis and to guide therapy.
Tubulointerstitial disease	Patients generally have a bland or relatively normal urinalysis but may have proteinuria, a concentrating defect, pyuria, casts, or radiologic abnormalities. Analgesic nephropathy, lead nephropathy, chronic obstruction, and reflux nephropathy are examples.
Vasculitis (see Chapter 97)	The clinical presentation depends on the type of blood vessels involved (small, medium, or large). Patients with small-vessel disease often have hematuria, proteinuria, and an associated systemic illness. Patients with vasculitis can present with a rapidly progressive glomerulonephritis. Hypertension is an example of medium-vessel disease and is the second leading cause of CKD in the United States. Hypertensive disease generally is slowly progressive, leading to stage 5 CKD in a minority of patients. Blacks have more aggressive CKD caused by hypertension. Renal artery stenosis is an example of large-vessel disease.
Renal cystic disease	Patients can have normal findings on urinalysis. Diagnosis usually is made by imaging techniques and family history. Simple renal cysts are common, particularly in older persons. Autosomal dominant polycystic disease types I and II are the most common forms.
Transplant-related kidney disease	CKD in the renal transplant recipient may be due to chronic rejection, drug toxicity, or recurrence of native kidney disease. A careful history and serum drug levels and often a kidney biopsy are required for diagnosis.

GFR = glomerular filtration rate; SLE = systemic lupus erythematosus.

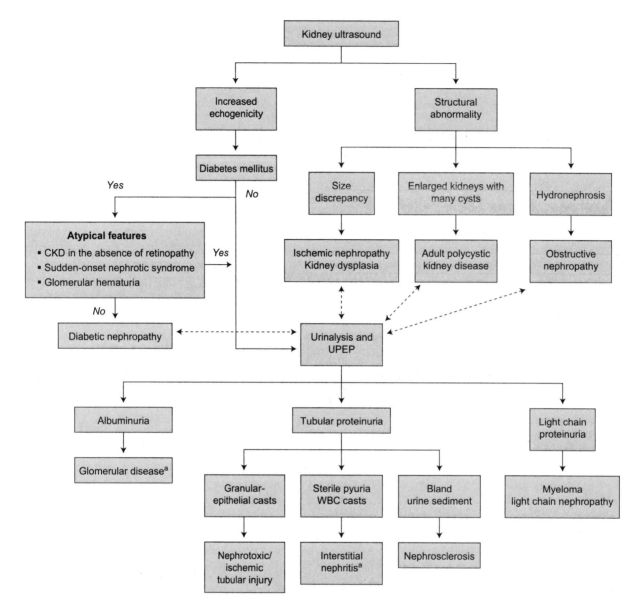

Figure 1. Diagnostic evaluation of chronic kidney disease. Dotted lines emphasize that urinalysis and urine sediment analysis should be performed in all patients. CKD = chronic kidney disease; UPEP = urine protein electrophoresis. [a]Consider kidney biopsy.

Obtain a detailed medication history; many medications may contribute to the development of CKD, and many require dose adjustment based on the eGFR. Specifically ask about NSAIDs, acetaminophen, and herbal preparations. Ask about symptoms of fluid retention. When eGFR declines to <20 mL/min/1.73 m^2, evaluate for symptoms of uremia, such as anorexia, nausea, vomiting, weight loss, or itching.

A thorough physical examination may identify important clinical consequences and comorbidities. Look for hypertension and signs of volume overload. Examine the fundi for evidence of hypertensive or diabetic retinopathy, and check for signs of uremia, such as asterixis or a pericardial rub.

To evaluate for kidney damage, obtain a protein-creatinine ratio and urine microscopy to look for erythrocytes, leukocytes, and casts. Also obtain a complete blood count, serum electrolytes,

a fasting lipid profile, kidney ultrasonography, and, in patients with stage 3 or higher CKD, serum albumin and intact parathyroid hormone levels (Table 2). Use the MDRD or Cockcroft-Gault equation to calculate eGFR and to stage CKD, then classify CKD as diabetic, nondiabetic, or transplant-related kidney disease (Table 3). In patients in whom glomerular disease is suspected or the diagnosis is uncertain, obtain a nephrology consultation for a renal biopsy (Figure 1).

Therapy

Management of CKD requires a multidisciplinary approach and involves treating underlying disease, attempting to delay disease progression, treating complications and symptoms of CKD, and preventing or treating cardiovascular disease.

CKD is associated with sodium and phosphorus retention and inability to excrete daily potassium load. Patients with CKD have salt-sensitive hypertension; dietary sodium restriction to <2.4 g/day is crucial in these patients. Recommend dietary potassium restriction to <2 g/day for patients with hyperkalemia, and recommend dietary phosphorus restriction to <1 g/day when serum phosphorus is >4.6 mg/dL (1.5 mmol/L). Recommend a low-protein diet (0.6 g/kg/day) for patients with stage 4 or 5 CKD, provided that caloric intake can be maintained at 35 kcal/kg/day. Consult a dietician to achieve these goals. Counsel patients about the importance of smoking cessation, limiting alcohol consumption, regular exercise, and maintaining ideal body weight. Instruct patients to avoid magnesium- and phosphorus-containing laxatives, NSAIDs, COX-2 inhibitors, and radiocontrast procedures including MRI with gadolinium due to the risk of nephrogenic systemic fibrosis.

In patients with diabetes, maintain HbA_{1c} levels at <7% to slow progression of CKD. Hypertension control is paramount to prevent progression of CKD and to decrease cardiovascular risk; control blood pressure to <130/80 mm Hg. Use ACE inhibitors or angiotensin II receptor blockers (ARBs) as first-line therapy in patients with diabetes and hypertension and in any patient with proteinuria. There is no specific eGFR to discontinue use of these agents. An increase in serum creatinine of ≤30% is acceptable. Measure blood pressure, eGFR, and serum potassium within 3 to 5 days of initiating or adjusting the dose of an ACE or ARB and every 2 to 3 months thereafter. CKD is a cause of resistant hypertension and often requires three or more drugs to control blood pressure. Patients usually are volume expanded, and diuretics should be titrated to optimal doses. Diuretics are first-line therapy in nondiabetic patients without proteinuria. Use thiazide diuretics when eGFR is >30 mL/min/1.73 m^2 and twice-daily loop diuretics when eGFR is <30 mL/min/1.73 m^2. Use other synergistic classes of medications as needed.

Proteinuria is associated with a progressive decline in renal function and an increase in cardiovascular risk; reduction in proteinuria is associated with slower progression of CKD. Initiate ACE inhibitors or ARB therapy to lower the protein-creatinine ratio to <500-1000 mg/g. If proteinuria persists, increase the dose of ACE inhibitors or ARBs as tolerated by blood pressure and serum potassium levels. The role of dual blockade of the renin-angiotensin system in patients with proteinuria is unclear. Combination therapies (i.e., ACE inhibitor plus ARB, ARB plus aliskiren, ACE inhibitor or ARB plus aldosterone antagonist) lower proteinuria greater than any monotherapy. However, data on disease progression are lacking. A recent cardiovascular trial suggests that combining ACE inhibitors and ARBs actually may be harmful. If dual blockade is considered, eGFR and serum potassium levels must be closely monitored. Add nondihydropyridine calcium channel blockers as second-line therapy to further lower blood pressure and reduce proteinuria.

As GFR declines, erythropoietin production diminishes and anemia results. Consider erythropoiesis-stimulating agents to correct anemia and to maintain hemoglobin levels at 10-12 g/dL. Higher levels may increase the risk of death and serious cardiovascular complications and should be avoided. Use oral or intravenous iron to maintain adequate iron stores (i.e., transferrin sat-

uration >20% and serum ferritin >100 ng/mL [100 µg/L]). Evaluate and rule out other causes of anemia (e.g., hemolysis, vitamin deficiencies), because CKD-associated anemia is a diagnosis of exclusion.

Alterations in bone mineral metabolism develop in CKD. Decreased renal mass leads to decreased phosphorus clearance and decreased 1,25-dihydroxyvitamin D$_3$ production. This results in hyperphosphatemia, hypocalcemia, and secondary hyperparathyroidism. Secondary hyperparathyroidism may result in renal osteodystrophy and increased cardiovascular morbidity and mortality by promoting vascular calcification. Renal osteodystrophy may manifest as osteitis fibrosa cystica, osteoporosis, osteomalacia, adynamic bone disease, mixed bone disease, or amyloidosis. Management requires multiple medications aimed at lowering serum phosphorus, correcting vitamin D deficiency, and suppressing parathyroid hormone (PTH) levels. Dietary restriction of phosphorus is recommended in patients with hyperphosphatemia. Give phosphate binders with meals to prevent gastrointestinal absorption of phosphorus. Calcium salts (e.g., calcium carbonate, calcium gluconate) can be used to maintain serum phosphorus levels between 2.7 and 4.6 mg/dL (0.9 and 1.5 mmol/L); however, the total dose of elemental calcium should not exceed 1500 mg/d. When serum calcium levels are elevated, use non–calcium-containing phosphate binders (e.g., lanthanum carbonate, sevelamer). Use of aluminum-containing antacids should be avoided due to the risk of aluminum toxicity. Use calcitriol or vitamin D analogs to maintain serum calcium levels within the normal range and to suppress elevated PTH levels. PTH suppression is indicated when values are >70 pg/mL (70 ng/L) in stage 3 CKD and >110 pg/mL (110 ng/L) in stage 4 CKD. 25-Hydroxyvitamin D$_3$ insufficiency/deficiency also is common in patients with CKD and is treated with vitamin D$_2$ (ergocalciferol). Cinacalcet (a calcimimetic agent) binds to the calcium-sensing receptor on the parathyroid gland and suppresses PTH and lowers calcium levels; however, cinacalcet is not approved for patients with CKD who are not on dialysis.

Hyperkalemia may develop in advanced CKD and in certain forms of renal tubular acidosis. Restrict dietary potassium, ensure adequate hydration, and use loop diuretics as necessary. Some patients require sodium polystyrene sulfonate to maintain serum potassium levels within normal range. Severe hyperkalemia (>6.0 meq/L [6.0 mmol/L]) is associated with life-threatening cardiac dysrhythmias; patients with severe hyperkalemia require hospitalization and referral to a nephrologist. Initially give intravenous calcium gluconate to stabilize the myocardium, intravenous glucose and insulin to shift potassium into the cells, and sodium polystyrene sulfonate to increase gastrointestinal clearance of potassium. Give intravenous fluids to patients who are intravascularly volume depleted. Consider hemodialysis if hyperkalemia is not decreased by these measures, especially in patients who are oliguric.

Metabolic acidosis commonly develops in advanced CKD, accelerating renal osteodystrophy and suppressing albumin synthesis; metabolic acidosis also is linked with malnutrition. Treating metabolic acidosis may slow progression of CKD. Use sodium bicarbonate to maintain serum carbon dioxide levels within the range of 22 to 26 meq/L (22 to 26 mmol/L).

Follow-Up

Patients with CKD require close follow-up with laboratory measurements initially every 3 to 4 months and more frequently as CKD becomes more advanced. Consult a nephrologist for patients with CKD before eGFR decreases to <30 mL/min/1.73 m^2. Ensure medications are dosed appropriately for the eGFR. If administration of iodinated contrast is essential, give sodium bicarbonate or isotonic saline intravenously and consider using *N*-acetylcysteine before and after the procedure, closely monitoring fluid and electrolyte status to decrease the risk of contrast-induced nephropathy.

At radiologic doses, gadolinium is not nephrotoxic but is associated with a nephrogenic systemic fibrosis (NSF). NSF is a disorder seen only in patients with kidney failure who are exposed to gadolinium. NSF causes thickening and hardening of the skin over the extremities and trunk but may involve other organ systems as well. NSF may cause severe disability and even death. Limit the amount of gadolinium used for MRI in patients with stage 3 CKD, and avoid gadolinium completely when eGFR is <30 mL/min/1.73 m^2 to prevent NSF. There is no treatment for NSF.

Patients with stage 5 CKD often become uremic and require renal replacement therapy (RRT). Options for RRT should be discussed when a patient reaches stage 4 CKD or 1 year before it is anticipated that the patient will reach stage 5 CKD. Options include outpatient hemodialysis, home hemodialysis, peritoneal dialysis, and renal transplantation. If hemodialysis is preferred, an arteriovenous fistula or graft should be placed well before initiation of RRT. RRT is indicated in patients with stage 5 CKD who have uremic signs or symptoms (Table 4). For patients without uremic signs or symptoms, the optimal timing of RRT is unknown. Patients requiring RRT have high rates of cardiovascular events and are at increased risk for infectious complications. Discuss advanced directives and end-of-life issues. Evaluate for and treat depression when indicated.

RRT in the United States is dominated by hemodialysis and is performed at outpatient centers three sessions per week for approximately 3.5 hours per session. Hemodialysis treatments are commonly associated with hypotension, nausea, vomiting, and chest pain. Other common symptoms during dialysis include pruritis, muscle cramping, and restless legs. Complications also include an increase in acquired renal cystic disease and renal cell carcinoma.

Table 4. Indications for Dialysis

Relative	Absolute
Nausea, vomiting, poor nutrition caused by decreased appetite	Uncontrollable hyperkalemia
Metabolic acidosis	Uncontrollable hypervolemia
Altered mental status (lethargy, malaise), asterixis	Altered mental status, somnolence
Worsening kidney function with GFR <15-20 mL/min/1.73 m^2	Pericarditis, bleeding diathesis from uremia-induced platelet dysfunction

GFR = glomerular filtration rate.

Transplantation is the treatment of choice for stage 5 CKD; however, donor organs are in short supply. Compared with hemodialysis, transplantation is associated with more favorable outcomes in all groups and allows for a more normal lifestyle. Refer patients early for transplantation evaluation to determine eligibility and to facilitate identification of potential living donors. Living donor kidneys afford better patient and graft survival. Furthermore, transplantation before or shortly after initiation of hemodialysis is associated with improved patient outcomes. Contraindications to transplantation include recent or advanced malignancy, current infection, severe irreversible extrarenal disease, nonadherence, active use of illicit drugs, and primary oxalosis without plans for liver transplantation. Immunosuppression with both induction and maintenance therapy is needed to prevent rejection of the transplanted organ. Patients who have received kidney transplants are at increased risk for coronary vascular disease, infection, malignancy, recurrent kidney disease, graft loss, and bone disease associated with prolonged corticosteroid use.

Book Enhancement

Go to www.acponline.org/essentials/nephrology-section.html. In *MKSAP for Students 5*, assess your knowledge with items 10-13 in the **Nephrology** section.

Bibliography

Abboud H, Henrich WL. Clinical practice. Stage IV chronic kidney disease. N Engl J Med. 2010;362:56-65. [PMID: 20054047]

Chapter 63

Acid-Base Disorders

Joseph Charles, MD

A systematic approach to acid-base problem solving involves an analysis of arterial blood gases and electrolytes focused on answering five questions:

- Is the patient acidemic or alkalemic?
- Is the acid-base disorder primarily metabolic or respiratory?
- Is there an anion gap?
- If a metabolic acidosis exists, is there an appropriate respiratory compensation?
- If an anion gap acidemia is present, is there an additional complicating metabolic disturbance?

Table 1 summarizes a differential diagnosis for the primary acid-base disorders.

Metabolic Acidosis

Metabolic acidosis is the most common acid-base disorder and can be life-threatening. It results from excessive cellular acid production, reduced acid secretion, or loss of body alkali. The body has two buffering mechanisms to counteract an increase in acid. The initial response is to increase carbon dioxide excretion by increasing ventilation. The second response is increased renal excretion of acids and renal regeneration of bicarbonate. The adequacy of compensation can be assessed by the quick check method or the Winter formula (Table 2).

Metabolic acidosis can be classified into two categories using the anion gap. Each category has a distinct differential diagnosis.

Table 1. Causes of Primary Acid-Base Disorders

Metabolic Acidosis ([bicarbonate]<22 meq/L [22 mmol/L]; pH <7.35)	**Metabolic Alkalosis** ([bicarbonate] >28 meq/L [28 mmol/L]; pH >7.45)
Increased serum anion gap (anion gap >12 meq/L [12 mmol/L])	Chloride responsive (urine [chloride] <10 meq/L [10 mmol/L])
• Ketoacidosis (diabetes, alcohol abuse, starvation)	• Vomiting
• Lactic acidosis (ischemia, sepsis, shock, drugs)	• Nasogastric suctioning
• Exogenous substances (methanol, ethylene glycol, salicylates, toluene)	• Thiazide and loop diuretic therapy
• Chronic kidney disease	• Contraction alkalosis
Normal serum anion gap (hyperchloremic)	• Exogenous bicarbonate in the setting of kidney dysfunction
• Positive urine anion gap	Chloride unresponsive (urine [chloride] >20 meq/L [20 mmol/L])
○ Type I RTA (normo- or hypokalemic)	• Elevated mineralocorticoid activity (primary hyperaldosteronism, Cushing syndrome)
○ Type II RTA (normo- or hypokalemic)	• Exogenous mineralocorticoid
○ Type IV RTA (hyperkalemic)	• Bartter, Gitelman, Liddle syndromes
• Negative urine anion gap	• Some forms of congenital adrenal hyperplasia
○ GI bicarbonate loss (severe diarrhea, ureterosigmoidostomy)	• Severe hypokalemia
○ Ingestion of acid	• Chronic licorice ingestion
Respiratory Acidosis (arterial P_{CO_2} >45 mm Hg [6 kPa]; pH <7.35)	**Respiratory Alkalosis** (arterial P_{CO_2} <35 mm Hg [4.7 kPa]; pH >7.45)
• Respiratory center depression (stroke, infection, tumor, drugs, COPD, OHS)	• CNS stimulation (stroke, infection, tumor, fever, pain)
• Neuromuscular failure (muscular dystrophy, ALS, Guillain-Barré syndrome, myasthenia gravis, COPD, OHS)	• Drugs (aspirin, progesterone, theophylline, caffeine)
• Decreased respiratory system compliance (kyphoscoliosis, interstitial lung disease)	• Anxiety, psychosis
• Increased airway resistance or obstruction (asthma, COPD, OHS)	• Hypoxemia (low atmospheric oxygen, severe anemia, lung disease, right-to-left shunt, heart failure)
• Increased dead space/ventilation-perfusion mismatch (pulmonary embolism, COPD, OHS)	• Pregnancy

ALS = amyotrophic lateral sclerosis; CNS = central nervous system; GI = gastrointestinal; OHS = obesity hypoventilation syndrome; RTA = renal tubular acidosis.

Table 2. Compensation in Acid-Base Disorders

Condition	Expected Compensation
Metabolic acidosis	Acute: $P_{CO_2} = (1.5 \times [\text{bicarbonate}]) + 8$
	Chronic: $P_{CO_2} = [\text{bicarbonate}] + 15$
	Quick check: P_{CO_2} value should approximate last two digits of pH
	Failure of P_{CO_2} to decrease to the expected value indicates complicating respiratory acidosis; excessive decrease of P_{CO_2} indicates complicating respiratory alkalosis.
Metabolic alkalosis	For each 1 meq/L increase in [bicarbonate], P_{CO_2} should increase 0.7 mm Hg.
Respiratory acidosis	Acute: 1 meq/L increase in [bicarbonate] for each 10 mm Hg increase in P_{CO_2}
	Failure of the bicarbonate concentration to increase to the expected value indicates complicating metabolic acidosis; excessive increase in the bicarbonate concentration indicates complicating metabolic alkalosis.
	Chronic: 3.5 meq/L increase in [bicarbonate] for each 10 mm Hg increase in P_{CO_2}
Respiratory alkalosis	Acute: 2 meq/L decrease in [bicarbonate] for each 10 mm Hg decrease in P_{CO_2}
	Chronic: 4-5 meq/L decrease in [bicarbonate] for each 10 mm Hg decrease in P_{CO_2}
	Failure of the bicarbonate concentration to decrease to the expected value indicates complicating metabolic alkalosis; excessive decrease in the bicarbonate concentration indicates complicating metabolic acidosis.
	Where P_{CO_2} is in mm Hg and [bicarbonate] in meq/L.

$$\text{Anion gap} = [\text{sodium}] - ([\text{chloride}] + [\text{bicarbonate}])$$

Normally, the anion gap is approximately 12 ± 2 meq/L (12 ± 2 mmol/L). Most unmeasured anions consist of albumin. Therefore, the presence of either a low albumin level or an unmeasured cationic light chain, which occurs in multiple myeloma, results in a low anion gap. Increased hydrogen ion concentration or decreased bicarbonate concentration will increase the gap. When the primary disturbance is a metabolic acidosis, the anion gap helps to narrow the diagnostic possibilities to a high anion gap acidosis or a normal anion gap acidosis.

High Anion Gap Metabolic Acidosis

Common causes include ketoacidosis (diabetes mellitus, alcohol abuse, starvation), lactic acidosis, chronic kidney disease, salicylate toxicity, and ethylene glycol and methanol poisoning. Diabetic ketoacidosis is the most common cause of a high anion gap acidosis, but a normal anion gap acidosis may be present early in the disease course when the extracellular fluid volume is nearly normal. Ketoacidosis also may develop in patients with a history of chronic alcohol abuse, decreased food intake, and (often) nausea and vomiting. The alcohol withdrawal, volume depletion, and starvation that occur in these patients significantly increase the levels of circulating catecholamines, which results in peripheral mobilization of fatty acids that is much greater than would be associated with starvation alone. Lactic acidosis develops when an imbalance occurs between the production and use of lactic acid and is most commonly associated with tissue ischemia. Lactic acidosis due to increased production of lactic acid may occur in patients who engage in extreme exercise or who have tonic-clonic seizures and usually is of short duration. Aspirin poisoning leads to increased lactic acid production; the accumulation of lactic acid, salicylic acid, ketoacids, and other organic acids results in an anion gap metabolic acidosis. Salicylate poisoning manifests as either a respiratory alkalosis or an anion gap metabolic acidosis in adults, whereas affected children usually have only an anion gap metabolic acidosis.

Ethylene glycol and methanol poisoning are characterized by a severe anion gap metabolic acidosis accompanied by an osmolal gap. An osmolal gap is present when the measured plasma osmolality exceeds the calculated plasma osmolality by >10 mosm/kg H_2O (10 mmol/kg H_2O). Plasma osmolality is calculated as:

$$\text{Plasma osmolality} = (2 \times [\text{sodium}]) + ([\text{glucose}]/18) + ([\text{BUN}]/2.8)$$

where glucose and BUN (blood urea nitrogen) are measured in mg/dL.

Ethylene glycol poisoning initially causes neurologic manifestations similar to those of alcohol intoxication, and seizures and coma can develop rapidly. Ethylene glycol poisoning also is associated with acute kidney injury and oxalate crystalluria. Clinical manifestations of methanol ingestion include acute inebriation followed by an asymptomatic period lasting 24 to 36 hours. Because formic acid, the metabolic end product of methanol, is toxic to the retina, blindness may result.

Normal Anion Gap Metabolic Acidosis

Normal anion gap metabolic acidosis is secondary to kidney or extrarenal disease. The clinical history usually helps to distinguish between kidney and extrarenal causes of metabolic acidosis, but the two categories can be reliably differentiated by measuring the urine anion gap:

$$\text{Urine anion gap} = (\text{urine}[\text{sodium}] + \text{urine}[\text{potassium}]) - [\text{urine chloride}]$$

The urine anion gap normally is 30-50 meq/L (30-50 mmol/L). Metabolic acidosis of extrarenal origin (usually gastrointestinal) is suggested by a large, negative urine anion gap caused by significantly increased urine ammonium excretion.

Metabolic acidosis of kidney origin is suggested by a positive urine anion gap related to minimal urine ammonium excretion. Severe diarrhea is the most common gastrointestinal cause. The most common kidney-related causes are renal tubular disorders causing renal tubular acidosis (RTA). Type 1 (distal) RTA, caused by impaired distal tubule acidification, should be considered in patients with a normal anion gap acidosis, hypokalemia, a positive urine anion gap, and a urine pH >5.5 in the setting of systemic acidosis; serum bicarbonate concentration may be as low as 10 meq/L (10 mmol/L). Type 2 (proximal) RTA is due to reduced proximal tubule bicarbonate reabsorption and should be suspected in patients with a normal anion gap metabolic acidosis, a normal urine anion gap, hypokalemia, and an intact ability to acidify the urine to a pH of <5.5 while in a steady state. The serum bicarbonate concentration usually is 16-18 meq/L (16-18 mmol/L). Type 4 RTA should be suspected in patients with a normal anion gap metabolic acidosis associated with hyperkalemia and a slightly positive urine anion gap. Type 4 RTA occurs most often in patients with diabetes who have mild to moderate kidney insufficiency; the disorder is due to hyporeninemic hypoaldosteronism, which is characterized by deficient angiotensin II production due to both decreased renin production and an intra-adrenal defect leading to aldosterone deficiency. Figure 1 outlines an approach to patients with a low serum bicarbonate concentration.

Mixed Metabolic Disorders

To determine whether a complicating metabolic disturbance is present along with an anion gap metabolic acidosis, it is necessary to calculate the corrected bicarbonate level. If the corrected bicar-

bonate level is less than 24 + 2 meq/L (24 + 2 mmol/L), a coexisting normal anion gap metabolic acidosis is present; conversely, if the corrected bicarbonate level is greater than 24 + 2 meq/L (24 + 2 mmol/L), a coexisting metabolic alkalosis is present. The corrected bicarbonate level is obtained using the following formula:

$$\text{Corrected [bicarbonate]} = \text{measured [bicarbonate]} + [\text{anion gap} - 12]$$

This formula is based on the assumption that the measured anion gap represents, in part, the bicarbonate that was consumed in attempting to compensate for the process producing the anion gap metabolic acidosis. If the measured anion gap is added to the measured bicarbonate concentration and the normal anion gap of 12 is subtracted, the result should represent the bicarbonate concentration if the anion gap acidosis were not present, hence the name "corrected bicarbonate."

Metabolic Alkalosis

A primary increase in bicarbonate concentration can result from loss of hydrogen chloride or, less commonly, addition of bicarbonate. Table 2 lists the expected respiratory compensation for metabolic alkalosis. Once generated, the metabolic alkalosis is corrected through urinary excretion of the excess bicarbonate. Alkalosis is maintained only when renal bicarbonate excretion is limited owing to a reduction in kidney function or stimulation of renal tubule bicarbonate reabsorption. Increased bicarbonate reabsorption is caused by extracellular fluid volume contraction, chloride depletion, hypokalemia, or elevated mineralocorticoid activi-

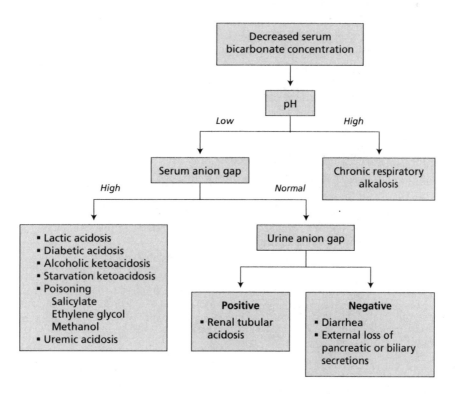

Figure 1. Approach to the patient with a decreased serum bicarbonate concentration.

ty. Persistent delivery of sodium chloride to the distal tubule in the presence of high levels of aldosterone results in urinary loss of potassium and hydrogen, which maintains the metabolic alkalosis.

The most common causes of metabolic alkalosis are vomiting, nasogastric suction, and diuretic therapy. In these cases, which are classified as *chloride responsive*, administration of sodium chloride fluid reverses the alkalosis by expanding the intravascular volume and reducing the activity of the renin-angiotensin-aldosterone axis. Low urine chloride concentration suggests vomiting or remote diuretic ingestion; in either case, sodium chloride volume expansion will correct the alkalosis.

Less commonly, metabolic alkalosis is maintained in the absence of volume depletion. This condition is recognized by a high urine chloride level (>20 meq/L [20 mmol/L]) related to elevated mineralocorticoid activity and does not correct with sodium chloride volume replacement. Consequently, these disorders are classified as *chloride-unresponsive* or *chloride-resistant metabolic alkaloses*. Examples are primary hyperaldosteronism and Cushing syndrome.

H_2-Receptor blockers (e.g., cimetidine) and proton pump inhibitors (e.g., omeprazole) may decrease hydrogen in patients with prolonged gastric aspiration or chronic vomiting. Potassium chloride almost always is indicated for hypokalemia, although potassium concentration may increase as the alkalosis is corrected.

Respiratory Acidosis

Primary respiratory acidosis develops as a result of ineffective alveolar ventilation and is suggested by an arterial P_{CO_2} >45 mm Hg (6.0 kPa). However, an arterial P_{CO_2} <45 mm Hg (6.0 kPa) may indicate respiratory acidosis in a patient with primary metabolic acidosis that is not adequately compensated by alveolar ventilation. This condition must be differentiated from primary respiratory acidosis (Table 1). Respiratory acidosis is due to a primary increase in arterial P_{CO_2}, which accumulates when ventilation is inadequate. Hypoventilation can result from neurologic disorders (e.g., stroke) or medications (e.g., opiates) that affect the central nervous system respiratory center, respiratory muscle weakness (e.g., myasthenia gravis, Guillain-Barré syndrome) or chest wall deformity (e.g., severe kyphoscoliosis), obstruction of airways (e.g., COPD), or ventilation-perfusion mismatch (e.g., pulmonary embolism). Respiratory acidosis may manifest as hypercapnic encephalopathy, a clinical syndrome that initially can present as irritability, headache, mental cloudiness, apathy, confusion, anxiety, and restlessness and can progress to asterixis, transient psychosis, delirium, somnolence, and coma. Severe hypercapnia may cause decreased myocardial contractility, arrhythmias, and peripheral vasodilatation, particularly when the serum pH decreases to <7.1. Patients with acute respiratory acidosis are primarily at risk for hypoxemia rather than hypercapnia or acidemia. Therefore, initial therapy should focus on establishing and maintaining a patent airway and improving ventilation in order to provide adequate oxygenation. Excessive oxygen may worsen hypoventilation in patients with chronic respiratory acidosis and should be avoided in this population.

Respiratory Alkalosis

Primary respiratory alkalosis is characterized by an arterial P_{CO_2} <35 mm Hg (4.7 kPa). Primary respiratory alkalosis must be differentiated from secondary respiratory alkalosis, which is a compensatory mechanism in the setting of primary metabolic acidosis (Table 2). To maintain a normal extracellular fluid volume in the setting of increased urinary loss of sodium bicarbonate, the kidney retains sodium chloride. Therefore, patients with chronic respiratory alkalosis typically have hyperchloremia.

Common causes of respiratory alkalosis can be sorted by underlying pathology. Those involving the pulmonary vasculature include pulmonary hypertension and pulmonary embolism. Pulmonary parenchymal diseases are represented by pulmonary fibrosis, heart failure, and pneumonia. In patients with asthma, acute exacerbations of bronchospasm trigger an increased respiratory rate. Respiratory alkalosis also can result from conditions affecting ventilatory control (e.g., anxiety, aspirin toxicity, sepsis, hypoxia, hepatic encephalopathy, pregnancy). Acute hypocapnia decreases cerebral blood flow and causes binding of free calcium to albumin in the blood. Mild respiratory alkalosis may cause lightheadedness and palpitations. More profound respiratory alkalosis may cause symptoms that resemble those of hypocalcemia, including paresthesias of the extremities and circumoral area and carpopedal spasm. Patients with ischemic heart disease may occasionally develop cardiac arrhythmias, ischemic electrocardiographic changes, and angina pectoris. In psychogenic hyperventilation, rebreathing air using a bag increases the systemic arterial P_{CO_2}. This method also may help to rapidly reduce the pH in patients with mixed, severe alkalosis.

Book Enhancement

Go to www.acponline.org/essentials/nephrology-section.html. In *MKSAP for Students 5*, assess your knowledge with items 14-19 in the **Nephrology** section.

Acknowledgment

We would like to thank Dr. Tomoko Tanabe, who contributed to an earlier version of this chapter.

Bibliography

Kraut JA, Madias NE. Approach to patients with acid-base disorders. Respir Care. 2001;46:392-403. [PMID: 11262558]

Chapter 64

Fluid and Electrolyte Disorders

Mary Jane Barchman, MD

Total body water (TBW) constitutes approximately 60% of body weight in males and 50% in females. Two thirds of TBW is intracellular fluid; the remaining third is extracellular fluid, which is distributed 25% as intravascular volume and 75% as interstitial volume. The osmolality of the various fluid compartments is similar, but the solutes dictating the osmolality are not; the main extracellular osmole is sodium, and the primary intracellular osmoles are potassium and phosphates. Plasma osmolality is calculated as:

$$\text{Plasma osmolality} = (2 \times [\text{sodium}]) + ([\text{glucose}]/18) + ([\text{blood urea nitrogen}]/2.8);$$
where blood urea nitrogen and glucose are mg/dL

Serum osmolality also can be measured indirectly by an osmometer, which determines freezing point of the specimen; the lower the temperature needed to freeze the serum, the higher the osmolality. The difference between the measured and calculated values is the osmolal gap (normal osmolal gap = 10-15 mosm/kg [mmol/kg]). A large osmolal gap suggests the presence of added unmeasured osmotically active particles. Typically, this calculation is used to screen for ethylene glycol ingestion, but in practice, the most common cause of an osmolal gap is ethanol toxicity.

Water Metabolism

Normal plasma osmolality (285-295 mosm/kg [285-295 mmol/kg]) is maintained by thirst, renal handling of water, and antidiuretic hormone (ADH). The thirst center is located in the hypothalamus and is stimulated or suppressed by changes in plasma osmolality and effective intravascular volume. Water is filtered at the glomerulus, and 80% is absorbed isotonically in the proximal tubule. Water is then passively reabsorbed throughout the descending limb of the loop of Henle in response to the increasing osmolality in the medullary interstitium; this segment of the tubule is impermeable to sodium chloride. The ascending limb of the loop of Henle constitutes the diluting segment of the nephron; sodium chloride is reabsorbed to maintain the medullary gradient but water is retained, resulting in a minimum urine osmolality of 50-100 mosm/kg [50-100 mmol/kg]. Water is reabsorbed in the distal tubule and cortical collecting duct under the influence of ADH. The hypothalamic osmostat has projections to the posterior pituitary gland, which stimulate or inhibit ADH release based on plasma osmolality and effective intravascular volume. Pain, nausea, emotional stress, psychosis, and several drugs also increase ADH levels. One of the most common drugs associated with hyponatremia is hydrochlorothiazide, which interferes with the function of the diluting segment of the nephron and causes mild intravascular volume depletion, leading to increased ADH release and thirst. The street drug "ecstasy" (3,4-methylenedioxymethamphetamine) stimulates ADH release and intense thirst and is increasingly being recognized as a cause of severe hyponatremia. When hypo-osmolality and hypovolemia occur together, low-volume stimulus overrides the inhibitory effect of the hypo-osmolality, and ADH secretion increases to protect volume preferentially.

Hyponatremia

Hyponatremia (serum sodium concentration <136 meq/L [136 mmol/L]) can be associated with high, normal, or low plasma osmolality. Hyponatremia with high plasma osmolality occurs with accumulation of solutes in the extracellular fluid, which, in turn, causes movement of water from the intracellular space to the extracellular space. Hyperglycemia is the most common cause of a high solute load, and measured sodium concentration can be corrected by the following calculation:

$$\text{Corrected } [\text{Na}^+] = \text{measured } [\text{Na}^+] + 0.016 \times (\text{glucose} - 100);$$
where glucose is mg/dL

Other solutes capable of this effect include mannitol, radiographic contrast media, sorbitol, and glycine (sorbitol and glycine are used as irrigants during bladder or uterine surgical procedures). Treatment is supportive until the solute is excreted; in extreme cases, dialysis may be required.

Hyponatremia with normal plasma osmolality (pseudohyponatremia) is characterized by a low serum sodium concentration due to measurement in a falsely large volume; an interfering substance displaces water in the sample, similar to ice cubes in a pitcher. The most common space-occupying substances are lipids (e.g., hyperlipidemia) and paraproteins (e.g., multiple myeloma).

Evaluation of volume status is the first step in determining the cause of hyponatremia with hypo-osmolality (Figure 1). The most common cause is volume overload due to heart failure, cirrhosis, or the nephrotic syndrome. In each of these edematous states, the kidney is conserving both sodium and water because renal perfusion is compromised (by poor cardiac output, arteriovenous shunting, or decreased intravascular oncotic pressure, respectively). Renal conservation of sodium and water is documented by a low urine sodium concentration (<10 meq/L [10 mmol/L]) and highly concentrated urine (>450 mosm/kg [450 mmol/kg]). This results in water overload that is greater than sodium overload, but both are present. Symptomatic hyponatremia is uncommon, and aggressive treatment to raise the serum sodium level usually is unnecessary. The general approach to management is treatment of the underlying cause, dietary sodium restriction to 2-3 g/day, water restriction to 1-1.5 L/day, and adjunctive use of loop diuretics.

Hypo-osmolal hyponatremia associated with volume depletion manifests as dry mucous membranes, hypotension, and tachycardia. Volume loss can be gastrointestinal or renal or due to third-space fluid shifts. The urine indices reflect renal sodium conservation (urine sodium concentration <10 meq/L [10 mmol/L]) and water conservation (urine osmolality >450 mosm/kg [450 mmol/kg]). If volume loss is due to vomiting, a low urine chloride concentration is corroborative. Treatment is intravenous normal saline as well as managing the condition that precipitated the volume loss. Hypertonic saline is reserved for symptomatic hyponatremia. As volume is restored, the stimulus for ADH release will decrease, potentially leading to correction of the serum sodium concentration too quickly; consequently, serum sodium levels must be monitored closely. Correcting hyponatremia too rapidly can lead to central pontine myelinolysis, which is characterized by flaccid paral-

ysis, dysarthria, and dysphagia. The rate of sodium correction must be ≤0.3-0.5 meq/L/h [0.3-0.5 mmol/L/h].

Hypo-osmolal hyponatremia with euvolemia is caused by either massive intake of water or inability of the kidney to excrete a free water load. The normal renal capacity for water excretion is approximately 15 L/day. A massive increase in water intake occurs in psychogenic polydipsia or, rarely, in hypothalamic diseases. Urine indices are compatible with adequate intravascular volume (urine sodium concentration >20 meq/L [20 mmol/L]), and the urine is maximally dilute (50-100 mosm/kg [mmol/kg]). Treatment is water restriction.

Hypothyroidism, adrenal insufficiency, reset osmostat, inadequate osmoles, and syndrome of inappropriate ADH secretion (SIADH) all are associated with hyponatremia due to a renal defect in excreting free water. Thyroid and cortisol deficiencies lead to increased ADH release. The most common physiologic stimulus for reset osmostat is pregnancy, which contributes to the increase in plasma volume. At least 50 mosm [50 mmol] are needed to excrete 1 L of water; malnourished patients may not have

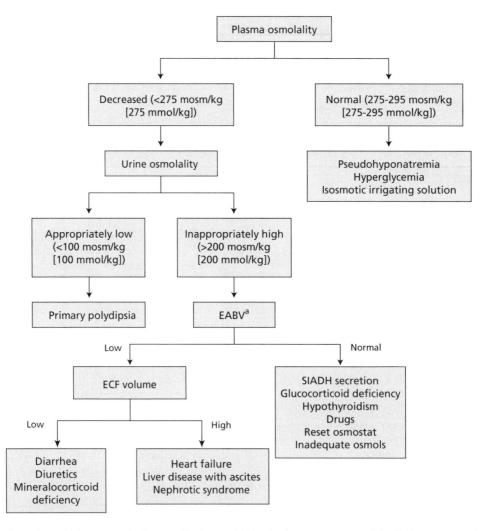

Figure 1. Approach to the patient with hyponatremia. EABV = effective arterial blood volume; ECF = extracellular fluid; SIADH = syndrome of inappropriate antidiuretic hormone secretion. ªThe clinical determination of EABV usually is straightforward. On physical examination, the best index of EABV is the pulse and blood pressure. Urine electrolyte levels also are extremely useful in assessing EABV. A low EABV is characterized by low urine sodium and chloride levels and low fractional excretion of sodium and chloride in the urine. In patients with normal serum creatinine levels, a high BUN (blood urea nitrogen) level suggests a low EABV, whereas a low BUN level suggests a high EABV.

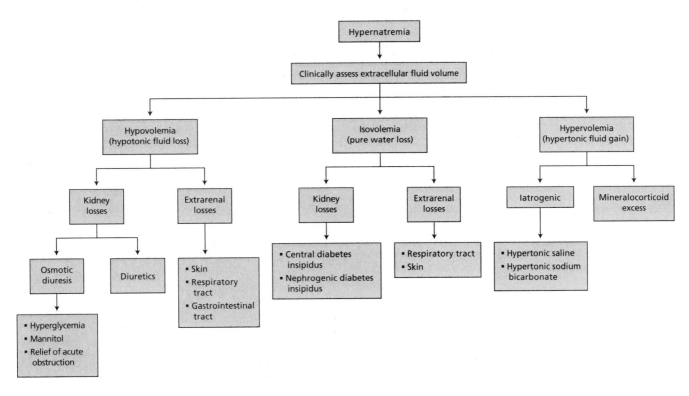

Figure 2. Approach to the patient with hypernatremia. All of these states are associated with impairment of thirst or access to water.

adequate osmoles to excrete excess free water. Treatment is water restriction until nutrition can be corrected. SIADH always is associated with hyponatremia but is a diagnosis of exclusion. Urine indices are compatible with euvolemia (urine sodium concentration >20 meq/L [20 mmol/L]), but the urine is inappropriately concentrated in the face of plasma hypo-osmolality. SIADH often is accompanied by very low serum uric acid and blood urea nitrogen levels, which help differentiate it from other causes of hyponatremia. Causes of SIADH include malignancy (e.g., small cell carcinoma of the lung), intracranial pathology, and pulmonary diseases, especially disorders that increase intrathoracic pressure and decrease venous return to the heart.

Symptoms occur at a serum sodium level of 110 meq/L (110 mmol/L) and include obtundation, coma, seizures, and death (if untreated). In general, symptoms tend to be worse when the hyponatremia develops quickly. Serum sodium level should be corrected to 120 meq/L (120 mmol/L) at a rate of 1-2 meq/L/h (1-2 mmol/L/h); once this level is achieved, the rate of correction is slowed to 0.3-0.5 meq/L/h (0.3-0.5 mmol/L). The quantity of sodium chloride required to increase the serum sodium concentration is calculated as:

$$\text{TBW (L)} \times (\text{desired serum [sodium]}$$
$$- \text{actual serum [sodium] where the desired [sodium]}$$
$$\text{is 120 meq/L (120 mmol/L)}$$

The intravenous vasopressin receptor antagonist conivaptan and the oral vasopressin receptor antagonist tolvaptan are approved for the treatment of euvolemic and hypervolemic hyponatremia. These agents should not be used to treat hypovolemic

hyponatremia. As with the administration of saline, care must be taken to prevent overly rapid correction of the serum sodium concentration. The efficacy of tolvaptan may be limited by stimulated thirst.

Hypernatremia

Hypernatremia is a serum sodium concentration >145 meq/L (145 mmol/L). All hypernatremia is associated with intracellular fluid contraction, and both thirst and ADH levels should be elevated. Therefore, severe hypernatremia indicates a defective thirst mechanism, inadequate access to water, and/or a renal concentrating defect. The brain generates idiogenic osmoles to protect the intracellular volume within 4 hours of development of hypernatremia, and the process stabilizes within 4 to 7 days. Symptoms of hypernatremia include weakness, lethargy, seizures, and coma. The approach to the patient with hypernatremia begins with assessment of volume status, as outlined in Figure 2. Hypernatremia associated with volume overload is unusual and often iatrogenic. Rarely, mild hypernatremia and volume overload occur with Cushing syndrome or primary hyperaldosteronism. Spontaneous diuresis often self-corrects volume overload hypernatremia, but on rare occasion, diuretic or dialysis therapy with simultaneous free water replacement is necessary.

Most commonly, hypernatremia is due to loss of hypotonic fluids with inadequate water replacement. Hypernatremia associated with volume depletion occurs with gastrointestinal, renal, cutaneous, or pulmonary losses. Therapy includes sodium chloride replacement, free water replacement, and correction of the underlying problem leading to hypotonic fluid loss. The water deficit is estimated by the formula:

$$\text{Water deficit} = TBW - (\text{desired [sodium]}/ \\ \text{current [sodium]}) \times TBW$$

Because of the presence of idiogenic osmoles created by the brain to protect intracellular fluid volume, correcting hypernatremia too quickly can lead to cerebral edema. Extreme care must be taken to correct serum sodium concentration at a rate ≤1 meq/L/h (1 mmol/L/h), with a goal of 50% correction at 24 to 36 hours and complete correction in 3 to 7 days.

Central diabetes insipidus is a partial or complete deficiency of ADH production and/or release, resulting in inadequate concentration of the urine. Provided the patient has access to water, the serum sodium concentration is normal. The presence of hypernatremia indicates loss of free water, and treatment is water replacement and administration of ADH (desmopressin, vasopressin). Nephrogenic diabetes insipidus is an insensitivity of the cortical collecting duct to circulating ADH and can be caused by drugs (e.g., lithium, foscarnet), hypokalemia, hypercalcemia, sickle cell disease and trait, and amyloidosis. Treatment requires adequate water intake, salt restriction, and, in some cases, a thiazide diuretic. Thiazide diuretics effectively block sodium reabsorption in the distal renal tubule, thereby causing natriuresis. Patients with an intact thirst mechanism do not develop significant hypernatremia unless their access to water is restricted by unconsciousness, immobility, or an altered mental status.

Potassium Metabolism

Serum potassium concentration is tightly regulated. Most of the body's potassium is intracellular and is maintained by the integrity of the cell membrane and sodium-potassium adenosine triphosphate (Na^+,K^+-ATPase). Because potassium is a steady-state ion, intake must equal output in order to maintain balance. Typical dietary intake of potassium is 50-100 meq/day (50-100 mmol/day), and renal excretion can be up to 1000 meq/day (1000 mmol/day). Potassium is excreted primarily (90%) by the kidneys. Normal renal handling of potassium depends on adequate glomerular filtration, aldosterone, intact distal tubular function, distal tubular flow, distal tubular sodium delivery, acid-base status, and intracellular potassium stores. Intracellular potassium balance is further affected by shifting of potassium between the intracellular fluid and extracellular fluid due to circulating insulin, catecholamines, acid-base status, and plasma osmolality.

Hypokalemia

Hypokalemia (serum potassium concentration <3.5 meq/L [3.5 mmol/L]) can result from potassium loss or intracellular shift in potassium; it is rarely due to inadequate potassium intake. The most common causes of potassium loss are gastrointestinal and renal (diuretics). Rare causes include primary aldosteronism, Bartter syndrome, Gitelman syndrome, and periodic paralysis. Bartter syndrome is caused by various genetic mutations in the sodium-potassium-chloride (Na^+-K^+-2Cl^-) cotransporter in the thick ascending limb of the loop of Henle, which produce a clin-

ical picture similar to that seen with chronic loop diuretic therapy (i.e., hypokalemia, hypomagnesemia, and varying degrees of hypocalcemia). Gitelman syndrome is a milder disorder caused by mutations in the sodium-potassium (Na^+-Cl^-) cotransporter in the distal convoluted tubule, which lead to hypokalemia, hypomagnesemia, and metabolic alkalosis. Bartter and Gitelman syndromes differ from primary hyperaldosteronism (another cause of hypokalemia) in that patients are not hypertensive. Hypokalemic periodic paralysis is caused by a genetic defect leading to mutations in voltage-sensitive calcium or sodium channels. These patients will have profound weakness, especially in proximal muscles, and are at risk for life-threatening cardiac arrhythmias due to hypokalemia caused by excessive intracellular shifting of potassium in response to a meal high in carbohydrates or sodium. Manifestations of hypokalemia are ileus, muscle cramps, paralysis, rhabdomyolysis, impaired insulin secretion, and cardiac arrhythmias. Electrocardiographic findings of hypokalemia include U waves and flat or inverted T waves (Figure 3). Hypomagnesemia should always be suspected in patients with hypokalemia, because these ions often are lost together and magnesium is necessary for renal conservation of potassium.

Hypokalemia is treated with oral or intravenous potassium salts. In severe cases, potassium is given intravenously at a rate ≤20-40 meq/h (20-40 mmol/h) and at a concentration ≤40 meq/L (40 mmol/L). Although total potassium deficits are difficult to predict, a serum potassium level of 3 meq/L (3 mmol/L) is equivalent to a deficit of 200-400 meq (200-400 mmol), and a serum potassium level of 2 meq/L (2 mmol/L) is equivalent to a deficit of 400-800 meq (400-800 mmol).

Hyperkalemia

Excessive dietary intake of potassium rarely is a cause of hyperkalemia unless there is coexisting kidney disease. Potassium may shift out of cells secondary to tissue injury (e.g., rhabdomyolysis, hemolysis), hyperosmolality, insulin deficiency, β-adrenergic blockade, metabolic acidosis, or inhibition of Na^+,K^+-ATPase activity (e.g., by digoxin toxicity) and cause hyperkalemia. Decreased renal potassium excretion occurs if there is reduced

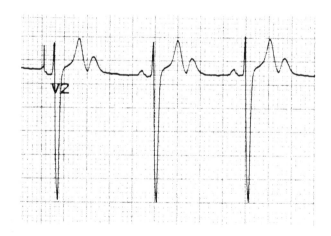

Figure 3. The characteristic electrocardiographic finding in hypokalemia is the appearance of a U wave after the T wave, eventually replacing the T wave.

glomerular filtration, poor distal tubular urine flow (e.g., hypovolemia or reduced effective circulating volume), aldosterone deficiency, or tubulointerstitial disease leading to aldosterone unresponsiveness. Several medications (e.g., ACE inhibitors, angiotensin II receptor blockers, NSAIDs, β-blockers) decrease aldosterone production by decreasing angiotensin II levels. Heparin and cyclosporine also decrease aldosterone production. Potassium-sparing diuretics that inhibit aldosterone effect (e.g., spironolactone) or block sodium channels in the collecting duct (e.g., triamterene, amiloride) can lead to hyperkalemia. Trimethoprim and pentamidine similarly block sodium channels and can cause hyperkalemia.

Hyporeninemic hypoaldosteronism commonly causes mild hyperkalemia and is characterized by deficient angiotensin II production due to both decreased renin production and an intra-adrenal defect leading to aldosterone deficiency. This syndrome most commonly is associated with diabetic nephropathy but also may occur in patients with chronic interstitial nephritis, renal transplant recipients taking cyclosporine, patients with HIV infection, and patients using NSAIDs. Severe hyperkalemia is uncommon unless there is also renal insufficiency.

Acute hyperkalemia causes muscle weakness or flaccid paralysis. The cardiac toxicity is associated with peaked T waves, flattened P waves, and widened QRS complexes on electrocardiography (Figure 4). Ventricular arrhythmias result from an increased resting membrane potential and are managed acutely with intravenous calcium, which raises the threshold for depolarization. Other measures include shifting potassium into cells with sodium bicarbonate, β-adrenergic agonists, or insulin and glucose, or augmenting excretion of potassium with loop diuretics (e.g., furosemide), cation-exchange resins (e.g., sodium polystyrene sul-

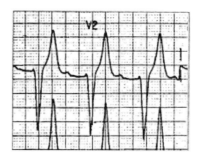

Figure 4. Electrocardiogram demonstrating tall, peaked T waves characteristic of hyperkalemia.

fonate), or dialysis. Chronic hyperkalemia is managed with a low-potassium diet, loop diuretics, and avoidance of drugs known to increase serum potassium levels.

Book Enhancement

Go to www.acponline.org/essentials/nephrology-section.html. In *MKSAP for Students 5*, assess your knowledge with items 20-25 in the **Nephrology** section.

Bibliography

Ellison DH, Berl T. Clinical practice. The syndrome of inappropriate antidiuresis. N Engl J Med. 2007;356:2064-2072. [PMID: 17507705]

Gennari FJ. Disorders of potassium homeostasis. Hypokalemia and hyperkalemia. Crit Care Clin. 2002;18:273-288, vi. [PMID: 12053834]

Lien YH, Shapiro JI. Hyponatremia: clinical diagnosis and management. Am J Med. 2007;120:653-658. [PMID: 17679119]

Chapter 65

Calcium and Phosphorus Metabolism

Mary Jane Barchman, MD

Calcium is a vital regulator of numerous cellular functions. An average daily diet contains 1000 mg of calcium, 200 to 400 mg of which is absorbed by the intestine when adequate vitamin D is present. The remainder is excreted in the urine and stool. Most of the total body calcium resides in bone. Calcium in the extracellular fluid exists in three forms: ionized (the metabolically active fraction), bound to protein (primarily albumin), and complexed with organic ions. The protein-bound calcium fraction increases with alkalosis (ionized calcium decreases) and decreases with acidosis (ionized calcium increases).

Phosphorus is a critical component of cellular energy metabolism and bone formation. Bone mineral accounts for approximately 90% of total body phosphorus; 10% of phosphorus exists in the intracellular fluid, and <1% is present in the extracellular fluid. Approximately 70% of blood phosphorus is contained in phospholipids. The remaining inorganic phosphorus exists as either protein-bound or free phosphorus or is complexed with circulating cations. Average daily dietary phosphorus intake varies between 800 and 1800 mg of phosphate, of which about half is absorbed in the small intestine.

Regulation of calcium and phosphorus metabolism are tightly linked through the action of parathyroid hormone (PTH), vitamin D, and, to a lesser extent, calcitonin (Figure 1). The primary role of PTH is to prevent hypocalcemia. The calcium-sensing receptor is located on cell membranes of the parathyroid gland and triggers release of preformed PTH into the circulation in response to low levels of ionized calcium. PTH returns ionized calcium levels to normal by rapidly mobilizing calcium and phosphate from bone stores and by increasing both gastrointestinal and renal absorption. PTH also up-regulates 1α-hydroxylase expression in the kidney, resulting in increased production of 1,25-dihydroxyvitamin D_3 ($1,25(OH)_2D_3$; calcitriol), the most active form of vitamin D, further increasing gastrointestinal absorption of calcium. Vitamin D_3 (cholecalciferol) is obtained from dietary sources but also is generated from cholesterol precursors by skin exposure to ultraviolet light, with ultimate conversion to 25-hydroxyvitamin D_3 ($25(OH)D_3$; calcidiol) by the liver. Measurement of serum $25(OH)D_2$ is the best indicator of total body vitamin D stores because of its long half-life. Calcitonin is secreted by thyroid parafollicular C cells in response to hypercalcemia and inhibits

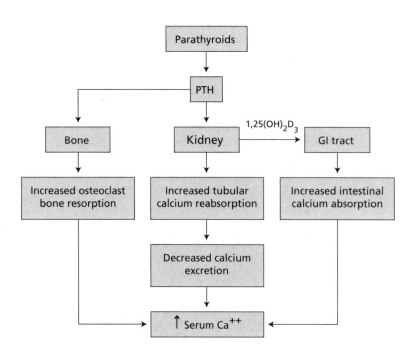

Figure 1. Overview of the metabolic systems that maintain calcium homeostasis. Ca^{++} = ionized calcium; GI = gastrointestinal; $1,25(OH)_2D_3$ = 1,25-dihydroxyvitamin D_3; PTH = parathyroid hormone; ↑ = increased.

osteoclast-mediated bone resorption. This effect is clinically insignificant in humans.

Hypocalcemia

Acute hypocalcemia leads to neuromuscular irritability (e.g., cramping, paresthesia, tetany, seizure, laryngospasm, prolonged QT interval). Mild hypocalcemia is well tolerated, especially if the reduction in ionized calcium has been gradual. Precipitous development of hypocalcemia is more likely to result in symptoms and may be detected by the presence of Chvostek sign (unilateral contraction of the facial muscles when the facial nerve is tapped just in front of the ear) and Trousseau sign (carpal spasm after occluding the brachial artery with an inflated blood pressure cuff).

In most cases, low total serum calcium levels are due to low albumin levels; the ionized calcium concentration is normal. In general, total calcium declines by 0.8 mg/dL (0.2 mmol/L) for each 1 g/dL (10 g/L) decrement in serum albumin concentration. The most common cause of acquired hypocalcemia is parathyroidectomy or vascular injury to the parathyroid glands. Other causes include autoimmune destruction and infiltrative diseases. Hypomagnesemia can cause hypocalcemia by impairing the release and activity of PTH. Patients who undergo subtotal parathyroidectomy may develop hungry bone syndrome, postoperatively characterized by hypocalcemia and hypophosphatemia. Vitamin D deficiency or resistance can cause mild hypocalcemia. Hyperphosphatemia due to chronic kidney disease, rhabdomyolysis, or tumor lysis syndrome may result in hypocalcemia caused by formation and deposition of calcium-phosphate complexes. Hypocalcemia also may complicate pancreatitis, when ionized calcium complexes with the free fatty acids are liberated by the action of pancreatic enzymes.

In patients with symptomatic hypocalcemia, treatment includes intravenous 10% calcium gluconate or calcium chloride. In less severe cases, calcium is replaced orally along with vitamin D; magnesium also must be replenished if serum values are low.

Hypercalcemia

Mild hypercalcemia (serum calcium level of 10.0-11.5 mg/dL [1.5-2.9 mmol/L]) usually is well tolerated and causes no symptoms. As serum calcium levels increase, more progressive symptoms occur, such as fatigue, weakness, polyuria, anorexia, nausea, vomiting, abdominal pain, pancreatitis, constipation, lethargy, and even coma. Serious cardiac dysrhythmias with a shortened QT interval may occur when serum calcium levels are >14 mg/dL (3.5 mmol/L). Chronic hypercalcemia due to hyperparathyroidism can lead to osteopenia, osteoporosis, nephrolithiasis, nephrocalcinosis, hypertension, progressive renal failure, and soft-tissue calcifications.

Causes for hypercalcemia are divided into PTH-mediated and non–PTH-mediated (Table 1). Non–PTH-mediated hypercalcemia is present when PTH is suppressed (<20 pg/mL [20 ng/L]). Malignancy is the most common cause and is responsible for most cases of hypercalcemia in hospitalized patients. The mechanism of hypercalcemia is related to humoral factors (PTH-related protein) or local osteolysis of bone. Granulomatous tissue

Table 1. Differential Diagnosis of Hypercalcemia

Disorder	Notes
Primary hyperparathyroidism	Often an incidental finding. Associated with elevated calcium, low phosphate, normal PTH (20%) or elevated PTH (80%), normal or elevated alkaline phosphatase, and normal or elevated urine calcium.
Humoral hypercalcemia of malignancy	Most common cause of hypercalcemia in patients with cancer, even in those with skeletal metastases. Associated with elevated calcium, normal or low phosphate (elevated if GFR <35 mL/min/1.73 m^2), suppressed PTH, normal or elevated PTHrP (not needed for diagnosis), normal or elevated alkaline phosphatase, and elevated urine calcium.
Metastatic bone disease	Hypercalciuria without hypercalcemia is most common. Associated with elevated calcium, normal or elevated phosphate, elevated alkaline phosphatase (most cases), suppressed PTH, and variable PTHrP.
Multiple myeloma	Common cause of hypercalcemia in patients with decreased GFR and anemia. Associated with elevated calcium, elevated phosphate, normal alkaline phosphatase, suppressed PTH, normal or low PTHrP, and abnormal serum protein immunoelectrophoresis.
Granulomatous disease (e.g., sarcoidosis, tuberculosis)	Associated with elevated calcium, elevated phosphate, elevated alkaline phosphatase (but may not be of skeletal origin), suppressed PTH, elevated urine calcium, and elevated vitamin D.
Milk-alkali syndrome	Consider in healthy persons in whom primary hyperparathyroidism has been excluded. Excessive ingestion of calcium-containing antacids may be present. Associated with elevated calcium, elevated phosphate, elevated creatinine, normal alkaline phosphatase, elevated bicarbonate, suppressed PTH, and variable urine calcium.
Benign familial hypocalciuric hypercalcemia	Constitutive overexpression of the calcium-sensing receptor gene. Elevated calcium, low phosphate, normal PTH, and a calcium-creatinine clearance ratio <0.01 [calculated as (urine calcium ÷ serum calcium) × (serum creatinine ÷ urine creatinine)].
Immobilization	Occurs in persons with high bone turnover before an immobilizing event (e.g., untreated primary hyperparathyroidism, hyperthyroidism, Paget disease of bone). Associated with elevated calcium, elevated phosphate, elevated alkaline phosphatase, suppressed PTH, and elevated urine calcium.
Hyperthyroidism	Hypercalcemia is a frequent incidental finding in hyperthyroidism, which results from direct stimulation of osteoclasts by thyroxine or tri-iodothyronine.

GFR = glomerular filtration rate; PTH = parathyroid hormone; PTHrP = parathyroid hormone–related protein.

(e.g., sarcoidosis, tuberculosis, leprosy) may express 1α-hydroxylase activity, resulting in excess vitamin D production with subsequent development of significant hypercalcemia.

Primary hyperparathyroidism is the most common cause of hypercalcemia in outpatients. Effects of excess PTH include increased $1,25(OH)_2D_3$ levels, increased osteoclast-mediated bone resorption, enhanced distal tubular reabsorption of calcium, decreased proximal tubular reabsorption of phosphorus, hypercalcemia, hypophosphatemia, and increased urine phosphate and calcium levels. Primary hyperparathyroidism is due to a solitary adenoma in about 85% of patients, with hyperplasia of all glands or multiple adenomas being less frequent. Multigland parathyroid hyperplasia should raise suspicion for multiple endocrine neoplasia types 1 and 2a. Surgical resection of a hyperfunctioning adenoma may be curative in those patients with primary hyperparathyroidism and manifestations of chronic hypercalcemia. Parathyroidectomy generally is indicated in asymptomatic patients with any of the following criteria: serum calcium level >1 mg/dL (0.25 mmol/L) above the upper limit of normal; creatinine clearance (calculated) <60 mL/min; reduction in bone mineral density of the femoral neck, lumbar spine, or distal radius >2.5 standard deviations below peak bone mass (T-score <−2.5); or age <50 years.

Secondary hyperparathyroidism is a normal physiologic response to chronically low calcium levels caused by chronic kidney disease, vitamin D deficiency, or gastrointestinal malabsorption. In secondary hyperparathyroidism, PTH is elevated, but calcium levels are low to low-normal.

Hypercalcemia requiring acute intervention is most common in the setting of malignancy. Due to the vasoconstrictive effects of calcium and a tendency toward nephrogenic diabetes insipidus with hypercalcemia, these patients usually are hypovolemic and require resuscitation with normal saline. Improved intravascular volume leads to improved glomerular filtration and increased sodium delivery to more distal nephron segments where calcium can be excreted. After generous volume resuscitation, calcium excretion can be further augmented by the addition of a loop diuretic; however, the variable utility and potential adverse effects of this measure (e.g., hypokalemia, aggravation of hypovolemia) and the availability of bisphosphonate therapy have led to a recent reappraisal of this approach. Bisphosphonates, given intravenously, may be used to decrease bone resorption and may have a prolonged effect. Calcitonin may be used to inhibit osteoclast-mediated bone resorption in hypercalcemia of malignancy but is of only modest benefit, and tachyphylaxis occurs quickly. The treatment of hypercalcemia due to granulomatous disease is directed at controlling the underlying process with corticosteroids or antimicrobial therapy as appropriate.

If a neoplastic process results in increased active vitamin D levels, oral corticosteroid therapy may be beneficial. In secondary hyperparathyroidism due to chronic kidney disease, a combination of calcitriol and phosphate binders is used to suppress serum PTH values to no more than 3 to 4 times the normal level. Tertiary hyperparathyroidism occasionally develops in these patients and is characterized by elevated serum PTH values despite elevated serum calcium levels. Cinacalcet is an agent for the treatment of secondary or tertiary hyperparathyroidism; the drug suppresses PTH secretion by acting primarily on the calcium-sensing receptor in the parathyroid glands. Cinacalcet may retard the development of renal bone disease while resulting in significantly less elevation in serum calcium and phosphorus levels. Its use is restricted to patients on hemodialysis.

Hyperphosphatemia

Hyperphosphatemia most often is due to phosphate retention caused by chronic kidney disease, but it also can occur with hypoparathyroidism, rhabdomyolysis, tumor lysis syndrome, acidosis, and overzealous phosphate administration. The symptoms of hyperphosphatemia are attributable to the attendant hypocalcemia. Most hyperphosphatemia is transient unless related to chronic kidney disease. Treatment of hyperphosphatemia associated with chronic kidney disease is a phosphorus-restricted diet, oral phosphate binders, saline diuresis, or dialysis (see Chapter 62).

Hypophosphatemia

Hypophosphatemia may result from impaired gastrointestinal absorption, increased renal excretion, or intracellular shift of phosphorus. Severe hypophosphatemia (serum phosphorus level <1 mg/dL [0.3 mmol/L]) usually indicates total body phosphate depletion and is characterized by muscle weakness, paresthesia, rhabdomyolysis, respiratory failure, heart failure, seizure, and coma; rarely, hemolysis, platelet dysfunction, and metabolic acidosis can occur. Moderate hypophosphatemia (serum phosphate level of 1.0-2.5 mg/dL [0.3-0.8 mmol/L]) is common in hospitalized patients but may not necessarily reflect total body phosphorus depletion. For example, insulin treatment of hyperglycemia will shift phosphate intracellularly. Refeeding syndrome is caused by a similar phenomenon; calories provided to a patient after a prolonged period of starvation serve as a stimulus for tissue growth, which consumes phosphorus in the form of phosphorylated intermediates such as adenosine triphosphate. Persons who chronically abuse alcohol frequently fall into this category, largely because of underlying poor nutrition. Acute respiratory alkalosis also can cause hypophosphatemia. Impaired absorption may be caused by excessive oral phosphate binders, chronic diarrhea/steatorrhea, and, rarely, inadequate intake. Persistent, moderate hypophosphatemia is treated with oral phosphorus replacement. Severe hypophosphatemia is treated with intravenous potassium phosphate or sodium phosphate. Patients who are hypophosphatemic often have associated hypokalemia and hypomagnesemia, which require correction.

Book Enhancement

Go to www.acponline.org/essentials/nephrology-section. In *MKSAP for Students 5*, assess your knowledge with items 26-29 in the **Nephrology** section.

Bibliography

Inzucchi SE. Management of hypercalcemia. Diagnostic workup, therapeutic options for hyperparathyroidism and other common causes. Postgrad Med. 2004;115:27-36. [PMID: 15171076]

Chapter 66

Approach to the Altered Mental State

Valerie J. Lang, MD

Normal consciousness is a state of awareness of self and the environment and the ability to interact with the environment. The normal conscious state requires that the brainstem reticular activating system and its cortical projections are intact and functioning. Alterations in mental status may range from a confused state with agitation or hypoactivity (delirium) to an unarousable, unresponsive state (coma), which may be followed by a persistent vegetative state. Delirium is an acute state of confusion, which may be characterized by a reduced level of consciousness, cognitive abnormalities, perceptual disturbances, and emotional disturbances. Because delirium is most common in the elderly, care should be taken not to confuse delirium with dementia. Coma is a sleeplike state in which the eyes are closed and the patient is unarousable even when vigorously stimulated. With the vegetative state, there is complete unawareness of self and surroundings but preserved sleep-wake cycles and at least partial preservation of hypothalamic and brainstem autonomic functions. The potential precipitating causes of altered mental status are broad and diverse (Table 1). Whether the patient has delirium, coma, or some mental state in between, each state represents a different stage of the same disease process and is investigated in the same manner.

Diagnosis

Coma

Coma is a medical emergency and requires rapid assessment and treatment. Cerebrovascular disease accounts for about 50% of cases of medical coma, and hypoxic injury accounts for another 20%. Toxic, metabolic, and infectious causes account for the remaining cases of coma. A focused history taken from family or bystanders may uncover important diagnostic clues.

The evaluation of coma should focus on finding the answer to three questions:

- Does the patient have meningitis?
- Are signs of a mass lesion present?
- Is this a diffuse syndrome of exogenous or endogenous metabolic cause?

A systematic physical examination often can answer these questions. The examination should be organized to collect information about level of consciousness, motor system activity, and cranial nerve reflexes. The Glasgow Coma Scale assesses the patient's level of consciousness and severity of neurologic deficit and is based on motor response, verbal response, and eye opening (Table 2).

Motor activity is assessed by observing the patient for spontaneous movement of the extremities (or following application of a noxious stimulus). Symmetric movement of the extremities suggests intact cerebral hemispheres and corticospinal tract. Asymmetric movement suggests a structural brain lesion, whereas no movement may attest to the depth of coma, bilateral cerebral dysfunction, or disruption of corticospinal tract at the level of the brainstem. Abnormal motor posturing (decorticate and decerebrate) may occur spontaneously or in response to noxious stimuli. Decorticate posturing consists of flexion of the elbows and wrists, adduction of the shoulders, and extension of the legs. Decerebrate posturing consists of extension of the legs and adduction of the shoulders, but the shoulders internally rotate, and the elbows and wrists extend. Patients with decorticate posturing generally have less severe neurologic injury and a better prognosis than patients with decerebrate posturing. The presence of myoclonic jerks strongly suggests a metabolic cause of coma, as does tremor and asterixis in the awake patient.

The most important brainstem reflexes are the pupillary light reflex, corneal reflex, and conjugate eye movements. Loss of the pupillary light reflex occurs with either brainstem herniation from an expanding temporal lobe mass or a primary brainstem lesion (e.g., stroke). Disparity in pupil size suggests a unilateral impingement on the third cranial nerve from temporal lobe herniation. Symmetric but small pupils may be an indication of overdose with opiates or sedative-hypnotic agents, whereas symmetric and large pupils may suggest overdose with cocaine or tricyclic antidepressants. In patients without structural brain lesions, the eyes will appear to be looking straight ahead. Eyes that deviate to one side suggest a large cerebral lesion; if hemiparesis has been detected, the eyes will look away from the paralyzed side. Spontaneous conjugate eye movement suggests that the third and sixth cranial nerves are intact, as is the medial longitudinal fasciculus connection between the nerves. If spontaneous movement is not present, the eyes are stimulated to move with the oculocephalic maneuver (i.e., by moving the patient's head quickly to the right or left). If the brainstem is intact, the eyes will rotate in the opposite direction of the head turn. This maneuver is performed in head trauma patients only after the integrity of the cervical spine has been confirmed with appropriate imaging studies. When head turning fails to elicit conjugate eye movement, the ear canal can be irrigated with cold water; a patient with an intact brainstem will have conjugate eye movement away from the irrigated ear. The corneal reflex is tested by touching the cornea with a wisp of cotton; the normal response is bilateral blinking.

Table 1. Precipitants of an Altered Mental State

Category	Notes
Metabolic	
Temperature	Fever or hypothermia (infection, environment, medication)
Hypernatremia	Diabetes insipidus, hypertonic fluid infusion
Hyponatremia	SIADH; thiazide diuretic; volume depletion; kidney, heart, or liver failure; CNS injury; psychogenic polydipsia
Hypercalcemia	Hyperparathyroidism, multiple myeloma, other cancer
Hypoglycemia	Medication (insulin, sulfonylurea), insulinoma (rarely)
Hyperosmolar	Type 2 diabetes mellitus (usually elderly patients), surgical use of hypertonic fluid (cystoscopy, hysteroscopy)
Hypothyroidism	Myxedema coma
Hyperthyroidism	Thyrotoxicosis, thyroid storm
Malnutrition	Advanced age, post–gastric bypass procedure
Thiamine deficiency	Wernicke encephalopathy (confabulation, ataxia, ophthalmoplegia)
Toxin	Illicit drug, alcohol, carbon monoxide
Medication	Centrally acting medication, polypharmacy (>6 total medications or >3 new medications increases delirium risk in elderly patients)
Dehydration	Decreased oral intake, diarrhea, diuretic
Structural brain lesion	Trauma, tumor, hemorrhage, abscess, ischemic infarction
Seizure	
Complex partial	Awake but with decreased responsiveness and awareness
Generalized	Characterized by loss of consciousness
Status epilepticus	Prolonged seizure (5-20 min) or repeated seizures without regaining consciousness between events
Postictal state	Prolonged somnolence, confusion, and headache following seizure
CNS infection	
Meningitis	Headache, meningismus, fever
Encephalitis	Headache, fever, focal neurologic findings
Subdural empyema	Fever, focal neurologic findings
Abscess	Fever, focal neurologic deficits, embolic or contiguous source
Delirium tremens (alcoholism)	Hallucinations, disorientation, tachycardia, hypertension, fever, agitation, and diaphoresis 48-72 h after last drink
Hypoxemia	Hypoventilation (narcotics), decreased oxygen-carrying capacity (anemia), lung disease, increased metabolic demand
Urinary retention	Bladder outlet obstruction (usually men), anticholinergic agent
Fecal impaction	Bed-bound elderly patient
Pain	Differentiate from side effects of opioid analgesic
Altered environment	Hospital admission, urinary catheter use, restraints, medication

CNS = central nervous system; SIADH = syndrome of inappropriate antidiuretic hormone secretion.

In brain death, patients are unresponsive and unarousable. There is no meaningful response to noxious stimuli, brainstem reflexes are absent, and there are no spontaneous respirations, while patients are off sedating medications and have no major metabolic disturbances, hypotension, or hypothermia.

Coma without focal signs, fever, or meningismus suggests a diffuse insult, such as hypoxia or a metabolic, toxic, drug-induced, infectious, or postictal state. In the case of coma after cardiac arrest, patients who lack pupillary and corneal reflexes at 24 hours and have no motor response at 72 hours have little chance of meaningful recovery. Coma without focal signs but with meningismus, with or without fever, suggests meningitis, meningoencephalitis, or subarachnoid hemorrhage. Coma with focal signs implies a structural lesion, such as stroke, hemorrhage, tumor, or abscess.

Patients with focal findings on examination or unexplained coma should have emergent imaging to exclude hemorrhage or mass lesion. Lumbar puncture is indicated when meningitis or subarachnoid hemorrhage is suspected but neuroimaging is normal. The possibility of nonconvulsive status epilepticus should be evaluated by emergent electroencephalography.

All patients should have a laboratory evaluation to assess for toxic and metabolic abnormalities, infection, or drug intoxication. Evaluation should include arterial blood gases, complete metabolic panel, complete blood count with differential, ammonia level, and drug and alcohol screen. More focused testing for salicylates, acetaminophen, or other specific drugs (e.g., tricyclic antidepressants) depends on the history and clinical suspicion.

Delirium

Delirium is associated with prolonged hospitalization, more frequent impairment of physical function, increased rates of institutionalization, subsequent development of dementia, and death. Delirium often results from both underlying vulnerability and acute precipitating factors. Predisposing factors include advanced age, cognitive impairment, multiple comorbidities, male gender, depression, alcohol abuse, and sensory impairment.

For patients with delirium, rapid detection, evaluation, and intervention are essential. Diagnosis of delirium is based on clinical information. The Confusion Assessment Method (Table 3) is a useful tool in diagnosing delirium (positive likelihood ratio = 9.6; negative likelihood ratio = 0.16). No laboratory tests, imaging studies, or other tests provide greater accuracy.

Look for association of the onset of delirium with other events, such as medication changes or development of physical symptoms. Also look for the presence of sensory deprivation (e.g., absence of glasses or hearing aids) or uncontrolled pain. Take a medication history with particular attention to sedative-hypnotic agents, barbiturates, alcohol, antidepressants, anticholinergic agents, opioid analgesics, antipsychotics, anticonvulsants, antihistamines, and antiparkinsonian agents, keeping in mind that drugs that are well tolerated in young patients can cause delirium in the elderly. The risk of delirium increases with the number of prescribed medications. Assess for signs of infection, heart failure, myocardial ischemia, dehydration, malnutrition, urinary retention, and fecal impaction. Tremor and asterixis are clues to metabolic encephalopathy secondary to liver or kidney failure.

Tailor the laboratory evaluation to the specific clinical situation (Table 4). In most patients, a complete blood count, basic metabolic panel (including sodium, calcium, bicarbonate, glucose, blood urea nitrogen, creatinine, and glucose), and urinalysis should be obtained. The yield of additional tests and procedures is low unless a specific condition is suggested by the history or physical examination. Brain imaging, although commonly used, usually is not helpful in the diagnosis of delirium unless there is a history of a fall or evidence of focal neurologic impairment.

Table 2. Glasgow Coma Scale

Best Motor Response	Score[a]
Obeying commands	6
Localizing to pain	5
Withdrawing to pain	4
Abnormal flexion (decorticate)	3
Extensor response (decerebrate)	2
None	1
Best Verbal Response	
Oriented	5
Confused conversation	4
Inappropriate words	3
Incomprehensible sounds	2
None	1
Eye Opening	
Spontaneous	4
To speech	3
To pain	2
None	1

[a]Scores are added and range from 3 to 15; lower scores indicate more severe deficits.

Table 3. Confusion Assessment Method for the Diagnosis of Delirium[a]

Feature	Assessment
1. Acute onset and fluctuating course	Usually obtained from a family member or nurse and shown by positive responses to the following questions:
	"Is there evidence of an acute change in mental status from the patient's baseline?"
	"Did the abnormal behavior fluctuate during the day, that is, tend to come and go, or increase and decrease in severity?"
2. Inattention	Shown by a positive response to the following question:
	"Did the patient have difficulty focusing attention, for example, being easily distracted or having difficulty keeping track of what was being said?"
3. Disorganized thinking	Shown by a positive response to the following question:
	"Was the patient's thinking disorganized or incoherent, such as rambling or irrelevant conversation, unclear or illogical flow of ideas, or unpredictable switching from subject to subject?"
4. Altered level of consciousness	Shown by any answer other than "alert" to the following question:
	"Overall, how would you rate this patient's level of consciousness?" (alert = normal; hyperalert = vigilant; drowsy, easily aroused = lethargic; difficult to arouse = stupor; unarousable = coma)

[a]The diagnosis of delirium requires the presence of features 1 and 2 plus either 3 or 4.
Adapted from Inouye SK, van Dyck CH, Alessi CA, Balkin S, Siegal AP, Horwitz RI. Clarifying confusion: the confusion assessment method. A new method for detection of delirium. Ann Intern Med. 1990;113:941-948. [PMID: 2240918]

Table 4. Laboratory and Other Studies for the Evaluation of Delirium

Test	Notes
Complete blood count	Screen for infection and anemia
Serum electrolytes, calcium	Screen for hypernatremia, hyponatremia, hypercalcemia, and acid-base abnormality
BUN, creatinine	Screen for dehydration and renal failure
Glucose	Screen for hypoglycemia, hyperglycemia, and hyperosmolar state
Urinalysis, culture	Screen for urinary tract infection
Aminotransferases, albumin, bilirubin, PT, ammonia	If liver failure and hepatic encephalopathy are suspected
Chest radiography	If pneumonia or heart failure is suspected or there is no obvious cause of delirium
Electrocardiography	If myocardial infarction or arrhythmia is suspected
Arterial blood gases	Helpful in patients with COPD, if hypercapnia or acid-base abnormality is suspected
Drug levels, toxin screen	If ingestion is suspected or patient is taking medication with narrow therapeutic window; keep in mind that delirium can occur with "normal" serum levels of a drug
Cerebral imaging	CT/MRI reserved for coma, patients with focal abnormalities on neurologic examination, head trauma, and other situations where suspicion is high or no cause is identified after initial evaluation
Lumbar puncture	Rarely helpful in the absence of high suspicion of meningitis, encephalitis, or subarachnoid hemorrhage
Electroencephalography	Rarely assists in the evaluation unless nonconvulsive status epilepticus is suspected

BUN = blood urea nitrogen; PT = prothrombin time.

Therapy

Coma

All patients with coma require the emergency ABCs of resuscitation (airway, breathing, circulation). In patients with unexplained coma, administer intravenous glucose (unless a rapid fingerstick glucose test determines normoglycemia) and thiamine for possible Wernicke encephalopathy. Administer naloxone if opiate overdose is a possibility. Flumazenil should be administered for benzodiazepine overdose; however, it can precipitate seizures in patients who take benzodiazepines chronically. Additional therapy is targeted to the specific underlying cause.

Delirium

Prevention of delirium includes interventions targeting specific risk factors, such as cognitive impairment, sleep deprivation, immobility, sensory impairment, and dehydration. Providing access to glasses and hearing aids; frequent reorientation to place, time, and date; minimizing nocturnal disruptions and increasing daytime stimulation to facilitate a normal sleep-wake cycle; and minimizing medication use can help prevent delirium. These measures also are instituted for patients with delirium, in addition to addressing the specific precipitants (e.g., hypoxemia, infection, pain) and managing the symptoms of delirium.

Antipsychotic agents should be used only when behavioral measures have been ineffective for symptom control and are necessary to prevent patient harm or to allow evaluation and treatment. Low-dose haloperidol, risperidone, and olanzapine are equally effective in treating agitation associated with delirium. However, both conventional and atypical antipsychotic agents are associated with increased risk of infection (most commonly pneumonia) and death when used in the elderly to treat delirium. All antipsychotic agents, and especially "typical" agents such as haloperidol, pose a risk of torsades de pointes and extrapyramidal side effects, as well as the neuroleptic malignant syndrome. Attempt to use the lowest dose of the least toxic agent that successfully controls the agitation. Use of benzodiazepines may worsen or prolong delirium and should be reserved for patients with alcohol withdrawal (treatment of choice).

Use of physical restraints generally is avoided, as these can increase patient agitation and the risk of patient injury. However, restraints can be used with caution if other measures to control a patient's behavior are ineffective and it seems likely that the patient, if unrestrained, may cause personal injury or injury to others.

Book Enhancement

Go to www.acponline.org/essentials/neurology-section. In *MKSAP for Students 5*, assess your knowledge with items 1-5 in the **Neurology** section.

Acknowledgment

We would like to thank Dr. Robert W. Neilson, Jr., who contributed to an earlier version of this chapter.

Bibliography

Booth CM, Boone RH, Tomlinson G, Detsky AS. Is this patient dead, vegetative, or severely neurologically impaired? Assessing outcome for comatose survivors of cardiac arrest. JAMA. 2004;291:870-879. [PMID: 14970067]

Young J, Murthy L, Westby M, Akunne A, O'Mahony R; Guideline Development Group. Diagnosis, prevention, and management of delirium: summary of NICE guidance. BMJ. 2010;341:c3704. doi: 10.1136/bmj.c3704. [PMID: 20667955]

Chapter 67

Headache

Eyad Al-Hibi, MD

Effective diagnosis and management of headache depend on: 1) recognizing the typical features, patterns, and prevalence of various headache syndromes; 2) attending to "red flags" in the history or physical examination; 3) using diagnostic studies wisely; and 4) developing an evidence-based strategy for treatment.

Primary headaches (e.g, migraine, tension-type headache, cluster headache) are headaches with no other known cause, whereas secondary headaches reflect an underlying structural, systemic, or infectious disorder (e.g., meningitis, giant cell arteritis). Features that suggest a secondary cause include the development of progressively frequent and severe headaches within 3 months; the presence of neurologic symptoms, focal or lateralizing neurologic signs, papilledema, or systemic symptoms (e.g., fever, night sweats, weight loss); headaches aggravated or relieved by postural changes; headaches precipitated by a Valsalva maneuver (cough, sneeze); history of sudden-onset headache; and headache onset after age 50 years. Most patients who are evaluated for headache have a primary headache disorder, and more than 90% of these patients have a type of migraine (Table 1).

Evaluation

Identify the pattern of headache and seek any "red flags" suggesting an underlying serious condition (tumor, aneurysm, infection). The odds of a significant abnormality on neuroimaging are increased if the patient reports rapidly increasing headache frequency, dizziness or lack of coordination, tingling, or awakening from sleep due to headache. Red flags on physical examination include focal or lateralizing neurologic findings, papilledema, fever, neck stiffness, meningeal signs, tenderness to palpation or diminished pulse over the temporal artery, diastolic blood pressure >120 mm Hg, and decreased visual acuity.

A neurologic abnormality on physical examination or any red flag symptom is an indication for neuroimaging. Noncontrast CT of the head is the procedure of choice when acute, sudden, severe headache suggests subarachnoid hemorrhage. A lumbar puncture is indicated if there is concern for meningitis (fever and neck stiffness) or encephalitis (focal neurologic signs, confusion, altered mental status) or if subarachnoid hemorrhage is suspected but

Table 1. Differential Diagnosis of Headache

Disorder	Notes
Tension-type headache	Lasts from 30 min to 7 d. Typically is bilateral, has a pressing or tightening quality, and is mild to moderate in intensity; not associated with nausea or vomiting. Headache is not aggravated by exertion and does not prohibit activity.
Migraine	Lasts from 4 to 72 h. May be unilateral, pulsating in quality, and moderate to severe in intensity; associated with nausea or vomiting, photophobia, and phonophobia.
Frontal sinusitis	Usually worse when lying down. Associated with nasal congestion. Tenderness overlies affected sinus.
Medication-overuse headache	Chronic headache with few features of migraine. Tends to occur daily in patients who frequently use headache medications.
Subarachnoid hemorrhage (see Chapter 71)	Sudden, explosive onset of severe headache ("worst headache of my life"). Sometimes preceded by "sentinel" headaches (10%).
Meningitis or encephalitis (see Chapter 70)	Meningitis is associated with fever and meningeal signs. Encephalitis is associated with neurologic abnormalities, confusion, altered mental state, or change in level of consciousness.
Benign intracranial hypertension (pseudotumor cerebri)	Often abrupt onset. Associated with nausea, vomiting, dizziness, blurred vision, and papilledema. Neurologic examination is normal but may reveal CN VI palsy. Headache aggravated by coughing, straining, or changing position. Cerebrospinal fluid pressure is elevated.
Intracranial neoplasm	Worse on awakening, generally progressive. Headache aggravated by coughing, straining, or changing position.
Temporal arteritis (see Chapter 97)	Occurs almost exclusively in patients aged >50 y. Associated with tenderness of the scalp and temporal artery, jaw claudication, and visual changes.
Trigeminal autonomic cephalalgias	Group of primary headache disorders characterized by excruciating unilateral headache that occurs in association with prominent cranial autonomic features (lacrimation, nasal congestion, rhinorrhea, conjunctival injection). Disorders include cluster headache, paroxysmal hemicrania, and SUNCT syndrome.
Cluster headache	Sudden-onset headache lasting minutes to hours. Sometimes occur several times per day (rare for migraine). Pattern repeats over a course of weeks, then disappears for months or years. Often associated with unilateral tearing and nasal congestion or rhinitis. Pain is severe, unilateral, and periorbital. More common in men but relatively uncommon overall (<1.0% prevalence).

CN = cranial nerve; SUNCT = short-lasting unilateral neuralgiform headache attacks with conjunctival injection and tearing.

imaging studies are normal. Lumbar puncture with measurement of the cerebrospinal fluid opening pressure is used to diagnose benign intracranial hypertension.

Migraine

Although tension-type headache is the most common type of headache reported in community-based surveys, migraine is the most common headache disorder seen in clinical practice and is frequently missed or misdiagnosed as another type of headache (i.e., tension-type or sinus headache). The criteria for diagnosis of migraine are well-established and can be recalled with the mnemonic POUND: Pulsatile quality (headache described as pounding or throbbing), One-day's duration (episode may last 4-72 hours if untreated), Unilateral in location, Nausea or vomiting, and Disabling intensity (altered usual daily activities during headache episode). The presence of ≥3 criteria is >90% predictive of migraine in patients consulting a physician for headache (Table 2). Fifteen percent to 20% of patients with migraine experience an aura. In >90% of these patients, the aura may consist of such visual symptoms as photopsia (sparks or flashes of light), fortification spectra (arcs of flashing light that often form a zigzag pattern), or a scotoma (an area of loss of vision surrounded by a normal field of vision). Paresthesia involving the hands, arms, and face or expressive or receptive language dysfunction also can occur.

Effective nonpharmacologic management strategies include avoidance of triggers, biofeedback, cognitive behavioral therapy, stress management, and relaxation therapy. Many patients with migraine can identify specific dietary triggers; elimination diets may decrease migraine symptoms substantially in some patients. Common dietary triggers include caffeine; nitrates or nitrites in preserved meats; phenylethylamine, tyramine, and xanthine in aged cheese, red wine, beer, champagne, and chocolate; monosodium glutamate (food additive); dairy products; and fatty foods. Relaxation training, thermal biofeedback with relaxation training, electromyographic biofeedback, and cognitive behavioral therapy reduce migraine frequency by 30% to 50%.

For acute attacks, treat as soon as possible to maximize the likelihood of rapid and sustained relief and to minimize the need for backup and rescue medication and subsequent emergency department visits. The treatment approach depends on several factors, including headache severity and frequency, associated symptoms (e.g., nausea, vomiting), and coexisting medical conditions. Intranasal and parenteral routes of drug administration should be used in patients with severe nausea or vomiting. Mild attacks are effectively treated with NSAIDs (including aspirin) or acetaminophen; more severe attacks are treated with a triptan (selective serotonin receptor agonist) medication. Triptans have the highest overall efficacy rates for moderate to severe migraine, but they are contraindicated in the presence of cardiovascular disease. Dihydroergotamine is an alternative to a triptan for acute migraine treatment but may not be as effective and is contraindicated in coronary artery disease and pregnancy. Dihydroergotamine should not be used concomitantly with a triptan. Acute therapies should not be taken more often than 2 to 3 days per week to avoid medication-overuse (rebound) headaches.

Taking a daily preventive medication typically reduces headache frequency by one third to half. Preventive therapy may be indicated for patients with frequent disabling headaches (usually ≥2 headaches per month), poor relief from appropriately used acute therapies, or uncommon migraine, such as basilar or hemiplegic migraine. Other appropriate candidates for preventive medications are patients with a contraindication to acute therapy, failure or overuse of acute therapy, adverse effects from acute therapy, or a preference for preventive therapy. Level I evidence supports the use of the following drugs, herbs, and nonpharmacologic approaches for migraine prevention: topiramate, valproic acid (divalproex sodium, sodium valproate), amitriptyline, metoprolol, propranolol, timolol, butterbur (root extract from the plant *Petasites hybridus*), relaxation therapy, and biofeedback. Efficacy can be maximized and side effects minimized by starting medications at a low dose and increasing slowly to the target dose.

Tension-Type Headache

Tension-type headaches have a 1-year prevalence of approximately 40%. Tension-type headaches may last minutes to days. Patients describe bilateral, pressing pain of mild to moderate intensity not aggravated by physical activities and without nausea. Chronic tension-type headache is present at least 50% of days and has a significant impact on the patient's daily life. Nonpharmacologic treatments include biofeedback training and cognitive behavioral therapy. Drug treatment usually begins with NSAIDs. Prophylaxis, often with a tricyclic antidepressant, may be needed.

Chronic Daily Headache

Chronic daily headache is a nonspecific term that refers to headache that is present >15 days per month for ≥3 months. The headache may be a primary or secondary headache. Risk factors for chronic daily headache include obesity, a history of >1 headache per week, caffeine consumption, and overuse of acute headache medications. Patients usually have significant disability secondary to pain, and many have depression, anxiety, panic disorder, or sleep disturbance requiring diagnosis and treatment.

Medication-Overuse Headache

Medication-overuse headache (previously referred to as analgesic rebound headache) is defined as daily or near-daily headache (≥15 days per month) in a patient with a primary headache disorder and

Table 2. Posttest Probability of Migraine

Number of Diagnostic Criteria[a]	Pretest Probability (%)[b]		
	20	50	80
0, 1, or 2	5	15	50
3	75	94	99
4 or 5	90	96	>99

[a]The 5 diagnostic criteria for migraine are: pulsatile quality, 1-day duration, unilateral location, nausea or vomiting, and disabling intensity.

[b]The pretest probability of migraine is 5%-20% among the general population but at least 50% among persons consulting a physician for headache. Additional factors (e.g., family history of headaches or migraine) can raise the pretest probability closer to 80%.

medication overuse. Overuse is defined as the use of acute headache medications on a regular basis for more than three months. Examples of overuse include simple analgesics (e.g., acetamonophen) or combination of drugs on ≥15 days a month. When the offending medication is withheld, "withdrawal" headaches ensue. There is agreement that opioids, butalbital combinations, isometheptene combinations, over-the-counter analgesic combinations, decongestants, ergotamine, and triptans can result in this pattern. Treatment is withdrawal of medication.

Cluster Headache

The trigeminal autonomic cephalalgias are a group of primary headache disorders characterized by excruciating unilateral headache that occurs in association with prominent cranial autonomic features, such as lacrimation, nasal congestion, rhinorrhea, and conjunctival injection. Cluster headache is the most common trigeminal cephalalgia, although it is much less common than migraine or tension-type headache. Prevalence is three times higher in men than in women.

Cluster headaches are characterized by unilateral, severe, boring pain that is usually orbital, supraorbital, and/or temporal in location. Onset to peak intensity is usually minutes, with the pain lasting 15 minutes to 3 hours. Frequency ranges from one headache every other day to eight per day. Accompanying autonomic symptoms include lacrimation, nasal congestion, rhinorrhea, miosis, ptosis, and conjunctival injection. The attacks occur in clusters that last weeks to months, with remissions lasting months to years. Oxygen inhalation delivered via a non-rebreather face mask at a flow rate of 7 L/min is often effective in terminating the attack. Subcutaneous sumatriptan is the other mainstay of acute therapy.

Book Enhancement

Go to www.acponline.org/essentials/neurology-section.html. In *MKSAP for Students 5*, assess your knowledge with items 6-9 in the **Neurology** section.

Bibliography

Wilson JF. In the clinic. Migraine. Ann Intern Med. 2007;147:ITC11-1-ITC11-16 [published erratum appears in Ann Intern Med. 2008; 148:408]. [PMID: 17975180]

Chapter 68

Dementia

Mark Allee, MD

Dementia is an acquired, persistent impairment of intellectual function with compromise in at least three of the following spheres of mental activity: language, memory, visuospatial skills, emotion or personality, and cognition (abstraction, calculation, judgment, executive function). This loss of function must be sufficiently severe to cause social or occupational disability. Advancing age is the major risk factor for dementia. Common causes include Alzheimer disease (50%-75%), vascular dementia (10%-20%), dementia with Lewy bodies (10%-15%), and frontotemporal dementia (5%-15%). Important conditions in the differential diagnosis of dementia are listed in Table 1. Dementia should be further differentiated from delirium, a state of mental confusion that develops quickly and usually fluctuates in intensity (Table 2; see Chapter 66). Dementia and delirium may coexist.

Dementia is the result of structural neuronal changes. The signature pathologic feature of Alzheimer disease is the deposition of insoluble, neurotoxic β-amyloid protein in extracellular parenchymal plaques. Another characteristic finding is the intracellular accumulation of neurofibrillary tangles composed of abnormal microtubule-associated tau protein; these tangles are quantitatively associated with the severity of dementia. The central cholinergic deficit associated with Alzheimer disease results from early degeneration of the basal forebrain and is the rationale behind cholinergic augmentation. Patients with Alzheimer disease have a normal neurologic examination except for characteristic broad-based cognitive impairment and prominent recent memory impairment.

Vascular dementia is causally related to cerebrovascular disease and may result from large-vessel occlusions, multiple small-vessel occlusions, or primary hemorrhagic processes; small-vessel cerebrovascular disease is the most common cause. In practice, at least one third of patients with vascular dementia experience an insidious disease onset and gradual decline. Many of these patients also lack both a clear history of stroke and focal neurologic signs on examination.

Dementia with Lewy bodies is a degenerative condition characterized by intraneuronal Lewy body inclusions in the cerebral cortex. Dementia with Lewy bodies is characterized by parkinsonism that is responsive to dopaminergic therapy, visual hallucinations, and/or fluctuating cognition.

Frontotemporal dementia is found in a variety of diseases associated with disproportionate atrophy of the frontal and anterior temporal brain regions, including Pick disease, and, occasionally, motor neuron disease. Many of these conditions are associated with the deposition of tau-positive inclusions in affected neurons; however, the cause of these tau deposits is not known. Patients

Table 1. Important Disorders in the Differential Diagnosis of Dementia

Disorder	Notes
Alzheimer disease	Gradual memory loss, preserved level of consciousness. Seizure, falls, tremor, weakness, and reflex abnormalities are not typical early in the disease. As the illness progresses, other cortical deficits (aphasia, apraxia, agnosia, inattention, left-right confusion) develop.
Creutzfeldt-Jakob disease	Rapid progression, early age at onset, prominent myoclonus, characteristic EEG pattern of triphasic sharp waves. CSF protein 14-3-3 has good diagnostic specificity, but diffusion-weighted MRI may be more sensitive and specific.
Delirium	Altered level of alertness and attention often in conjunction with globally impaired cognition. Onset may be abrupt. Fluctuating level of alertness is common.
Dementia with Lewy bodies	Mild parkinsonism, hallucinations, and delusions early in the illness course.
Depression	Low mood, reduced enjoyment of activities, diminished sense of self-worth or confidence, hopelessness, decreased appetite, decreased libido, disturbed sleep. May have increased somatic complaints, irritability, and wishes for death.
Frontotemporal dementia (including Pick disease)	Onset often before age 60 y. Language difficulties are common, as are behavioral disturbances, impulsivity, aggression, and apathy. Functional neuroimaging often shows diminished function in frontal and/or temporal lobes.
Mild cognitive impairment	Objective memory impairment in the absence of other cognitive deficits and intact ADL. Patients with mild cognitive impairment progress to dementia at a rate of about 12%-15% per year.
Normal pressure hydrocephalus	Triad of dementia, gait abnormality, and urinary incontinence associated with psychomotor slowing and apathy. Ventriculoperitoneal shunting may be curative.
Vascular dementia	Loss of function may be temporally correlated with cerebrovascular events. May be associated with "silent" strokes, multiple small strokes, or presence of cerebrovascular risk factors.

ADL = activities of daily living; CSF = cerebrospinal fluid; EEG = electroencephalogram.

Table 2. Delirium and Dementia

Feature	Delirium	Dementia
Onset	Abrupt, with identifiable date	Gradual, cannot be dated
Duration	Acute, generally lasting days to weeks (rarely months)	Long duration, progresses over years
Clinical course	Usually reversible, often completely	Chronically progressive
Disorientation	Early finding	Late finding
Mental status	Variable moment to moment	Generally stable from day to day
Memory	Both short- and long-term loss	Short-term loss is greatest
Vital signs	Prominent physiologic changes	Typically normal
Attention span	Strikingly short	Usually reduced
Sleep-wake cycle	Hour-to-hour variation	Day-night reversal
Psychomotor activity	Early psychomotor changes (hyper- or hypoactive)	Late psychomotor changes

with frontotemporal dementia demonstrate early changes in executive function and personality.

Prevention

Treatment and control of hypertension, hyperlipidemia, and diabetes mellitus reduces the incidence of vascular dementia. Specific lifestyle modifications, such as smoking cessation, engaging in regular physical exercise and mental activities (solving puzzles), and avoiding head trauma, also may be beneficial.

Screening

Although there is insufficient evidence of a benefit for dementia screening in the general population, consider screening patients aged >70 years and younger patients with risk factors for cerebrovascular disease, a history of stroke, or other neurologic conditions. If screening is undertaken, use a standardized cognitive screening test and interview a family member or caregiver. The Mini–Mental State Examination (MMSE) is the most well-known and validated screening test; it has a sensitivity of 87% and a specificity of 82% in discriminating patients with Alzheimer disease from normal controls, using a cutoff score of 24 (of a maximum 30 points). The MMSE is sensitive to cognitive change over time, but it may be insensitive for mild dementia.

Diagnosis

Specifically inquire about memory loss, getting lost, word-finding difficulties, and difficulties with dressing, grooming, and housework. Mild dementia (MMSE score of 20-23) implies that cognitive loss has progressed to a point of causing problems with normal daily activities, such as misplacing items, becoming lost in familiar places, and experiencing deterioration in personal care. Moderate dementia (MMSE score of 10-19) is characterized by impaired cognitive abilities (e.g., language) and disability in performing basic daily activities such as running a household. Patients with severe dementia (MMSE score of 0-9) require assistance with all basic activities of daily living. Changes in the patient's emotional state could indicate underlying depression. Perform a compre-

hensive neurologic examination to look for concurrent central nervous system disease. Look for evidence of gait abnormalities, falls, weakness, clumsiness, sensory abnormalities, incontinence, and rigidity. Perform a mental status examination (e.g., MMSE) to evaluate level of alertness, orientation, concentration, abstract reasoning, memory, and mood.

Diagnostic testing may disclose a reversible cause of the dementia (Table 3). Obtain CT or MRI scans of the head in all patients. Features that may predict a radiographic abnormality include symptoms of <3 years' duration, rapid progression, early age at onset, focal neurologic deficits, cerebrovascular disease risk factors, recent history of head trauma or central nervous system infection, and a clinical picture atypical for Alzheimer disease. Consider other studies (lumbar puncture, electroencephalogram, neuropsychological testing) only when the clinical picture suggests a specific underlying disease or the clinical course is unusual. Patients with chronic dementia presenting with acute to subacute deterioration need further assessment for a reversible cause. The differential diagnosis of this deterioration can include cerebral ischemia (stroke, vasculitis), infection (urinary tract infection, meningitis, pneumonia), metabolic conditions (hyperglycemia, hepatic insufficiency, kidney disease), intoxications (alcohol, medication side effect or overdose), trauma (concussion, subdural hematoma), and structural lesions (brain mass, obstructive hydrocephalus).

Therapy

Adopt a proactive approach to maximize patients' functional status by assessing and treating psychiatric and behavioral symptoms with nonpharmacologic interventions. Educate patients and their caregivers about sleep hygiene, specifically addressing sleep scheduling, nap restriction, daily physical activity, reduction of caffeine intake, and evaluation of nocturia. Local and national organizations such as the Alzheimer's Association (www.alz.org) may be useful to clinicians and families.

The major goal of pharmacotherapy is to delay cognitive and functional decline and to treat symptoms. Cholinesterase inhibitors are indicated for Alzheimer disease, dementia with Lewy bodies, and mixed Alzheimer disease and vascular dementia. These

Table 3. Laboratory and Other Studies for Dementia

Test	Notes
Recommended Studies in All Patients	
MRI or CT scan	Numerous expert consensus statements recommend neuroimaging to discover unsuspected structural lesions.
Complete blood count	Leukocytosis, anemia, or thrombocytopenia may indicate a condition related to cognitive problems.
Metabolic profile	Abnormal sodium, calcium, glucose, and liver or kidney function can be related to cognitive problems.
Thyroid-stimulating hormone	Thyroid disease can cause cognitive problems.
Vitamin B_{12}	If low-normal, measure methylmalonic acid and homocysteine (see Chapter 42).
Rapid plasma reagin (RPR)	Tertiary syphilis can cause dementia.
Suggested Studies in Selected Patients	
HIV antibody	Advanced HIV disease can lead to dementia.
Toxicology screen	Screen for benzodiazepines.
Erythrocyte sedimentation rate	Consider vasculitis and systemic rheumatologic diseases, including systemic lupus erythematosus.
Heavy metal screen	Useful when there is environmental exposure.
Folate	Consider in the setting of very poor nutrition.
Urinalysis	Look for infection, malignancy, or other systemic diseases.
Lumbar puncture	Consider in the setting of a reactive RPR; patient aged <55 y; rapidly progressive dementia; immunosuppression; possible CNS metastatic cancer, infection, or vasculitis; possible hydrocephalus or Creutzfeldt-Jakob disease.
Electroencephalogram	Obtain in the setting of delirium, seizures, encephalitis, or possible Creutzfeldt-Jakob disease.
Neuropsychologic testing	May be helpful in the differential diagnosis of Alzheimer disease, to distinguish from frontotemporal dementia, major depression, mild cognitive impairment, or normal aging.

CNS = central nervous system.

agents are approved for the treatment of mild to moderate dementia. Commonly used cholinesterase inhibitors include donepezil, galantamine, and rivastigmine. These medications are initiated once the diagnosis has been made and the patient is medically and psychiatrically stable. As a class, cholinesterase inhibitors may modestly improve deficits and in some instances produce temporary partial improvement. The treatment must be continuous, without lengthy interruptions. Memantine, a noncompetitive NMDA (N-methyl-D-aspartate)-receptor antagonist used in the treatment of moderate to severe dementia, can be added to a stable dose of a cholinesterase inhibitor or used alone. In patients with vascular dementia, aggressively control hypertension, hyperlipidemia, hypothyroidism, vitamin B_{12} deficiency, and diabetes. Aspirin may help to stabilize or improve cognition in patients with vascular dementia by preventing further cerebrovascular events.

Treat concomitant depression but avoid antidepressants with anticholinergic side effects, such as tricyclic antidepressants (amitriptyline, nortriptyline). Consider using an antipsychotic medication in the treatment of hallucinations and delusions or behavioral disturbances (aggression, severe irritability, agitation, explosiveness), if there is risk of harm to the patient or others or if patient distress is significant and nonpharmacologic treatments have been ineffective. Atypical neuroleptic agents (risperidone, olanzapine, quetiapine) may be beneficial and should be initiated at low doses. The FDA has issued a black box warning for all six atypical antipsychotic agents. This warning is in response to an increased risk of mortality due to cardiovascular events or infections, usually pneumonia. Clinicians need to weigh the potential benefits of drug treatment, including the suffering and morbidity due to untreated psychosis and behavioral disturbances.

Avoid the use of sedative-hypnotics, antihistamines, or benzodiazepines for sleep induction in patients with dementia due to side effects and potential hazards, including exacerbation of delirium.

Follow-Up

Each visit should include the evaluation of general health and hygiene and the patient's ability to drive. Inquire about dental or denture care, bathing and skin care, sensory aids (glasses, hearing aids), sleep hygiene, eating routine, and scheduled toileting. Inquire about motor vehicle accidents or near accidents and changes in driving habits or patterns. Patients who show driving impairment must no longer drive. Patients who have received the diagnosis of dementia but have not yet shown any difficulties with driving should undergo a driving evaluation and refrain from driving before completion of the evaluation.

Book Enhancement

Go to www.acponline.org/essentials/neurology-section.html. In *MKSAP for Students 5*, assess your knowledge with items 10-13 in the **Neurology** section.

Bibliography

Blass DM, Rabins PV. In the clinic. Dementia. Ann Intern Med. 2008; 148:ITC4-1-ITC4-16. [PMID: 18378944]

Chapter 69

Approach to Selected Movement Disorders

Bryan Ho, MD

Movement disorder refers to the category of neurologic disease that leads to abnormalities in movement specifically due to dysfunction in the extrapyramidal motor system. Depending on the type and degree of dysfunction, patients can present with a variety of clinical syndromes of too much movement (hyperkinesia) or too little movement (hypokinesia).

Hyperkinetic disorders include tremor, chorea, dystonia, myoclonus, and tics. Tremor refers to involuntary oscillatory movements of a body part over a fixed axis, usually but not always a joint. Tremor is described in terms of its amplitude and frequency and the presence of resting, postural, or action components. Tremor is the most common type of movement disorder encountered in general clinical practice and can be a primary disorder or secondary to a variety of drugs and metabolic conditions.

Chorea refers to involuntary, random, purposeless movements that can involve the limbs, face, or trunk. Chorea is derived from the Greek word "to dance," and patients may have strikingly abnormal gaits due to random interruptions of voluntary movement as they walk. Patients with chorea have difficulty sustaining a fixed posture, such as tongue protrusion or persistent hand grip. Chorea can be due to neurodegenerative diseases (e.g., Huntington disease), autoimmune diseases (e.g., systemic lupus erythematosus), and medications, particularly drugs involved in dopamine pathways (e.g., antipsychotic agents).

Dystonia refers to involuntary, sustained contraction of agonist/antagonist muscles, which often can lead to uncomfortable or even painful twisting, bizarre-looking postures. Dystonia can be classified as focal (involving only one body part), segmental (two or more contiguous body parts), multifocal (two or more noncontiguous body parts), hemidystonic (one side of the body), or generalized. Primary dystonias are rare. Secondary dystonias are more common and can be due to drugs that block dopamine pathways.

Myoclonus refers to rapid, jerk-like movements due to either sudden muscle contractions (positive myoclonus) or sudden interruption of sustained muscle contractions leading to loss of tone (negative myoclonus), as seen in asterixis. Similar to dystonia, myoclonus is classified by its distribution in the body (focal, segmental, multifocal, generalized). Most people have some degree of physiologic myoclonus that can occur when falling asleep. Myoclonus may be a clinical component of epilepsy (i.e., juvenile myoclonic epilepsy, myoclonic epileptic syndromes). Myoclonus can also be caused by toxic-metabolic derangements (e.g., hepatic encephalopathy), severe anoxic brain injury, and certain medication exposures (e.g., serotonin syndrome).

Tics refer to movements that are stereotyped in nature but are temporarily suppressible. Generally, when suppressing these movements, patients describe a buildup of anxiety or internal discomfort that is released when the movements are allowed to occur. Tics are commonly associated with Tourette syndrome but can also be part of other hyperkinetic movement disorders.

Parkinson Disease

One of the more common neurodegenerative disorders, Parkinson disease is associated with dopamine depletion from the basal ganglia. Loss of dopamine causes major disruptions in the connections to the thalamus and motor cortex, leading to the characteristic signs and symptoms of Parkinson disease. Most cases are idiopathic, although familial cases due to genetic mutations have been documented.

Parkinson disease is a clinical diagnosis based on three cardinal clinical features: bradykinesia, resting tremor, and postural instability. The diagnosis is established by the presence of bradykinesia and at least one other cardinal feature. Parkinson disease presents asymmetrically, with clinical features more prominent on one side. Findings that suggest an alternative diagnosis include symmetric symptoms or signs, early falling, rapid progression, poor response to levodopa, early dementia, early autonomic failure, and ataxia. The differential diagnosis of parkinsonism is summarized in Table 1.

The mainstay of drug therapy for Parkinson disease is dopamine replacement with levodopa or dopamine agonists. Levodopa is the most effective drug for symptom management. However, over time, patients on levodopa will inevitably develop motor fluctuations, including dyskinesia (excessive movements similar to chorea) and "wearing-off" effect (sudden return of symptoms and gait freezing as a result of the levodopa losing effect before the next dose). Levodopa is always given in combination with carbidopa, which acts as a peripheral inhibitor of levodopa breakdown, allowing more of the drug to enter the central nervous system. Dopamine agonists (e.g., ropinirole, pramipexole) also are effective for treating symptoms, although their effect is generally not as robust as that of levodopa. These agents are less likely to confer motor fluctuations, making them a good option for early disease. Side effects include somnolence, nausea, hallucinations, psychosis, and impulsive behavior.

Essential Tremor

Essential tremor is an upper extremity, high-frequency tremor that is present with both limb movement and sustained posture of the involved extremities. The tremor is characteristically bilateral, but there can be mild to moderate asymmetry. Tremor amplitude can

Table 1. Differential Diagnosis of Parkinsonism

Disorder	Notes
Degenerative parkinsonism	
Idiopathic Parkinson disease	Rest tremor, rigidity, bradykinesia, and gait disturbance
Multiple system atrophy	Ataxia, dysautonomia
Progressive supranuclear palsy	Early falls, impaired vertical eye movement
Corticobasal degeneration	Asymmetric spasticity and rigidity, alien limb movement, myoclonus
Dementia with Lewy bodies	Dementia, hallucinations
Secondary parkinsonism	
Drug (antipsychotic agents, antiemetics, metoclopramide, reserpine, lithium, tetrabenazine, flunarizine)	Exposure history
Toxin (manganese, MPTP, mercury, methanol, ethanol, carbon monoxide)	Exposure history
Cerebrovascular disease	History; MRI showing stroke
Head trauma (including pugilistic encephalopathy)	History of head trauma
Hydrocephalus	Lower body parkinsonism; MRI showing possible contusion
Creutzfeldt-Jakob disease	Rapidly progressive; signs/symptoms of ataxia, dementia, myoclonus, dystonia
Paraneoplastic syndrome	Rapidly progressive; signs/symptoms of ataxia, encephalopathy, myoclonus
Hepatocerebral degeneration	History of liver disease; MRI changes in basal ganglia
Hypothyroidism	Rare; resolves with treatment
Selected Hereditary Disorders Associated with Parkinsonism	
Wilson disease	Must be ruled out in patients aged <50 y; hepatic and psychiatric disease; tremor, dystonia, ataxia
Familial amyotrophy-dementia-parkinsonism	Cognitive/behavioral change; extremity weakness, atrophy; rigidity, bradykinesia
Spinocerebellar ataxia	Autosomal dominant; begins in early life; ataxia predominates
Huntington disease	Chorea, dystonia, psychiatric symptoms, dementia, ataxia
Fragile X–associated tremor/ataxia syndrome	Ataxia, tremor, dementia

MPTP= 1-methyl-4-phenyl-1,2,3,6-tetrahydropyridine

worsen over time and become so severe as to interfere with writing, drinking, and other activities requiring smooth, coordinated upper limb movements. Many patients report improvement in the tremor with ingestion of alcohol. Diagnosis of essential tremor is based on clinical features and the elimination of secondary causes. Patients with mild tremor may not require treatment. For more serious tremor, propranolol and primidone are first-line agents. Either drug may be initiated if the tremor interferes with activities of daily living or causes psychological distress.

Dystonia

All medications that block D_2 dopamine receptors can cause acute dystonic reactions. These movements most often affect the ocular muscles (oculogyric crisis) and the face, jaw, tongue, neck, and trunk. The limbs rarely are affected. Neuroleptic, antiemetic, and serotoninergic agents have been implicated. Treatment consists of parenteral diphenhydramine, benztropine mesylate, or biperiden.

Cervical dystonia, formerly known as torticollis, is the most commonly encountered primary dystonia. It is a focal dystonia that involves the cervical musculature and causes abnormal postures of the head, neck, and shoulders. Quick, nonrhythmic, repetitive movements, usually in a "no-no" pattern, also can occur and can be mistaken for tremor. The diagnosis is based on clinical features. Mild symptoms of cervical dystonia may not require therapy. However, dystonic movements that interfere with social or occupational functioning should be considered for pharmacotherapy or botulinum toxin injections. Botulinum toxin therapy, which has been reported to be beneficial in 60% to 85% of patients with cervical dystonia, is the treatment of choice. Anticholinergic medications result in improvement in 39% of patients with cervical dystonia but can be limited by systemic side effects.

Book Enhancement

Go to www.acponline.org/essentials/neurology-section. In *MKSAP for Students 5*, assess your knowledge with items 14-16 in the **Neurology** section.

Bibliography

Rao G, Fisch L, Srinivasan S, et al. Does this patient have Parkinson disease? JAMA. 2003;289:347-353. [PMID: 12525236]

Chapter 70

Approach to Meningitis and Encephalitis

Fred A. Lopez, MD

Central nervous system infections are medical emergencies classified by anatomic location and include the syndromes of meningitis (infection of tissues surrounding the cerebral cortex) and encephalitis (infection of the cerebral cortex). Bacterial meningitis requires early clinical recognition, an understanding of microbial causes, and an expedient diagnostic and therapeutic approach. Encephalitis is almost always caused by viral infection. Approximately 20,000 cases of encephalitis occur in the United States each year, with the predominant endemic cause being herpes simplex virus (HSV).

Bacterial Meningitis

More than 75% of cases of bacterial meningitis are due to either *Streptococcus pneumoniae* or *Neisseria meningitidis*. *S. pneumoniae* is the most common cause and may occur in patients with other foci of infection (e.g., pneumonia, otitis media, mastoiditis, sinusitis, endocarditis) or following head trauma with leakage of cerebrospinal fluid (CSF). The pneumococcal conjugate vaccine (children) and the pneumococcal polyvalent polysaccharide vaccine (adults) are effective in prevention of invasive disease.

N. meningitidis is the second most common cause of bacterial meningitis in the United States, occurring primarily in children and young adults. An associated rash—often petechial, maculopapular, or purpuric in appearance and usually sparing the soles and palms—is characteristic. Patients with deficiencies in the terminal complement components (C5-C9) are at increased risk for recurrent infection by *N. meningitidis*. An unconjugated polysaccharide meningococcal vaccine against serogroups A, C, Y, and W-135 is available, and a meningococcal polysaccharide diphtheria toxoid conjugate vaccine was approved by the FDA in 2005. Neither vaccine affords protection against serogroup B, the causative agent in up to one third of cases of bacterial meningitis in the United States.

Meningitis caused by *Listeria monocytogenes* is associated with extremes of age (neonates and adults aged >50 years), alcoholism, malignancy, immunosuppression, diabetes mellitus, hepatic failure, kidney failure, iron overload, collagen vascular disorders, and HIV infection. Group B streptococci, an important cause of meningitis in neonates, is seen in adults with underlying conditions such as diabetes, pregnancy, cardiac disease, malignancy, collagen vascular disorders, alcoholism, hepatic failure, kidney failure, corticosteroid use, and HIV infection. Aerobic gram-negative bacilli (*Klebsiella* species, *Escherichia coli*, *Serratia marcescens*, *Pseudomonas aeruginosa*), *Staphylococcus aureus*, and *Staphylococcus epidermidis* may cause meningitis in patients with head trauma or CSF shunts or following neurosurgical procedures. The differential diagnosis of bacterial meningitis is broad and includes other microbial agents (Table 1).

Diagnosis

Look for fever, headache, neck stiffness, and altered mental status; the absence of these findings essentially rules out the diagnosis. Jolt accentuation of headache elicited with horizontal movement of the head is more sensitive for the diagnosis of meningitis than the Kernig or Brudzinski sign.

The clinical presentations of viral and bacterial meningitis are similar. The diagnosis is established by CSF analysis (Table 2). Although some clinicians routinely perform CT prior to doing a lumbar puncture in suspected bacterial meningitis in order to reduce the risk of brain herniation, this procedure should not delay empiric antibiotic therapy based on the patient's age and underlying condition. The sensitivity and specificity of the CSF Gram stain for diagnosing bacterial meningitis range from 56% to 90% and 97% to 100%, respectively.

In the evaluation of patients with acute bacterial or viral meningitis, CSF findings that predict bacterial etiology with ≥ 99% certainty include:

- Protein concentration >220 mg/dL (2200 mg/L)
- Glucose concentration <34 mg/dL (1.9 mmol/L)
- CSF-blood glucose ratio <0.23
- Leukocyte count >2000/μL (2000 x 10^6/L)
- Neutrophil count >1180/μL (1180 x 10^6/L)

Consider CSF polymerase chain reaction (PCR) testing for non-poliovirus enteroviruses (echoviruses, coxsackieviruses) and HSV as well as IgM antibody-capture enzyme-linked immunosorbent assay (ELISA) testing for arboviruses (West Nile virus, St. Louis encephalitis virus, California encephalitis virus, eastern equine encephalitis virus) in patients with CSF findings consistent with aseptic meningitis (meningeal inflammation with negative bacterial cultures), encephalitis, or both when no bacterial agents are identified on Gram stain. Fungal, mycobacterial, HIV, and spirochetal testing should be performed when clinically indicated (immunosuppression, exposure history).

Treatment

If CSF examination reveals purulent meningitis, and a positive Gram stain suggests a specific etiology, targeted antibacterial therapy is initiated. If the Gram stain is negative, empiric antibiotic therapy is initiated, based on the patient's age and underlying conditions (Table 3). Administration of dexamethasone should be strongly considered in patients with acute bacterial meningitis.

Table 1. Differential Diagnosis of Meningitis

Disorder	Notes
Bacterial meningitis	Fever, severe headache, stiff neck, photophobia, drowsiness or confusion, nausea, vomiting. Neutrophil predominance on CSF evaluation.
Enteroviral infection	Fever, severe headache, stiff neck, photophobia, drowsiness or confusion, nausea, vomiting. Lymphocyte predominance on CSF evaluation. Most cases occur in the summer and early fall. Children are most often affected. Most frequently identified cause of aseptic meningitis. Primarily echovirus and coxsackievirus. PCR for enterovirus is available.
Arboviral infection	Most often presents as encephalitis but can present as meningitis or meningoencephalitis. Seen in patients living in or traveling to areas of arboviral activity or epidemic. St. Louis encephalitis virus, California encephalitis virus, and West Nile virus are most common. Most cases occur in warmer months and when contact with mosquito vectors is most likely.
HSV infection	HSV-1 most often presents as temporal lobe encephalitis; HSV-2 causes aseptic meningitis. HSV meningitis often is associated with primary genital infection. HSV accounts for approximately 0.5%-3% of all cases of aseptic meningitis. HSV meningitis often is self-limiting and does not require antiviral treatment. HSV encephalitis does require antiviral treatment.
HIV infection	HIV-associated aseptic meningitis generally follows a mononucleosis-like syndrome. Most commonly seen in acute HIV infection. Viral load should be obtained to exclude acute HIV. Always a consideration in young adults and patients with high-risk behaviors.
Tubercular meningitis	Headache, nausea, vomiting, fever, mental status changes lasting more than 2 weeks. CSF abnormalities are nonspecific and generally show normal to slightly decreased glucose, elevated protein, and moderate pleocytosis with variable differential. CSF culture for *Mycobacterium tuberculosis* is low yield and may take several weeks to become positive. A negative TB PCR result on CSF evaluation does not exclude diagnosis of tubercular meningitis.
Lyme disease (*Borrelia burgdorferi*)	Associated with rash (erythema migrans) early, followed by aseptic meningitis approximately 4 wk after initial signs of disease. Vector tick is endemic to northeastern United States and Great Lakes area. Occurs most frequently in summer and autumn.
Cryptococcal meningitis	Subacute or chronic presentation. Half of cases occur in HIV-negative patients. CSF pleocytosis of 40-400 cells/µL (40-400 x 10^6/L) with lymphocyte predominance and slightly low glucose is typical. India ink stain of CSF has limited sensitivity. CSF is positive for cryptococcal polysaccharide antigen in 90% of patients.

CSF = cerebrospinal fluid; HSV = herpes simplex virus; HSV-1 = HSV type 1; HSV-2 = HSV type 2; PCR = polymerase chain reaction; TB = tuberculosis.

Table 2. Typical Cerebrospinal Fluid (CSF) Findings in Patients with Acute Meningitis

CSF Parameter	Bacterial Meningitis	Viral Meningitis[a]
Opening pressure	200-500 mm H_2O[b]	≤250 mm H_2O
Leukocyte count	1000-5000/µL (1000-5000 × 10^6/L)[c]	50-1000/µL (50-1000 × 10^6/L)
Leukocyte differential	Neutrophils	Lymphocytes[d]
Glucose	<40 mg/dL (2.2 mmol/L)[e]	>45 mg/dL (2.5 mmol/L)
Protein	100-500 mg/dL (1000-5000 mg/L)	<200 mg/dL (2000 mg/L)
Gram stain	Positive in 60%-90%[f]	Negative
Culture	Positive in 70%-85%	Negative

[a]Primarily non-poliovirus enteroviruses (echoviruses, coxsackieviruses).
[b]Values >600 mm H_2O suggest cerebral edema, intracranial suppurative foci, or communicating hydrocephalus.
[c]Range may be <100 to >10,000 cells/µL (100-10,000 × 10^6/L).
[d]Neutrophil predominance may occur early in infection but gives way to lymphocyte predominance over the first 6-48 h.
[e]The CSF-blood glucose ratio is ≤0.40 in most patients.
[f]Likelihood of a positive Gram stain correlates with number of bacteria in CSF.

Clinical trials have established the benefit of adjunctive dexamethasone on adverse outcomes and death in adults with suspected or proven pneumococcal meningitis. Dexamethasone administered with or just prior to the first dose of antimicrobial therapy attenuates the inflammatory response following antimicrobial-induced lysis of meningeal pathogens. There are insufficient data in adults with pneumococcal meningitis to know whether dexamethasone administration after antimicrobial therapy offers any outcome benefit. Once an etiologic agent is identified and antimicrobial susceptibility has been performed, specific antibacterial therapy should be started (Table 4).

Viral Encephalitis

Viral encephalitis presents as an acute-onset, febrile illness associated with headache, altered level of consciousness, and, occasionally, focal neurologic signs. Arboviral diseases such as eastern equine encephalitis, St. Louis encephalitis, and others have occurred in humans in the United States for years. Although these infections may be fatal or have significant morbidity, the prevalence in humans has been low, and effective treatments and vaccines have not been developed. Lack of attention to viral encephalitis changed in 1999 when the first cases of West Nile

Table 3. Empiric Antibiotic Therapy for Purulent Meningitis Based on Patient Age and Underlying Condition

Predisposing Factor	Common Pathogens	Antibiotic Therapy
Age 0-4 wk	*Streptococcus agalactiae, Escherichia coli, Listeria monocytogenes, Klebsiella* species	Ampicillin + cefotaxime **or** ampicillin + aminoglycoside
Age 1-23 mo	*Streptococcus pneumoniae, Haemophilus influenzae, S. agalactiae, Neisseria meningitidis, E. coli*	Vancomycin + third-generation cephalosporin[a,b,c]
Age 2-50 y	*S. pneumoniae, N. meningitidis*	Vancomycin + third-generation cephalosporin[a,b,c]
Age >50 y	*S. pneumoniae, N. meningitidis, L. monocytogenes*, gram-negative bacilli	Vancomycin + ampicillin + third generation cephalosporin[a,b]
Basilar skull fracture	*S. pneumoniae, H. influenzae*, group A β-hemolytic streptococci	Vancomycin + third-generation cephalosporin[a]
Neurosurgery or head trauma	*Staphylococcus aureus*, coagulase-negative staphylococci (especially *Staphylococcus epidermidis*), gram-negative bacilli (including *Pseudomonas aeruginosa*)	Vancomycin + ceftazidime **or** cefepime **or** meropenem
Cerebrospinal fluid shunt	*S. aureus*, coagulase-negative staphylococci (especially *S. epidermidis*), gram-negative bacilli (including *P. aeruginosa*), diphtheroids (including *Propionibacterium acnes*)	Vancomycin + ceftazidime **or** cefepime **or** meropenem

[a]Cefotaxime or ceftriaxone.
[b]Some experts would add rifampin if dexamethasone is given.
[c]Add ampicillin if the patient has risk factors for *L. monocytogenes* or infection with this organism is suspected.

Table 4. Recommended Specific Antibiotic Therapy for Bacterial Meningitis Based on Pathogen and In Vitro Susceptibility Testing

Pathogen	Standard Therapy	Alternative Therapies
Streptococcus pneumoniae		
Penicillin MIC <0.1 µg/mL	Penicillin G or ampicillin	Third-generation cephalosporin,[a] chloramphenicol
Penicillin MIC 0.1-1.0 µg/mL	Third-generation cephalosporin[a]	Meropenem, cefepime
Penicillin MIC ≥2.0 µg/mL **or** cefotaxime or ceftriaxone MIC ≥1.0 µg/mL	Vancomycin + third-generation cephalosporin[a,b]	Fluoroquinolone[c]
Neisseria meningitidis		
Penicillin MIC <0.1 µg/mL	Penicillin G or ampicillin	Third-generation cephalosporin,[a] chloramphenicol
Penicillin MIC 0.1-1.0 µg/mL	Third-generation cephalosporin[a]	Chloramphenicol, fluoroquinolone, meropenem
Listeria monocytogenes	Ampicillin or penicillin G[d]	Trimethoprim-sulfamethoxazole
Streptococcus agalactiae	Ampicillin or penicillin G[d]	Third-generation cephalosporin,[a] vancomycin
Haemophilus influenzae		
β-Lactamase–negative	Ampicillin	Third-generation cephalosporin,[a] cefepime, chloramphenicol, fluoroquinolone, aztreonam
β-Lactamase–positive	Third-generation cephalosporin[a]	Chloramphenicol, cefepime, fluoroquinolone, aztreonam
Escherichia coli and other Enterobacteriaceae[e]	Third-generation cephalosporin[a]	Aztreonam, meropenem, fluoroquinolone, trimethoprim-sulfamethoxazole
Pseudomonas aeruginosa	Ceftazidime[d] or cefepime[d]	Aztreonam,[d] meropenem,[d] fluoroquinolone[d]
Staphylococcus aureus		
Methicillin-sensitive	Nafcillin or oxacillin	Vancomycin, meropenem
Methicillin-resistant	Vancomycin[f]	Trimethoprim-sulfamethoxazole, linezolid, daptomycin
Staphylococcus epidermidis	Vancomycin[f]	Linezolid

MIC = minimum inhibitory concentration.
[a]Cefotaxime or ceftriaxone.
[b]Addition of rifampin should be considered if the organism is sensitive and if the ceftriaxone MIC is >2 µg/mL.
[c]No clinical data available; would use newer fluoroquinolones with in vitro activity against *S. pneumoniae* (e.g., moxifloxacin). Many experts would not use a fluoroquinolone as single-agent therapy but would combine with vancomycin or a third-generation cephalosporin such as cefotaxime or ceftriaxone.
[d]Addition of an aminoglycoside should be considered.
[e]Choice of specific antimicrobial therapy should be guided by in vitro susceptibility test results.
[f]Consider addition of rifampin.

encephalitis occurred in the United States. The virus spread throughout the United States and is now diagnosed in thousands of patients annually. West Nile encephalitis is most severe in older patients, and the highest mortality and morbidity rates occur in those aged ≥65 years. The most common manifestations are encephalitis, meningitis, flaccid paralysis, and fever.

HSV is one of the most common causes of identified sporadic encephalitis worldwide, accounting for 5% to 10% of cases. HSV type 1 occurs more commonly in adults, and HSV type 2 occurs more commonly in neonates. The encephalitis in adults results from reactivation of the latent virus in the trigeminal ganglion, which leads to inflammatory necrotic lesions in the temporal cortex and limbic system. Most cases occur in the absence of an antecedent illness.

Diagnosis

Obtain CSF analysis (including PCR testing for HSV and arbovirus-associated IgM antibody capture ELISA), MRI, and an electroencephalogram (EEG). CSF analysis usually reveals an increased opening pressure, a lymphocytic pleocytosis, a modestly elevated protein level, and a normal or slightly low glucose level. The CSF may be completely normal in about 3% to 5% of patients with viral encephalitis. CSF cultures for HSV and arboviruses usually are negative, but PCR for HSV and IgM antibody capture ELISA for arboviruses both have a sensitivity exceeding 90%.

In HSV encephalitis, MRI demonstrates unilateral or bilateral abnormalities in the medial and inferior temporal lobes, which may extend into the frontal lobe. EEG findings include focal delta activity over the temporal lobes, typically occurring between 2 and 14 days after symptom onset; periodic lateralizing epileptiform discharges (PLEDs) also may be noted. Brain biopsy is reserved for patients who do not respond to acyclovir.

In patients with encephalitis caused by flaviviruses (Japanese encephalitis virus, St. Louis encephalitis virus, West Nile virus) or eastern equine encephalitis virus, MRI may display a characteristic pattern of mixed-intensity or hypodense lesions on T1-weighted images in the thalamus, basal ganglia, and midbrain; the lesions are hyperintense on T2-weighted and fluid-attenuated inversion recovery (FLAIR) imaging. These neuroimaging findings occur in about 30% of patients with West Nile encephalitis.

Therapy

Although various viruses may cause encephalitis, specific antiviral therapy is generally limited to disease caused by the herpes viruses, particularly HSV. In HSV encephalitis, prompt acyclovir reduces mortality to approximately 25% in adults and older children; however, >50% of patients who survive will have neurologic sequelae. There is no reliably effective therapy available for arborvirus-associated encephalitis.

Book Enhancement

Go to www.acponline.org/essentials/neurology-section.html. In *MKSAP for Students 5,* assess your knowledge with items 17-20 in the **Neurology** section.

Bibliography

Spanos A, Harrell FE Jr, Durack DT. Differential diagnosis of acute meningitis. An analysis of the predictive value of initial observations. JAMA. 1989;262:2700-2707. [PMID: 2810603]

van de Beek D, de Gans J, Tunkel AR, Wijdicks EF. Community-acquired bacterial meningitis in adults. N Engl J Med. 2006;354:44-53. [PMID: 16394301]

Chapter 71

Stroke and Transient Ischemic Attack

Jane P. Gagliardi, MD

Stroke—irreversible neurologic symptoms caused by disrupted cerebral blood flow and cerebral ischemia—is the third leading cause of death in the United States and an important cause of disability. Most strokes are ischemic, resulting from thrombosis, embolism, or hypertensive vasospasm. Hemorrhagic stroke results from rupture of a blood vessel (in the case of subarachnoid hemorrhage) or from hypertensive or amyloid changes (in the case of intracranial hemorrhage). Transient ischemic attack (TIA) results from temporary disruption of cerebral blood flow; TIA mimics stroke but usually resolves within 30 minutes and is not associated with ischemic changes on brain imaging. Up to 40% of patients with TIA will eventually have a stroke; up to 20% will have a stroke within 90 days. Within the first minutes to hours after the onset of cerebral ischemia, an irreversibly damaged area of brain develops (the "infarct core"). Potentially viable brain tissue (the "ischemic penumbra") surrounds, and will eventually become part of the infarct core, if blood flow is not restored quickly or even if blood pressure is lowered. The penumbra is the target of acute ischemic stroke therapy. Most damage occurs in the first 3 to 6 hours poststroke, so stroke is a time-critical medical emergency. The differential diagnosis of stroke includes seizure, hypoglycemia, metabolic abnormalities, complicated migraine, rapidly growing mass or brain tumor, and functional illness (Table 1).

Prevention

It is important to educate patients and families about symptoms of stroke and the critical need for immediate evaluation if these symptoms occur. Modifiable risk factors (e.g., smoking, hypertension, hyperlipidemia) should be addressed with appropriate management strategies, including ACE inhibitors for hypertension and statins for hyperlipidemia. Discontinue hormone replacement therapy in postmenopausal women. For patients whose 10-year absolute risk of a first coronary artery event is ≥10% (see Chapter 2), it is reasonable to consider aspirin for primary prevention of stroke, provided there is no contraindication. Begin anticoagulation for atrial fibrillation unless bleeding risks outweigh potential benefits, in which case, start antiplatelet therapy. Asymptomatic carotid bruits are common, and their prevalence increases with age. The presence of a carotid bruit cannot be used to rule in, and its absence cannot rule out, surgically amenable carotid artery stenosis. Among patients aged <75 years with >60% carotid stenosis, carotid endarterectomy performed by a surgeon with low surgical morbidity (i.e., <3% perioperative stroke or mortality rate) can reduce annual stroke risk by half.

Table 1. Differential Diagnosis of Stroke and Transient Ischemic Attack (TIA)

Disorder	Notes
Stroke	Abrupt onset. Fixed focal findings referable to arterial distribution (i.e., hemiparesis of face, arm, or leg ± aphasia). Cannot distinguish stroke subtypes or infarct from hemorrhage without brain imaging.
TIA	Same clinical features as for stroke, but lasting <30 min.
Seizure	Abrupt onset and termination of ictus; usually decreased responsiveness during ictus; often involuntary movements during ictus; usually postictal lethargy or confusion; sometimes postictal focal findings that resolve over 24 h. May accompany stroke.
Hypoglycemia	May look like stroke or TIA. Almost always a diabetic patient taking hypoglycemic medications. May or may not be accompanied by seizure.
Complicated migraine (see Chapter 67)	Similar onset and focal findings as in stroke. Usually severe headache preceding or following attack. Sensory and visual disturbances often prominent; sensory symptoms often spread over affected area. Suspect in younger patients, more often women with history of severe headache. MRI usually normal. Stroke may accompany migraine.
Mass lesion (tumor, abscess, subdural hematoma)	Focal symptoms occur over days, not minutes; may not be in one vascular territory. Primary cancer, fever, immunosuppression, and history of trauma often present. Can be distinguished from stroke by brain imaging.
Encephalitis (see Chapter 70)	Onset over days, not minutes. Fever, followed by headache, possibly meningeal signs, and photophobia. Structural involvement suggested by mental status change
Functional	May look like stroke, but findings nonanatomic or inconsistent; normal MRI.

CT = computed tomography; MRI = magnetic resonance imaging; TIA = transient ischemic attack

Table 2. Cerebrovascular Territories and Syndromes

Artery	Major Clinical Features
Anterior cerebral artery	Contralateral leg weakness
Middle cerebral artery	Contralateral face and arm weakness greater than leg weakness; sensory loss, field cut, aphasia or neglect (depending on side)
Posterior cerebral artery	Contralateral field cut
Deep penetrating arteries	Contralateral motor or sensory deficit without cortical signs (e.g., aphasia, apraxia, neglect, normal higher cognitive functions)
Basilar artery	Oculomotor deficits and/or ataxia with "crossed" sensory/motor deficits. Crossed signs include sensory or motor deficit on one side of the face and the opposite side of the body.
Basilar artery (ventral pons)	Quadriplegia and speechlessness due to severe dysarthria with preserved consciousness; able to move eyes and wink
Vertebral artery	Lower cranial nerve deficits (e.g., dysphagia, dysarthria, tongue or palate deviation) and/or ataxia with crossed sensory deficits

Diagnosis

Successful stroke treatment requires rapid diagnosis. The abrupt or sudden onset of focal neurologic symptoms is a possible indicator of ischemic stroke or intracerebral hemorrhage. In the case of intracerebral hemorrhage, the sudden focal deficit will progress over minutes to hours and may evolve to include symptoms of increased intracranial pressure, such as headache, nausea, vomiting, and decreased level of consciousness. A sudden severe headache suggests subarachnoid hemorrhage; up to 40% of patients will have experienced a "thunderclap" or sentinel headache in the days to weeks leading up to the bleed. If the patient presents with a sudden severe headache and CT is negative for evidence of bleeding, it is necessary to perform lumbar puncture to assess the cerebrospinal fluid for evidence of erythrocytes or xanthochromia; 5% of patients presenting with an acute subarachnoid hemorrhage may have a negative head CT scan, and management of subarachnoid hemorrhage is quite different from management of ischemic stroke.

A thorough neurologic examination is performed to localize the ischemic region (Table 2). The presence of facial paresis, arm drift, or abnormal speech is highly suggestive of stroke. Small, deep penetrating arteries that arise from the larger vessels also may be affected by stroke. Occlusion of these vessels may cause small infarctions with stereotypical "lacunar" syndromes, such as pure motor hemiparesis, pure sensory stroke, dysarthria–clumsy hand syndrome, and ataxic hemiparesis.

Neuroimaging is essential to rule out hemorrhage and plan appropriate treatment. Obtain head CT or brain MRI within 30 minutes of the patient's arrival to the emergency department to rule out hemorrhage. Perform duplex ultrasonography of the carotid arteries within the first 2 days to assess for stenosis warranting consideration of carotid endarterectomy; the carotid arteries are not adequately assessed by MRI. Up to 40% of strokes may be idiopathic; up to 50% of these may be caused by an atrial septal defect or patent foramen ovale. Echocardiography with testing for right-to-left shunting across the atrial septum is recommended in patients with stroke or in patients aged >45 years in whom an alternative explanation for TIA cannot be identified. Obtain laboratory values to define potential underlying conditions as dictated by the history and physical examination (Table 3).

Therapy

Patients with suspected stroke, high risk for stroke, or TIA lasting >10 minutes (which conveys a high risk for recurrent events, particularly if accompanied by limb weakness, speech disturbances, presence of diabetes mellitus, or age >60 years) should be hospitalized, preferably in a dedicated stroke unit with a multidisciplinary stroke team, unless monitoring in an intensive care unit is required. Stroke patients treated in specialized stroke units experience lower mortality and morbidity than patients treated in conventional ward settings. Initiate cardiac, vital signs, blood glucose, and oxygen monitoring. Given the risk of aspiration pneumonia and subsequent death, it is important to do a bedside swallow evaluation to rule out evidence of dysphagia before permitting any oral intake.

Hypertension is common in patients presenting with acute stroke, even in those without a history of hypertension. Any rapid decrease in blood pressure can impair cerebral blood flow and lead to increased risk of cerebral ischemia. For this reason, in the setting of acute stroke, do not treat hypertension unless blood pressure exceeds 220/120 mm Hg or there is another acute indication for lowering blood pressure, such as acute coronary syndrome, heart failure, aortic dissection, hypertensive encephalopathy, or acute kidney injury. In these cases, gradually lower blood pressure by 15% over the first 24 hours and cautiously thereafter with intravenous nicardipine or labetalol. If the patient is otherwise a candidate for thrombolytic therapy, blood pressure must be stabilized and lowered to <185/110 mm Hg before initiation of thrombolysis and maintained at <180/105 mm Hg after initiation of therapy.

The thrombolytic agent alteplase (recombinant tissue-type plasminogen activator [r-tPA]) increases the chance of recovery from ischemic stroke when administered intravenously within 3 hours of symptom onset, or within 3 hours of when patient was last seen awake and without symptoms. Brain imaging must be negative for hemorrhage. Thrombolysis is contraindicated in patients with mean arterial pressure >130 mm Hg, systolic blood pressure >185 mm Hg, diastolic blood pressure >110 mm Hg, or intracerebral hemorrhage; mean arterial pressure is estimated as diastolic blood pressure plus one third of the pulse pressure (where pulse pressure is the difference between systolic and diastolic blood

Table 3. Laboratory Studies for Transient Ischemic Attack and Stroke

Test	Rationale/Notes
Complete blood count	Ensure adequate oxygen-carrying capacity
Prothrombin time and partial thromboplastin time	Baseline studies in anticipation of possible anticoagulation
Lupus anticoagulant, anticardiolipin antibody, factor V Leiden, protein C, protein S, antithrombin III (selected patients)	Screening for hypercoagulable states
Blood glucose, creatinine, and lipid profile	Define underlying risk factors
Blood cultures (selected patients)	Obtain if patient is febrile, especially if endocarditis is suspected
Antinuclear antibody and related serologic studies, erythrocyte sedimentation rate	Obtain if vasculitis is suspected
RPR or VDRL (selected patients)	Neurosyphilis may present as acute stroke
Hemoglobin electrophoresis (selected patients)	Identify hemoglobinopathies causing stroke
Serum protein electrophoresis (selected patients)	Useful in defining lymphoproliferative diseases predisposing to brain hemorrhage

RPR = rapid plasma reagin.

pressures). If thrombolytic therapy is administered after 3 hours, risk of hemorrhage and death increases. It is important to hold aspirin and anticoagulants for 24 hours after thrombolytic therapy to prevent bleeding.

Antiplatelet therapy (aspirin or aspirin-dipyridamole) should be initiated within 48 hours for stroke and TIA to reduce subsequent stroke risk. Antiplatelet therapy may be the only therapy initiated when patients present outside the 3-hour window for thrombolytic therapy. Clopidogrel is an alternative therapy for patients who cannot tolerate aspirin; routine combination of clopidogrel and aspirin is not recommended due to increased risk of major bleeding. As the small decrease in ischemia is completely offset by an increased risk of hemorrhage, even in instances of presumed cardioembolism (as with atrial fibrillation, intracardiac thrombus, or dilated cardiomyopathy), urgent anticoagulation with heparin is not recommended for patients with ischemic stroke unless cerebral venous thrombosis, basilar occlusion/stenosis, or extracranial arterial dissection is suspected.

Use antipyretics to keep core body temperature <38.0°C (100.4°F). Use supplemental oxygen to maintain oxygen saturation at >95%. Persistent hyperglycemia during the first 24 hours after stroke is associated with poor outcomes; thus, patients with glucose levels >140 mg/dL (7.8 mmol/L) should be given insulin. To avoid exacerbation of hyperglycemia, use normal saline (0.9%) for intravenous fluid hydration rather than dextrose-containing fluids. Prevent decubitus ulcers and deep venous thrombosis through frequent repositioning and use of subcutaneous heparin or graduated or pneumatic compression stockings. Hold oral nutrition until swallowing is evaluated, and consider early nasogastric tube feeding if risk of aspiration is suspected or confirmed. Consult with physical, occupational, and speech therapists.

Symptomatic patients with >70% carotid stenosis may benefit from carotid endarterectomy to decrease the risk of recurrent stroke; in one study, 2-year stroke risk decreased from 26% to 9% in those who underwent carotid endarterectomy. There may be some benefit from carotid endarterectomy among selected symptomatic patients with 50% to 69% carotid stenosis (e.g., patients

with a life expectancy >5 years); there is no clear benefit from carotid endarterectomy in patients with <50% carotid stenosis.

Follow-Up

Prognosis after intracerebral hemorrhage is related to the volume of the hemorrhage and the patient's level of consciousness. Prognosis after subarachnoid hemorrhage is related to severity of symptoms as well as localization and securing of the vascular anomaly (usually an aneurysm) within 72 hours. Studies support early mobilization of ischemic stroke patients to prevent complications. Refer patients for intensive rehabilitation (at home or in a facility) to improve function. Recognize and treat poststroke depression, which is common and can contribute to cognitive, functional, and social difficulties that impair rehabilitative efforts. Antihypertensive treatment with diuretics and ACE inhibitors is recommended for hypertensive patients beyond the hyperacute period to prevent recurrent stroke. Patients with elevated cholesterol levels should be treated with statins, with a target serum low-density lipoprotein (LDL) cholesterol level of <100 mg/dL (2.6 mmol/L); an optional LDL cholesterol goal of <70 mg/dL (1.8 mmol/L) is reasonable for high-risk patients with multiple risk factors. Modifiable risk factors that should be addressed include cigarette smoking, excessive alcohol consumption, obesity, and lack of physical activity.

Book Enhancement

Go to www.acponline.org/essentials/neurology-section.html. In *MKSAP for Students 5*, assess your knowledge with items 21-24 in the **Neurology** section.

Bibliography

Goldstein LB, Simel DL. Is this patient having a stroke? JAMA. 2005;293:2391-2402. [PMID: 15900010]

van der Worp HB, van Gijn J. Clinical practice. Acute ischemic stroke. N Engl J Med. 2007;357:572-579. [PMID: 17687132]

Chapter 72

Peripheral Neuropathy

Christopher A. Klipstein, MD

Peripheral neuropathy is a general term for any disorder affecting the peripheral nerves. Peripheral neuropathies are common and may involve a single nerve (mononeuropathy), two or more nerves in different sites (mononeuropathy multiplex), or many nerves over a wide area, leading to a more generalized disorder (polyneuropathy). Clinical manifestations include various combinations of altered sensation, pain, weakness, and autonomic dysfunction. The history and examination, in combination with electrodiagnostic studies, are used to determine the type of neuropathy present, thereby narrowing the list of possible causes.

Differential Diagnosis

Mononeuropathies most often are caused by nerve entrapment or compression. Two common mononeuropathies include carpal tunnel syndrome and Bell palsy. Carpal tunnel syndrome involves median nerve compression at the wrist. Patients report paresthesias, pain, and, occasionally, weakness in the hand and wrist. Symptoms can at times radiate up the forearm. The paresthesias often are worse at night or when holding a book or steering a car. Pain and decreased grip strength can make it difficult to make a fist or to grasp small objects. Examination may show sensory loss over the palmar surface of the first three digits (median nerve distribution), weakness of thumb abduction and opposition, and atrophy of the thenar eminence.

Bell palsy refers to unilateral facial muscle weakness due to acute dysfunction of the facial nerve. Growing evidence implicates facial nerve inflammation due to viral infection (especially herpes simplex virus type 1 infection) in the pathogenesis of Bell palsy. Symptoms typically begin suddenly and peak over 1 to 2 days. Paralysis of the upper and lower face distinguishes Bell palsy from facial paralysis caused by stroke, which affects only the lower facial muscles (sparing the forehead and eye).

Mononeuropathy multiplex refers to simultaneous involvement of two or more separate, noncontiguous peripheral nerves. Mononeuropathy multiplex often is the result of a systemic disease (e.g., diabetes mellitus, amyloidosis, vasculitis, sarcoidosis); the mechanism of nerve injury may be a combination of compressive, ischemic, metabolic, and inflammatory factors. When successive acute involvement of individual nerves is accompanied by pain, suspect a vasculitis as the cause.

Polyneuropathy refers to diffuse, generalized, usually symmetric involvement of the peripheral nerves. Polyneuropathy often is a manifestation of systemic disease or exposure to a toxin or medication. Polyneuropathy presents in variable ways, depending on the pathophysiology of the underlying cause. Polyneuropathies can be characterized as axonal or demyelinating. Axonal polyneuropathies result from dysfunction of peripheral nerve cells and their axons, usually from metabolic or toxic causes (e.g., diabetes, alcohol). Demyelinating polyneuropathies are due to dysfunction of the myelin sheath that encases many peripheral nerves.

Axonal polyneuropathies typically present as symmetric distal sensory loss, with or without burning, tingling, or muscle weakness. Because the longest nerves are affected earliest and most severely, initial symptoms usually are in the feet, beginning with numbness and paresthesias in the toes that gradually proceed up the limb, eventually resulting in depressed ankle jerks and atrophy of the intrinsic foot muscles. As the sensory symptoms ascend, the fingers and hands become involved, resulting in the classic "stocking-glove" pattern of sensory loss. Common causes of axonal polyneuropathies include diabetes (or impaired glucose tolerance), alcoholism, vitamin B_{12} deficiency, and uremia.

In contrast, most patients with a demyelinating polyneuropathy initially present with motor symptoms. Symmetric proximal weakness suggests an acquired demyelinating polyneuropathy, such as Guillain-Barré syndrome or chronic inflammatory demyelinating polyneuropathy. Guillain-Barré syndrome is caused by an immune-mediated attack against a component of peripheral nerve myelin. The syndrome is characterized by rapid-onset symmetric weakness in all limbs, which progresses over several days to weeks; deep tendon reflexes are diminished or absent. Patients usually note weakness in the legs first, more often proximal than distal, and symptoms spread in an ascending fashion. Although patients frequently report paresthesias with onset of symptoms, objective sensory loss is unusual. Most patients have a preceding history of infection, trauma, or surgery. The most frequent precipitating factor is a diarrheal syndrome caused by *Campylobacter jejuni* infection. Patients with chronic inflammatory demyelinating polyneuropathy present with slowly progressive, relatively symmetric limb weakness and sensory disturbances. The symptoms typically progress for several months, and symptom severity can fluctuate over many years.

A variety of other disorders may cause symptoms similar to those of a peripheral neuropathy. Myopathies (muscle disease) can cause muscle weakness, and diseases of the brain (e.g., stroke, tumor, multiple sclerosis) or spinal cord (e.g., herniated disc, spinal stenosis) can cause sensory or motor symptoms or signs. Although the pattern of sensory and motor symptoms— along with the presence or absence of upper motor neuron signs (e.g., hyperreflexia, Babinski sign, clonus)—can often identify the location of the pathology, electrodiagnostic and neuroimaging studies may be needed to distinguish muscle and central nervous system disorders from peripheral neuropathies.

Evaluation

For patients with a peripheral neuropathy, use the distribution of symptoms, combined with the characterization of the pathology (axonal or demyelinating), to identify potential causes (Table 1). Patients with severe or rapidly progressive symptoms or with no clear cause warrant prompt evaluation. Despite extensive diagnostic evaluation, no cause is found in approximately 20% of cases of polyneuropathy.

Focus the initial history on the distribution, time course, and nature of the deficit (sensory, motor, or both). In addition, ask about symptoms of systemic diseases that are associated with neuropathy (diabetes, uremia), exposure to medications (Table 2) or toxins that can cause a peripheral neuropathy (alcohol, heavy metals), and any family history of neuropathy. In the appropriate clinical context, inquire about recent viral illnesses, HIV risk factors, foreign travel (leprosy), and the possibility of a tick bite (Lyme disease). Use the review of systems to look for evidence of other organ involvement and symptoms of an underlying malignancy.

Use the physical examination to confirm the distribution of nerve involvement and to determine the extent of motor and/or sensory involvement. Abnormalities detected in the distribution of a single nerve indicate a mononeuropathy. Measure strength in all major muscle groups, and test all sensory modalities (i.e., light touch, pinprick, temperature, vibration, and proprioception). Assess deep tendon reflexes; remember that hyporeflexia suggests peripheral pathology, whereas hyperactive reflexes imply a central cause. Observe the patient's gait, and perform a Romberg test (afferent sensory pathways and posterior spinal column). In addition, look for evidence of systemic disease (lymphadenopathy, organomegaly, rash, arthritis).

Electromyography and nerve conduction studies often are the most useful tests in the evaluation of peripheral neuropathies. These tests augment the ability of the history and physical examination to distinguish neuropathies from myopathies and to differentiate mononeuropathies from polyneuropathies. For patients with polyneuropathies, electromyography and nerve conduction studies provide information as to the type of fibers involved (motor, sensory, or both) and characterize the pathologic process as primarily axonal or demyelinating.

Laboratory tests for the most common causes of an axonal polyneuropathy often include fasting blood glucose, hemoglobin A_{1c}, serum creatinine, thyroid-stimulating hormone, vitamin B_{12} level, complete blood count, erythrocyte sedimentation rate, serum protein electrophoresis, and urinalysis. In specific clinical contexts, other studies are potentially useful, including an antinuclear antibody test, HIV test, Lyme titer, and heavy metal screen.

When electromyography and nerve conduction findings suggest an acquired demyelinating neuropathy, the most common causes are Guillain-Barré syndrome and chronic inflammatory

Table 2. Drugs Associated with Peripheral Neuropathies

Amiodarone
Cisplatin
Colchicine
Dapsone
HIV drugs
    Didanosine
    Zalcitabine
    Stavudine
Hydralazine
Isoniazid
Metronidazole
Nitrofurantoin
Paclitaxel
Phenytoin
Vincristine

Table 1. Classification of Peripheral Neuropathies

Category	Distribution/Pattern	Examples	Mechanism
Mononeuropathy	Focal (single nerve)	Carpal tunnel syndrome, Bell palsy	Entrapment, inflammation
Mononeuropathy multiplex	Asymmetric, multifocal (several noncontiguous nerves)	Vasculitis, diabetes mellitus, lymphoma, amyloidosis, sarcoidosis, Lyme disease, acute HIV infection, leprosy	Ischemia, infiltration, inflammation
Axonal polyneuropathy	Symmetric, distal, predominantly sensory symptoms, sometimes also motor symptoms	Alcohol, drugs, chronic arsenic exposure, diabetes mellitus, uremia, low vitamin B_{12} or folate, hypothyroidism, paraproteinemia, paraneoplastic syndrome, chronic HIV infection, Charcot-Marie-Tooth disease	Toxin, metabolic, neoplasm, hereditary defect, inflammation
Demyelinating polyneuropathy	Symmetric, often proximal, predominantly motor symptoms, spreading in ascending fashion	Acute arsenic toxicity, Guillain-Barré syndrome, chronic inflammatory demyelinating polyneuropathy, paraproteinemia	Toxin, immunologic dysfunction, neoplasm

demyelinating polyneuropathy. Diagnosis is based on clinical recognition of progressive muscle weakness and reduced deep tendon reflexes, combined with abnormal electrodiagnostic studies and a cerebrospinal fluid evaluation showing a high protein level with few or no leukocytes (albuminocytologic dissociation).

Nerve biopsy (usually sural nerve) is indicated only for investigation of possible vasculitis, amyloidosis, sarcoidosis, leprosy, or tumor infiltration. Molecular genetic tests are commercially available for several hereditary neuropathies.

Therapy

Conservative treatment options for carpal tunnel syndrome include wrist splints and corticosteroid injections. Surgery should be considered for patients with severe sensory loss, hand weakness, moderate to severe electrodiagnostic findings, or failure to respond to conservative therapy.

Treatment of Bell palsy involves eye patching and lubrication to protect the cornea. Patients treated with prednisone within 72 hours of symptom onset have improved outcomes. Evidence-based studies have not clearly demonstrated benefit with antiviral therapy. The prognosis is related to the severity of the initial symptoms; although most patients experience excellent recovery, those who present with complete unilateral facial paralysis may not recover full function of the facial nerve.

Treatment of axonal polyneuropathies is centered on removal of the toxic agent (e.g., alcohol) or improvement of the underlying metabolic condition (e.g., diabetes, vitamin B_{12} deficiency), which often halts the progression of symptoms. Treat pain and dysesthesias symptomatically using agents such as tricyclic antidepressants, gabapentin, pregabalin, or duloxetine. Educate patients with diminished distal sensation about appropriate foot care to decrease the risk of foot ulcers and infections.

Vasculitic mononeuropathies and acute demyelinating polyneuropathies require prompt recognition and treatment with immunomodulating agents. Treat nonambulatory patients with Guillain-Barré syndrome with plasmapheresis or intravenous immune globulin. There is no evidence that corticosteroids shorten the course or reduce residual deficits in Guillain-Barré syndrome. Ventilatory support (needed in up to 30% of cases), infection surveillance, prophylaxis of venous thrombosis, pain management, and nutritional and psychological support contribute to reduced morbidity and mortality. The overall prognosis in patients with Guillain-Barré syndrome is good, with 80% of patients achieving recovery with little or no disability. Poor prognostic features include rapidly progressive weakness and the need for mechanical ventilation.

In addition to plasmapheresis and intravenous immune globulin, corticosteroids are effective for chronic inflammatory demyelinating polyneuropathy. Most patients need long-term treatment with plasmapheresis or intravenous immune globulin every 4 to 6 weeks to prevent relapse.

Book Enhancement

Go to www.acponline.org/essentials/neurology-section.html. In *MKSAP for Students 5,* assess your knowledge with items 25-28 in the **Neurology** section.

Bibliography

Pascuzzi RM. Peripheral neuropathy. Med Clin North Am. 2009;93:317-342, vii-viii. [PMID: 19272511]

Chapter 73

Breast Cancer

Kathleen F. Ryan, MD

Breast cancer is the most frequently diagnosed cancer and the second most common cause of cancer death in women. Each year, >200,000 people are diagnosed with invasive breast cancer; >39,000 of these people will die from their disease. Most cases involve women, but nearly 2000 cases each year involve men. In women, the main risk factor for breast cancer is age. Other risk factors are inherited mutations of the *BRCA1* or *BRCA2* gene, personal history of breast cancer, family history of breast cancer (particularly in first-degree relatives), prior biopsy showing atypical ductal or lobar hyperplasia, and prolonged estrogen exposure (i.e., early menarche, late menopause, nulliparity). Only age shows a strong enough correlation to target women for screening.

Prevention

Routine screening for *BRCA1* and *BRCA2* mutations is not recommended in women who are at low risk for developing breast cancer. Although *BRCA1* and BRCA2 mutations are highly associated with cancer risk (>60% by age 50 years), they account for only a small percentage of all breast cancers (<5%). Any woman with a family history of breast or ovarian cancer that includes a relative with a *known BRCA1* or *BRCA2* mutation should be referred for genetic counseling.

Prevention strategies are available for women at high risk for breast cancer. One option is a 5-year course of an antiestrogen medication (e.g., tamoxifen, raloxifene) to reduce the risk of developing estrogen receptor (ER)-positive cancer. The risks of these medications are not insignificant and include thrombosis, endometrial cancer, and hot flashes. Due to these possible side effects, cancer risk must be calculated to determine whether the benefits outweigh the risks of treatment. The Breast Cancer Risk Assessment Tool (Gail model), available at the National Cancer Institute Web site (www.cancer.gov/bcrisktool), was developed to estimate a woman's risk of developing invasive breast cancer within the next 5 years. The Gail model incorporates factors such as current age, age at menarche, age at first live birth, breast cancer in first-degree relatives, previous breast biopsy, and ethnicity. Women with a calculated 5-year risk ≥1.7% (risk of an average 60-year-old woman) are classified as being at high risk. Consider offering antiestrogen therapy to women aged 35 to 60 years at high risk for breast cancer in the next 5 years, based on the Gail model.

Prophylactic mastectomy is another option for women at increased risk for breast cancer, especially women found to have a genetic predisposition. Women with a known *BRCA1* or *BRCA2* mutation should be referred to a genetic counselor for discussion of the risks and benefits of prophylactic mastectomy and oophorectomy.

Screening

There are differing screening recommendations for breast cancer. The American Cancer Society (ACS) recommends that all women aged ≥20 years should be taught and encouraged to perform breast self-examination (BSE) and to report any breast changes to their health care provider. The ACS also recommends that women should have a clinical breast examination (CBE) performed by a health professional every 3 years between age 20 and age 39 years and annually after age 40. It is important to note that BSE has not been shown to improve cancer-specific or all-cause mortality, and the U.S. Preventive Services Task Force (USPSTF) cites insufficient evidence to determine whether CBE affects breast cancer mortality. The USPSTF recommends screening all women aged 50 to 74 years every other year using mammography, with or without a CBE. In women aged 40 to 49 years, clinicians should periodically assess individual risk for breast cancer and patient-specific values to help guide decisions about screening mammography.

There is no consensus on what age to stop screening, because shortened life expectancy results in less benefit from breast cancer screening. It is reasonable to continue screening for breast cancer as long as life expectancy is ≥10 years. For women with known *BRCA1* or *BRCA2* mutations, consider starting screening at age 25 years. Specialized breast imaging techniques (e.g., ultrasonography, scintigraphy with technetium 99m sestamibi, MRI) should be reserved for women with abnormal or inconclusive mammograms or clinical examinations.

Diagnosis

Women reporting new breast symptoms or new abnormalities on BSE should be carefully evaluated. The history should include an assessment of risk factors (age, family history of breast or ovarian cancer, use of hormone replacement therapy or oral contraceptives, age at menarche, number of pregnancies, menopausal status) and a detailed account of the patient's symptoms and concerns. Inquire about breast pain, nipple discharge, abdominal discomfort, bone pain, and respiratory or neurologic symptoms. Knowing the results of prior imaging studies or biopsies also is important.

The physical examination should include a detailed examination of both breasts and complete lymph node evaluation. Most often, breast cancer presents as a new lump, nipple discharge, or skin changes (retraction, dimpling). Erythema, scaliness, and edema with enlargement of pores and change in skin color (peau d'orange) are signs of inflammatory breast cancer, which often is misdiagnosed as eczema or mastitis. Younger women may have

Table 1. Evaluation of Clinical Breast Abnormalities

Breast Abnormality	Diagnostic Approach
Palpable lump or mass (patient aged <30 y)	Consider observation to assess for resolution within 1 or 2 menstrual cycles. If persistent, perform ultrasonography. If asymptomatic and cystic on ultrasonography, observe. If symptomatic or not clearly cystic on ultrasonography, aspirate. If aspirate fluid is bloody or a mass persists following aspiration, biopsy or excise for diagnosis. If solid on ultrasonography, obtain mammogram and tissue diagnosis (fine-needle aspiration, core biopsy, or surgical excision). If not visualized on ultrasonography, obtain mammogram and tissue diagnosis.
Palpable lump or mass (patient aged ≥30 y)	Obtain mammogram. If BI-RADS category 1-3,[a] perform ultrasonography and follow protocol described for patient aged <30 y. If BI-RADS category 4-5, obtain tissue diagnosis.
Nipple discharge, no mass (any age)	If discharge is bilateral and milky, perform pregnancy test. If test is negative, conduct endocrine evaluation. If discharge is persistent, spontaneous, unilateral, or serous/bloody or involves one duct, obtain mammogram and surgical referral for duct exploration; cytology is optional.
Thickening or asymmetry (patient aged <30 y)	Consider unilateral mammogram. If normal, reassess in 3-6 mo. If abnormal, obtain tissue diagnosis.
Thickening or asymmetry (patient age ≥30 y)	Obtain bilateral mammogram. If normal, reassess in 3-6 mo. If abnormal, obtain tissue diagnosis.
Skin changes[b] (patient aged <30 y)	Consider mastitis and treat with antibiotics (if appropriate) and reevaluate in 2 wk. Otherwise, evaluate as described for patient aged ≥30 y.
Skin changes[b] (patient aged ≥30 y)	Obtain bilateral mammogram. If normal, obtain skin biopsy. If abnormal or indeterminate, obtain needle biopsy or excision (also consider skin punch biopsy).

BI-RADS = Breast Imaging Reporting and Data System.
[a] BI-RADS 1 = negative. BI-RADS 2 = benign finding. BI-RADS 3 = probably benign finding; short-interval follow-up suggested. BI-RADS 4 = suspicious abnormality; consider biopsy. BI-RADS 5 = highly suggests malignancy; take appropriate action.
[b] Erythema, peau d'orange, scaling, nipple excoriation, eczema.

denser breasts, making detection of a mass more challenging than in older women, who tend to have more fat content in their breasts. Standardization of the CBE improves examiner accuracy. Four variables important for proper examination of the breast are: proper positioning of the patient (to flatten the breast against the chest), accurate identification of breast boundaries, finger position (palpating along vertical strips) and palpation pressure, and duration of the examination (3 minute per breast). Axillary adenopathy may indicate more advanced disease, whereas supraclavicular or cervical adenopathy usually means metastatic disease.

For nipple discharge, cytology is an excellent diagnostic tool. All patients with new breast symptoms or abnormal CBE findings should undergo mammography or ultrasonography. Women aged <40 years are likely to have benign findings; following the abnormality through one menstrual cycle rather than imaging immediately is a reasonable option. Obtain a tissue diagnosis in women with a suspicious abnormality on mammography and in all women with a suspicious palpable mass, even if an imaging study is not abnormal (Table 1). The differential diagnosis of a breast mass is summarized in Table 2.

If surgery is planned to treat confirmed breast cancer, a preoperative evaluation consisting of bilateral mammography, chest radiography, and laboratory studies based on age and comorbidities is performed. Evaluation of ER and progesterone receptor (PR) status is important, as it predicts benefit from endocrine therapy. HER1-4 (human epidermal growth factor receptors 1-4) is a family of membrane-bound proteins with tyrosine kinase activity, which act as epidermal growth factors. Overexpression of HER2 occurs in up to 40% of breast cancers and is associated with a poorer prognosis.

Staging of breast cancer is based on the TNM staging system, which is based on tumor size (T), axillary node status (N), and presence or absence of metastatic disease (M). Staging determines prognosis and therapeutic options. The two most important prognostic factors are tumor size and axillary node status. In the future, genomic testing may replace staging systems.

Breast cancer usually metastasizes locally to axillary lymph nodes. Breast cancer also commonly spreads to the bones, lungs, liver, or brain. Some women have been found to have cancer of unknown primary origin and have adenocarcinoma or poorly differentiated carcinoma in the axillary lymph nodes and no evident primary breast lesions or distant disease spread after completion of the routine staging evaluation. These patients have been found to be potentially curable when managed according to standard guidelines for stage II breast cancer.

Therapy

Surgery is a mainstay of treatment for breast cancer. Lumpectomy (breast-conserving surgery) followed by radiation is an option for patients with focal disease (tumor <5 cm) or ductal carcinoma in situ; survival rates are similar to mastectomy. For more extensive ductal carcinoma, modified radical mastectomy with radiation is the best option to lower recurrence rates. Mastectomy is indicated for patients with very large tumors or with contraindications to radiation (e.g., prior radiation). Radiation does carry the risk of future cardiovascular damage and lymphoma. Surgery may be used as palliative therapy for metastatic disease (e.g., to prevent complications such as infection).

Lymph node sampling is done as part of staging. Because aggressive removal of all axillary nodes does not improve survival and leads to limb lymphedema, sentinel node dissection often is used instead. Dye or tracer is injected into the tumor, and the first draining lymph node is biopsied and examined for tumor presence. If tumor is absent, no further dissection is needed; if tumor is noted, further lymph node dissection is performed.

Table 2. Differential Diagnosis of a Breast Mass

Disorder	Notes
Fibrocystic changes of the breast	Excessive nodularity and general lumpiness. Pain may be exacerbated premenstrually.
Fibroadenoma	Tender, discrete, mobile, well-circumscribed mass. Confirmed by examination, ultrasonography, and fine-needle aspiration biopsy.
Breast cyst	Severe localized pain associated with rapid expansion of a cyst. Ultrasonography usually is diagnostic and is the test of choice in women aged <40 y.
Breast hematoma	Tender mass, usually in association with breast trauma or after biopsy.
Breast cancer	Pain in 5%-20% of patients. Firm, irregular mass and axillary nodes may be present. Skin thickening and erythema suggest an underlying neoplasm or inflammation. Examination, mammography, ultrasonography, and fine-needle aspiration are indicated. Associated bloody discharge is more suggestive of cancer.
Breast abscess	Erythema, pain, and fever. More common in lactating breast.
Ductal papilloma	Unilateral bloody discharge. Mass may not be detectable. Refer for duct exploration.

Adjuvant systemic therapy is indicated for patients with early-stage breast cancer at significant risk for recurrence in a distant metastatic site. The purpose of adjuvant systemic therapy is to reduce the burden of clinically undetectable, distant micro-metastatic disease. The most important prognostic factors used to determine the need for adjuvant therapy in patients with breast cancer are lymph node involvement and tumor size. Endocrine therapy is beneficial only in patients with ER- or PR-positive tumors. In premenopausal women with ER- or PR-positive tumors, 5 years of tamoxifen is the standard adjuvant endocrine therapeutic regimen; treatment longer than 5 years is not recommended.

Aromatase inhibitors (e.g, anastrozole, letrozole, exemestane) appear to be more effective than tamoxifen in reducing risk for breast cancer recurrence in postmenopausal women with ER-positive breast cancer. Although aromatase inhibitors do not increase the risk for thromboembolic disease or endometrial cancer, they are associated with postmenopausal symptoms (hot flashes), musculoskeletal symptoms (arthralgia), and an increased risk for osteoporosis. The American Society of Clinical Oncology has suggested including an aromatase inhibitor as adjuvant therapy for postmenopausal women with hormone receptor–positive breast cancer to lower the risk of tumor recurrence. However, the optimal strategy—primary therapy with an aromatase inhibitor or sequential therapy with tamoxifen followed by an aromatase inhibitor—is currently unclear. Aromatase inhibitors are contraindicated in premenopausal women, because reduced feedback of estrogen to the hypothalamus and pituitary gland leads to an increase in gonadotropin secretion, with potential adverse effects. Trastuzumab is a humanized monoclonal antibody to the HER2 receptor. In patients with HER2-positive tumors, adjuvant trastuzumab therapy reduces the risk for breast cancer recurrence by approximately 50% and may reduce mortality by as much as 30%.

The decision to use systemic chemotherapy is based on the risk for recurrent disease. The presence of invasive disease within the biopsy is the most powerful prognostic factor for recurrence.

Typical chemotherapy regimens include methotrexate, cyclophosphamide, doxorubicin or epirubicin, and 5-fluorouracil. Chemotherapy may cause short- and long-term side effects. Short-term effects include hair loss, mouth sores, vomiting, diarrhea, anorexia, fatigue, increased risk of infection, and easy bruising and bleeding. Long-term side effects include infertility, peripheral neuropathy, osteoporosis, myocardial damage (with doxorubicin or trastuzumab), decreased cognitive function, and leukemia.

For patients with metastatic disease, therapy is palliative. Patients with ER/PR-receptor–positive tumors and bone or visceral disease are initially treated with tamoxifen. Aromatase inhibitors are used in postmenopausal women with tamoxifen-resistant disease. For patients with lytic bone disease, radiation therapy is used to reduce pain or prevent pathologic fractures. Bisphosphonates, such as pamidronate, clodronate, risedronate (given orally) and zoledronate (given intravenously), are used to treat hypercalcemia from bone involvement in breast cancer. Bisphosphonate-related osteonecrosis of the jaw has been associated with high-dose bisphosphonate use in cancer patients.

Follow-Up

Breast cancer survivors should undergo annual mammography of the preserved and contralateral breast. In the absence of specific symptoms, routine blood tests or imaging procedures looking for metastatic disease should not be performed.

Book Enhancement

Go to www.acponline.org/essentials/oncology-section.html. In *MKSAP for Students 5*, assess your knowledge with items 1-5 in the **Oncology** section.

Bibliography

Maughan KL, Lutterbie MA, Ham PS. Treatment of breast cancer. Am Fam Physician. 2010;81:1339-1346. [PMID: 20521754]

Chapter 74

Colorectal Cancer

Kathleen F. Ryan, MD

Colorectal cancer is the second leading cause of cancer death in the United States. Each year, >102,000 new cases of colorectal cancer are diagnosed and >51,000 people die from the disease. Death is preventable by using effective, safe, and relatively inexpensive screening methods.

Colorectal cancer arises from adenomatous polyps, and polyp removal reduces the risk of colorectal cancer. The main risk factors for malignant transformation are polyp size (>1.0 cm), number, and histologic type.

It is important to note that approximately 75% of colorectal cancers arise in individuals who have no obvious cancer risk. In some cases, however, these cancers are genetically linked. Genes implicated in the development of colorectal cancer fall into three categories: oncogenes, tumor suppressor genes, and DNA nucleotide mismatch repair genes. Oncogenes promote cell growth and replication, and their normal suppression in the healthy cell prevents cancer; mutations of oncogenes are oncogenic. In most sporadic cancers and some familial syndromes, mutations occur in the *APC* gene—an important tumor suppression gene. When both copies (alleles) of *APC* within a cell are mutated, cell growth becomes dysregulated. *APC* mutations, which tend to occur early in the process of colon carcinogenesis, are the cause of most cases of familial adenomatous polyposis. Mismatch repair genes assist in the repair of errors in DNA that occur during replication. When these genes are defective, small abnormal sequences of DNA called *microsatellites* are inserted into the genetic code, resulting in microsatellite instability, which predisposes the cell to malignant transformation.

Inherited colon cancer syndromes include autosomal dominant familial adenomatous polyposis (FAP) and its variants, autosomal dominant hereditary nonpolyposis colorectal cancer (HNPCC [also called Lynch syndrome]), and the autosomal dominant hamartomatous polyposis syndromes (e.g., Peutz-Jegher syndrome, juvenile polyposis). FAP accounts for 1% of all colorectal cancers; in FAP, the mucosa of the colon is covered with polyps. HNPCC accounts for 5% to 10% of colorectal cancers, is seen in younger patients, and usually involves the right colon. Patients with HNPCC also have an increased risk of other cancers (endometrial, ovarian, urologic, gastric, small bowel, pancreatic, biliary, skin, brain). Lastly, the very rare hamartomatous polyposis syndromes present in children and are associated with pigmentation of the lips.

Prevention

Although the precise pathologic mechanisms of colorectal cancer have not been identified, patients should be counseled to stop smoking, avoid excess alcohol intake, maintain a normal body weight, keep physically active, and eat red meat in moderation. A diet rich in fresh fruits and vegetables can be recommended for general health purposes, but definitive evidence linking such a diet with colorectal cancer prevention is lacking.

Screening

Screening recommendations are based on risk. All adults aged >50 years at average risk for colorectal cancer can be screened by one of several acceptable methods (Table 1). Persons at high risk are screened more intensely with colonoscopy, usually beginning at

Table 1. Screening Recommendations for Average-Risk Persons

Screening Tool	USPSTF 2008 (adults 50-75 y)	ACS 2010 (adults ≥50 y)	ACG 2008 (adults ≥50 y)
FOBT (two samples each from 3 spontaneously passed stools)	Annually	Annually	Annually
FIT	Annually	Annually	Annually
Fecal DNA testing (entire stool required)	No recommendation	Interval uncertain	Every 3 y
Sigmoidoscopy	Every 5 y	Every 5 y	Every 5-10 y
FOBT or FIT combined with sigmoidoscopy	Stool study (FOBT or FIT) every 3 y plus sigmoidoscopy every 5 y	No recommendation	No recommendation
Double-contrast barium enema	No recommendation	Every 5 y	No recommendation
Colonoscopy	Every 10 y	Every 10 y	Every 10 y (start at age 45 y in black persons)
CT colonography	No recommendation	Every 5 y	Every 5 y

ACG = American College of Gastroenterology; ACS = American Cancer Society; FOBT = fecal occult blood test; FIT = fecal immunochemical test; USPSTF = U.S. Preventive Services Task Force.

Table 2. Screening Recommendations For High-Risk Persons

Risk	Recommendation
Second- or third-degree relatives with colorectal cancer	Screen as described for average-risk person (see Table 1).
First-degree relative with colorectal cancer or adenomatous polyps at age ≥60 y	Screen as described for average-risk patient (see Table 1), beginning at age 40 y.
Two or more first-degree relatives with colorectal cancer or one first-degree relative with colorectal cancer or adenomatous polyps at age <60 y	Colonoscopy every 5 y, beginning at age 40 y or 10 years younger than the earliest diagnosis in the family, whichever comes first. Double-contrast barium enema may be substituted, but colonoscopy is preferred.
Personal history of inflammatory bowel disease	Begin surveillance colonoscopy every 1-2 y, starting 8-10 y after disease onset. If dysplasia is discovered on random biopsy, colectomy is recommended.

age 40 years and every 5 years thereafter (Table 2). High risk is defined as having multiple first-degree relatives with colorectal cancer or a first-degree relative diagnosed with colonic adenomatous polyps or colorectal cancer at age <60 years. Persons with a personal history of an adenomatous polyp larger than 1.0 cm require a repeat colonoscopy within 3 years. Serum carcinoembryonic antigen (CEA) should not be used as a screening test for colorectal cancer due to its poor sensitivity and specificity. Computed tomographic colonography ("virtual colonoscopy") is a new screening modality that uses helical CT to capture two-dimensional axial images that can be converted into a three-dimensional view. Studies are underway to determine its effectiveness in screening populations. When fecal occult blood testing (FOBT) is used, a positive reading in even one slide window should be evaluated with colonoscopy.

Diagnosis

Common signs and symptoms of colorectal cancer are influenced by the site of the primary tumor and may include a change in bowel habits, diarrhea, constipation, a feeling that the bowel does not empty completely, bright red blood in the stool or melanotic stools, and stools that are narrower in caliber than usual. Other signs include general abdominal discomfort (frequent gas pains,

bloating, fullness, cramping), unintentional weight loss, fatigue, and vomiting. Findings of iron deficiency anemia in persons aged >40 years require careful evaluation for colorectal cancer (Table 3). Colonoscopy is performed when colorectal cancer is suspected. The sensitivity and specificity of colonoscopy are each >95%, and colonoscopy is the reference standard for detecting cancer or polyps. If colonoscopy is unavailable, a double-contrast barium enema can be used; sensitivity and specificity are 85% and 80%, respectively, for detecting cancer, but the test is much less sensitive in detecting polyps. If an inherited colorectal cancer syndrome is suspected when there is a dominant pattern of cancer occurrence in family members, both the patient and family members should be referred for genetic testing. Also suspect an inherited syndrome if hamartomatous polyps or >10 adenomatous polyps are found on colonoscopy. If undetected, colorectal cancer can spread to the liver, lungs, pleural space, bone, or brain.

Therapy

Surgery is an integral component of colorectal cancer treatment. Surgery usually is followed by chemotherapy in cases of advanced-stage colon cancer and in most cases of rectal cancers. There is debate over the usefulness of preoperative staging, but many experts agree that the initial evaluation should include a

Table 3. Differential Diagnosis of Colorectal Cancer

Clinical Finding	Notes
Hematochezia (see Chapter 23)	Blood on toilet tissue and bright red or maroon stool characterizes hemorrhoids; diverticulosis and arteriovenous malformations usually exhibit massive bleeding. These nonmalignant conditions account for more than 95% of visible rectal bleeding, although evaluation to rule out cancer is always necessary.
Positive FOBT	Approximately 3%-5% of persons with a positive FOBT will have colorectal cancer; up to 50% will have polyps. Other causes of positive FOBT include NSAIDs, upper GI lesions, and false-positive results.
Iron deficiency anemia (see Chapter 42)	Menstrual blood loss is a frequent cause of iron loss in women of childbearing age but should not be presumed to be the diagnosis. Other causes include IBD, GERD, and causes listed for positive FOBT. Sprue causes iron malabsorption and is characterized by diarrhea and fat malabsorption. A substantial fraction of persons aged >50 y with iron deficiency anemia will be found to have colorectal cancer.
Change in bowel habits	IBS is characterized by abdominal pain plus diarrhea, constipation, or both. Changes in diet and bed rest may decrease bowel frequency. Many medications affect bowel frequency. Colorectal cancer accounts for <5% of cases of change in bowel habits but nonetheless must be considered.
Abdominal mass or hepatomegaly	Abdominal masses found on physical examination may have many causes. Abdominal and bowel imaging are the next steps. These findings are extremely rare presentations of colon cancer, although a rectal mass on rectal examination is quite specific for colon cancer or polyp.
Hypogastric abdominal pain (see Chapter 15)	Consider IBS, diverticulitis, IBD, ischemic colitis, colonic volvulus, and uterine or ovarian disease. Bowel, abdominal, and genitourinary imaging should follow physical examination for evaluating these possible conditions and for ruling out colon cancer. Colon cancer accounts for abdominal pain in <5% of patients.

FOBT = fecal occult blood test; GERD = gastroesophageal reflux disease; GI = gastrointestinal; IBD = inflammatory bowel disease; IBS = irritable bowel syndrome.

Table 4. Staging, Treatment, and Survival for Patients with Colon Cancer

AJCC Stage	Definition	Treatment	5-Year Survival (%)
I	Confined to muscularis propria	Resection for cure	92
II	Extends into subserosa or directly invades other structures	Resection for cure	73
III	Metastatic to regional lymph nodes	Resection and adjuvant chemotherapy	56
IV	Distant metastases	Palliative resection, multi-agent chemotherapy	8

AJCC = American Joint Committee on Cancer.

complete blood count, serum CEA and aminotransaminase measurements, chest radiography, and abdominal and pelvic CT. In rectal cancer, endoscopic ultrasonography is done to determine depth of tumor invasion.

For stage I or stage II colonl cancer, tumor resection is performed for cure (Table 4). For stage III disease, the cancer is resected, and adjuvant chemotherapy is initiated. For advanced metastatic disease (stage IV), removal of the primary tumor is indicated for palliative relief of obstruction or to stop bleeding. Isolated hepatic metastases can be resected, depending on the patient's overall functional status.

For rectal cancers beyond stage I, radiation therapy in addition to surgery (with or without chemotherapy) is first-line treatment. The addition of radiation therapy to surgery and chemotherapy has been shown to decrease the risk of recurrence and death.

Chemotherapy is used as both adjuvant and palliative therapy in colon and rectal cancer after surgery to decrease relapses and increase survival. First-line agents for stage III colorectal cancer include 5-fluorouracil, leucovorin, and, possibly, oxaliplatin. In metastatic colorectal cancer, multi-agent chemotherapy increases median survival compared with standard chemotherapy. Agents include oxaliplatin or irinotecan combined with a fluoropyrimidine. The addition of bevacizumab, an antiangiogenesis monoclonal antibody, further increases the efficacy of chemotherapy. The monoclonal antibodies cetuximab and panitumumab are epidermal growth factor receptor inhibitors that have been approved to treat metastatic colorectal cancer.

In advanced disease, palliative surgical resection is sometimes needed to prevent obstruction. In addition, a palliative care consult can be helpful in assisting with pain management, navigation of the complex health care system, and psychosocial support for the patient and family.

Follow-Up

Colorectal cancer survivors are at increased risk for future adenomatous polyps and new colorectal cancers. The most common sites of recurrence of colorectal cancer are the site of initial removal as well as the liver, bone, and brain. Follow-up examinations allow removal of polyps and prevention of cancer. If a noninvasive cancerous polyp was removed, follow-up colonoscopies are recommended at 3 and 6 months, 1 year, and 2 years. If an invasive cancer was resected, repeat colonoscopy at 3 years is performed to examine the anastomotic site and to look for new neoplasms.

Five to twenty percent of patients with stage I or II colorectal cancer will develop metastases. Some metastatic disease can be surgically resected (salvage surgery), resulting in a substantial cure rate. When a curative approach is not appropriate, palliative care is instituted. Patients with stage III disease are followed for both recurrence of the tumor and adverse effects of chemotherapy. Periodic serum aminotransaminase and CEA measurements and chest radiography are often done but have not been shown to improve survival.

Book Enhancement

Go to www.acponline.org/essentials/oncology-section.html. In *MKSAP for Students 5*, assess your knowledge with items 6-9 in the **Oncology** section.

Bibliography

Ballinger AB, Anggiansah C. Colorectal cancer. BMJ. 2007;335:715-718. [PMID: 17916855]

Rex DK, Johnson DA, Anderson JC, Schoenfeld PS, Burke CA, Inadomi JM; American College of Gastroenterology. American College of Gastroenterology guidelines for colorectal cancer screening 2009 [corrected]. Am J Gastroenterol. 2009;104:739-750 [published erratum appears in Am J Gastroenterol. 2009;104:1613]. [PMID: 19240699]

Chapter 75

Lung Cancer

Alyssa C. Perroy, MD

Lung cancer is the leading cause of cancer-related death in both men and women in the United States. Despite being less common, lung cancer accounts for more cancer deaths than the three most common cancers (breast, prostate, and colon) combined. Lung cancer mortality correlates with prevalence of cigarette smoking, and lung cancer will occur in 15% of lifetime smokers.

Prevention

Abstinence from smoking remains the best method of preventing lung cancer. All patients should be screened for current or prior tobacco use; current smokers should be encouraged to stop smoking, and all patients should be advised to avoid second-hand smoke exposure. Smoking cessation could prevent up to 90% of all lung cancers. Retinol (vitamin A), β-carotene, N-acetylcysteine, and selenium supplementation do not prevent lung cancer.

Screening

There is no proven role for routine screening for lung cancer. Recent reports of high survival rates among patients with lung cancer detected by chest CT appear promising; however, results may be due to lead time bias. Currently, screening with chest radiography or CT is not recommended but is under study in a large randomized clinical trial. Outcome data will inform future recommendations as to whether screening via chest imaging in current or former smokers leads to a mortality benefit.

Diagnosis

Carefully evaluate new pulmonary or chest complaints, particularly in smokers or former smokers. Be alert for symptoms such as hemoptysis, pulmonary infections, dyspnea, cough, or chest pain. Patients with small cell lung cancer often present with metastatic disease and paraneoplastic syndromes (Table 1).

In patients with new or persistent pulmonary symptoms, look for findings suggestive of a primary tumor (abnormal lung findings), intrathoracic spread (hoarse voice, Horner syndrome, brachial plexopathy, chest wall tenderness), extrathoracic spread (wasting, lymphadenopathy, focal neurologic findings, bone tenderness, skin nodules, hepatomegaly), and paraneoplastic syndromes. Obtain a chest radiograph to look for masses, lymphadenopathy, and pleural effusions. Smaller lung cancers may require CT for detection.

Histologic confirmation is necessary for diagnosis. To guide patient management, tissue should be obtained by an approach that furthers disease staging. For example, the best approach to a patient with a lung mass in the setting of weight loss and unilateral supraclavicular lymph node enlargement is to obtain a peripheral node biopsy, which will simultaneously diagnose and stage the lung cancer. Alternatively, tissue can be obtained by percutaneous lung biopsy, pleural cytology, or transbronchial biopsy. Sputum cytology is reserved for patients with poor pulmonary function who cannot tolerate invasive procedures. Treatment and prognosis vary based on whether the patient has non–small cell lung cancer (adenocar-

Table 1. Paraneoplastic and Other Syndromes Associated with Lung Cancer

Syndrome	Notes
Acromegaly	Growth hormone–releasing hormone (small cell carcinoma)
Cushing syndrome	Adrenocorticotropic hormone (small cell carcinoma)
Eaton-Lambert syndrome	Proximal limb weakness and fatigue due to antibodies to voltage-gated calcium channels (small cell carcinoma)
Hypercalcemia	Parathyroid hormone–related peptide (small cell carcinoma)
Hypertrophic pulmonary osteoarthropathy	Painful, new periosteal bone growth and clubbing (most common with adenocarcinoma)
Hyponatremia	Arginine vasopressin and atrial natriuretic peptide (small cell carcinoma)
Pancoast syndrome (superior sulcus tumor)	Shoulder pain, lower brachial plexopathy, and Horner syndrome from apical lung tumor
Superior vena cava syndrome	External compression of superior vena cava causing face and arm swelling
Trousseau syndrome	Hypercoagulable state (most common with adenocarcinoma)
Vocal cord paralysis	Entrapment of recurrent laryngeal nerve

cinoma, large cell carcinoma, or squamous cell carcinoma) or, less commonly, small cell lung cancer.

In staging non–small cell lung cancer, the task is to find evidence of metastatic disease, which eliminates surgery as a therapeutic option. The staging evaluation should include CT of the chest and abdomen and a combined positron emission tomography and CT (PET-CT) scan to assess for malignant mediastinal lymphadenopathy. PET-CT may identify advanced disease and can preclude unnecessary thoracotomy in approximately 1 in 5 patients. When aggressive therapy is considered in a patient with clinical disease stage II or higher (Table 2), brain MRI is indicated to rule out occult intracranial involvement. If the patient is not otherwise a candidate for aggressive therapy, brain imaging is indicated only to evaluate neurologic signs or symptoms. A bone scan is indicated if there is bone pain or an elevated serum calcium or alkaline phosphatase level. A complete blood count and serum calcium, alkaline phosphatase, and aminotransferase levels are obtained to detect advanced disease.

Small cell lung cancer generally is viewed as a systemic disease at diagnosis, as most patients have widespread organ involvement. Small cell tumors are exquisitely sensitive to radiation and chemotherapy. A simplified and accepted method of staging is described in terms of whether a tumor is limited to inclusion within a tolerable radiation therapy field. For example, a small cell tumor localized to one hemithorax, which could safely be radiated in one "port site," is termed limited-stage disease in contrast to the usual presentation of extensive-stage disease (more than one "port site"). Extensive-stage disease typically is associated with metastases involving the liver, bone, bone marrow, brain, adrenal glands, retroperitoneal lymph nodes, pancreas, and subcutaneous soft tissues. In patients who are eligible for treatment, perform chest radiography, CT of the chest and abdomen, MRI of the brain, PET-CT scan, and bone scan (optional if PET-CT scan is obtained). Obtain electrolytes and serum calcium, aminotransferase, and lactate dehydrogenase levels.

Incidentally discovered pulmonary nodules are common. Incidental pulmonary nodules are defined as an asymptomatic, discrete radiographic density ≤3 cm that is completely surrounded by aerated lung. Two features characterize benign pulmonary nodules: (1) no growth in 2 years and (2) calcification in a diffuse, central, or laminar pattern. Malignant nodules typically are >2 cm,

have spiculated edges, and are located in the upper lobes. The probability of malignancy increases with age >40 years, past or current smoking status, asbestos or radon exposure, and previous diagnosis of cancer. The general approach to management of pulmonary nodules is to determine behavior over time and stratify risk. If possible, obtain prior chest radiographs or imaging scans to determine stability over time. No follow-up is recommended for nodules that are ≤4 mm in patients who have never smoked and who have no other known risk factors for malignancy (history of a first-degree relative with lung cancer or significant radon or asbestos exposure). Nodules >4 mm in any patient require follow-up at an interval determined by whether the patient is considered to be at high or low risk for malignancy. Solid nodules ≥1.5 to 2.0 cm in high-risk patients require consideration for immediate biopsy; close interval CT scanning is another option in low-risk patients. Dynamic CT performed with contrast further aids in predicting a benign pulmonary nodule; a multicenter study showed a 97% negative predictive value for nonenhancing nodules with a density of ≤15 Hounsfield units.

Therapy

Tumor staging dictates prognosis and management of any lung cancer. For non–small cell lung cancer, tumor size (T), regional node status (N), and presence or absence of metastatic disease (M) are used to assign patients to a stage of I to IV (Table 2). Surgery is the mainstay of treatment for patients with stage I or II disease and select patients with stage III disease; the use of adjuvant chemotherapy has improved survival for patients with stage IB and higher disease. The use of adjuvant radiation therapy in patients with early-stage non–small cell lung cancer has not been associated with a survival benefit, but radiation therapy can be considered as primary local treatment for patients with early-stage but inoperable disease. Patients with stage III disease represent a heterogeneous group. Most have mediastinal lymphadenopathy, and survival rates depend on extent of mediastinal disease. For patients with minimal mediastinal lymphadenopathy and potentially resectable cancer, neoadjuvant chemotherapy (with or without radiation) often is administered to shrink the tumor prior to surgery. For patients with unresectable disease, chemoradiation is superior to radiation alone. Encourage all patients who smoke to

Table 2. Staging, Treatment, and Prognosis for Patients with Non–Small Cell Lung Cancer

Stage	Definition	Treatment	Prognosis
I	Tumor surrounded by lung or pleura, more than 2 cm from carina	Surgery and, in selected cases, adjuvant chemotherapy; radiotherapy if not a surgical candidate; intent is cure	60% to 70% long-term disease-free survival
II	Locally advanced disease, without mediastinal involvement	Surgery and adjuvant chemotherapy, radiotherapy if not a surgical candidate; intent is cure	40% to 50% long-term disease-free survival
III	Mediastinal involvement, or two separate tumor nodules in same lobe without mediastinal involvement	Combined modalities of chemotherapy, radiotherapy, and/or surgery	5% to 20% long-term disease-free survival
IV	Metastatic	Chemotherapy	Median survival 4 months

quit smoking before surgery or radiation to improve lung function and reduce iatrogenic morbidity.

Metastatic (inoperable) non–small cell lung cancer necessitates consideration of a combined treatment approach including local radiation for a symptomatic mass or metastatic sites and/or palliative chemotherapy. Patients with good performance status but disease progression after one chemotherapy regimen may benefit from treatment with alternate single-agent regimens. Treatment is not shown to be beneficial in patients with poor performance status (e.g., patients who are bed bound, have weight loss >10%, or have severe symptoms). Monthly intravenous bisphosphonate therapy with pamidronate or zolendronate decreases skeletal complications in patients with bony metastases.

For small cell lung cancer, combination chemotherapy with a platinum agent (e.g., cisplatin) and etoposide is the mainstay of treatment; tumor radiation is given concurrently or sequentially. Treatment markedly improves survival; even elderly patients with poor initial performance status may tolerate standard regimens. If small cell tumors respond to initial therapy, subsequent prophylactic cranial irradiation increases survival and decreases symptomatic brain involvement. Unfortunately, despite initial response to chemotherapy and radiotherapy, most patients relapse and die of their disease. In patients with good performance status despite documented relapse, consider second-line chemotherapy while educating the patient and family that tumor response is often short-lived.

Palliative treatment is important in cases of advanced disease (see Chapter 79). Severe pain typically requires scheduled administration of opioid analgesics. Use corticosteroids for patients with brain metastases to decrease intracranial edema. Use thoracic radiation for airway obstruction or superior vena cava syndrome. Use targeted radiation to relieve bone pain, visceral pain secondary to capsular distention, or pain due to nerve compression or spinal cord metastases. Early referral to comprehensive palliative care services along with standard oncologic care has been shown to lengthen overall survival in patients with metastatic non–small cell lung cancer, improve quality of life, and lower rates of depression.

Follow-Up

Continue comprehensive, ongoing follow-up of patients for detection of recurrence, management of disease and treatment complications, and symptom palliation. Most patients with lung cancer will develop recurrent disease. In long-term survivors, surveillance may lead to the detection of a second primary tumor, most commonly of the lung. Schedule follow-up at frequent intervals, and evaluate for recurrent disease using clinical examination and laboratory testing. Patients with advanced, metastatic disease should be seen monthly to assess for and address new symptoms.

Book Enhancement

Go to www.acponline.org/essentials/oncology-section.html. In *MKSAP for Students 5*, assess your knowledge with items 10-13 in the **Oncology** section.

Bibliography

Sculier JP, Berghmans T, Meert AP. Update in lung cancer and mesothelioma 2009. Am J Respir Crit Care Med. 2010;181:773-781. [PMID: 20382800]

Chapter 76

Prostate Cancer

Eric H. Green, MD

Prostate cancer is the most common cancer in men and is second only to lung cancer as a cause of cancer-related deaths. Tumor growth can be slow or moderate in pace but occasionally is quite rapid. Prostate cancer is strongly associated with age, its incidence rising from near zero in patients younger than 40 years to 1 in 12 men in their seventies. Prostate cancer also is more common in black men and in men with a family history of the disease. Although the lifetime risk of developing prostate cancer is 1 in 6, the risk of death from prostate cancer is 1 in 30. Given the older age at which many patients are diagnosed and the slowly progressive nature of low-grade tumors, many patients with prostate cancer die of other illnesses.

Prevention

Because prostate cancer is common, slow-growing, and usually dependent on testosterone for growth, it is a potentially good target for chemoprophylaxis. Prophylactic use of 5α-reductase inhibitors (finasteride, dutasteride)—agents that inhibit conversion of testosterone to the more active dihydrotestosterone—reduces the incidence of prostate cancer. The cancers that do develop may be of a higher grade, although the clinical importance of these observations is unclear. Importantly, overall prostate cancer mortality is unchanged with 5α-reductase inhibitors. Furthermore, these agents have significant side effects, including decreased libido, erectile dysfunction, and gynecomastia. Thus, these drugs should not be used routinely for chemoprophylaxis, although they can be considered after a discussion with the patient of risks and benefits.

Screening

Although prostate cancer would seem to be an ideal disease for screening, given a presumed prolonged treatable preclinical disease state, screening is controversial because of the imperfect sensitivity and specificity of the screening test (serum prostate-specific antigen [PSA] measurement) and the unclear natural history of untreated disease. There is conflicting evidence from both large randomized controlled trials and epidemiologic studies regarding the efficacy of prostate cancer screening. Screening should be done only after a detailed discussion with the patient outlining both the potential benefits and known harms of screening. This discussion should include information regarding:

- The indolent nature of many prostate cancers, which suggests that early detection may not change outcomes
- The relatively low specificity and positive predictive value of current tests

- The likely need for multiple biopsies after an abnormal test
- The morbidity associated with current treatment strategies

Patients who elect screening receive both a serum PSA measurement and a digital rectal examination. Screening, if done, starts at age 50 years (or age 45 years, if the person is black or has a positive family history of prostate cancer) and continues until age 75 years or until the patient has a life expectancy of <10 years.

Diagnosis

Early prostate cancer usually is asymptomatic, although some patients may present with hematospermia, painful ejaculation, or symptoms of bladder outlet obstruction, such as urinary hesitancy and frequency. Patients with metastatic disease may present with bone pain, back pain, weight loss, or fatigue. Digital rectal examination can be used to detect prostate cancer. Although it has low sensitivity, digital rectal examination is inexpensive, without risk, and easy to perform. Any abnormality on digital rectal examination requires biopsy, regardless of serum PSA level. More advanced disease may present as signs of metastatic spread, including pelvic lymphadenopathy or signs of spinal cord compression. In addition, men with metastatic disease from an unknown primary source should be evaluated for the possibility of prostate cancer. Table 1 describes important conditions in the differential diagnosis of prostate cancer.

Serum PSA measurement is the best available noninvasive test to diagnose prostate cancer. The normal range of PSA values varies with age and race, with older men and white men having higher PSA values. PSA testing is avoided immediately after a urinary tract infection or prostatitis, both of which can raise PSA levels for up to 4 to 8 weeks. Although digital rectal examination also can elevate PSA values, this change rarely is clinically significant. Serum PSA values >4.0 ng/mL (4 µg/L) generally are considered abnormal. Serum PSA measurement has imperfect sensitivity: only 25% of men with PSA values between 4.0 (4 µg/L) and 10.0 ng/mL (10 µg/L) have prostate cancer, although most of these cancers are early stage and, therefore, potentially curable. Because the PSA value rises very slowly over time, an increase of >0.75 ng/mL (0.75 µg/L) in 1 year, regardless of the initial value, is considered abnormal.

Refer any patient with an abnormal PSA value for transrectal ultrasound-guided prostate biopsy. This outpatient procedure usually consists of six random needle biopsies. Random biopsies have a high false-positive rate and often need to be repeated if negative. Tumors detected on these biopsies are further classified according to their histology, using the Gleason score. In the Gleason histologic scoring system, tumors are graded from 1 to 5 based on the

Table 1. Differential Diagnosis of Prostate Cancer

Disorder	Notes
Abnormal Findings on Prostate Examination	
Benign prostatic hyperplasia (BPH)	BPH is characterized by symptoms of urinary outflow obstruction (nocturia, urinary urgency and hesitancy) and may result in elevated serum PSA levels. Prostate cancer and BPH can coexist, but there is no causal association between the diseases. BPH results in a generalized and symmetric enlargement of the prostate, whereas prostate cancer may manifest as a palpable lump, induration, or asymmetric enlargement. Biopsy distinguishes between the two entities.
Acute prostatitis	Acute prostatitis can result in elevated serum PSA levels but also fever, chills, dysuria, pelvic or perineal pain, and possible obstructive symptoms (dribbling, hesitancy, anuria). DRE reveals edematous and tender prostate. Urine shows pyuria and positive urine culture.
Metastatic Skeletal Disease	
Osteomyelitis	Osteomyelitis results in increased uptake on bone scans and can be confused with metastatic disease. Osteomyelitis is not associated with an elevated serum PSA level, and metastatic prostate cancer in the context of a normal PSA level is very unusual. Metastatic prostate cancer tends to be multifocal, whereas osteomyelitis tends to be unifocal. Prostate cancer and osteomyelitis have very different appearances on CT and MRI scans.
Paget disease	Paget disease of the bone can look like sclerotic bone metastases. Paget disease is not associated with an elevated serum PSA level.
Other cancers	Many other cancers spread to the pelvic and retroperitoneal lymph nodes and the bones, including bladder cancer, colorectal cancer, testicular cancer, renal cell carcinoma, carcinoma of the ureter and renal pelvis, and penile cancer. Prostate cancer can generally be distinguished from other malignancies on the basis of histopathologic examination of biopsy specimens.

DRE = digital rectal examination; PSA = prostate-specific antigen.

degree of glandular differentiation and structural architecture. The composite Gleason score is derived by adding together the two most prevalent differentiation patterns (a primary and a secondary grade) and is the best predictor of the biology of the tumor. Gleason score >7, serum PSA level >15 ng/mL (15 µg/L), large tumors, or the presence of bone pain requires a bone scan and abdominal and pelvic CT to evaluate for metastatic disease. Table 2 reviews laboratory and other studies for prostate cancer.

Therapy

Three major treatment strategies exist for localized prostate cancer: surgery, radiation therapy, and active surveillance. To date, the optimal treatment is not defined, and the choice should be governed by both the tumor risk score (a combination of TMN staging, PSA value, and Gleason score) and anticipated life expectancy, with more aggressive therapy offered to patients with either long life expectancy or high-risk tumors. Radical prostatectomy usually is reserved for patients with at least a 10-year life expectancy. Radical prostatectomy usually is curative in patients whose disease is confined to the prostate (stage T0-T2) and who lack high-risk features, such as a high serum PSA level or Gleason score. Historically, radical prostatectomy was associated with a high rate of erectile dysfunction, but surgical advances, including robotic assistance, have reduced this risk considerably.

Radiation therapy can be delivered using external beam radiation or by implanting radioactive "seeds" around the prostate (brachytherapy). Radiation therapy has a similar cure rate as surgery for localized disease. In comparison to surgery, radiation carries lower risks of urinary incontinence and erectile dysfunction at the expense of risks for radiation proctitis and cystitis. Radiation therapy also does not confer the added risks of general anesthesia and surgery, although therapy may take months to complete. External beam radiation often is combined with androgen deprivation therapy (ADT) to treat locally advanced disease (defined by tumor size, a high serum PSA level, or high Gleason score). Palliative external beam radiation is effective for painful bone metastases.

Active surveillance without immediate therapy is a reasonable treatment modality for some patients, especially patients with low-grade, prostate-confined disease. This treatment strategy capitalizes on the slow-growing nature of most prostate cancers; the natural history of prostate cancer often confers a 10- to 15-year lag before metastatic spread. Patients receive continued evaluation of their prostate cancer, with the options of surgery or radiation therapy if there is cancer progression. Observation also is used for men with a reduced life expectancy, although in these patients, progressive prostate cancer often is treated palliatively.

Prostate cancers are dependent on testosterone for growth; thus, ADT often is used to treat higher-risk localized cancers, advanced disease, and local treatment failures (defined by a rise in serum PSA level after surgery or radiation therapy). Although some patients undergo surgical orchiectomy, most rely on a luteinizing hormone-releasing hormone analog (e.g., leuprolide, goserelin) for "chemical castration." When these agents are initiated, there often is a transient testosterone surge, and patients with painful bone metastases or epidural metastases need additional short-term androgen blockade (usually using bicalutamide or flutamide). ADT has significant side effects, including hot flashes, loss of libido, gynecomastia, impotence, and osteoporosis. Patients with progressive disease despite ADT often are treated with added androgen blockade, diethylstilbestrol, or ketoconazole. Patients whose disease continues to progress may require chemotherapy. In patients with prostate cancer metastatic to bone, annual infusions of the bisphosphonate zoledronate can decrease the risk for skeletal complications.

Table 2. Laboratory and Other Studies for Prostate Cancer

Test	Notes
Prostate-specific antigen (PSA)	A serum PSA level >4.0 ng/mL (4 µg/L) has a PPV for prostate cancer of 30%-37%; most men with PSA level of 4-10 ng/mL (4-10 µg/L) do not have prostate cancer. BPH, prostatitis, urinary tract infection, prostatic stones, manipulation of the prostate or lower urinary tract, and ejaculation can result in elevated serum PSA level. A serum PSA level >50 ng/mL (50 µg/L) has a PPV for prostate cancer of 98%-99%. In men with prostate cancer, the initial PSA level carries important prognostic information, with lower levels predicting localized and less aggressive tumors.
Bone alkaline phosphatase	Not used in diagnosing prostate cancer. Elevated levels in patients with prostate cancer suggest bone metastases.
Transrectal ultrasonography	Transrectal ultrasonography has a PPV of 7%-34% and a NPV of 85%. The test is used to guide prostate biopsies; it is not used to screen for or stage prostate cancer.
Prostate biopsy	Biopsy is the only way to definitively diagnose prostate cancer.
CBC	Metastatic cancer to the bone marrow is common and can result in anemia.
Abdominal and pelvic CT	CT is helpful in evaluating for pelvic or retroperitoneal lymph node metastases or bone metastases. Bone or lymph node metastases are rare in men with serum PSA levels <20 ng/mL (20 µg/L), especially if the Gleason score is <8.
Bone scan	Bone is the most common site of metastatic prostate cancer, and bone scans are useful for detection. Osteoarthritis, other degenerative changes, trauma or fracture, osteomyelitis, and Paget disease also can result in increased uptake on bone scans. Ambiguous bone scan results often lead to additional bone imaging studies (radiography, CT, MRI). A biopsy is performed for ambiguous radiologic imaging results.

BPH = benign prostatic hyperplasia; CBC = complete blood count; NPV = negative predictive value; PPV = positive predictive value.

Follow-Up

Patients are monitored at least annually for recurrent disease after definitive local therapy. Evaluation includes serum PSA levels and an interval history and examination to evaluate for signs or symptoms of relapse. Patients undergoing active surveillance are reevaluated more frequently, with PSA measurements sometimes done at 3-month intervals. Digital rectal examinations or imaging studies (e.g., bone scan, CT) are not routinely performed unless specifically indicated by signs or symptoms of recurrence. Patients undergoing ADT should receive supplemental calcium and vitamin D and undergo surveillance for osteoporosis with bone density scans. Bisphosphonates can be used in patients who develop osteoporosis. The primary complication of prostate cancer is metastatic spread, most commonly to regional lymph nodes and bone. Bone metastases can cause severe pain as well as spinal cord compression. Back pain in a patient with prostate cancer may represent the first sign of spinal cord compression from epidural metastases and requires urgent evaluation with a spine MRI.

Book Enhancement

Go to www.acponline.org/essentials/oncology-section.html. In *MKSAP for Students 5*, assess your knowledge with items 14-17 in the **Oncology** section.

Bibliography

Damber JE, Aus G. Prostate cancer. Lancet. 2008;371:1710-1721. [PMID: 18486743]

Chapter 77

Cervical Cancer

Asra R. Khan, MD

Cervical cancer is the most common cancer in women worldwide and the seventh most common cancer in the United States. Women in their teens to age 30 years typically present with dysplasia, whereas invasive cancer is more commonly seen after age 45 years. Persistent infection with high-risk human papillomavirus (HPV) subtypes (HPV-16 and HPV-18) can cause cervical dysplasia, and subsequently, cancer. Dysplastic lesions can progress to cellular intraepithelial neoplasia, which in turn can evolve into well-differentiated low-grade lesions and then undifferentiated high-grade lesions. These precancerous lesions may regress spontaneously at any point or may progress to invasive cancer.

Prevention

HPV infection is sexually transmitted and can cause cervical dysplasia and cervical cancer. Having multiple sexual partners increases exposure to HPV, and intercourse at an early age exposes the cervix to HPV when it is most vulnerable to infection. Using condoms helps decrease exposure to HPV. Therefore, patients should be advised to limit their number of sexual partners, avoid intercourse at an early age (age <13-15 years), and use condoms to decrease the risk of acquiring HPV infection. Patients who smoke should also be advised about smoking cessation; women who smoke have an increased risk of developing cervical dysplasia and cancer because of the carcinogenic and immunosuppressive effects of smoking.

A quadrivalent vaccine against HPV has been approved for females aged 9 to 26 years and is recommended for girls aged 11 to 12 years and females aged 13 to 26 years who have not received or completed the vaccine series. The vaccine protects against high-risk HPV subtypes (HPV-16 and HPV-18) and subtypes that cause genital warts (HPV-6 and HPV-11). The vaccine consists of three doses; the second dose is given 2 months after the initial dose, and the third dose is given 6 months after the initial dose. Ideally, the vaccine should be administered prior to the onset of sexual activity. Pregnant women should not receive the vaccine, because there is a lack of safety data in this population. In 2010, the Advisory Committee on Immunization Practices stated that males aged 9 to 26 years may be considered for immunization with the quadrivalent vaccine to reduce their likelihood of acquiring genital warts.

The vaccine is very effective against HPV-16 and HPV-18; however, it does not protect against all types of HPV. It also does not treat existing HPV-related infections, warts, or precancerous lesions. Roughly 30% of cervical cancers will not be prevented by the vaccine, so women should continue to get regular Pap smears.

Moreover, the length of immunity is not yet known, so a booster may be needed.

Screening

Annual Pap smears decrease the risk of death from cervical cancer by 95%. Screening is initiated at age 21 years or within 3 years of onset of vaginal intercourse. The screening interval may be decreased to every 2 to 3 years in women aged >30 years who have had three consecutive satisfactory, normal smears, unless there is a history of diethylstilbestrol exposure or the patient is HIV-positive or immunocompromised. These high-risk women should undergo screening every 6 to 12 months. Alternatively, low-risk women aged >30 years can be screened with a combined Pap smear and HPV DNA test. If both tests are negative, the screening interval can be increased to every 3 years; if the cytology is negative but high-risk HPV DNA testing is positive, both tests should be repeated at 6 to 12 months. Discontinue screening at age 65 to 70 years if the patient has been adequately screened, has had normal Pap smears, and has no other risk factors. Also, discontinue screening patients who have had a total hysterectomy (with removal of the cervix) for benign disease.

Results of cervical cytology are reported using the standard 2001 Bethesda System. Pap smears are reported as satisfactory if they contain an adequate sample, including an endocervical component. If the cytology result is unsatisfactory, usually due to scant cellularity, a Pap test should be repeated at the earliest convenient time. If the cytology result is atypical squamous cells of undetermined significance (ASC-US), there are three alternative management strategies. Patients may be referred immediately for colposcopy; however, this may not be convenient for patients and is not cost-effective. The colposcope is a low-powered magnification device that permits the identification of mucosal abnormalities characteristic of dysplasia or invasive cancer and guides selection of tissue for biopsy. The second strategy is to repeat the Pap smear at 6 and 12 months. If both subsequent Pap smears are normal, the patient may return to routine screening. If any subsequent test result is ASC-US or a higher-grade lesion, the patient should be referred for colposcopy. Finally, the most cost-effective and convenient way to manage ASC-US is to order an HPV test when obtaining a Pap smear (called "reflex HPV testing"). The lab will then check for HPV on any Pap smear that is reported as ASC-US. If results are positive for high-risk HPV, the patient is referred for colposcopy. If results are negative for the high-risk subtypes, the Pap smear is repeated in 1 year. The preceding recommendations apply to both pre- and postmenopausal women with ASC-US. For females aged ≤20 years with ASC-US or low-grade squamous intraepithelial lesion (LSIL), repeat the Pap test in 1 year instead of following the adult recommendations. The following cytology findings in pre- or postmenopausal women should be referred for colposcopy or further evaluation, even if HPV testing is negative: LSIL, high-grade squamous intraepithelial lesion (HSIL), atypical squamous cells/cannot exclude HSIL (ASC-H), squamous cell cancer, adenocarcinoma, atypical glandular cells, or endometrial cells in women aged >40 years (Table 1).

Diagnosis

Table 2 summarizes the differential diagnosis of cervical cancer. Symptoms of cervical cancer may include postcoital bleeding, foul-smelling vaginal discharge, change in urinary or bowel habits, right upper quadrant abdominal pain, back pain, or leg swelling. The first symptom often is bleeding after intercourse. Large exophytic tumors and large ulcerative lesions can become necrotic and produce a foul-smelling vaginal discharge. Advanced cervical cancer may impinge on the urinary bladder, ureters, or rectosigmoid colon, causing change in urinary or bowel habits. Cancer can invade through the parametrium to the pelvic sidewall and obstruct the ureter, infiltrate nerves along the uterosacral ligament and sacrum, and compress the iliac vessels. The "terrible triad" of advanced cervical cancer is sciatic back pain, hydroureter, and leg swelling.

On physical examination, look for an exophytic or ulcerative lesion on the cervix, foul-smelling vaginal discharge, firmness in the parametrium, leg swelling, and supraclavicular lymphadeno-

pathy (Virchow node). Metastatic disease to the liver may present as tenderness or a mass in the right upper quadrant.

A Pap smear can detect cervical dysplasia and microinvasive and small invasive cancers of the cervix; a Pap test is indicated for any patient with postcoital bleeding. Cervical dysplasia and some early cancers are not visible to the naked eye and require colposcopic examination of the cervix for detection. Biopsies are taken of any grossly visible abnormality of the cervix to determine the histologic diagnosis and to exclude invasive cancer.

The following tests should be obtained in all patients with cervical cancer: chest radiography, abdominal and pelvic CT, and pelvic examination under anesthesia with cystoscopy and proctoscopy (Table 3). Proper staging of cervical cancer (FIGO [International Federation of Obstetrics and Gynecology] system) helps with prognosis and tailoring of treatment and gives a small survival advantage.

Therapy

Stage 1A1 cancers (microscopic, confined to cervix, depth of invasion <3 mm, horizontal spread <7 mm) have a small chance of recurrence and lymph node metastasis. Women with this diagnosis who wish to retain fertility may be treated with a loop electrosurgical excision procedure (LEEP) or cervical conization instead of hysterectomy, to preserve childbearing potential. Women who do not wish to retain fertility may undergo vaginal, abdominal, or modified radical hysterectomy to decrease the chance of recurrence. Once cervical cancer has extended to stage 1A2 (microscopic, confined to cervix, depth of invasion 3-5 mm, horizontal spread <7 mm) or beyond, LEEP, cervical conization, or abdominal or vaginal hysterectomy alone cannot cure the patient; these patients require modified radical hysterectomy. If a tumor is stage 1B or 2A (microscopic cancer with dimensions >stage 1A2, any gross cervical lesion, or cancer extending to the upper two thirds of the vagina), a radical hysterectomy is required to ensure that the tumor is removed en bloc with an adequate margin and regional lymph nodes.

Patients with early cervical cancer who are not surgical candidates or who do not wish surgery may undergo primary radiation therapy. Once a tumor has grown into the parametrium or lower vagina (stages 2B to 4A), adequate margins cannot be obtained by surgery and radiation therapy is required. Total pelvic exenteration consists of resection of the uterus, vagina, bladder, and rectosigmoid colon and is reserved for patients with recurrent or persistent cancer after radiation therapy, provided the patients are good surgical candidates with no evidence of metastatic disease. Chemotherapy is not effective following high-dose radiation, because radiation fibrosis prevents adequate drug delivery.

Of cancers occurring during pregnancy, cervical cancer is one of the most common. Treatment is based on stage, but the timing of treatment is influenced by the duration of the pregnancy.

Radiation-sensitizing chemotherapy increases the response to radiation by facilitating additional tumor cell killing. Because of the direct killing of tumor cells by chemotherapy, the tumor tends to shrink more rapidly, and thus the hypoxic tumor cells (which are relatively resistant to radiation) receive more blood supply and oxygenation, becoming more sensitive to radiation. Radiation-

Table 1. The 2001 Bethesda System for Reporting Results of Cervical Cytology

Specimen adequacy

Satisfactory

Unsatisfactory

Interpretation/result

Negative for intraepithelial lesion or malignancy

Epithelial cell abnormalities

  Squamous cell

    ASC-US

    ASC-H

    LSIL

    HSIL

    Squamous cell carcinoma

  Glandular cell

    Atypical glandular cells

    Atypical glandular cells, favor neoplastic

    Endocervical adenocarcinoma in situ

    Adenocarcinoma

    Other malignant neoplasms

ASC-H = atypical squamous cells/cannot exclude a high-grade squamous intraepithelial lesion; ASC-US = atypical squamous cells of undetermined significance; HSIL = high-grade squamous intraepithelial lesion; LSIL = low-grade squamous intraepithelial lesion.
http://nih.techriver.net/bethesdaTable.php.

Table 2. Differential Diagnosis of Cervical Cancer

Disorder	Notes
Dysplasia	Abnormal Pap test result. Needs colposcopy and biopsy.
Nabothian cysts[a]	Nabothian cysts are formed when glandular tissue is covered by squamous epithelium. Nabothian cysts are common and can become quite large. If diagnosis is questionable, needs biopsy.
Cervicitis (see Chapter 53)	May cause postcoital bleeding. There are no discrete lesions on the cervix, but the cervix is red and inflamed. Needs biopsy if Pap smear result is abnormal.
Cervical ectopy[a]	Presence of columnar epithelium on the ectocervix is a normal variant appearing as a red, beefy area; occasionally mistaken for cervicitis. Close inspection reveals the demarcation where the squamous epithelium begins.
Cervical atrophy	May cause postcoital bleeding. Vagina and cervix tend to be pale and atrophic. Obtain Pap smear.
Cervical polyp[a]	Finger-like mass protruding from os. Needs biopsy or excision.
Cervical cysts	Tend to be well-circumscribed bubble-like lesions on the cervix. If diagnosis is questionable, needs biopsy.

[a]Go to www.acponline.org/essentials/oncology-section.html to see images of these findings.

Table 3. Laboratory and Other Studies for Cervical Cancer

Test	Notes
Pap smear	Annual Pap smears reduce the risk of death from cervical cancer by 95%.
HPV DNA	Testing for high-risk HPV DNA identifies more women with high-grade dysplasia than does Pap smear.
Colposcopy	Used to direct cervical biopsies after Pap smear that shows high-grade squamous intraepithelial lesion or cancer.
Cervical biopsy	Helps differentiate cervical dysplasia from microinvasive and invasive cancer.
Chest radiography	Used in staging to detect asymptomatic lung metastasis (1%).
Kidney ultrasonography	Used to detect hydroureter in patients with pelvic spread of cancer.
Abdominal and pelvic CT	May be used to help direct therapy but is not used as a part of staging.
Examination under anesthesia, with cystoscopy and proctoscopy	Used to detect regional spread to help determine stage.

HPV = human papillomavirus

sensitizing chemotherapy is not regarded as an adequate systemic chemotherapy, because the drugs are given in too low a dose and over too short a time period.

Once cervical cancer has spread from the pelvis, pelvic surgery and radiation therapy are no longer options, and chemotherapy is needed to treat distant disease. Cisplatin is the most active chemotherapeutic agent with which to treat cervical cancer.

Follow-Up

Routine examination may allow for early detection of cancer recurrence. Schedule regular follow-up visits every 3 months for the first year, every 4 months for the second year, and every 6 months until 5 years. At follow-up visits, include history, physical examination, and Pap smear of the vaginal cuff. Patients with advanced disease may require chest radiography and abdominal and pelvic CT.

Book Enhancement

Go to www.acponline.org/essentials/oncology-section.html. In *MKSAP for Students 5*, assess your knowledge with items 18-21 in the **Oncology** section.

Bibliography

Apgar BS, Kittendorf AL, Bettcher CM, Wong J, Kaufman AJ. Update on ASCCP consensus guidelines for abnormal cervical screening tests and cervical histology. Am Fam Physician. 2009;80:147-155. [PMID: 19621855]

Chapter 78

Skin Cancer

Monica Ann Shaw, MD

More than 1 million cases of the most common skin cancers (basal cell carcinoma and squamous cell carcinoma) are diagnosed annually in the United States. The incidence of melanoma, the most serious form of skin cancer, is increasing at a rate of 3% to 6% annually. The lifetime risk of melanoma in the United States for persons with light skin is estimated to be 1 in 50. Melanoma is the most common cancer among people aged 25 to 29 years.

Prevention

Ultraviolet (UV) radiation from sunlight and man-made sources (tanning beds) is the most important environmental factor predisposing to skin cancer. Children and adults should limit sun exposure and prevent sunburn by wearing protective clothing, avoiding exposure during peak hours, and wearing sunscreen with SPF 15 or greater. Nonmelanoma skin cancers, particularly squamous cell carcinoma, are associated with cumulative sun exposure and occur more frequently in areas maximally exposed to the sun, such as the face, forearms, and back of the hands. Melanomas are associated with intense intermittent sun exposure and tend to occur in areas exposed to the sun sporadically, such as the lower legs in women and the back in men. Studies suggest that sunscreen has a direct protective effect against acute UV-related skin damage and nonmelanoma skin cancer, but studies have failed to find any association between the use of sunscreen and the incidence of melanoma. Studies have shown that exposure to UV radiation from indoor tanning devices is associated with an increased risk of melanoma, particularly with exposure before age 35 years. The increased risk is reported to be as high as 75%. Studies also demonstrate an increased risk of squamous cell and basal cell carcinomas with tanning bed use.

Screening

The U.S. Preventive Services Task Force has not found sufficient evidence to recommend for or against screening (by clinical examination) to prevent skin cancer but have concluded that counseling in primary care settings can increase behaviors that reduce sun exposure and the use of indoor tanning. Patients can examine their own skin for changes in moles (nevi) and have regular clinical examinations. Individuals at high risk for melanoma benefit most from clinical examinations. Risk factors for melanoma include UV radiation exposure, large number (≥50) of nevi, dysplastic nevi, history of blistering sunburns, poor tanning ability (fair skin, freckles, blonde or red hair, blue eyes), and personal or family history of melanoma. Approximately 10% of melanomas are familial. In the United States, the incidence of melanoma is at least 10 to 20 times greater in white populations than in black populations. Among white individuals, rates are >50% higher in men than in women. The trunk is the most common primary tumor site for persons who are white or American Indian, whereas the lower extremity is the most common primary site for persons who are Hispanic, black, Asian, or Pacific Islander.

Risk factors for basal cell carcinoma include chronic exposure to UV radiation, fair skin, immunosuppression, exposure to ionizing radiation, chronic arsenic exposure, previous basal cell carcinoma, and basal cell nevus syndrome. For white individuals in the United States, the lifetime risk of developing basal cell carcinoma is 30%.

The most important risk factors for squamous cell carcinoma include cumulative UV radiation exposure and increasing age. Other risk factors include skin that does not tan, exposure to ionizing radiation, immunosuppression, chronic inflamed skin resulting from scars or burns, arsenic exposure, family history, smoking, and inherited skin disorders (e.g., xeroderma pigmentosum, epidermolysis bullosa, albinism). Actinic keratoses are precursors of squamous cell carcinoma; the lesions present as 1- to 3-mm, tan to red, raised, scaling "rough spots" on sun-exposed areas (e.g., head, neck, dorsum of forearms and hands, legs). Patients with risk factors, sun-damaged skin, and actinic keratoses should be screened for basal cell and squamous cell cancers.

Diagnosis

Diagnose melanoma by carefully evaluating any skin lesion that is new, suspicious, or changing in size, shape, or color (Table 1, Plate

Table 1. ABCDE of Melanoma

Asymmetry: a lesion that is not regularly round or oval.

Border irregularity: a lesion with notching, scalloping, or poorly defined margins.

Color variegation: a lesion with shades of brown, tan, red, white, or blue-black, or combinations thereof.

Diameter: a lesion >6 mm in diameter; although a high level of suspicion exists for a lesion >6 mm in diameter, early melanomas may be diagnosed at a smaller size.

Evolution: a lesion that changes in size, shape, symptoms (itching, tenderness), surface (bleeding), or shade of color.

Table 2. Major Subtypes of Melanoma

Subtype	Notes
Superficial spreading melanoma (see Plate 55); ~70% of cases	Presents as a variably pigmented plaque with an irregular border and expanding diameter ranging from a few millimeters to several centimeters. Can occur at any age and anywhere on the body, although most commonly seen on the back in men and on the legs in women. Most superficial spreading melanomas appear to arise de novo.
Nodular melanoma (see Plate 56); ~15% of cases	Presents as a dark blue or black "berry-like" lesion that expands vertically (penetrating skin). Most commonly arises from normal skin. Most often found in people aged ≥60 y. Often fails to fulfill the ABCDE criteria (Table 1).
Lentigo maligna melanoma (see Plate 57); ~10% of cases	Presents initially as a freckle-like, tan-brown patch. When confined to the epidermis, the lesion is called "lentigo maligna type." May be present for many years before it expands and becomes more variegated in color. Once it invades the dermis, it becomes melanoma. Most often arises in sun-damaged areas (face, upper trunk) in older people.
Acral lentiginous melanoma (see Plate 58); ~5% of cases	Presents as an unevenly darkly pigmented patch. Can appear as a bruise or nail streak. Most often arises on the palmar, plantar, or subungual surfaces. Most common type among Asian and dark-skinned people, with a predilection for the soles of the feet.

Table 3. Differential Diagnosis of Melanoma[a]

Lesion	Notes
Common nevi (moles)	Tend to be small macules or papules; most are <5 mm. Border is regular, smooth, and well defined. Coloration is homogeneous; usually no more than 2 shades of brown. Can be found at any site.
Dysplastic nevi	Occur predominantly on the trunk. Usually >5 mm, with a flat component. Border is characteristically fuzzy and ill defined. Shape can be round, oval, or asymmetric. Color usually is brown but can be mottled with dark brown, pink, and tan. Some individuals have only 1-5 lesions, whereas others have >100 lesions. Some clinical features of dysplastic nevi are similar to those of melanoma. Significant asymmetry and heterogeneity of color should prompt a biopsy to rule out melanoma. Recognized as a precursor to melanoma.
Melanoma	Often >10 mm. Border is more irregular. Significant heterogeneity of color ranging from tan-brown, dark brown, or black to pink, red, gray, blue, or white. Can be found at any site.

[a] Go to www.acponline.org/essentials/oncology-section.html to see images of these skin lesions.

54). Review the history of the lesion and the patient's risk factors, and perform a complete skin examination. An increase in lesion size and a change in lesion color are the most common signs of melanoma.

There are four major subtypes of melanoma (Table 2, Plates 55, 56, 57, 58). Biopsy is the gold standard to diagnose melanoma and to distinguish it from other pigmented lesions (Table 3). The biopsy must include sufficient tissue to establish the diagnosis and to allow accurate assessment of tumor thickness/extension, tumor ulceration, and adequacy of surgical margins. An excisional biopsy is preferred for all subtypes of melanoma with the exception of lentigo maligna, for which a paper-thin shave biopsy offers the highest yield. For undiagnosed pigmented lesions, removal/destruction by laser, cryosurgery, or electrodessication is inappropriate, because the ability to diagnose and stage a potentially lethal skin cancer is lost. After diagnosis of melanoma, staging involves a complete history and physical examination, emphasizing complete skin and regional node examination to determine the extent of disease and presence or absence of metastases.

Sentinel lymph node biopsy should be considered in patients with primary melanomas >1 mm thick. Although currently there is no evidence of a survivor benefit from sentinel lymph node mapping, sentinel node involvement is a powerful prognostic indicator and stratifies patients for trials of adjuvant therapy. In patients with advanced disease (e.g., node involvement), evaluation includes a complete blood count, liver chemistry studies, serum lactate dehydrogenase measurement, chest radiography, and CT of the chest and abdomen, although the yield of routine imaging is low. Staging is based on tumor thickness (T), regional lymph node involvement (N), and presence or absence of metastatic disease (M). Proper staging is important for guiding further management.

To assess for potential basal cell or squamous cell carcinomas, ask about skin lesions that fail to heal or that bleed, itch, are painful, or are slowly enlarging. A basal cell cancer classically presents as a pink, pearly or translucent, dome-shaped papule with telangiectasias, but it can also appear as a flat or scar-like lesion (Plate 59). The most readily recognized clue to the diagnosis of basal cell carcinoma is a changing skin lesion that spontaneously bleeds (Table 4).

Cutaneous squamous cell carcinoma presents as a firm, isolated, slowly evolving, keratotic macule or patch, commonly on the scalp, neck, pinna, or lip (Plate 60). Keratoacanthoma is a rapidly growing skin cancer thought to be a form of squamous cell cancer. Early lesions present as solitary, round nodules that grow rapidly. As the lesions mature, a central keratotic plug becomes visible, and the lesion becomes crater-like. Keratoacanthoma rarely progresses to invasive or metastatic cancer and often involutes within months (Plate 61).

Table 4. Differential Diagnosis of Basal Cell Carcinoma (BCC)[a]

Lesion	Notes
Nodular BCC (~60% of BCC)	A skin-toned to pink, pearly translucent, firm papule with telangiectasias. May have rolled borders and a central depression with ulceration. Often found on the head or neck.
Superficial BCC (~30% of BCC)	A well-defined, erythematous, scaling plaque or occasional papules with a thin pearly border. Larger lesions often have hemorrhagic crusts and occur predominately on the trunk. A complete skin examination to find other similar plaques may help distinguish the solitary lesion of superficial BCC from psoriasis.
Morpheaform BCC (~5-10% of BCC)	A skin-colored, waxy, scar-like area that slowly enlarges. Usually develops on the head or neck of an older person. So-named because it resembles morphea (scleroderma).
Common nevi (moles)	Nevi can become elevated and may be irritated by clothing, causing inflammation and bleeding. Nevi can undergo progressive loss of color over time. By age 60 y, nevi may be flesh-colored, dome-shaped, soft papules. Even inflamed nevi do not have overlying telangiectasias.
Sebaceous hyperplasia	Benign, 2- to 4-mm papules with a characteristic yellow color and central umbilication. Occur in clusters on the face without telangiectasia or bleeding.
Actinic keratosis	Early lesions (1-3 mm) often are felt, not seen, and have a rough sandpaper texture. Color ranges from skin-colored to pink to red to brown. Occur on sun-damaged skin. Early superficial BCC may look like early actinic keratoses. With time, superficial BCC develops a rolled border and actinic keratoses get a thicker keratotic scale.
Bowen disease (SCC in situ)	A solitary, sharply demarcated, pink to fiery red scaly plaque that resembles superficial BCC, psoriasis, or eczema. May have a keratotic surface. Most commonly occurs on sun-exposed areas.
Psoriasis	In the early phase, the sharply demarcated erythematous plaques with slight scale may resemble superficial BCC. As the psoriatic area matures, a silvery-white scale develops that has characteristic pinpoint bleeding when removed.
Nummular eczema	Round, well-demarcated, eczematous patches (1-3 cm) found on the extremities. Pruritus may be intense, which results in scratching. The scratch marks may be the best way to discriminate nummular eczema from superficial BCC.
Tinea	Scaly patch with central clearing and an active border of erythema, papules, and vesicles. Tinea is more erythematous than BCC and usually has a larger area of central clearing.

[a] Go to www.acponline.org/essentials/oncology-section.html to see images of these lesions.

Therapy

Surgery is the mainstay of therapy for patients with melanoma. Because melanoma cells extend beyond the visible borders of the tumor, wide excision is necessary to ensure that all melanoma is removed. The extent of surgery depends on the thickness of the primary melanoma. Several studies show that 80% of patients with melanoma are cured with wide-margin surgical resection. Melanomas that are <1 mm thick are associated with a 90% long-term overall survival. Patients with melanomas between 1 and 4 mm thick have a long-term survival that ranges from 50% to 85%.

Node dissection is performed in patients with clinically palpable regional lymph nodes. Patients with node-positive disease have potentially curable melanoma and should be treated aggressively with surgery. Tumor thickness and number of positive nodes are the most important prognostic factors in patients with melanoma. Many patients with melanoma are at low risk for recurrence (primary tumor <4 mm thick or negative nodes) and do not require postsurgical treatment. For patients with primary melanomas >4 mm thick or positive nodes, adjuvant treatment with high-dose interferon therapy is beneficial, but toxicity is considerable. Interferon is the only adjuvant therapy approved by the FDA for the treatment of high-risk patients to prevent disease recurrence and possibly improve overall survival rates. Metastatic melanoma (i.e., melanoma that has spread beyond regional lymph nodes) is an incurable disease, and there is no evidence that treatment of metastatic disease prolongs overall survival. Palliation of symptoms may be possible with chemotherapy or immunotherapy.

Patients with metastatic melanoma have an estimated 5-year overall survival between 6% and 10%. Median survival is 8.5 months. Melanoma can metastasize to virtually any organ of the body.

Nonmelanoma skin cancers can be categorized as low-risk or high-risk based on lesion and host characteristics. Lesion characteristics include anatomic location, size, cell type, border (well- or ill-defined), and whether the tumor is primary or recurrent; host characteristics include history of previous radiation therapy to the tumor site and immunosuppression. Basal cell carcinoma rarely metastasizes, but its growth and treatment can be a source of morbidity. With squamous cell cancer, the thickness of the lesion is an important prognostic indicator. Squamous cell cancer metastases are seen in 1% to 5% of cases and are associated with a poor prognosis.

Surgery is the mainstay of therapy for nonmelanoma skin cancers. The goal is complete excision with cosmetic preservation. For actinic keratoses and low-risk basal cell or squamous cell skin cancers, treatment options include cryosurgery, electrodessication and curettage, topical therapy with fluorouracil or imiquimod, and surgical excision. For high-risk skin cancers, traditional surgical excision or Mohs surgery is preferred. Mohs micrographic surgery is the treatment of choice for many high-risk situations (e.g., cancers with risk factors for recurrence, tumors located in the central face or periorificial area, tumor recurrence following previous treatment, incompletely excised tumor, high-risk pathology, large tumor, tumor with poorly defined borders). Mohs surgery involves excision of the tumor and immediate preparation of tissue to allow histologic examination at the time of the procedure to ensure that all margins are clear of tumor, thus reducing the chance of recurrence. Radiation therapy can be an option in older patients who cannot tolerate surgery or with large tumors.

Follow-Up

Patients with a history of melanoma have a 4% to 6% increased risk of developing a second primary melanoma as well as an increased risk of developing a basal cell or squamous cell cancer. Patients need education about skin self-examination, sun exposure, and careful lifelong surveillance. Most recurrences of melanoma occur within 10 years.

Patients with squamous cell or basal cell carcinoma are at an increased lifelong risk of developing another skin cancer. Approximately 50% of patients with one nonmelanoma skin cancer develop another in the next 5 years. Patients need to do skin self-examination, reduce sun exposure, and have follow-up clinical examinations.

Book Enhancement

Go to www.acponline.org/essentials/oncology-section.html. In *MKSAP for Students 5*, assess your knowledge with items 22-26 in the **Oncology** section.

Bibliography

Madan V, Lear JT, Szeimies RM. Non-melanoma skin cancer. Lancet. 2010;375:673-685. [PMID: 20171403]

Thompson JF, Scolyer RA, Kefford RF. Cutaneous melanoma. Lancet. 2005;365:687-701. [PMID: 15721476]

Chapter 79

Palliative Care

Patrick C. Alguire, MD

In palliative care, physicians focus on short-term outcomes designed to improve patient comfort and quality of life. The most common patient symptoms encountered are pain, dyspnea, anorexia and weight loss, and depression.

Pain

The World Health Organization's three-step analgesic "ladder" represents a useful framework for pharmacologic treatment of pain (Figure 1). Mild pain (a score of 1-3 on the 0-10 pain intensity scale) is treated with nonnarcotic pain relievers (e.g., aspirin, acetaminophen, NSAIDs). Moderate pain (pain score of 4-6) is treated with a combination of nonnarcotic pain relievers and opioid analgesics. Severe pain (pain score 7-10) is treated mainly with opioid analgesics. If an opioid medication and acetaminophen are combined in a single pill, care must be taken to avoid inadvertent overdosing of the acetaminophen component if the need for the opioid ingredient increases; the maximum daily dose of acetaminophen for adults is 4 g. Adjuvant therapies can be used at all levels of the ladder (see Figure 1).

Starting doses of common opioid pain medications, given in morphine equivalents, are detailed in Table 1; morphine equivalents can also be used to convert dosages of one opioid to another and to convert oral and parenteral dosages. Oral administration is the preferred route for opioid analgesics because of its convenience, low cost, and ability to produce stable opioid blood levels. Intramuscular injections are not recommended because of the associated pain, unreliable absorption, and relatively long interval to peak drug concentrations. If a parenteral route is needed, intravenous or subcutaneous administration is preferred. Intravenous administration is associated with the most rapid onset of analgesia

but also the shortest duration of action. A transdermal opioid patch is available for the treatment of chronic pain but should never be used in the management of acute pain due to its slow onset of analgesia and the inability to rapidly titrate an effective dose. Long- and short-acting morphine remains one of the most cost-effective choices for palliative pain relief. Codeine, tramadol, and morphine can accumulate in patients with kidney failure and should be used with caution in this setting.

If a patient begins having pain constantly and uses opioid analgesics the entire day, a shift in treatment strategy is required. Typically, a longer-acting opioid medication is started to ensure basal pain relief for the entire day. The three most common long-acting narcotic agents are extended-release morphine, oxycodone, and transdermal fentanyl (oral transmucosal fentanyl also is available as a solid sweetened lozenge or buccal patch). A shorter-acting opioid (e.g., morphine) with or without a nonopioid analgesic is used for breakthrough pain relief (rescue therapy). To avoid overmedication, a typical starting dose of long-acting basal pain medication is 30% to 50% (based on morphine equivalents) of the patient's average 24-hour narcotic dosage. The long-acting narcotic can be titrated upward every 3 to 4 days to avoid frequent administration of the breakthrough medication. A typical starting dose for rescue therapy is 10% of the patient's total daily narcotic need. As these medications may take 1 to 3 days to take full effect, the patient must be followed carefully for sedation. Ideally, to allow ease of dose titration, the same agents should be used for rescue and basal pain relief. Bone metastases represent a special situation in which adjuvant therapies, such as radiation therapy and bisphosphonates, may provide additional pain relief.

Several narcotic analgesics should be avoided when treating chronic pain. Meperidine is rarely appropriate for oral use, owing

Table 1. Dosing and Conversion Chart for Opioid Analgesics

Drug	Equianalgesic Oral Dose	Equianalgesic Parenteral Dose
Morphine[1]	30 mg q 3-4 h	10 mg q 3-4 h
Codeine[2]	130 mg q 3-4 h	75 mg q 3-4 h
Hydromorphone	7.5 mg q 3-4 h	1.5 mg q 3-4 h
Hydrocodone	30 mg q 3-4 h	Not available
Levorphanol	4 mg q 6-8 h	2 mg q 6-8 h
Oxycodone	20 mg q 3-4 h	Not available
Oxymorphone	Not available	1 mg q 3-4 h

[1] For morphine, hydromorphone, and oxymorphone, rectal administration is an alternate route for patients unable to take oral medications, but equianalgesic doses may differ from oral and parenteral doses because of pharmacokinetic differences.
[2] Caution: Codeine doses above 65 mg often are not appropriate, due to diminishing incremental analgesia with increasing doses but continually increasing constipation and other side effects.

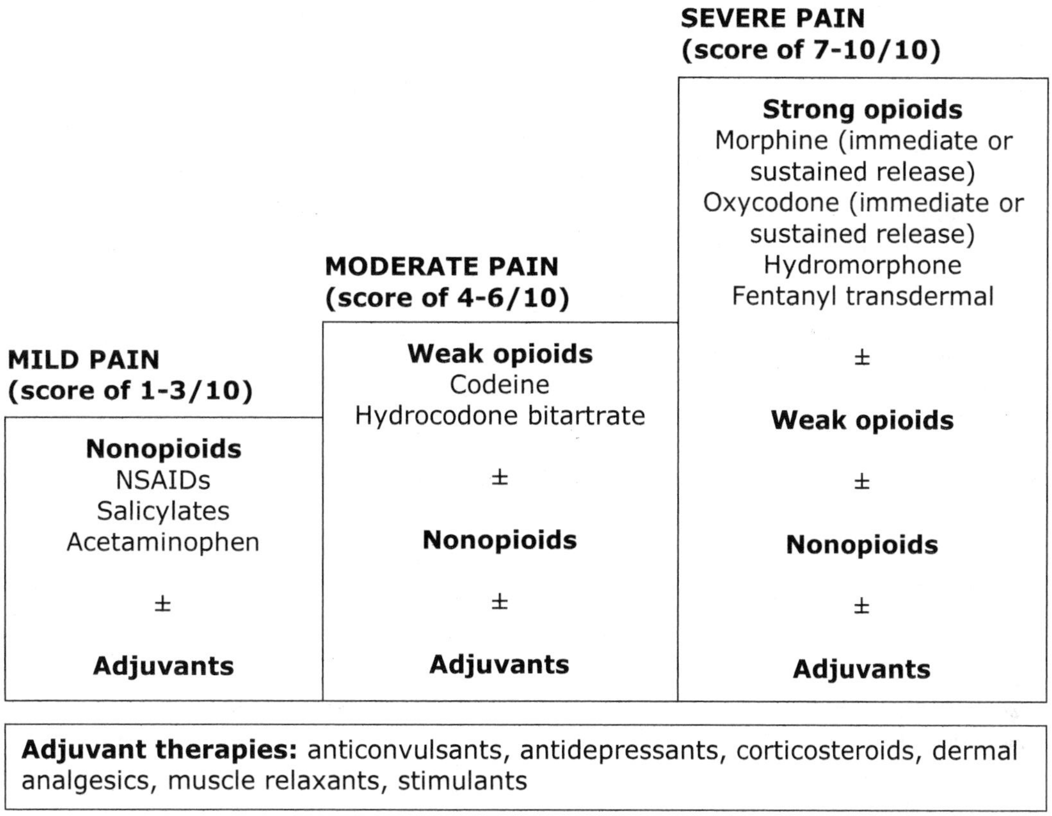

**SEVERE PAIN
(score of 7-10/10)**

Strong opioids
Morphine (immediate or
sustained release)
Oxycodone (immediate or
sustained release)
Hydromorphone
Fentanyl transdermal

±

Weak opioids

±

Nonopioids

±

Adjuvants

**MODERATE PAIN
(score of 4-6/10)**

Weak opioids
Codeine
Hydrocodone bitartrate

±

Nonopioids

±

Adjuvants

**MILD PAIN
(score of 1-3/10)**

Nonopioids
NSAIDs
Salicylates
Acetaminophen

±

Adjuvants

Adjuvant therapies: anticonvulsants, antidepressants, corticosteroids, dermal
analgesics, muscle relaxants, stimulants

Figure 1. World Health Organization three-step analgesic ladder.

to variable oral bioavailability and the accumulation of active metabolites with prolonged use at high doses or in kidney failure. Such accumulation lowers the seizure threshold and causes central nervous system symptoms, such as tremor, twitching, and nervousness. Partial opioid receptor agonists and agonist/antagonist agents (e.g., buprenorphine, dezocine, nalbuphine, pentazocine, butorphanol) may cause delirium and provide less incremental analgesia when used alone. Methadone is difficult to titrate, as its onset of action is far shorter than its half-life. For this reason, methadone should be administered only by providers experienced in its use.

Opioid analgesics have several side effects, including nausea, constipation, pruritus, and sedation. Mild sedation usually dissipates as the patient builds tolerance to the medication, and more significant sedation usually is reversible with dose reduction. Constipation is one of the most common side effects of opioid medications. Stool softeners and laxatives should be prescribed for patients who use opioid medications daily. A combination of docusate as a stool softener and senna or bisacodyl as a mild laxative is a popular initial prophylactic therapy. Osmotic laxatives, such as magnesium citrate, lactulose, and polyethylene glycol, are used if the prophylactic regimen does not produce daily bowel movements. Opioid-related itching and urticaria are due to the release of histamine. For these patients, an antihistamine is useful. Switching to an opioid agent that does not release histamine (oxymorphone, fentanyl) also can be considered. Opioid-induced

nausea can be treated with metoclopramide, meclizine, or another phenothiazine medication.

Neuropathic pain usually is caused by direct pathologic changes to the central or peripheral nervous system. In terminally ill patients, this is most often related to a malignancy causing nerve root compression or encroachment on a plexus of nerve fibers. Neuropathic pain may be constant or episodic and usually is characterized as burning, tingling, lancinating, or shooting in nature. Several therapies are effective for neuropathic pain. Tricyclic antidepressants, venlafaxine, and duloxetine may be especially useful in patients with both neuropathic pain and depression. Tramadol, gabapentin, and pregabalin also are effective for neuropathic pain. Corticosteroids can reduce edema and lyse certain tumors, thereby enhancing the analgesic effect of nonopioid and opioid drugs. Corticosteroids are effective in the management of malignant infiltration of the brachial or lumbar plexus and spinal cord compression, as well as headache pain due to brain tumors.

Dyspnea

Dyspnea is one of the most common symptoms encountered in palliative care. Dyspnea most often is the result of direct cardiothoracic pathology (e.g., pleural effusion, heart failure, chronic obstructive pulmonary disease, pulmonary embolism, pneumonia, lung metastasis) but can also be caused by systemic conditions (e.g., anemia, muscle weakness, conditions causing abdominal distention). The patient's self-report of discomfort should be the driving factor for treatment and often has little correlation with respiration rate, arterial blood gas levels, oxygen saturation, or use of accessory musculature.

Patients with underlying lung disease who are on broncho-dilator therapy should continue this therapy to maintain comfort. Opioid analgesics are effective in reducing dyspnea in patients with underlying cardiopulmonary disease and malignancy. In patients already receiving opioid medications, using the pain rescue dose for dyspnea as well and increasing this dose by 25% if not fully effective may be helpful. A 5-mg dose of oral morphine given four times daily has been shown to help relieve dyspnea in patients with end-stage heart failure. Low-dose (20 mg) extended-release morphine given daily has been used to relieve dyspnea in patients with advanced chronic obstructive pulmonary disease.

Oxygen may be useful for relieving dyspnea in terminally ill patients with hypoxemia, but it has limited value for symptom relief in patients without hypoxemia. If severe anemia is uncovered as a cause of dyspnea, a blood transfusion may help relieve symptoms.

Nutrition

Reduced appetite and weight loss are common symptoms in patients dying of cancer or chronic disease. A lack of interest in food and poor nutrition are viewed with distress by many families. Patient and caregiver education about how the disease process may cause anorexia and cachexia often helps to relieve guilt and to promote acceptance of a dying patient's altered eating habits. A realistic discussion regarding nutrition and hydration advance directives is also useful.

If prognosis is uncertain and death is not imminent, appetite stimulants may be considered. In cancer-related anorexia, the most commonly studied medications are progestins, such as megestrol (in doses of 400-800 mg/day) or medroxyprogesterone (typically 500 mg twice daily). These medications improve anorexia and promote weight gain but have an uncertain impact on quality of life. Side effects include an increased incidence of thromboembolic disease, hyperglycemia, adrenal suppression, and vaginal bleeding. Prokinetic agents (e.g., metoclopramide) significantly reduce nausea but have no impact on weight or anorexia. Short-term corticosteroids improve nausea and anorexia in advanced cancer patients, but little is known about corticosteroid use in palliative care populations.

The use of enteral and parenteral feeding in terminally ill patients is controversial. The benefits of these modalities are most pronounced in patients with good functional status and with gastrointestinal disease affecting nutritional intake. There is scant evidence for improved quality of life in patients with anorexia and weight loss due to terminal disease. In addition, there are important risks associated with enteral and parenteral feeding, such as line infection or dislodgement, hyperglycemia, electrolyte imbalances, and fluid overload. Discussing patient nutrition preferences before extreme weight loss and anorexia occur is important to avoid emotional distress for the patient and family.

Depression

The diagnosis of depression in terminally ill patients often can be problematic. First, it is difficult to separate symptoms traditionally associated with depression (e.g., anorexia, weight loss) from the patient's underlying disease, and both patients and providers may have the misconception that depression is a normal or untreatable symptom of terminal disease.

Techniques to screen for depression may require modification in the palliative care setting. The presence of low mood and low interest has been found to be 91% sensitive and 86% specific for the diagnosis of depression in this setting. Given the low risk of short-term complications of therapy and the potential benefit of improving the patient's remaining quality of life, physicians should have a low threshold for initiating depression therapy in this setting.

Tricyclic antidepressants, selective serotonin reuptake inhibitors, and psychotherapy are all effective in improving symptoms of depression in patients who are terminally ill. In patients with a prognosis of less than 1 month, some experts recommend psychostimulant medications, owing to their short onset of action compared with antidepressant medications.

Book Enhancement

Go to www.acponline.org/essentials/oncology-section. In *MKSAP for Students 5*, assess your knowledge with items 27-30 in the **Oncology** section.

Bibliography

Qaseem A, Snow V, Shekelle P, et al; Clinical Efficacy Assessment Subcommittee of the American College of Physicians. Evidence-based interventions to improve the palliative care of pain, dyspnea, and depression at the end of life: a clinical practice guideline from the American College of Physicians. Ann Intern Med. 2008;148:141-146. [PMID:18195338]

Chapter 80

Interpretation of Pulmonary Function Tests

Mysti D.W. Schott, MD

Pulmonary function tests are measurements of lung function used for diagnosing lung disease and managing patients with known pulmonary disorders. Although pulmonary function tests are effort-dependent, they are more precise than using symptoms or physical examination findings to gauge the severity of underlying lung disease. Specific indications for pulmonary function tests include (1) assessment of patients at risk for lung disease; (2) evaluation of respiratory symptoms, such as cough, wheezing, or dyspnea; (3) monitoring the benefits and risks of therapeutic interventions; and (4) assessment of pulmonary risk before surgery.

The four pulmonary function tests commonly used to measure lung function are spirometry, lung volumes, flow-volume loops, and diffusing capacity for carbon monoxide (DLCO). Spirometry can be performed in the office, but measurement of lung volumes, flow-volume loops, and DLCO requires a pulmonary function laboratory (Table 1).

Spirometry

Spirometry measures airflow rate and expired volume over time during forced breathing. Spirometry can help differentiate obstructive from restrictive lung disease (Table 2). Spirometry results are compared with reference values that are stratified by

height, weight, sex, and ethnicity, with the measured value expressed as a "percent of predicted" (i.e., percent of the predicted value for persons with similar characteristics). The most useful measures of expired volume over time are the forced vital capacity (FVC) and the forced expiratory volume in 1 second (FEV_1). FVC is the volume of air held by the lungs, measured from peak inspiration to maximum expiration. The FEV_1 is the volume of air exhaled in the first second of the FVC maneuver. FEV_1 and FVC values ≥80% of predicted are considered normal. The ratio of the absolute (not percent of predicted) values for FEV_1 and FVC is calculated. Patients with normal airflow will have a FEV_1/FVC

Table 2. Common Causes of Obstructive and Restrictive Lung Disease

Obstructive Lung Disease	Restrictive Lung Disease
Asthma	Chest wall deformities
Bronchiectasis	Interstitial disease
Chronic bronchitis	Neuromuscular disease
Emphysema	Obesity, pregnancy, ascites
Upper airway obstruction	Pain
	Pleural effusion

Table 1. Pulmonary Function Tests

Test	Notes
Spirometry	FEV_1 and FVC are the main measures. FEV_1/FVC ratio distinguishes obstructive from restrictive airway disease. A reduced ratio suggests obstructive disease (e.g., asthma, COPD); a normal ratio suggests restrictive disease (e.g., IPF) if lung volumes are reduced.
Lung volumes	Reduced lung volumes suggest restrictive airway disease if FEV_1/FVC ratio is normal. Increased lung volumes suggest obstructive airway disease if FEV_1/FVC ratio is decreased. Mixed restrictive and obstructive disease can occur and is diagnosed with spirometry and lung volumes.
Diffusing capacity for carbon monoxide (DLCO)	Decreased DLCO and restrictive pattern on spirometry suggests intrinsic lung disease (e.g., IPF), whereas normal DLCO accompanied by restrictive pattern on spirometry suggests a nonpulmonary cause of restriction (e.g., severe kyphoscoliosis, morbid obesity). Markedly decreased DLCO and obstructive spirometry pattern suggests emphysema, whereas normal or mildly decreased DLCO suggests other obstructive airway disease (e.g., COPD).
Flow-volume loops	Flow-volume loops can identify upper airway obstruction. A characteristic limitation of flow (i.e., a flattening of the loop) during inhalation suggests variable extrathoracic obstruction (e.g., vocal cord dysfunction); limitation of flow during forced exhalation suggests variable intrathoracic obstruction (e.g., asthma, COPD). Fixed upper airway obstruction (e.g., tracheal tumor) causes flow limitation during both forced inhalation and forced exhalation.
Maximal inspiratory and expiratory pressures	These measurements are used to detect respiratory muscle weakness.
Pulse oximetry	Use in patients with dyspnea on exertion or other limitation of exercise to screen for oxygen desaturation. A decrease >4% indicates significant desaturation.

FEV_1 = forced expiratory volume in 1 second; FVC = forced vital capacity; IPF = idiopathic pulmonary fibrosis.

ratio of approximately 75%. Spirometry also directly measures airflow as a function of time, with the most useful measure being the peak expiratory flow rate (PEFR), which is the maximum flow rate generated by the patient during the FVC maneuver.

If initial spirometry results are abnormal and suggest obstructive disease, the test is repeated following administration of an inhaled bronchodilator. An increase in FEV_1 of >12% and a minimum of 200 mL increase in FEV_1 after bronchodilator use establishes the presence of airflow reversibility and the diagnosis of asthma. A lack of response to bronchodilators is compatible with COPD but does not preclude a therapeutic trial of bronchodilator therapy.

Patients with a history suggestive of asthma (e.g., dyspnea, cough) but with normal spirometry findings can be evaluated for reactive airway disease with a methacholine challenge test. Spirometry is repeated following inhalation of the cholinergic agent methacholine. A ≥20% decrease in at least two flow parameters establishes the diagnosis of asthma. Methacholine challenge is not performed in patients with known obstructive lung disease. Other contraindications include recent myocardial infarction or stroke, aortic or cerebral aneurysm, and uncontrolled hypertension.

Lung Volumes

Lung volumes are static measurements obtained through a dilution technique involving breathing either helium or nitrogen in a closed system or through body plethysmography with the patient in a sealed box. The most useful lung volume measurements are total lung capacity (TLC) and residual volume (RV). The TLC is the total amount of air in the lungs. It is equal to the vital capacity (VC) plus RV. The RV is the air remaining in the lungs after a full exhalation. Like spirometry measurements, lung volume measurements are compared to reference values and reported as percent of predicted values. TLC and RV values between 80% and 120% of predicted are considered normal.

Flow-Volume Loops

Flow-volume loops plot forced inspiratory and expiratory flow in liters per second (y-axis) as a function of volume (x-axis). The normal expiratory portion of the flow-volume loop (above the x-axis) is characterized by a rapid rise to the peak flow rate, followed by a nearly linear fall in flow as the patient exhales. The inspiratory curve (below the x-axis) appears as a semicircle. If the flow-volume

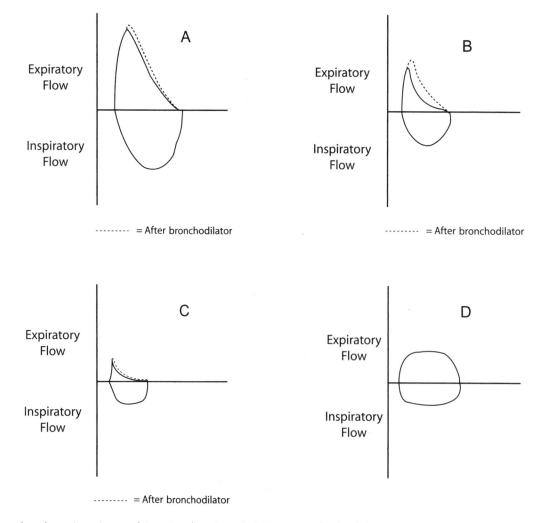

Figure 1. Flow-volume loops. Loop A: normal. Loop B: asthma. Loop C: COPD. Loop D: fixed extrathoracic obstruction.

Table 3. Interpreting Pulmonary Function Tests

Measurement	Normal Range	Obstructive/ Parenchymal (e.g., COPD)	Obstructive/ Nonparenchymal (e.g., asthma)	Restrictive/ Parenchymal (e.g., pulmonary fibrosis)	Restrictive/ Nonparenchymal (e.g., obesity)
FEV_1	≥80% of predicted	Decreased	Decreased	Decreased	Decreased
FVC	≥80% of predicted	Normal or decreased	Normal or decreased	Decreased	Decreased
FEV_1/FVC ratio	75%	≤70%	≤70%	>75%	>75%
TLC	80%-120% of predicted	Normal or increased	Normal or increased	Decreased	Decreased
RV	80%-120% of predicted	Normal or increased	Normal or increased	Decreased	Decreased
DLCO	≥80% of predicted	Decreased	Normal	Decreased	Normal

DLCO = diffusing capacity for carbon monoxide; FEV_1 = forced expiratory volume in 1 second; FVC = forced vital capacity; RV = residual volume; TLC = total lung capacity.

loop appears normal and FVC is normal, pulmonary function almost always is normal. Patients with obstructive disease have a "scooped out" expiratory curve (nonlinear) with a reduced slope. If the slope of the expiratory flow-volume loop appears normal or increased but FVC is reduced, restriction may be present. Flow-volume loops also are useful in assessing upper airway obstruction, which causes a plateau (flattening) in the expiratory curve. Flow-volume loops demonstrating a decrease in both inspiratory and expiratory flow (flattened curves above and below the x-axis) are compatible with fixed obstruction outside the chest (e.g., tracheal stenosis). An isolated decreased peak inspiratory flow (flattened curve below the x-axis) is compatible with an obstruction within the chest (e.g., tumor, mediastinal mass). Figure 1 shows examples of normal and abnormal flow-volume loops.

Diffusing Capacity for Carbon Monoxide

The DLCO is a measurement of the rate of diffusion of carbon monoxide across the alveolar-capillary membrane. The patient inhales a minute amount of carbon monoxide, some of which diffuses across the membrane while the patient holds his or her breath for a specified amount of time, typically 10 seconds. The remaining carbon monoxide is exhaled and measured to determine the diffusing capacity (difference between inhaled and exhaled carbon monoxide). This value is compared to a standard and reported as a percent of predicted value. A DLCO value ≥80% of predicted is considered normal.

DLCO is used to determine the possible presence of parenchymal lung disease. DLCO is normal in conditions associated with abnormal spirometry measurements and lung volumes but normal lung parenchyma (e.g., asthma, neuromuscular disease). DLCO is reduced in diseases associated with decreased alveolar-capillary membrane surface area (e.g., emphysema) and thickened alveolar-capillary membranes (e.g., interstitial lung disease, pulmonary fibrosis). Extrapulmonary conditions such as anemia (fewer red blood cells to transport carbon monoxide), pulmonary embolism (ventilation-perfusion mismatch), and pulmonary edema (interstitial edema is a barrier to gas flow) are associated with a decreased DLCO.

Diagnostic Use of Pulmonary Function Tests

Obstructive lung disease results in a reduced ability to move air out of the lungs. This can be due to actual airway resistance or loss of elastic recoil. Obstructive lung disease causes a marked reduction in FEV_1 and a lesser reduction in FVC, resulting in a reduced FEV_1/FVC ratio. The inability to move air out of the lungs results in hyperinflation, causing an increase in TLC and RV.

Restrictive lung disease results in a reduced ability to maintain normal lung volumes due to reduced movement of air into the lungs. This can be due to parenchymal lung disease (infiltrative disease, fibrosis), abnormalities of the chest wall (scoliosis, extreme obesity), or muscle weakness (neuromuscular disease). Restrictive lung disease causes a proportional reduction in FEV_1 and FVC, a normal or elevated FEV_1/FVC ratio, and a reduction in TLC and RV. DLCO is decreased in parenchymal lung disease; DLCO is normal in conditions affecting the chest wall and in neuromuscular disorders. Patients with mixed obstructive and restrictive disease will have a decreased FEV_1/FVC ratio and reduced lung volumes. Table 3 summarizes the diagnostic use of pulmonary function tests.

Book Enhancement

Go to www.acponline.org/essentials/pulmonary-section.html. In *MKSAP for Students 5*, assess your knowledge with items 1-4 in the **Pulmonary Medicine** section.

Acknowledgment

We would like to thank Dr. Kevin D. Whittle, who contributed to an earlier version of this chapter.

Bibliography

Pellegrino R, Viegi G, Brusasco V, et al. Interpretative strategies for lung function tests. Eur Respir J. 2005;26:948-968. [PMID: 16264058]

Chapter 81

Approach to Dyspnea

Mark D. Holden, MD

Dyspnea may be acute or chronic. Primary cardiovascular causes are associated with decreased cardiac output, elevated left atrial pressure, increased pulmonary capillary pressure, or poor oxygen delivery. Respiratory causes are related to central control of respiration, abnormalities of the ventilatory pump, pleural disease, or disturbance of airflow or the gas exchange process. Anemia also can cause dyspnea due to reduced oxygen carrying capacity of the blood.

The pathophysiology of dyspnea is complex and incompletely understood. The brainstem and higher brain centers receive afferent sensory information from various chemoreceptors and mechanoreceptors. Central and peripheral chemoreceptors sense changes in arterial Pco_2 and Po_2. Mechanoreceptors, such as pulmonary stretch receptors, muscle spindles, and diaphragmatic tendon organs, sense expansion of the lungs and chest wall, contraction of respiratory muscles, and airflow. Information from these receptors is integrated by the central nervous system to modulate the perception of dyspnea. Efferent impulses from the medullary respiratory center to the ventilatory muscles also signal higher cortical centers, providing awareness of respiratory drive. Dyspnea is associated with increased efferent output to respiratory muscles, impaired chest expansion, bronchoconstriction, and stimulation of pulmonary vagal receptors. The sensation of dyspnea also may occur when there is an imbalance of efferent respiratory motor signals and resultant afferent receptor responses, reflecting the ineffectiveness of ventilation.

Acute Dyspnea

Acute dyspnea occurs rapidly over minutes to 24 hours and has a limited differential diagnosis. Cardiovascular causes are related to acute decreases in left ventricular function or any event that increases pulmonary capillary pressure (acute coronary syndrome, tachycardia, cardiac tamponade). Respiratory causes are related to airway dysfunction (bronchospasm, aspiration, obstruction), disruption of the gas exchange system by parenchymal disease (pneumonia, acute respiratory distress syndrome), vascular disease (pulmonary embolism), or disturbance of the ventilatory pump (pleural effusion, pneumothorax, respiratory muscle weakness). Panic disorder and hyperventilation syndrome are relatively uncommon causes of dyspnea.

The history and physical examination provide important clues to the differential diagnosis of acute dyspnea (Table 1). Some conditions are associated with well-defined, predictive findings that should be specifically sought. For example, paroxysmal nocturnal dyspnea (positive likelihood ratio = 2.6) and a history of heart failure (positive likelihood ratio = 5.8) increase the probability of heart failure as the cause of dyspnea. Pulsus paradoxus >10 mm Hg in the setting of a pericardial effusion suggests cardiac tamponade (positive likelihood ratio = 3.3). The presence of an S_3 strongly supports the diagnosis of heart failure (positive likelihood ratio = 11). Panic disorder involves recurrent episodes of abrupt onset of chest pain, dyspnea, palpitations, diaphoresis, trembling, dizziness, paresthesias, hot flushes, or fear of dying or losing control. Symptoms typically peak within 10 minutes of onset, and attacks usually last from 15 to 60 minutes. Diagnosis of panic disorder requires that one or more of the attacks be followed by at least 1 month of (1) persistent concern about having another attack, (2) worry about the implications of the attack or its consequences, or (3) significant change in behavior related to the attacks.

Pulse oximetry should routinely be used to assess oxygen saturation. Low oxygen saturation suggests a problem with respiratory gas exchange and points to processes such as asthma, acute exacerbation of COPD, acute respiratory distress syndrome, heart failure, pulmonary fibrosis, or pulmonary vascular disease.

Chest radiography is the key diagnostic tool. Focal infiltrates suggest pneumonia, air or fluid in the pleural space indicates pneumothorax or hydrothorax, and cardiomegaly and vascular congestion support heart failure (positive likelihood ratio = 12). Depending on the clinical situation, other helpful diagnostic tests may include spiral CT of the chest, ventilation-perfusion lung scan, or pulmonary angiography to diagnose pulmonary embolism. High-resolution CT might be useful when chest radiography is normal but suspicion for an infiltrative lung disease is high. Atrial fibrillation on electrocardiogram (ECG) supports heart failure (positive likelihood ratio = 3.8). Serum B-type natriuretic peptide (BNP) level <100 pg/mL helps exclude heart failure (negative likelihood ratio = 0.1) in the setting of acute dyspnea. Laryngoscopy and bronchoscopy are useful in the diagnosis of suspected foreign body aspiration, airway obstruction, and vocal cord dysfunction and in certain cases of pneumonia.

Chronic Dyspnea

Dyspnea becomes chronic when symptoms persist longer than 1 month. In two thirds of patients, chronic dyspnea results from COPD, asthma, interstitial lung disease, or heart failure. Less common causes include pulmonary vascular disorders, valvular and pericardial heart disease, anemia, and thyroid disease (Table 2).

The history includes detailed exploration of the quality and severity of the dyspnea, precipitating and positional factors, timing of symptoms, associated features, and cardiopulmonary risk fac-

Table 1. Selected Differential Diagnosis of Acute Dyspnea

Disorder	History Clues	Physical Examination Clues
Pulmonary Causes		
Anaphylaxis	Allergen exposure	Urticaria, facial edema, wheezing
Asthma (may also present as chronic dyspnea)	Episodic cough, chest tightness; related to exercise; nocturnal symptoms	Wheezing
Pneumonia	Fever, cough, sputum	Fever, crackles, dullness to percussion
Pneumothorax	History of trauma, pleuritic chest pain	Absent breath sounds, deviated trachea (tension pneumothorax)
Pleural effusion/hemothorax	History of trauma or pneumonia	Dullness to percussion, absent breath sounds
Pulmonary embolism	Risk factors for thromboembolism, pleuritic chest pain, hemoptysis	Normal examination, possible leg swelling
Cardiovascular Causes		
Heart failure (acute)	Cardiovascular risk factors, paroxysmal nocturnal dyspnea	Jugular venous distention, S_3, pulmonary crackles, possible murmur, edema
Myocardial infarction	Cardiovascular risk factors, chest pain, nausea, diaphoresis	S_3 and/or S_4, jugular venous distention, possible mitral regurgitant murmur, pulmonary crackles
Pericardial tamponade	History of trauma, preceding "flu" symptoms, collagen vascular disease	Jugular venous distention, clear lungs, pulsus paradoxus
Upper Airway Causes		
Tracheal stenosis, tracheomalacia	Prolonged mechanical ventilation and intubation	Stridor, clear lungs, normal cardiac examination
Vocal cord dysfunction	Previous normal spirometry results	Single frequency wheezing localized to throat
Vocal cord paralysis	History of thyroid or neck surgery	Single frequency wheezing localized to throat, dysphonia
Psychiatric Causes		
Panic attack	Rapid onset of chest pain, dyspnea that resolve without specific treatment	Normal cardiac and pulmonary examinations

tors. Patients with dyspnea due to chronic heart failure tend to characterize their dyspnea as air hunger or suffocating, whereas those with asthma often describe chest tightness. Review in detail all medical problems, prescription and nonprescription medications, substance use, hobbies, and occupational/environmental exposures. Physical examination focuses on the cardiovascular and respiratory systems but must also include a search for abnormalities related to the thyroid, liver, nervous system, and musculoskeletal system.

Findings from the history and physical examination direct the selection of diagnostic testing, which may include chest radiography, electrocardiography, pulmonary function testing, and echocardiography. Laboratory tests should include a complete blood count and assessment of thyroid function. Results of these initial tests may suggest further investigation with CT or bronchoscopy. Lung biopsy may be necessary to evaluate parenchymal lung disease of uncertain cause.

Supportive evidence for COPD includes smoking longer than 40 pack-years (positive likelihood ratio = 8.3), self-reported history of COPD (positive likelihood ratio = 7.3), laryngeal height (distance between the top of the thyroid cartilage and the suprasternal notch) ≤4 cm (positive likelihood ratio = 2.8), and age ≥45 years (positive likelihood ratio = 1.3). The presence of all four signs is associated with a positive likelihood ratio of 220. Physical findings of advanced disease include hyperresonance to percussion, decreased breath sounds, prolonged expiration, and

wheezing. Nonspecific radiographic signs of emphysema are flattening of the diaphragm, irregular lung lucency, and reduction or absence of vasculature. Spirometry demonstrates airflow obstruction, with a forced expiratory flow in 1 second to forced vital capacity (FEV_1/FVC) ratio <70%. Other causes of chronic airway obstruction include bronchiectasis and cystic fibrosis; voluminous sputum production with frequent purulent exacerbations suggests bronchiectasis, whereas chronic obstructive pulmonary symptoms beginning at an early age in the absence of a smoking history may indicate cystic fibrosis.

Patients with asthma have intermittent dyspnea with episodic airway obstruction and often have a personal or family history of atopic disease. Patients may describe chest tightness, wheezing, sputum production, dry cough, or exacerbations with exercise or exposure to airway irritants or cold air. Physical examination during exacerbations may reveal diminished breath sounds, wheezing, and prolonged expiration. Chest radiography often is normal but may show hyperinflation. Spirometry during an attack will show obstruction that typically improves following bronchodilator administration, but normal spirometry results do not exclude asthma. Asthma that is suspected despite normal spirometry measurements may require provocative testing with methacholine to establish the diagnosis. Rare mimics of asthma include upper airway obstruction due to vocal cord paralysis, tumors of the trachea, tracheal stenosis, tracheomalacia, and vocal cord dysfunction (paradoxical adduction during inspiration). The flow-volume loop

Table 2. Selected Differential Diagnosis of Chronic Dyspnea

Disorder	History Clues	Physical Examination Clues
Pulmonary Causes		
COPD	Smoking history, cough, sputum	Diminished breath sounds, wheezing, prolonged expiration, large chest
Interstitial lung disease	Possible exposure history (silica, asbestos, smoking); collagen vascular disease (scleroderma)	Possible clubbing (pulmonary fibrosis), Velcro-like crackles (pulmonary fibrosis)
Pulmonary hypertension	May be idiopathic or related to other disease, such as interstitial lung disease (scleroderma) or cardiac shunts (atrial septal defect)	Jugular venous distention, increased P_2, fixed split S_2, tricuspid regurgitant murmur, clear lungs or crackles depending on cause
Pleural effusion/hemothorax	History of cancer, possible chest pain	Dullness to percussion, absent breath sounds
Hepatopulmonary syndrome	Cirrhosis, platypnea (dyspnea sitting up, relieved lying down)	Findings of chronic liver disease, normal pulmonary examination
Cardiovascular Causes		
Aortic stenosis	History of heart murmur, chest pain, syncope, dyspnea; history of rheumatic fever; history of aortic coarctation	Crescendo-decrescendo systolic murmur at right upper sternal border cardiac base with radiation to carotid arteries
Mitral stenosis	History of rheumatic fever, heart murmur	Opening snap followed by diastolic murmur with presystolic accentuation
Mitral regurgitation	History of heart murmur, mitral valve prolapse, or myocardial infarction	Holosystolic murmur at cardiac base
Chronic constrictive pericarditis	History of pericarditis, possible chest pain	Elevated jugular venous pressure, clear lungs, edema, tricuspid regurgitation, pulsatile liver
Other Causes		
Anemia	History of blood loss or hemolytic disease	Conjunctival pallor
Thyrotoxicosis	Heat intolerance, weight loss, nervousness	Possible goiter
Neuromuscular disease	Known neuromuscular disease	Normal cardiac and pulmonary examinations, neuromuscular findings
Deconditioning	Situations leading to decreased exercise tolerance	Normal cardiac and pulmonary examinations

P_2 = pulmonic component of S_2.

usually shows a characteristic plateau in the expiratory or inspiratory curve or in both curves (see Chapter 80). Diagnosis usually requires CT, MRI, or direct endoscopic visualization of the airway, depending on the suspected nature of the diagnosis.

Interstitial lung disease presents as progressive dyspnea on exertion and cough but may be associated with other symptoms related to the specific cause. The history may identify occupational or environmental exposures or symptoms of systemic disease. Physical examination findings are nonspecific and may include dry crackles. The examination includes a careful search for extrapulmonary involvement (skin, joint, and neurologic findings) suggesting underlying systemic illness. Chest radiographs may be normal or show reticular, nodular, or alveolar infiltrates or pleural effusion. High-resolution CT scans may provide evidence of interstitial disease when chest radiographs are normal. Pulmonary function testing typically shows evidence of restriction and decreased diffusing capacity for carbon dioxide. Arterial blood gas abnormalities include resting hypoxemia or hypoxemia on exercise testing. Specialized procedures (e.g., bronchoalveolar lavage, transbronchial lung biopsy via bronchoscopy, video-assisted thoracoscopic lung biopsy, open lung biopsy) may be necessary to confirm a diagnosis.

Exertional dyspnea is a common symptom in patients with pulmonary arterial hypertension, which may be idiopathic, familial, or associated with collagen vascular disease, portal hypertension, and many other conditions. Chronic thromboembolic disease and hypoventilation also may cause pulmonary hypertension and dyspnea. Physical examination in chronic pulmonary hypertension may reveal parasternal heave, right-sided S_4, loud pulmonic component of S_2 with fixed splitting, and holosystolic murmur of tricuspid regurgitation. Also look for clues of collagen vascular disease (skin and musculoskeletal changes, Raynaud phenomenon) and portal hypertension. Chest radiographs may show enlarged pulmonary arteries centrally. ECG may show right axis deviation, right ventricular hypertrophy, and right atrial enlargement. Echocardiography can assess for valvular heart disease and right ventricular hypertrophy or enlargement and can estimate pulmonary artery systolic pressure.

Heart failure may manifest as chronic dyspnea along with orthopnea, paroxysmal nocturnal dyspnea, edema, increased central venous pressure, crackles, S_3, vascular congestion on chest radiography, and elevated BNP level. Other cardiac conditions associated with chronic dyspnea include arrhythmias (atrial fibrillation), diastolic dysfunction, valvular heart disease, pericardial disease, and cardiomyopathies. Echocardiography is helpful in evaluating these cardiac conditions.

Patients with advanced liver disease may have chronic dyspnea from several causes, including hydrothorax, ascites, and hepatopulmonary syndrome characterized by pulmonary vascular dilatation, ventilation-perfusion mismatch, and intrapulmonary shunting resulting in hypoxemia. Dyspnea may occur at rest or with exertion and may worsen upon sitting upright (platypnea). The history may reveal risk factors for liver disease or evidence of ascites or other complications. On physical examination, look for spider nevi, digital clubbing, cyanosis, and other manifestations of chronic liver disease.

Patients with neuromuscular disease may present with dyspnea as well as other extrapulmonary symptoms, including difficulty rising from a chair or climbing stairs (proximal muscle weakness), diplopia (myasthenia gravis), and muscle fasciculations (amyotrophic lateral sclerosis). Cardiopulmonary examination typically is normal early in the course of these diseases. Pulmonary function testing may indicate inspiratory muscle weakness, with inability to generate a maximum inspiratory pressure more negative than –60 mm Hg.

Dyspnea of Obscure Cause

When no diagnosis can be made after evaluation for cardiac, pulmonary, and neuromuscular disorders, cardiopulmonary exercise testing can be used to evaluate cardiac performance, ventilatory capacity, and gas exchange during exercise. Cardiopulmonary exercise testing quantifies the patient's exercise tolerance and provides evidence of abnormal cardiac or pulmonary responses to exercise that may suggest a diagnosis. While the patient exercises on a treadmill or stationary bicycle, exhaled gases are collected and continuous oximetry and electrocardiography are performed. An indwelling arterial line can be placed for arterial blood gas measurements. Low maximum oxygen uptake in the absence of an identifiable abnormality often indicates deconditioning.

Book Enhancement

Go to www.acponline.org/essentials/pulmonary-section.html. In *MKSAP for Students 5*, assess your knowledge with items 5-9 in the **Pulmonary Medicine** section.

Bibliography

Lepor NE, McCullough PA. Differential diagnosis and overlap of acute chest discomfort and dyspnea in the emergency department. Rev Cardiovasc Med. 2010;11 Suppl 2:S13-23. [PMID: 20700098]

Wills CP, Young M, White DW. Pitfalls in the evaluation of shortness of breath. Emerg Med Clin North Am. 2010;28:163-181, ix. [PMID: 19945605]

Chapter 82

Pleural Effusion

Dario M. Torre, MD

A pleural effusion is created by an imbalance between the production and removal of fluid from the pleural space. Two major mechanisms lead to the accumulation of excessive fluid in the pleural space: increased capillary hydrostatic pressure (e.g., heart failure, superior vena cava syndrome, constrictive pericarditis) and/or decreased plasma oncotic pressure (e.g., cirrhosis, nephrotic syndrome, hypoalbuminemia). Pleural effusions may be caused by various disease processes, including heart failure, cirrhosis, nephrosis, infection, cancer, trauma, collagen vascular disease, venous thromboembolism, or aortic rupture.

The evaluation of pleural effusion requires a systematic history and physical examination and pertinent laboratory and imaging tests. The leading causes of pleural effusion in the United States are heart failure, pneumonia, and cancer.

Diagnosis

Symptoms of pleural effusion may include fever, dyspnea, and chest pain. Fever suggests an underlying infection, malignancy, or associated collagen vascular disease. Chest pain and dyspnea may be caused by the space-occupying effect of a large effusion or associated parenchymal lung disease. Small pleural effusions, such as those caused by nephrotic syndrome or rheumatoid arthritis, often are asymptomatic. Large accumulations of fluid in the pleural space block transmission of sound between the lung and the chest wall; percussion over an effusion is dull, and tactile (vocal) fremitus is diminished or absent. On auscultation, the most common findings are decreased to absent breath sounds over the effusion and bronchial breath sounds toward the top of the effusion. A pleural friction rub (harsh, rubbing, scratchy sound heard predominantly during expiration) may be auscultated.

Chest radiography is the first diagnostic test for pleural effusion (Figure 1). Chest radiography can identify and quantify the amount of fluid and may demonstrate underlying diseases responsible for the effusion (e.g., pneumonia, cancer) or suggest aortic dissection (widened mediastinum). Approximately 250 mL of pleural fluid is needed to blunt the costophrenic angle on a chest radiograph; greater amounts of fluid opacify the lower thorax and create a "meniscus sign."

After documenting the presence of an effusion, obtain decubitus films to evaluate whether the effusion is free-flowing or loc-

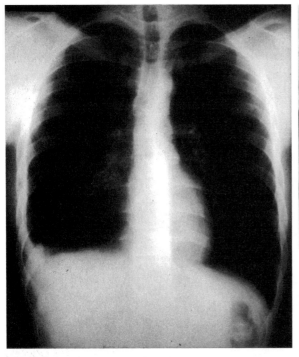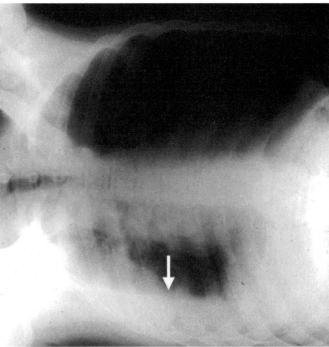

Figure 1. Chest radiograph showing a right-sided pleural effusion (*left panel*) that layers out along the right thorax when the radiograph is repeated with the patient in the right lateral decubitus position (*right panel*).

ulated and whether a sufficient quantity of fluid is present to perform thoracentesis. A 1-cm distance measured from the pleural fluid line to the chest wall on a decubitus radiograph is indicative of enough pleural fluid to perform thoracentesis. Chest CT is a valuable adjunct to chest radiography, because it can more effectively define the size and location of the pleural effusion and distinguish parenchymal from pleural disease. A spiral chest CT with contrast is highly sensitive for pulmonary embolism and may be indicated if the pretest probability of pulmonary embolism is moderate to high. Ultrasonography can be used to detect loculations, guide thoracentesis, and detect pleural abnormalities that are not apparent on chest radiographs.

A massive effusion, occupying the entire hemithorax, increases the likelihood of an underlying lung cancer or pleural mesothelioma. Bilateral transudative effusions are commonly associated with heart or liver failure. Bilateral exudative effusions suggest malignancy but also occur in patients with pleuritis due to systemic lupus erythematosus and other collagen vascular diseases. An empyema is suggested by the presence of a loculated (non–free-flowing) effusion on upright and decubitus chest radiography or by obvious loculation on chest CT.

Electrocardiography and echocardiography can be useful to exclude pericardial disease or right ventricular strain and dilatation caused by a moderate- to large-sized pulmonary embolism. Antinuclear antibody and rheumatoid factor testing, erythrocyte sedimentation rate, and complement levels may be useful if other signs and symptoms suggest collagen vascular disease.

Perform thoracentesis in all patients with a newly discovered pleural effusion to assist in diagnosis and management. Pneumothorax is the major complication of thoracentesis. Most pleural fluid analyses narrow the diagnostic possibilities but are not definitive by themselves. Pleural fluid evaluation should include pH, glucose, lactate dehydrogenase, protein, bacterial and acid-fast bacilli stains and culture, and leukocyte count with differential. If tuberculosis is suspected based on clinical presentation and lymphocytic predominance on leukocyte count, adenosine deaminase activity and polymerase chain reaction assays can be useful adjuncts to diagnosis. Gross pus in the pleural space is diagnostic of empyema.

Exudative pleural effusions are predominantly caused by inflammatory, infectious, and malignant conditions and less commonly by collagen vascular disease, intra-abdominal processes, and hypothyroidism. Venous thromboembolic disease may cause either an exudative (particularly in the case of pulmonary infarction) or, less commonly, a transudative effusion. Transudative pleural effusions are associated more commonly with heart failure and cirrhosis and less commonly with nephrotic syndrome and constrictive pericarditis. Table 1 summarizes causes of transudative effusions.

The most likely diagnoses associated with a pleural fluid leukocyte count >10,000/μL (10 x 10^9/L) include parapneumonic effusion; acute pancreatitis; splenic infarction; and subphrenic, hepatic, and splenic abscesses. A pleural fluid leukocyte count >50,000/μL (50 x 10^9/L) always is associated with complicated parapneumonic effusions and empyema but occasionally occurs with acute pancreatitis and pulmonary infarction. Malignant disease and tuberculosis typically present as a lymphocyte-predominant exudate.

Normal pleural fluid pH is 7.60 to 7.66. Transudates are associated with a pleural fluid pH of 7.45 to 7.55. A limited number of diagnoses are associated with a pleural fluid pH <7.30; the most common causes are complicated parapneumonic effusion or empyema, tuberculous pleurisy, esophageal rupture, rheumatoid pleuritis, and malignancy.

Pleural fluid amylase should be measured only when pancreatic disease, esophageal rupture, or malignancy is considered. A chylous effusion (milky white fluid) is highly likely if the serum triglyceride level is >110 mg/dL (1.2 mmol/L). A chylous effusion (chylothorax) is commonly caused by leakage of lymph, rich in triglycerides, from the thoracic duct due to trauma or obstruc-

Table 1. Causes of Transudative Effusions

Cause	Notes
Atelectasis	Small effusion caused by increased negative intrapleural pressure; common in patients in the intensive care unit
Constrictive pericarditis	Bilateral effusions with normal heart size; jugular venous distention present in 95% of cases
Duropleural fistula	Cerebrospinal fluid in the pleural space; caused by trauma and surgery
Extravascular migration of central venous catheter	With saline or dextrose infusion
Glycinothorax	High pleural fluid to serum glycine ratio following bladder irrigation with rupture
Heart failure	Most common cause of transudates; diuresis can increase pleural fluid protein and lactate dehydrogenase, resulting in discordant exudate
Hepatic hydrothorax	Occurs in 6% of patients with cirrhosis and clinical ascites; up to 20% do not have clinical ascites
Hypoalbuminemia	Small bilateral effusions; edema fluid rarely isolated to pleural space
Nephrotic syndrome	Typically small and bilateral effusions; unilateral effusion with chest pain suggests pulmonary embolism
Peritoneal dialysis	Small bilateral effusions common; rarely, large right effusion develops within 72 h of initiating dialysis
Superior vena cava obstruction	Acute systemic venous hypertension
Trapped lung	Unexpandable lung; unilateral effusion as a result of imbalance in hydrostatic pressures from remote inflammation
Urinothorax	Unilateral effusion caused by ipsilateral obstructive uropathy

tion (e.g., lymphoma). When malignancy is suspected but initial thoracentesis is nondiagnostic, cytologic evaluation of a second, large-volume pleural fluid sample may be helpful. Figure 2 and Table 2 summarize a diagnostic approach and ancillary tests that can be used to evaluate the causes of pleural effusion.

The sensitivity of cytologic analysis of pleural fluid ranges from 40% to 90% in patients with known malignancy. One reason for the variation is that the effusion may be associated with the malignancy, but malignant cells are not detected in the pleural fluid; these are termed paramalignant effusions, the causes of which include impaired lymphatic drainage, postobstructive pneumonia, and pulmonary embolism. Other factors affecting the sensitivity of pleural fluid cytology include the type of tumor (high positivity with adenocarcinoma and low positivity with Hodgkin lym-

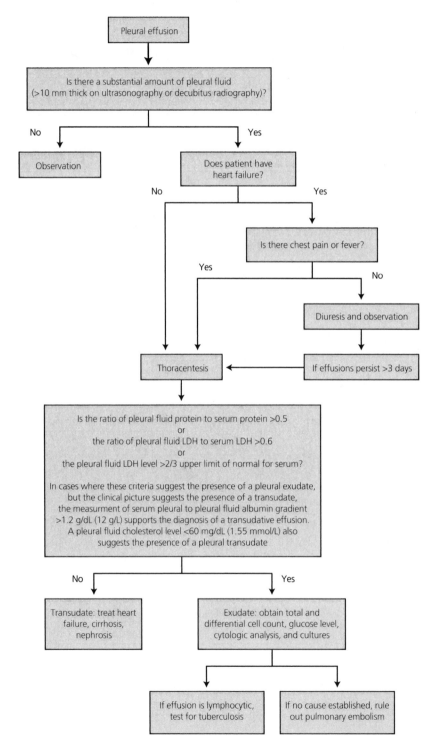

Figure 2. Evaluation of a patient with pleural effusion. (Adapted from Light RW. Clinical practice. Pleural effusion. N Engl J Med. 2002;346:1971-77; with permission. Copyright © 2002 Massachusetts Medical Society.)

Table 2. Additional Pleural Fluid Tests

Test	Notes
Erythrocyte count	>100,000/μL (100 x 10^9/L): malignancy, trauma, parapneumonic effusion, pulmonary embolism
Leukocyte count	>50,000/μL (10 x 10^9/L): complicated para-pneumonic effusion or empyema
Neutrophils	>50%: parapneumonic effusion, pulmonary embolism, abdominal disease
Lymphocytes	>80%: tuberculosis (most common), lymphoma, coronary artery bypass surgery, rheumatoid pleuritis, sarcoidosis
pH	<7.20: complicated parapneumonic effusion or empyema, malignancy (<10%), tuberculosis (<10%), esophageal rupture
Glucose	<60 mg/dL (3.3 mmol/L): complicated parapneumonic effusion or empyema, tuberculosis (20%), malignancy (<10%), rheumatoid arthritis
Adenosine deaminase	>40 U/L: tuberculosis (>90%), complicated parapneumonic effusion (30%) or empyema (60%), malignancy (5%)
Cytology	Positive: malignancy
Culture	Positive: infection
Useful in certain circumstances	
Hematocrit fluid to blood ratio	≥0.5: hemothorax
Amylase	>upper limit of normal for serum: malignancy, pancreatic disease, esophageal rupture
Triglycerides	>110 mg/dL (1.2 mmol/L): chylothorax

phoma), the number of specimens submitted, the stage of pleural involvement (the more advanced the stage, the higher the sensitivity), and the expertise of the cytopathologist.

Approximately 25% of pleural effusions remain undiagnosed after analysis of one or more pleural fluid samples. Additional diagnostic evaluations are undertaken if the effusion is persistently symptomatic or if a progressive disease is suspected, such as malignancy, tuberculosis, or pulmonary embolism.

Therapy

Treatment of pleural effusions is dictated by the underlying cause. However, large effusions should be evacuated. For massive effusions associated with mediastinal shift, 2.0 L or more can be removed safely in one setting. Otherwise, therapeutic thoracentesis is limited to removal of 1.0 to 1.5 L at a time to minimize the likelihood of reexpansion pulmonary edema.

In pleural effusions associated with pneumonia, the presence of loculated pleural fluid, pleural fluid pH <7.20, pleural fluid glucose level <60 mg/dL (3.3 mmol/L), positive pleural fluid Gram stain or culture, or the presence of gross pus in the pleural space predicts a poor response to antibiotics alone; such pleural effusions are treated with drainage of the fluid through a catheter or chest tube. Thoracic empyema (pus in the pleural space) develops when antibiotics are not given and the pleural space is not drained in a timely manner. In this case, video-assisted thoracoscopic surgery is indicated to break down loculations and drain pus from the pleural cavity.

Patients with recurrent, symptomatic malignant pleural effusions not responsive to chemotherapy require drainage for relief of dyspnea. Drainage can be accomplished either by placing a chronic indwelling pleural catheter or by performing chemical pleurodesis (typically an inpatient procedure) using a chemical agent (e.g., large-particle talc) as a slurry through a chest tube.

Book Enhancement

Go to www.acponline.org/essentials/pulmonary-section.html. In *MKSAP for Students 5*, assess your knowledge with items 10-13 in the **Pulmonary Medicine** section.

Bibliography

Hooper C, Lee YC, Maskell N; BTS Pleural Guideline Group. Investigation of a unilateral pleural effusion in adults: British Thoracic Society Pleural Disease Guideline 2010. Thorax. 2010;65 Suppl 2:ii4-ii17. [PMID: 20696692]

Chapter 83

Asthma

Patricia Short, MD

Asthma is a disease of intermittent and reversible airway obstruction associated with chronic inflammation and a disordered immune response. Asthma affects 5% to 10% of the U.S. population and is steadily increasing in prevalence. The underlying cause of asthma remains unknown. Eosinophils are increased in the airway of patients with asthma, especially those with active disease, and neutrophils are increased during exacerbations and in severe disease; the role of neutrophils in the pathogenesis remains unclear. Th2 cells, a subtype of CD4 T cells, appear to play a central role in activation of the inflammatory response in asthma. Airway inflammation contributes to airway hyperresponsiveness and narrowing. Structural alterations occur in the lungs of some patients (a process known as *airway remodeling*) and consist of subepithelial fibrosis, increased smooth muscle mass, angiogenesis, and hyperplasia of mucous gland and goblet cells. Effective management of asthma involves use of objective measures of lung function to assess disease severity and to monitor therapeutic efficacy, identification and avoidance of environmental triggers that exacerbate symptoms, long-term use of medications that decrease airway inflammation, and use of medications to treat acute exacerbations.

Diagnosis

The diagnosis of asthma is based on episodic symptoms of airflow limitation and/or airway inflammation, evidence of reversible airflow obstruction, and exclusion of alternative diagnoses. Symptoms of airflow obstruction include wheezing, dyspnea, cough, and chest tightness. Symptoms that are intermittent and worsen in the presence of aeroallergens, irritants, cold air, or exercise are typical, as are nighttime symptoms that awaken the patient from sleep. The diagnosis of asthma should be considered in all patients with a chronic cough, especially if the cough is nocturnal, seasonal, or related to a workplace or an activity; coughing may be the only manifestation of asthma. A history of atopic dermatitis or eczema and a family history of asthma are additional risk factors for development of the disease.

Physical examination may be normal in the absence of an acute exacerbation. Findings of asthma may include wheezing during normal breathing or with forced expiration, chest hyperexpansion, and prolonged expiratory phase. Accessory muscle use may be seen during an acute exacerbation. Additional findings may include nasal mucosal thickening, nasal polyps, or rhinitis manifested by cobblestoning of the oropharynx. Patients also may have evidence of atopic dermatitis or eczema on skin examination.

Perform spirometry in all patients suspected of having asthma (Table 1). Spirometry measurements, including forced expiratory volume in 1 second (FEV_1) and forced vital capacity (FVC), are taken before and after bronchodilator use. A reduced FEV_1 or a reduced FEV_1/FVC ratio documents airflow obstruction. An increase in FEV_1 of >12% with a minimum increase of 200 mL in FEV_1 after bronchodilator use establishes the presence of airflow

Table 1. Laboratory and Other Studies for Asthma

Test	Notes
Spirometry	Abnormal spirometry results (reversible obstruction) can help to confirm an asthma diagnosis, but normal results do not exclude asthma.
Peak flow variability	A patient with normal spirometry results but marked diurnal variability (based on a peak-flow diary kept for >2 wk) may have asthma and may warrant an empiric trial of asthma medications or bronchoprovocation testing.
Bronchoprovocation testing	In a patient with a highly suggestive history of asthma and normal baseline spirometry results, a low PC_{20} (concentration of inhaled methacholine needed to cause a 20% drop in FEV_1) on methacholine challenge testing supports a diagnosis of asthma. A normal bronchoprovocation test essentially excludes asthma.
Chest radiography	Chest radiography may be needed to exclude other diagnoses but is not recommended as a routine test in the initial evaluation of asthma.
CBC with differential	A CBC is not helpful in the diagnosis of asthma.
Sputum evaluation	Routine sputum evaluation is not helpful in the diagnosis of asthma.
Serum IgE level	Routine serum IgE is not helpful in the diagnosis of asthma.
Quantitative IgE antibody assays	Specific IgE immunoassays (e.g., RAST) are not useful in the diagnosis of asthma.
Skin testing	There is a strong association between allergen sensitization, exposure, and asthma. Allergy testing is the only reliable way to detect the presence of specific IgE to allergens. Skin testing (or in vitro testing) may be indicated to guide the management of asthma in selected patients, but results are not useful in establishing the diagnosis of asthma.

CBC = complete blood count; FEV_1 = forced expiratory volume in 1 second; RAST = radioallergosorbent test.

reversibility and the diagnosis of asthma. However, normal measurements do not exclude the diagnosis. Patients suspected of having asthma who have normal spirometry results should proceed with a bronchoprovocation test, such as a methacholine challenge. The lower the concentration of inhaled methacholine needed to cause a 20% drop in FEV_1, the more likely the patient has asthma. Methacholine challenge has a high sensitivity and a high negative predictive value for the diagnosis of asthma. Other bronchoprovocation tests include histamine and exercise; however, methacholine challenge remains the test of choice in patients for whom there is clinical suspicion for asthma despite normal spirometry results.

For patients with a smoking history who present with respiratory complaints consistent with asthma, consider obtaining a diffusing capacity for carbon monoxide (DLco) to differentiate between asthma and COPD (i.e., chronic bronchitis, emphysema). DLco is normal or increased in asthma and decreased in COPD. Patients with COPD also do not demonstrate reversibility with bronchodilators on spirometry.

Exposure to high-level irritants (e.g., chlorine gas, bleach, ammonia) can result in significant airway injury, which can lead to persistent airway inflammation and dysfunction with airway hyperresponsiveness and obstruction. A chronic cough, shortness of breath, and chest tightness may develop—a condition known as reactive airways dysfunction syndrome (RADS). The symptoms of RADS may resolve with time but can persist for years in some patients.

Occupational asthma is an important consideration in patients with asthma symptoms. Patients should be asked about exposure to irritants, sensitizing chemicals, and allergens. Improvement of symptoms during weekends or vacations is an important historical clue in making this diagnosis.

Alternative diagnoses should be considered when symptoms are difficult to control or if signs and symptoms are atypical. Vocal cord dysfunction, COPD, heart failure, interstitial lung disease, pulmonary hypertension, cystic fibrosis, Churg-Strauss syndrome, allergic bronchopulmonary aspergillosis, mechanical obstruction of the airway (endobronchial tumor or foreign body), obstructive sleep apnea, and medication-induced symptoms (particularly ACE inhibitor use) are in the differential diagnosis of asthma (Table 2).

Therapy

The goal of asthma therapy is to achieve good long-term control, which is defined as infrequent asthma symptoms, unrestricted level of activity, normal or near-normal lung function, and rare asthma attacks requiring emergency care.

Encourage patients with asthma to reduce exposure to factors that worsen their asthma. Advise those who are allergic to dust mites to use measures to reduce mite allergen exposure at home, including (1) covering mattresses and pillows in allergen-proof fabric and laundering all bedding materials weekly in hot water (≥54.4°C [130°F]), (2) using air conditioning to maintain humidity at <50%, (3) removing carpets, and (4) limiting fabric-covered items (e.g., upholstered furniture, drapes, soft toys). Sensitive individuals may also benefit from other environmental control measures aimed at reducing potential reservoirs of common allergens in the home, such as exterminating cockroaches, removing cats, and reducing dampness. Advise patients to minimize exposure to

Table 2. Differential Diagnosis of Asthma

Disorder	Notes
COPD (see Chapter 84)	Less reversibility of airflow obstruction; associated with a history of tobacco use. COPD may coexist with asthma in adults.
Vocal cord dysfunction	Abrupt onset of severe symptoms, often with rapid improvement. Monophonic wheeze heard loudest during either inspiration or expiration. The preferred diagnostic test is direct visualization of the vocal cords during symptoms. May closely mimic asthma, particularly in young adults.
Heart failure (see Chapter 7)	Spirometry results may or may not be normal; wheezing may be a sentinel manifestation. Consider when there is not prompt improvement with asthma therapy. Heart failure always is a consideration for persons with underlying cardiac disease.
Medication side effect	Chronic cough may occur with certain medications (e.g., ACE inhibitors).
Bronchiectasis	Voluminous sputum production, often purulent and sometimes blood tinged. Suspect if physical examination reveals crackles with wheezing or clubbing or if chest radiograph shows peribronchial thickening.
Pulmonary infiltrates with eosinophilia (ABPA, Churg-Strauss syndrome, Loeffler syndrome, chronic eosinophilic pneumonia)	Wheezing may be seen in ABPA, chronic eosinophilic pneumonia, and Churg-Strauss syndrome. Note that in uncomplicated asthma, chest radiographs are normal. Findings of infiltrates, striking peripheral blood eosinophilia, and constitutional symptoms (e.g., fever, weight loss) suggest chronic eosinophilic pneumonia. Asthma with eosinophilia, markedly high serum IgE levels, and intermittent pulmonary infiltrates is characteristic of ABPA. Difficult-to-treat asthma, upper airway and sinus disease, and multisystem organ dysfunction suggest Churg-Strauss syndrome.
Obstructive sleep apnea (see Chapter 85)	Excessive snoring and daytime fatigue; the patient's sleep partner may offer a history of noisy, labored, or erratic breathing. Obstructive sleep apnea is more common in obese patients.
Mechanical airway obstruction	Respiratory noises may be more pronounced in the inspiratory or expiratory phase of respiration, depending on location of obstruction. Diagnosed via flow-volume loop.
Cystic fibrosis	Associated with thick, purulent sputum containing bacteria and with GI symptoms due to pancreatic insufficiency. Recurrent respiratory infections may be present without GI or other system involvement.

ABPA = allergic bronchopulmonary aspergillosis; GI = gastrointestinal.

tobacco smoke, wood-burning stoves, fireplaces, and unvented gas stoves. Other irritants to avoid include perfume, cleaning agents, sprays, dust, and vapors. There is no clear evidence regarding the value of high-efficiency particulate air filters (HEPA filters), air duct cleaning, or dehumidifiers in the control of asthma. Dehumidifiers may actually increase allergen levels if they are not properly cleaned and maintained.

Up to 20% of people may experience bronchoconstriction after taking aspirin or NSAIDs. Patients with a history of nasal polyps are at increased risk, and aspirin and NSAIDs must be avoided if sensitivity to these medications exists. β-Blockers, even topical β-blockers, may exacerbate symptoms in susceptible individuals. Sulfite-containing foods (e.g., processed potatoes, shrimp, dried fruit, beer, wine) should be avoided in patients with a history of sulfite sensitivity.

Medical management of asthma uses a step-wise approach based on asthma severity. Asthma severity is classified, based on spirometry measurements and frequency of symptoms, into one of four categories: intermittent, mild persistent, moderate persistent, or severe persistent (Table 3). Each category is defined by frequency of rescue inhaler use and nighttime symptoms as well as FEV_1 or peak expiratory flow rate (PEFR) measurement.

Regardless of disease severity, all patients are prescribed a short-acting, inhaled β-agonist medication. Short-acting β-agonists are the drugs of choice for reversal of acute symptoms of bronchoconstriction and are safe, well tolerated, and easy to use. All patients should be instructed on proper use of meter-dosed inhalers and be advised to have the medication available at all times

in case symptoms arise. Patients with intermittent asthma do not need daily controller medication and are treated as needed with a short-acting β-agonist. If short-acting bronchodilators are needed for symptom relief more than twice a week for daytime symptoms or twice a month for nighttime awakenings, a long-acting controller medication is indicated. Use of more than one canister of short-acting β-agonist per month may be a clue to poor control of asthma and warrants further investigation.

Mild persistent asthma is treated with a single long-term controller medication. Patients with this level of disease activity are more prone to disease exacerbations and have underlying inflammation. A low-dose inhaled corticosteroid is the preferred long-term controller medication; alternatives include a mast cell stabilizer, leukotriene modifier, or sustained-release methylxanthine. Inhaled corticosteroids reduce bronchial hyperresponsiveness, decrease use of short-acting β-agonists, and control symptoms. Patients should be advised to rinse their mouth carefully after using inhaled corticosteroids to reduce the risk of complications (thrush, dysphonia, cough, sore throat). Patients with moderate to severe disease should be taught how to use a peak-flow meter to self-monitor disease severity.

Moderate persistent asthma is treated with one or two long-term controller medications. Use either low doses of inhaled corticosteroid and a long-acting β-agonist (preferred) or medium doses of a single long-term controller medication. In patients who remain symptomatic while taking medium doses of inhaled corticosteroids, the addition of a long-acting bronchodilator (e.g., salmeterol) results in improved lung physiology, decreased use of

Table 3. Classification of Asthma Severity

Components of Severity	Intermittent	Persistent		
		Mild	Moderate	Severe
Impairment[a]				
Symptoms	≤2 days/week	>2 days/week but not daily	Daily	Throughout the day
Nighttime awakenings	≤2 ×/month	3-4 ×/month	>1 ×/week but not nightly	Often 7 ×/week
SABA use for symptom control (not prevention of EIB)	≤2 days/week	>2 days/week but not more than 1 ×/d	Daily	Several times a day
Interference with normal activity	None	Minor limitation	Some limitation	Extremely limited
Lung function	Normal FEV_1 between exacerbations FEV_1 >80% of predicted FEV_1/FVC normal	FEV_1 >80% of predicted FEV_1/FVC normal	FEV_1 >60% but <80% of predicted FEV_1/FVC reduced 5%	FEV_1 <60% of predicted FEV_1/FVC reduced >5%
Risk				
Exacerbations (consider frequency and severity)[b,c]	0-2/year		>2/year	
Recommended step for initiating treatment [d]	Step 1	Step 2	Step 3; consider short courses of systemic corticosteroids	Step 4 or 5; consider short courses of systemic corticosteroids

EIB = exercise-induced bronchospasm; SABA = short-acting β-agonist.

[a]Normal FEV_1/FVC: 8-19 years old, 85%; 20-39 years old, 80%; 40-59 years old, 75%; 60-80 years old, 70%.

[b]Frequency and severity may fluctuate over time for patients in any severity category.

[c]Relative annual risk for exacerbations may be related to FEV_1.

[d]In 2 to 6 weeks, evaluate the level of asthma control that is achieved and adjust therapy accordingly.

U.S. Department of Health and Human Services, National Institutes of Health. Expert Panel Report 3 (EPR-3): Guidelines for the Diagnosis and Management of Asthma–Summary Report 2007. www.nhlbi.nih.gov/guidelines/asthma/asthsumm.pdf. Published October, 2007. Accessed July 15, 2009.

short-acting β-agonists, and reduced symptoms when compared with doubling the dose of inhaled corticosteroid. Patients on long-acting β-agonists seem to obtain the same quick relief from a short-acting β-agonist when needed, although some mild tachyphylaxis does occur. However, a long-acting β-agonist should not be used alone; it should be used in conjunction with an inhaled corticosteroid based on studies suggesting increased mortality associated with long-acting β-agonist monotherapy for asthma, including exercise-induced asthma.

Patients with severe persistent asthma may require at least three daily medications to manage their disease (i.e., high doses of an inhaled corticosteroid plus a long-acting bronchodilator and possibly oral corticosteroids). These patients are highly prone to disease exacerbations and have underlying inflammation. The addition of a leukotriene modifier can improve FEV_1, decrease daytime symptom scores, and reduce nighttime awakenings. Patients with asthma who are obese, smoke cigarettes, or have aspirin sensitivity also may benefit from the use of a leukotriene modifier.

Omalizumab is a monoclonal antibody that binds to IgE and is useful for patients with severe persistent asthma to reduce exacerbations. Severe anaphylaxis has been reported up to 24 hours after injection and can occur even after prolonged use; therefore, patients should carry an epinephrine-containing auto-injector as a precaution.

Asthma treatment should continue during pregnancy. Short-acting β-agonists are safe during pregnancy. Inhaled corticosteroids also are considered safe and should be used for long-term control of asthma during pregnancy; cromolyn sodium, montelukast, zafirlukast, and theophylline can be used if necessary but are considered less-preferred alternatives to inhaled corticosteroids for daily control. For acute severe asthma exacerbations during pregnancy, oral corticosteroids are recommended, even though a small risk of congenital malformations has been reported.

Exercise-induced bronchospasm typically begins at the start of exercise and peaks 5 to 10 minutes after exercise. Several therapeutic options are available for patients with asthma symptoms during exercise, particularly vigorous exercise in cold, dry air. Patients should be advised to use a short-acting β-agonist such as albuterol 15 to 30 minutes before the start of exercise. Cromolyn sodium or nedocromil 15 to 30 minutes before exertion also can be used. Leukotriene modifiers are useful for patients with chronic asthma and exercise-induced asthma. Patients with chronic asthma and poorly controlled exercise-induced asthma are candidates for a long-acting β-agonist added to an inhaled beta corticosteroid or leukotriene modifier.

Management of comorbid conditions such as gastroesophageal reflux disease (GERD), allergic rhinitis, and chronic sinusitis may result in improved asthma control. Allergy tests, nasal examination, and assessment for GERD should be considered in all patients with asthma, particularly those who remain poorly controlled on long-term medications. Immunotherapy can be useful in patients with allergic rhinitis or insect hypersensitivity. Patients may need a "step up" in controller therapy during an acute upper respiratory infection.

When evaluating a patient for an acute asthma exacerbation, look for historical features that identify high risk for a difficult course or complications, including (1) a history of intubation, intensive care unit admission, or unscheduled hospital admission for asthma; (2) β-agonist dispensing frequency exceeding one canister per month; (3) poor adherence to inhaled corticosteroids; or (4) a history of depression, substance abuse, personality disorder, unemployment, or recent bereavement. Objective features that raise a red flag include FEV_1 <50% of predicted, PEFR <50% of predicted, pulse oximetry <95%, arterial P_{CO_2} >40 mm Hg (5.3 kPa), arterial P_{O_2} <75 mm Hg (10 kPa), theophylline level >12 µg/mL (66.6 µmol/L), leukocyte count with >5% eosinophils or a total eosinophil count >1000 to 1500/µL (1000 to 1500 × 10^6/L), respiration rate >30/min, and pulse rate >120/min. These patients are more prone to respiratory compromise and may require more intensive monitoring.

Follow-Up

Patients should be reassessed regularly (experts suggest every 3 to 6 months) to determine whether their asthma classification has changed and whether therapy with controller medications should be increased ("stepped up") or decreased ("stepped down"). Monitor pregnant patients with asthma more frequently, as asthma symptoms can improve, worsen, or stay the same during pregnancy. Ensuring good asthma control during pregnancy is important, as pregnancy-related complications (preeclampsia, low birth weight or intrauterine growth restriction, premature labor, infant mortality) are more common in patients with severe, poorly controlled disease.

For all patients, develop individual self-management plans, taking into consideration the patient's underlying disease severity and ability to adapt to self-management. Have all patients demonstrate proper use of prescribed inhaler devices; improper use can be a cause of difficult to control asthma. For patients with intermittent or mild persistent asthma, provide a simple plan outlining how to handle exacerbations, including health care contacts in cases of emergency. Patients with moderate to severe persistent asthma should keep a daily diary and have a detailed written action plan with specific objective or subjective markers for self-directed changes in therapy. Ensure that all patients with moderate to severe persistent asthma have a peak-flow meter at home and know how to use it. Provide instruction in symptom-based monitoring to patients who are not using a peak-flow meter.

Book Enhancement

Go to www.acponline.org/essentials/pulmonary-section.html. In *MKSAP for Students 5*, assess your knowledge with items 14-18 in the **Pulmonary Medicine** section.

Bibliography

Panettieri RA Jr. In the clinic. Asthma. Ann Intern Med. 2007;146:ITC6-1-ITC6-16. [PMID: 17548407]

Chapter 84

Chronic Obstructive Pulmonary Disease

Carlos Palacio, MD

COPD is characterized by airflow limitation that is not fully reversible. Chronic bronchitis and emphysema are the predominant conditions included in COPD; either or both may be present in a given patient. Chronic bronchitis is defined as a productive cough for 3 months in each of 2 successive years in a patient in whom other causes of chronic sputum production have been excluded. Chronic bronchitis is associated with an increase in the volume of tissue in the bronchiolar wall and an accumulation of inflammatory exudate in the airway lumen. Emphysema is defined as permanent enlargement of airspaces distal to the terminal bronchioles, with destruction of the bronchiolar walls without obvious fibrosis. Loss of alveolar attachments and elasticity contributes to small airway collapse during expiration. Chronic bronchitis and emphysema both result in peripheral airway obstruction, parenchymal destruction, and pulmonary vascular abnormalities that reduce the capacity for gas exchange, producing arterial hypoxemia, hypercapnia, and cor pulmonale. Hyperinflation causes respiratory muscle inefficiency and increased work of breathing.

Other conditions characterized by airflow limitation that is not fully reversible (e.g., bronchiectasis, cystic fibrosis, bronchiolitis) should be differentiated from COPD (Table 1). The distinction between COPD and asthma can be challenging, as some overlap may be seen.

Risk factors for COPD include host factors and environmental exposures. Hereditary deficiency of α_1-antitrypsin (AAT) is the best-documented genetic risk factor. AAT is an antiproteolytic enzyme that neutralizes neutrophil elastase. AAT deficiency results in excessive amounts of neutrophil elastase in the lung, which destroys elastin, causing early-onset obstructive pulmonary disease, typically panacinar emphysema. Some individuals with AAT deficiency may develop liver and skin disorders. Also implicated in COPD are genes responsible for the production of enzymes involved in detoxification of cigarette smoke (e.g., microsomal epoxide hydrolase, glutathione S-transferase). Developmental risk factors (e.g., low birth weight) and childhood illness have a profound effect on lung growth. Important environmental exposures include tobacco smoke, occupational dust, chemical agents, and air pollution.

Prevention

Eighty percent to 90% of the risk of developing COPD is attributable to cigarette smoking. Cigarette smoke is responsible for the development of bronchial mucous gland hypertrophy and goblet cell metaplasia with inflammatory cell infiltrates. Airway changes include squamous epithelial metaplasia, ciliary loss and dysfunction, and increased proliferation of smooth muscle and connective tissue. These smoking-related changes result in an accelerated decline in lung function. Smoking cessation slows the accelerated decline in forced expiratory volume in 1 second (FEV_1) and reduces all-cause mortality. Advise patients not to start smoking and to stop if they have started.

Screening

Screening for airway obstruction in asymptomatic patients is not recommended, as there is little evidence that making the diagnosis in this setting is beneficial. Patients with early-onset COPD (age ≤45 years) and patients with a strong family history of lung or liver disease should be screened for AAT deficiency.

Table 1. Differential Diagnosis of COPD

Disorder	Notes
Asthma	Onset typically in childhood, although may occur at any age; history of allergy often is present. Lability of symptoms, with overt wheezing and rapid response to β-agonist bronchodilators, is typical. Asthma may be present in ~10% of cases of COPD.
Bronchiectasis	Often associated with excessive sputum production with purulent exacerbations. Chest radiograph and CT scan may be diagnostic, showing thickened and cystic airways. Often a specific inciting event may be recognized, such as pneumonia in childhood.
Cystic fibrosis	Onset usually at birth but in rare cases may be in adulthood. Positive sweat chloride test; cystic fibrosis transmembrane conductance regulator test is abnormal in many cases.
Bronchiolitis	Onset often follows respiratory infection; may be idiopathic or associated with other diseases (e.g., rheumatoid arthritis). Postviral bronchiolitis usually is self-limited over a period of up to 3 mo. Bronchiolitis is poorly responsive to bronchodilators; oral corticosteroids may be helpful in some cases.
α_1-Antitrypsin deficiency	Early-onset COPD, usually age <45 y. Family history of COPD; COPD and liver disease; emphysema affecting the lower lobes. Measure α_1-antitrypsin levels.

Diagnosis

Assess for the presence of cough, sputum production, and dyspnea. Inquire about exercise tolerance, energy level, and frequency and severity of exacerbations. A detailed smoking history is essential, and a history of exposure to other inhalation exposures should be noted. Self-reported history of COPD, >40 pack-year smoking history, age ≥45 years, and maximum laryngeal height ≤4 cm are most predictive of COPD (positive likelihood ratio >200). Laryngeal height is the distance between the top of the thyroid cartilage and the suprasternal notch.

Look for signs of hyperinflation, including barrel chest, hyperresonant percussion note, distant breath sounds, and prolonged expiratory time. Pursed lip breathing, paradoxical chest or abdominal wall movements, and use of accessory muscles are all signs of severe airflow limitation. Cardiac examination may show cor pulmonale (increased intensity of the pulmonic sound, persistently split S_2, and a parasternal lift due to right ventricular hypertrophy). Extracardiac signs of cor pulmonale include neck vein distention, liver enlargement, and peripheral edema. Nonspecific radiographic signs of emphysema are flattening of the diaphragms, irregular lung lucency, and reduction or absence of pulmonary vascular markings.

COPD is confirmed and staged with spirometry (Table 2). The presence of a postbronchodilator FEV_1 <80% of predicted and an FEV_1 to forced vital capacity (FEV_1/FVC) ratio <70% confirms the presence of nonreversible airflow obstruction. Severity of COPD also can be graded using the BODE index, which consists of BMI, airflow obstruction, dyspnea, and exercise capacity (the 6-minute walk distance); higher BODE scores are associated with a greater risk of death (www.acponline.org/acp_press/essentials/pulmonary-section.html).

Static lung volumes, including total lung capacity, residual volume, and functional residual capacity, are increased in advanced COPD. Diffusing capacity for carbon dioxide is reduced, particularly in emphysema. Obtain an oxygen saturation measurement and arterial blood gas measurement if oximetry testing suggests hypoxemia (<94% on ambient air) or if there is suspicion of hypercapnia.

AAT deficiency predisposes to early-onset COPD, especially panacinar emphysema, which is suggested by increased basilar radiolucency. When suspected, measure the serum AAT level; severe deficiency of AAT is associated with serum AAT levels <50 to 80 mg/dL (0.5 to 0.8 g/L).

Therapy

Stable COPD

Smoking cessation slows the decline in pulmonary function and should be reinforced at each visit. Administer annual influenza vaccine to all patients unless contraindicated because of hypersensitivity to egg protein. Administer pneumococcal vaccine to all patients and revaccinate those aged ≥65 years who were immunized more than 5 years ago and were younger than age of 65 years at the time of vaccination.

Management of stable COPD is characterized by a stepwise increase in treatment based on spirometry results (see Table 2). Medications are used to alleviate symptoms, improve pulmonary function, and prevent complications (Table 3). Inhaled therapy is preferred over systemic agents. A metered-dose inhaler (MDI), with proper instruction and good technique, is as effective as a nebulizer. A spacer device, which holds the medicine in a chamber and allows the patient to inhale the drug fully, reduces oropharyngeal deposition of the drug and decreases subsequent local side effects. Nebulizers may be helpful for patients who cannot use MDIs because of severe dyspnea, difficulties with coordination, or physical problems such as arthritis.

Three types of bronchodilators are used to treat patients with stable COPD: β-agonists, anticholinergic agents, and methylxanthine products (e.g., theophylline). These medications all work by relaxing airway smooth muscle, thereby improving lung ventilation.

Short-acting β-agonists (e.g., albuterol, levalbuterol)—also known as "rescue" medications—act within a few minutes of administration, and their effect lasts approximately 4 to 6 hours. Give these medications as needed for relief of persistent or worsening symptoms and to improve exercise tolerance. Long-acting β-agonists (e.g., salmeterol, formoterol, arformoterol) achieve sustained and more predictable improvement in lung function than the short-acting agents. They improve health status, reduce symptoms, decrease the need for rescue medication, and increase the time interval between exacerbations. Long-acting β-agonists, which typically are given every 12 hours, can be used as monotherapy or combined with other bronchodilators and/or inhaled corticosteroids for better control of chronic symptoms. The most common side effects of β-agonist therapy are increased heart rate and tremor.

Vagal stimulation in the lung is mediated via muscarinic receptors. Anticholinergic drugs used to treat COPD include short-acting inhaled agents (e.g., ipratropium) and tiotropium, a long-act-

Table 2. Classification and Management of COPD[a]

Stage	Characteristics
I: Mild	• FEV_1/FVC <70%; FEV_1 ≥80% of predicted • With or without chronic symptoms (cough, sputum production) • Add short-acting bronchodilator when needed
II: Moderate	• FEV_1/FVC <70%; 50% ≤FEV_1 <80% of predicted • With or without chronic symptoms (cough, sputum production) • Add regular treatment with one or more long-acting bronchodilators; add pulmonary rehabilitation
III: Severe	• FEV_1/FVC <70%; 30% ≤FEV_1 <50% of predicted • With or without chronic symptoms (cough, sputum production) • Add inhaled corticosteroids if repeated exacerbations
IV: Very severe	• FEV_1/FVC <70%; FEV_1 <30% of predicted **or** FEV_1 <50% of predicted plus chronic respiratory failure • Add long-term oxygen therapy if chronic respiratory failure; consider surgical treatments

FEV_1 = forced expiratory volume in 1 second; FVC = forced vital capacity.

[a] Classification based on postbronchodilator FEV_1.

Reproduced from the Global Initiative for Chronic Obstructive Pulmonary Disease, Executive Summary: Global Strategy for the Diagnosis, Management, and Prevention of COPD, 2006, www.goldcopd.com (Accessed February 16, 2011).

Table 3. Treatment of COPD

Agent	Notes
Inhaled short-acting β-agonists	Bronchodilators; alleviate symptoms and improve pulmonary function. Generally used as needed.
Inhaled short- and long-acting anticholinergic agents	Bronchodilators; alleviate symptoms and improve pulmonary function. Used as scheduled maintenance. Do not combine short- and long-acting anticholinergic drugs.
Inhaled long-acting β-agonists	Bronchodilators; alleviate symptoms and improve pulmonary function. Used as scheduled maintenance.
Oral theophylline, aminophylline[a]	Bronchodilators; alleviate symptoms and improve pulmonary function; possibly improve respiratory muscle function. Used as scheduled maintenance. Maintain serum levels at 5-12 µg/mL (27.7-66.6 µmol/L).
Oral β-agonists	Bronchodilators; alleviate symptoms and improve pulmonary function. Used as scheduled maintenance. Rarely used because of side effects but may benefit patients who cannot use inhalers.
α_1-Antitrypsin augmentation therapy for AAT deficiency	Antiproteolytic enzyme; possibly reduces decline in pulmonary function and reduces mortality; life-long therapy. Most effective in patients with FEV_1 35%-60% of predicted. May be used in patients receiving lung transplants for AAT deficiency.
Inhaled corticosteroids	Anti-inflammatory agents; alleviate symptoms; improve pulmonary function in 10%-20% of patients, with symptoms and exacerbations reduced in a larger percentage; no effect on decline in pulmonary function. Used as scheduled maintenance. High doses are best studied in patients with a history of frequent exacerbations.
Systemic corticosteroids	Anti-inflammatory agents; alleviate symptoms and improve pulmonary function. Avoid use in stable chronic disease. Intravenous or oral corticosteroids are effective for acute exacerbations.
Supplemental oxygen	Improves tissue oxygenation; improves quality of life; prolongs life. Patients must qualify for use on the basis of arterial Po_2 or arterial oxygen saturation level.
Antibiotics	Used in treatment of acute exacerbations; may alleviate symptoms and reduce severity of exacerbation.

AAT = α_1-antitrypsin; FEV_1 = forced expiratory volume in 1 second.

[a] These agents are administered intravenously in the emergency department.

ing inhaled bronchodilator used in stable outpatients. Tiotropium selectively blocks the M3 muscarinic receptor. Short-acting anticholinergic agents are less potent than long-acting β-agonist or long-acting anticholinergic agents. Anticholinergic agents are especially useful in COPD when combined with short- or long-acting β-agonists and/or theophylline. Tiotropium should not be combined with short-acting anticholinergic drugs. The primary side effect of the inhaled anticholinergic agents used for COPD is dry mouth. Anticholinergic agents should be used with caution in patients with urinary obstruction and narrow-angle glaucoma.

Theophylline is a nonspecific phosphodiesterase inhibitor that increases intracellular cyclic adenosine monophosphate within airway smooth muscle and inhibits intracellular calcium release. Theophylline also increases histone deacetylase activity, which may improve the efficacy of corticosteroids. The role of theophylline in treatment of COPD exacerbations is controversial; it may be used as an adjunct to inhaled bronchodilators and inhaled corticosteroids. Some patients with COPD may benefit from a trial of theophylline for 1 to 2 months. Theophylline has a narrow therapeutic index, and toxicity therefore is a risk; maintain serum theophylline levels at 5 to 12 µg/mL (27.8 to 66.6 µmol/L). Sustained-release theophylline must be monitored carefully, particularly in elderly patients. Side effects include nausea, vomiting, and cardiac arrhythmias. Discontinue theophylline if side effects develop or objective benefit is not evident within several weeks.

The role of corticosteroids in the management of stable COPD is limited. However, regular use of inhaled corticosteroids in patients with recurrent exacerbations reduces the frequency of further exacerbations. Inhaled corticosteroids should not be used alone. Combinations of inhaled corticosteroids and long-acting bronchodilators are more effective than either therapy alone in

reducing exacerbations and improving health status. The long-term safety of inhaled corticosteroids in COPD is unknown. The use of inhaled corticosteroids in elderly patients must be carefully monitored because of the risk of adverse effects such as osteopenia, cataracts, hyperglycemia, and pneumonia, all which may be particularly debilitating in older patients with compromised health and comorbidities frequently associated with COPD.

Oxygen therapy is a major component of therapy for very severe (stage IV) COPD and usually is prescribed for patients with arterial Po_2 ≤55 mm Hg (7.3 kPa) or oxygen saturation ≤88% with or without hypercapnia. Patients with arterial Po_2 of ≤59 mm Hg (7.8 kPa) or oxygen saturation ≤89% also qualify for oxygen therapy if they have pulmonary hypertension, evidence of cor pulmonale or edema as a result of right-sided heart failure, or a hematocrit <55%. Oxygen treatment should be administered ≥15 hours per day. Long-term oxygen therapy improves survival in patients with chronic respiratory failure and has a beneficial effect on hemodynamics, exercise capacity, and mental status.

Pulmonary rehabilitation improves quality of life in patients with moderate to severe symptoms that persist despite optimal medical management. Exercise improves cardiovascular conditioning and increases ability to perform daily activities. Intensive counseling improves patient adherence and reinforces the proper use of pulmonary medications. Early pulmonary rehabilitation after hospitalization for an exacerbation leads to improved exercise capacity and health status.

Surgical interventions, including bullectomy, lung volume reduction surgery, and lung transplantation, may improve symptoms. Lung volume reduction surgery improves exercise capacity, lung function, dyspnea, and quality of life but does not confer an overall survival advantage. Patients with predominantly upper lobe emphysema and low baseline exercise capacity may have improved survival.

COPD Exacerbation

COPD exacerbation is characterized by a sudden change in the patient's baseline dyspnea, cough, and/or sputum production that is beyond the typical day-to-day variation in symptoms. Various nonspecific signs and symptoms also may be present, such as fatigue, insomnia, depression, and confusion. Exacerbations commonly are caused by infection and air pollution. Mild to moderate exacerbations can be managed at home. Mild exacerbations require treatment with short-acting bronchodilators; moderate exacerbations require short-acting bronchodilators and systemic corticosteroids and/or antibiotics. Severe exacerbations are treated in the hospital; severe exacerbations are characterized by loss of alertness or a combination of two or more of the following parameters: dyspnea at rest, respiration rate ≥25/min, pulse rate ≥110/min, or use of accessory respiratory muscles.

Oxygen therapy is the cornerstone of hospital management of COPD exacerbations, with a goal of adequate levels of oxygenation (arterial Po_2 >60 mm Hg [8.0 pKa] or oxygen saturation >90%). Arterial blood gas levels should be measured 30 to 60 minutes after oxygen therapy is started to ensure that oxygenation is adequate without carbon dioxide retention or acidosis.

Bronchodilator therapy with short-acting β-agonists is preferred for treating exacerbations. An anticholinergic agent should be added if the patient does not respond promptly to the β-agonist. In addition, systemic (oral or intravenous) corticosteroids are used for hospital management of acute exacerbations of COPD to improve symptoms and lung function and to reduce the length of hospitalization. The effective dose is unknown, but high doses are associated with a significant risk of side effects. Prolonged treatment does not result in greater efficacy and increases the risk of side effects.

There is a significant benefit to using antibiotics in patients who have moderate or severe COPD exacerbations. The predominant bacteria recovered are *Haemophilus influenzae*, *Streptococcus pneumoniae*, and *Moraxella catarrhalis*. Generally, antibiotic regimens for community-acquired infection include coverage with a third-generation cephalosporin in combination with a macrolide or monotherapy with a fluoroquinolone. Sputum Gram stain and culture usually is unnecessary.

In patients with COPD exacerbations, adjunctive nonpharmacologic therapies help alleviate dyspnea and decrease sputum production. The following interventions may be considered:

- Percussion, vibration, and postural drainage to enhance clearance of sputum
- Relaxation techniques to reduce anxiety from dyspnea
- Control of breathing, pursed lip breathing, and diaphragmatic breathing to alleviate dyspnea

Noninvasive intermittent ventilation alleviates respiratory acidosis and decreases respiration rate, severity of dyspnea, and length of hospital stay; importantly, mortality also is reduced. Indications for noninvasive ventilation include moderate to severe dyspnea with the use of accessory muscles of breathing and paradoxical abdominal motion, moderate to severe acidosis (pH <7.35) and/or hypercapnia (arterial Pco_2 >45 mm Hg [6.0 kPa]), and respiration rate >25/min. Exclusion criteria include respiratory arrest, cardiovascular instability (hypotension, arrhythmias, myocardial infarction), change in mental status (lack of cooperation), high aspiration risk, viscous or copious secretions, recent facial or gastroesophageal surgery, craniofacial trauma, fixed nasopharyngeal abnormalities, burns, and extreme obesity.

Invasive mechanical ventilation is indicated for patients who cannot tolerate noninvasive ventilation and patients with severe dyspnea with a respiration rate >35/min, life-threatening hypoxia, severe acidosis (pH <7.25) and/or hypercapnia (arterial Pco_2 >60 mm Hg [8.0 kPa]), respiratory arrest, somnolence or impaired mental status, cardiovascular complications (hypotension, shock), or other complications (e.g., metabolic abnormalities, sepsis, pneumonia, pulmonary embolism, barotrauma, massive pleural effusion).

Follow-Up

After severe acute exacerbation, most patients experience reduced quality of life, and nearly 50% are readmitted more than once in the ensuing 6 months. Therefore, the goal is to reduce the number and severity of exacerbations through smoking cessation, preventive vaccination, adherence with maintenance medications, and early attention to mild exacerbations.

Ensure that patients participate in disease self-management by understanding the causes, management, course, and prognosis of COPD. At follow-up visits, observe patients' use of inhalers and reinforce proper inhaler technique. Monitor pulmonary function periodically to determine the need for a change in or addition to treatment, including possible oxygen therapy.

Book Enhancement

Go to www.acponline.org/essentials/pulmonary-section.html. In *MKSAP for Students 5*, assess your knowledge with items 19-24 in the **Pulmonary Medicine** section.

Bibliography

Littner MR. In the clinic. Chronic obstructive pulmonary disease. Ann Intern Med. 2008;148:ITC3-1-ITC3-16. [PMID: 18316750]

Chapter 85

Obstructive Sleep Apnea

Arlina Ahluwalia, MD

Although more than 70 primary disorders of sleep have been identified, these conditions remain undiagnosed in a large proportion of patients. Within the subgroup of chronic respiratory sleep disorders, obstructive sleep apnea (OSA) is the most common diagnosis. OSA is characterized by recurrent episodes of partial or complete airway obstruction during sleep. Manifestations include limited attention and memory and significantly increased risk of motor vehicle accidents. The pathophysiology of pharyngeal collapse during sleep is not entirely understood. However, patients with OSA have smaller upper airways and substantial decrements in pharyngeal dilator muscle activity during sleep. Recurrent arousals from sleep, in addition to hypoxemia and hypercapnia, constitute the likely physiologic mechanism for the characteristic daytime somnolence and sequelae of the disorder. Symptomatic OSA contributes to secondary hypertension, likely related to peripheral vasoconstriction from arousal-prompted sympathetic discharge. In addition, patients with severe OSA accompanied by marked hypoxemia may develop secondary polycythemia and related complications. Hemodynamic consequences include increased left and right ventricular afterload, decreased left ventricular compliance, and increased myocardial oxygen demand; heart failure and stroke are important sequelae of OSA.

Diagnosis

Excessive daytime sleepiness is the most common manifestation of OSA, but patients may have many other symptoms related to OSA (Table 1). Obtain a sleep history from the patient and bed partner. Specifically address disruptive snoring, witnessed apnea, excessive

Table 1. Clinical Features of Obstructive Sleep Apnea

Symptoms	Physical Findings
Habitual snoring	Obesity
Reports of witnessed apnea	Large neck circumference
Nighttime awakening with gasping or choking	Nasal obstruction
Insomnia	Enlarged tonsils
Nighttime diaphoresis	Low-lying soft palate
Morning headaches	Narrow oropharynx
Erectile dysfunction	Macroglossia
Daytime fatigue or sleepiness	Retro- or micrognathia
Alterations in mood	
Neurocognitive decline	

daytime sleepiness (including while driving), fatigue, nasal congestion, weight gain, morning headaches, and number of hours slept per night (to rule out contributing sleep deprivation). Patients often do not report excessive daytime sleepiness, because they accommodate to the symptom complex. Consider using a validated questionnaire, which can be useful in assessing the need for diagnostic testing for sleep disorders (www.acponline.org/essentials/pulmonary-section.html).

Although prevalence is higher in men, OSA is likely underdiagnosed and undertreated in women. Obesity, the most common risk factor, is associated with an 8- to 12-fold increased risk of OSA in middle-aged adults. However, thinner, especially Asian, patients also may be affected. Other anatomic features associated with OSA include increased waist-hip ratio, self-reported large neck circumference (e.g., >40 cm [18 in]), crowded pharynx (due to long, low-lying uvula/soft palate, macroglossia, or enlarged tonsils), nasal obstruction, retrognathia, or overbite. Further physical examination findings may include systemic hypertension, decreased oxygen saturation, nasal congestion, wheezing, an accentuated pulmonic component of S_2 (suggesting pulmonary hypertension), or S_3 (suggesting heart failure).

Obtain a formal polysomnogram, with an electroencephalogram for sleep staging, to most accurately confirm the diagnosis, as clinical features are neither sufficiently sensitive nor specific for the diagnosis of OSA. This sleep study measures respiratory events and hours of sleep, from which the apnea-hypopnea index (AHI) is derived. An AHI of >5 per hour confirms OSA, and a combination of AHI, degree of sleepiness, and presence or absence of cardiovascular problems (e.g., hypertension, stroke, heart failure) determines the severity of disease. The use of alternative home respiratory tests, even when interpreted by a certified sleep specialist, may provide less accurate results. Continuous positive airway pressure (CPAP) titration, if indicated, may be conducted in the same session as diagnostic polysomnography.

Consider additional testing to assess for possible contributing factors or complications (Table 2). Order tests of thyroid function to exclude hypothyroidism, screen for acromegaly if clinically suspected, and obtain a complete blood count to assess for polycythemia that may accompany severe OSA. Perform daytime awake pulse oximetry; if a patient with suspected OSA demonstrates hypoxemia in this setting, measure arterial blood gases to assess for obesity hypoventilation syndrome (awake PCO_2 >45 mmHg [6.0 kPa]). Consider chest radiography or electrocardiography if cardiac complications are suspected.

The broad differential diagnosis of OSA includes other primary sleep disorders (e.g., central sleep apnea, periodic limb movements of sleep, narcolepsy) and conditions or factors that can disturb sleep (Table 3), such as medical conditions (e.g., obstructive lung disease, drug use, heart failure), depression, and neurologic disorders (e.g., stroke, movement disorder, seizure).

Therapy

Treatment of OSA aims to improve daytime sleepiness and cognitive performance and to prevent sequelae. Lifestyle changes and CPAP form the cornerstone of therapy; oral (dental) devices or upper airway surgical procedures may play a role in selected cases. Advise patients to defer driving or other potentially dangerous activities until OSA and alertness improve.

Crucial lifestyle changes include weight loss of at least 10% in obese patients (to increase airway size), avoidance of alcohol and sedatives 3 to 4 hours before bedtime (to maintain muscle tone of airway dilators), and lateral sleeping position (to render airways less collapsible). If nasal obstruction or congestion continues after

Table 2. Laboratory and Other Studies for Obstructive Sleep Apnea (OSA)

Test	Notes
Polysomnography	Considered the gold standard test for OSA.
Reduced channel polysomnography (usually includes respiratory monitoring and oximetry)	Sensitivity 82%-94%, specificity 82%-100%. Less expensive and less accurate than polysomnography but may offer increased access to diagnosis.
Overnight oximetry	Sensitivity 87%, specificity 65%. Overnight oximetry is not an accurate test for OSA.
Serum TSH level	Obtain in patients with recent weight gain and fatigue. TSH level is elevated in 2%-3% of patients with OSA.
Complete blood count	Polycythemia can be a complication of severe OSA with accompanying severe hypoxemia.
Chest radiography	Obtain if coexisting heart failure is suspected based on physical examination. Heart failure can be a complication of OSA.
Electrocardiography	Obtain if coexisting heart failure is suspected based on physical examination.
Arterial blood gas analysis	Obtain if obesity hypoventilation syndrome is suspected, to look for hypercapnia and hypoxemia.

TSH = thyroid-stimulating hormone.

Table 3. Differential Diagnosis of Obstructive Sleep Apnea (OSA)

Disorder	Notes
Central sleep apnea	Most commonly seen in patients with heart failure and stroke. Polysomnogram shows an absence of respiratory effort during apnea, distinguishing central from obstructive apnea. Central sleep apnea sometimes is induced by narcotics.
Upper airway resistance syndrome	Most commonly seen in loud snorers who complain of excessive sleepiness. Polysomnogram with EEG shows a normal AHI (<5/hr) and reveals that increased respiratory effort is causing frequent EEG interruptions during sleep. Symptoms and treatment are the same as for OSA.
Periodic limb movements of sleep	A neurologic disorder of unknown cause, characterized by frequent episodes of leg kicking during sleep. Most common in patients on dialysis. Limb movements are not associated with respiratory events on polysomnogram.
Narcolepsy	Severe excessive sleepiness and cataplexy (episodes of muscle weakness in response to emotion); onset peaks at age 15-25 y. Polysomnogram does not show OSA or periodic limb movements, but multiple sleep latency tests are abnormal (patient falls asleep quickly and has REM sleep during short naps).
Obstructive or restrictive lung disease (see Chapters 85 and Chapter 86)	Shortness of breath or cough may disturb sleep. Pulmonary function tests establish the diagnosis and can guide specific therapy.
GERD (see Chapter 20)	Cough or choking may disturb sleep. Acid or burning taste in the throat is helpful but may be absent. A successful trial of empiric GERD therapy may confirm the diagnosis.
Sinusitis	Cough and drainage may disturb sleep. Clinical symptoms (nasal congestion, postnasal drip) suggest the diagnosis.
Heart failure (see Chapter 7)	Dyspnea and cough may disturb sleep. Symptoms and examination usually suggest heart disease. Central sleep apnea may be seen in patients with severe heart failure and indicates a worse prognosis.
Epilepsy	Seizures may occur only at night, with or without motor activity. Obtain neurology consultation and EEG.
Sleep deprivation or short sleep schedule	Inadequate hours of sleep can cause daytime sleepiness; naps usually are refreshing, which is not typical for OSA. Review of sleep schedule is essential, and a trial of longer sleep hours may be helpful.
Hypothyroidism (see Chapter 12)	Only 2%-3% of patients with OSA have hypothyroidism. Suspect in patients with weight gain and fatigue, and screen with a serum TSH level.
Acromegaly	Screen patients with compatible signs and symptoms. Treatment of acromegaly may significantly reduce OSA severity.

AHI = apnea-hypopnea index; EEG = electroencephalogram; GERD = gastroesophageal reflux disease; REM = rapid eye movement; TSH = thyroid-stimulating hormone.

treatment with nasal corticosteroids and decongestants for rhinitis, consider surgical procedures to restore nasal patency.

If moderate to severe OSA persists despite these interventions, or if the changes cannot be instituted, nightly continuous positive airway pressure (CPAP) is instituted. This most consistently effective therapy pneumatically splints the entire airway, preventing collapse during sleep. CPAP raises intraluminal airway pressure and increases functional residual capacity. Regular use of CPAP may dramatically improve quality of life by increasing daytime alertness, decreasing hypertension, and eliminating apneic episodes. However, adherence to CPAP is particularly challenging; measures shown to improve adherence include early patient education, follow-up, heated humidification, and establishing a comfortable interface for the CPAP device (nasal mask or nasal pillows). Patients still uncomfortable with CPAP (or with hypoventilation) may benefit from a trial of bilevel positive airway pressure (BiPAP) nasal ventilation; allowing higher inspiratory and lower expiratory pressure settings or auto-titrating positive pressure devices also may be helpful. The precise role of supplemental oxygen is not yet determined.

Consider oral appliances or surgical intervention as alternative therapies in patients who are unable or unwilling to use CPAP. Resection of enlarged, obstructing tonsils may be beneficial. Oral appliances aim to open the posterior airway space, usually by protruding the lower jaw or holding the tongue forward; however, these devices eliminate the need for CPAP in only mild to moderate disease. Surgical procedures for OSA, most commonly uvulopalatopharyngoplasty, are designed to alleviate retropalatal and retroglossal obstruction of the hypoglossal space. Surgical procedures have variable success rates depending on complex factors, including BMI, severity of OSA, and individual anatomy. A follow-up polysomnogram is recommended to document the effect of an oral appliance or a surgical procedure.

Follow-Up

Arrange follow-up at 1 month and then 6 month intervals to assess adherence to treatment and change in symptoms, particularly daytime sleepiness, and to emphasize weight loss in obese patients. Nonadherence, erroneously titrated CPAP, failure to wear CPAP every night, or coexisting periodic limb movements in sleep may contribute to persistent sleepiness. Perform a repeat sleep study if significant lifestyle goals have been attained, to assess whether OSA is resolved or if CPAP should be adjusted. Monitor patients with moderate to severe OSA for potentially related cognitive, cardiovascular, or obesity-related or metabolic conditions.

Book Enhancement

Go to www.acponline.org/essentials/pulmonary-section.html. In *MKSAP for Students 5*, assess your knowledge with items 25-27 in the **Pulmonary Medicine** section.

Bibliography

Basner RC. Continuous positive airway pressure for obstructive sleep apnea. N Engl J Med. 2007;356:1751-1758. [PMID: 17460229]

Guilleminault C, Abad VC. Obstructive sleep apnea syndromes. Med Clin North Am. 2004;88:611-630, viii. [PMID: 15087207]

Chapter 86

Infiltrative and Fibrotic Lung Diseases

Amy W. Shaheen, MD

The term *diffuse parenchymal lung disease* (DPLD) encompasses more than 200 distinct disorders that cause infiltration of the gas exchange components of the lungs. DPLD is characterized clinically by dyspnea on exertion, cough, and radiographic findings of diffuse pulmonary infiltrates. Although "diffuse" suggests widespread involvement of the lungs, the process may not affect the lung uniformly, and some areas may be spared. Alveolar filling processes are included with DPLD because of the similarity in presentation.

Recent guidelines for the classification of DPLD recommend grouping the disorders into four categories:

- DPLD of known cause, such as systemic illness (e.g., collagen vascular disease), environmental exposure, infection, or neoplasm
- Granulomatous DPLD (e.g., sarcoidosis, hypersensitivity pneumonitis)
- Rare DPLD with well-defined features (e.g., eosinophilic pneumonia, lymphangioleiomyomatosis, Langerhans cell histiocytosis, pulmonary alveolar proteinosis)
- Idiopathic interstitial pneumonias

The idiopathic interstitial pneumonias are further classified into groups of disorders with distinct clinical and pathologic features. Idiopathic pulmonary fibrosis (IPF), sarcoidosis, DPLD associated with collagen vascular disease, and hypersensitivity pneumonitis account for approximately 80% of DPLD. Key features of selected forms of DPLD are summarized in Table 1.

Evaluation

The process of determining a specific diagnosis when faced with such a broad spectrum of disorders can be daunting. Important features to keep in mind are clinical history and physical findings, tempo of disease progression, and radiographic distribution and pattern of the infiltrate. Depending on these factors, a tentative diagnosis may be confirmed with appropriate diagnostic testing, which may include biopsy.

The patient history should include age, sex, smoking history, current and previous illnesses, immunocompromising conditions including HIV infection, prescription and nonprescription medications, environmental and occupational exposures, travel, and family history. For example, patients with a history of malignancy may present with DPLD when there is lymphangitic spread. Common drugs that can cause pulmonary toxicity include antibiotics (e.g., nitrofurantoin), anti-inflammatory drugs (e.g., methotrexate), antiarrhythmic agents (e.g., amiodarone), and chemotherapeutic agents (e.g., bleomycin). Updated and referenced information regarding drugs that can cause pulmonary disease can be found at www.pneumotox.com. Environmental exposures, such as asbestos, may be remote or subtle and may not be considered important by the patient. Exposure to low-molecular-weight organic antigens from sources such as moldy hay, bird feathers, or mycobacteria found in hot tubs can cause acute or chronic forms of hypersensitivity pneumonitis.

Systemic illnesses may have specific features that provide clues. For example, pleuritic chest pain suggests collagen vascular diseases such as systemic lupus erythematosus or rheumatoid arthritis, and hemoptysis suggests alveolar hemorrhage due to Goodpasture syndrome. Some unusual causes of DPLD occur in specific patient populations. Lymphangioleiomyomatosis, a disorder of smooth muscle proliferation in the lung, primarily affects young women. Other disorders such as respiratory bronchiolitis–associated interstitial lung disease or Langerhans cell histiocytosis are seen predominantly in heavy smokers. Some DPLD may be genetic, as in familial forms of sarcoidosis, interstitial pulmonary fibrosis, or Hermansky-Pudlak syndrome.

Determining the onset of symptoms or radiographic changes is helpful in making a diagnosis. Symptoms may be insidious in onset, occurring over months to years, as in many of the idiopathic interstitial pneumonias or pneumoconioses. Alternatively, rapidly progressive symptoms of dyspnea and radiographic changes occurring over days to weeks may indicate an acute process, such as heart failure, allergy, acute interstitial pneumonia, or drug reaction. A patient with cryptogenic organizing pneumonia may describe an antecedent flu-like illness or may have been treated appropriately for a suspected bacterial infection in the 4 to 8 weeks prior to presentation but not improved on treatment. A pneumothorax suggests lymphangioleiomyomatosis in a young woman or Langerhans cell histiocytosis in a man who smokes. Radiation to the head, neck, or chest in the previous 6 months may suggest radiation pneumonitis.

Physical examination findings of DPLD often are nonspecific and may include basilar Velcro-like crackles. Velcro-like crackles are common in patients with interstitial lung disease and frequently are heard in patients with IPF; they rarely are present in patients with sarcoidosis. Similarly, clubbing has been described in as many as two thirds of patients with IPF (Plate 62) but is rare in patients with sarcoidosis. Evidence of right-sided heart failure (e.g., jugular venous distention, prominent pulmonic component of S_2, right ventricular heave) may be seen in advanced lung disease. The examination should include a careful search for extrapulmonary involvement (e.g., skin, joint, and neurologic findings) suggesting an underlying systemic illness (Table 2).

Table 1. Distinguishing Features of Select Forms of Diffuse Parenchymal Lung Disease (DPLD)

Disorder	Notes
DPLD of Known Cause	
Drug toxicity	Examples: amiodarone, nitrofurantoin, bleomycin, sulfasalazine (see www.pneumotox.com for a complete listing)
Infection	Examples: viruses, atypical bacteria (*Mycloplasma pneumoniae, Legionella pneumophila, Chlamydophila pneumoniae*), fungi (*Pneumocystis*), mycobacteria
Malignancy	Lymphangitic carcinomatosis (breast, stomach, lung, pancreas) is associated with insidious onset of cough and dyspnea.
Pneumoconioses	Asbestosis: pleural plaques on chest radiograph. Silicosis: "eggshell calcification" on chest radiograph.
Rheumatoid arthritis	Pleural effusions, pulmonary nodules, and interstitial disease; 10%-20% of patients with rheumatoid arthritis (mostly men) are affected.
Scleroderma	Nonspecific interstitial pneumonia pathology; antibody to Scl-70 or pulmonary hypertension portends a poorer prognosis.
Dermatomyositis/polymyositis	Many different types of histology; poor prognosis.
Systemic lupus erythematosus	Shrinking lung syndrome, fever, dyspnea, effusions, or atelectasis.
Other collagen vascular diseases	Behçet disease, Sjögren syndrome.
Idiopathic Interstitial Pneumonias	
Idiopathic pulmonary fibrosis (IPF)	Chronic, insidious onset of cough and dyspnea, usually in a patient aged >50 y. Usual interstitial pneumonia pathology (honeycombing, bibasilar infiltrates with fibrosis). Diagnosis of exclusion.
Nonspecific interstitial pneumonia	Subacute presentation; patient usually is younger than in IPF and more likely to be female. Ground-glass opacities. May respond to immunomodulating drugs.
Diffuse interstitial pneumonia or respiratory bronchiolitis–associated interstitial lung disease	"Smokers" bronchiolitis characterized by gradual onset of persistent cough and dyspnea. Radiograph shows ground-glass opacities and thickened interstitium. Smoking cessation improves prognosis.
Acute interstitial pneumonia	Dense bilateral acute lung injury similar to acute respiratory distress syndrome; 50% mortality rate.
Cryptogenic organizing pneumonia	May be preceded by flu-like illness. Radiograph shows focal areas of consolidation that may migrate from one location to another.
Granulomatous DPLD	
Sarcoidosis	Variable clinical presentation, ranging from asymptomatic to multiorgan involvement. Stage 1: hilar adenopathy. Stage 2: hilar adenopathy plus interstitial lung disease. Stage 3: interstitial lung disease. Stage 4: fibrosis.
Hypersensitivity pneumonitis	Allergic reaction to an inhaled low-molecular-weight antigen; may be acute, subacute, or chronic. Noncaseating granulomas are hallmarks. Chronic hypersensitivity pneumonitis has a poor prognosis.
Rare DPLD with Well-Defined Features	
Lymphangioleiomyomatosis	Affects women in their 30s and 40s. Associated with spontaneous pneumothorax. Chest CT shows cystic disease.
Langerhans cell histiocytosis	Affects younger men who smoke. Improves with smoking cessation.
Goodpasture syndrome	Associated with anti-glomerular basement membrane antibody. Hemoptysis and glomerular disease are hallmarks.
Hermansky-Pudlak syndrome	Autosomal recessive disorder associated with oculocutaneous albinism, bleeding diathesis, and pulmonary disease.
Chronic eosinophilic pneumonia	Chest radiograph shows "radiographic negative" of heart failure, with peripheral alveolar infiltrates predominating. Other findings may include peripheral blood eosinophilia and eosinophilia on bronchoalveolar lavage.
Pulmonary alveolar proteinosis	Slowly progressive disorder affecting patients in their 20s to 50s (predominantly men). Diagnosed via broncho-alveolar lavage, which shows abundant protein in the airspaces. Chest CT shows "crazy paving" pattern.

Laboratory evaluation should include a complete blood count with differential, a standard metabolic panel, antinuclear antibody and rheumatoid factor assays, and urinalysis. Where indicated, additional helpful tests may include electrocardiography, echocardiography, or serologic assays for autoantibodies to extractable nuclear antigens, anti–double-stranded DNA antibody, anti-neutrophil cytoplasmic antibody, or anti–glomerular basement membrane antibody (Table 3).

Obtain chest radiography, CT, and high-resolution CT. High-resolution CT should be used when interstitial or parenchymal disease is suspected, as the images will provide detail about the distribution and extent of disease and may reveal characteristic findings that, in the right clinical context, confirm a specific diagnosis. For example, "honeycomb" fibrosis (characterized by clusters or rows of cysts with shared walls) typically is associated with end-stage refractory disease, whereas a "ground-glass" appearance (hazy opacity indicating filling of alveoli or thickening of the interstitium) is associated with active inflammation that may be amenable to therapy, as is the case in acute hypersensitivity pneumonitis. Certain radiographic patterns are suggestive of specific

Table 2. Clinical Clues to Causes of Diffuse Parenchymal Lung Disease

Finding or Factor	Notes
Patient age	Interstitial lung disease often occurs in patients aged >60 y, but interstitial lung disease with collagen vascular disease, sarcoidosis, lymphangioleiomyomatosis, and Langerhans cell histiocytosis usually occurs in patients aged 20-40 y.
Female sex	Lymphangioleiomyomatosis and tuberous sclerosis.
Smoking history	Associated with respiratory bronchiolitis–associated interstitial lung disease, diffuse interstitial pneumonitis, and Langerhans cell histiocytosis.
Exposure history	Consider asbestosis and silicosis if occupational exposure. Consider hypersensitivity pneumonitis if exposure to birds, hay, or mold.
Acute onset (days to weeks)	Consider acute interstitial pneumonia, acute eosinophilic pneumonia, cryptogenic organizing pneumonia, drug-induced interstitial lung disease, and diffuse alveolar hemorrhage syndrome.
Velcro-like crackles	Present in >80% of patients with idiopathic pulmonary fibrosis but common in many interstitial lung diseases.
Signs of pulmonary hypertension[a]	May occur secondary to advanced interstitial lung disease or as a specific feature of an underlying cause of lung disease (e.g., scleroderma).
Clubbing	Common in idiopathic pulmonary fibrosis (30%). Rare in respiratory bronchiolitis–associated interstitial lung disease, cryptogenic organizing pneumonia, and collagen vascular disease.
Erythema nodosum	Associated with sarcoidosis, Behçet disease, ankylosing spondylitis, and inflammatory bowel disease.
Uveitis/conjunctivitis	Associated with sarcoidosis, Behçet disease, ankylosing spondylitis, and inflammatory bowel disease.
Lacrimal/salivary gland enlargement	Associated with sarcoidosis and Sjögren syndrome.
Lymphadenopathy, hepatosplenomegaly	Associated with sarcoidosis and amyloidosis.
Arthritis	Associated with collagen vascular disease, sarcoidosis, Behçet disease, ankylosing spondylitis, and inflammatory bowel disease.
Muscle weakness	Associated with polymyositis and dermatomyositis.
Neurologic abnormalities	Associated with sarcoidosis, tuberous sclerosis, and lymphomatoid granulomatosis.
Response to corticosteroids	Associated with cryptogenic organizing pneumonia and lymphoid interstitial pneumonia.

[a] May include increased pulmonic valve sound, right ventricular lift, tricuspid regurgitation murmur, and elevated central venous pressure.

Table 3. Laboratory Findings in Diffuse Parenchymal Lung Disease (DPLD)

Finding	Notes
Eosinophilia	May be seen in eosinophilic pneumonia, sarcoidosis, systemic vasculitis, and drug-induced DPLD.
Hemolytic anemia	May be seen in collagen vascular disease, sarcoidosis, lymphoma, and drug-induced DPLD.
Normocytic anemia	May be seen in diffuse alveolar hemorrhage syndromes, collagen vascular disease , and lymphangitic carcinomatosis.
Urinary sediment abnormalities	May be seen in systemic vasculitis (Wegener granulomatosis, Goodpasture syndrome) and drug-induced DPLD.
Hypogammaglobulinemia	May be seen in lymphocytic interstitial pneumonitis and common variable immunodeficiency.
Serum angiotensin-converting enzyme elevation	May be seen in sarcoidosis, hypersensitivity pneumonitis, silicosis, and Gaucher disease.
Antinuclear antibody (ANA), rheumatoid factor (RF)	Low-titer ANA and RF may be present in 10%-20% of patients with idiopathic pulmonary fibrosis.
Anti–glomerular basement membrane antibody	Diagnostic of Goodpasture syndrome in patients with alveolar hemorrhage.
Anti-neutrophil cytoplasmic antibody	May be present in Wegener granulomatosis, Churg-Strauss syndrome, and microscopic polyangiitis.
Serum precipitating antibodies	May indicate hypersensitivity pneumonitis.

diseases, with high correlation between the histologic and radiographic appearances for many forms of DPLD. For example, reticular lower lobe infiltrates with peripheral involvement, traction bronchiectasis, and honeycombing suggest IPF (Figure 1); a reverse heart failure pattern suggests chronic eosinophilic pneumonia; diffuse cystic disease suggests lymphangioleiomyomatosis or Langerhans cell histiocytosis; and nodules may indicate metastatic disease or miliary tuberculosis. Migrating, bibasilar, peripheral infiltrates in a subacutely ill patient may indicate cryptogenic organizing pneumonia.

Obtain spirometry, lung volumes, and diffusing capacity for carbon monoxide (D$_{LCO}$). Patients with DPLD frequently have evidence of restriction, with a decreased D$_{LCO}$. Arterial blood gas abnormalities typically include resting or exercise hypoxemia.

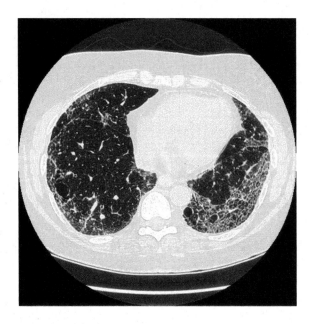

Figure 1. High-resolution thin-section CT scan showing extensive parenchymal involvement with fibrotic and honeycomb-like changes.

Bronchoalveolar lavage may help exclude infection and is of little risk. The procedure involves "washing" segments of lung during bronchoscopy and then collecting and analyzing the lavage fluid. Bronchoalveolar lavage can be diagnostic for lymphangitic carcinomatosis, pulmonary alveolar proteinosis, and pulmonary infiltrates with eosinophilia syndromes. Tissue biopsy (transbronchial lung biopsy via bronchoscopy, video-assisted thoracoscopic lung biopsy, or open lung biopsy) may be necessary to confirm a diagnosis. Surgical lung biopsy carries greater risk, and benefits should be weighed against the potential for harm.

The most common form of DPLD is IPF (also called cryptogenic fibrosing alveolitis), which accounts for up to 35% of DPLD cases. A definitive diagnosis requires a biopsy specimen showing histologic evidence of usual interstitial pneumonia (UIP). UIP is characterized by patchy collagen fibrosis and scarring in a peripheral pattern with subpleural, fibrotic honeycomb-like changes. Because UIP is not specific for IPF, the diagnosis is one of exclusion. The diagnosis may be made presumptively in the appropriate clinical setting, such as an older patient with gradually worsening dyspnea, Velcro-like crackles, restrictive pattern on pulmonary function tests, diminished D_{LCO}, and a high-resolution CT scan showing reticular subpleural infiltrates and predominantly basilar honeycomb-like fibrosis. The other interstitial pneumonias may have a different histologic pattern or different characteristics on CT scan, affect other patient types (e.g., smokers in respiratory bronchiolitis–associated interstitial lung disease and diffuse interstitial pneumonia, young women in nonspecific interstitial pneumonia), or have a different time course (e.g., acute interstitial pneumonia, cryptogenic organizing pneumonia).

Sarcoidosis, a multisystem disorder of unknown cause, is the second most common DPLD. The hallmark of sarcoidosis is noncaseating epithelioid cell granulomas in the absence of infection or malignancy. Patients with sarcoidosis usually are aged <40 years.

There are many variants ranging from Löfgren syndrome (hilar adenopathy, erythema nodosum, arthralgia, fever), which has an excellent prognosis (85% of patients have spontaneous remission in 2 years), to fibrotic lung disease, which carries a poor prognosis. Chest radiography commonly demonstrates mediastinal and bilateral hilar lymphadenopathy with or without parenchymal involvement. High-resolution CT may reveal nodular infiltrates in a perilymphatic distribution with a mid to upper lung field predominance; in IPF, the infiltrates are more peripheral and basilar. Pleural effusions are uncommon. Bronchoscopy with biopsy is helpful in the diagnosis of sarcoidosis.

Therapy

Encourage all patients who smoke to stop smoking and provide supportive care, including oxygen, symptomatic treatment for reactive airways or cough, maintenance of nutrition and fitness, and treatment of infections. Whenever possible, suspected causative exposures should be eliminated. In these cases, the DPLD may remit. Smoking cessation may result in stabilization or remission of Langerhans cell histiocytosis or respiratory bronchiolitis–associated interstitial lung disease. In patients with DPLD due to collagen vascular disease, the underlying disease is treated. Sarcoidosis often remits spontaneously, and the need for therapy is controversial. Cryptogenic organizing pneumonia responds to high-dose, prolonged tapers of corticosteroid therapy. Acute hypersensitivity pneumonia responds to removal from the antigenic stimulus and corticosteroid therapy; treatment of chronic hypersensitivity pneumonitis is less clear. Radiation pneumonitis responds to corticosteroid therapy.

Acute decompensation in a patient with DPLD most often is due to infection or edema. Treatment of the cause of acute decompensation should result in improvement. However, in patients with IPF, acute exacerbation of the underlying fibrosing process can occur. This is a catastrophic event characterized by unexplained and severe worsening of dyspnea and hypoxemia within 30 days of presentation, for which there is no effective treatment and a high mortality rate. Supportive care should be offered.

Immunosuppressive agents and corticosteroids have limited efficacy in the treatment of IPF, and side effects often complicate their use. Patients aged <60 years may be candidates for lung transplantation and should be referred early to appropriate centers.

Book Enhancement

Go to www.acponline.org/essentials/pulmonary-section.html. In *MKSAP for Students 5*, assess your knowledge with items 28-31 in the **Pulmonary Medicine** section.

Acknowledgment

We would like to thank Dr. Janet N. Myers, who contributed to an earlier version of this chapter.

Bibliography

Morgenthau AS, Padilla ML. Spectrum of fibrosing diffuse parenchymal lung disease. Mt Sinai J Med. 2009;76:2-23. [PMID: 19170214]

Chapter 87

Venous Thromboembolism

Alpesh N. Amin, MD

Pulmonary embolism (PE) and deep venous thrombosis (DVT) are different manifestations of the same disease, often collectively referred to as venous thromboembolism (VTE). An estimated 2 million cases of DVT, 600,000 cases of symptomatic PE, and 300,000 VTE-related deaths occur annually in the United States. Venous stasis, hypercoagulability, and endothelial damage are the underlying predisposing conditions for VTE. PE is the result of DVT formation and subsequent embolization into the pulmonary arteries. The thrombotic material obstructing blood flow through the pulmonary arteries has several physiologic consequences, including ventilation-perfusion aberrations and relative ischemia of the peripheral lung tissues. The most important clinical effect, however, is an acute increase in pulmonary vascular resistance, which increases the demand on the right ventricle and may lower cardiac output. In its extreme form, this combination of effects can cause right ventricular dysfunction, infarction, and even cardiac arrest. The differential diagnosis of VTE is reviewed in Table 1.

Prevention

Consider VTE prophylaxis for all patients admitted to the hospital, especially medical patients who are immobilized, most surgical patients, and patients who have had major trauma. Prevention strategies include the following:

- Low-dose, subcutaneous unfractionated heparin or low-molecular-weight heparin in high-risk medical patients and in surgical patients, except those at highest risk for bleeding
- Warfarin or low-molecular-weight heparin in patients undergoing hip or knee replacement, patients aged >40 years undergoing general surgery for malignancy, and patients with a thrombophilic state
- Fondaparinux (inactivates factor Xa) in patients undergoing hip or knee replacement and in at-risk medical patients
- Pneumatic compression with graduated compression stockings for patients at high risk for bleeding with anticoagulation and for patients at highest risk requiring dual therapy
- Low-molecular-weight heparin in patients with cancer

Screening

Do not routinely screen for DVT in high-risk asymptomatic patients. Noninvasive diagnostic tests are not recommended, because they are insensitive and are not associated with improved clinical outcomes.

Diagnosis

The diagnosis of VTE begins with a detailed history of risk factors, including current malignancy, past history of VTE, recent immobilization, hospitalization, major surgery, advanced age, obesity, trauma, smoking, acute myocardial infarction, heart failure, coagulopathy, pregnancy, postpartum state, and estrogen therapy.

Deep Venous Thrombosis

The most common symptom associated with DVT is calf pain, but many patients are asymptomatic. On physical examination, look for posterior calf tenderness and leg edema. Because signs and symptoms of DVT are nonspecific, clinical prediction rules assist in identifying patients who require further diagnostic testing. The best-known predictive model is that of Wells. According to the Wells criteria, each of the following characteristics earns 1 point: active cancer, paralysis or recent plaster cast, recent immobilization or major surgery, tenderness along the deep veins, swelling of the whole leg, >3-cm difference in calf circumference compared with other leg, pitting edema, and collateral superficial veins. Patients in whom an alternative diagnosis is likely earn -2 points. A Wells score >3 indicates a high pretest probability of DVT, a score of 1 to 2 indicates moderate probability, and a score ≤0 indicates a low pretest probability of DVT. Select lower extremity venous ultrasonography in patients with a moderate or high probability of DVT. Measure D-dimer levels in patients with a low probability of DVT; if D-dimer results are abnormal, perform lower extremity ultrasonography (Table 2).

Pulmonary Embolism

The most common symptoms of PE are dyspnea, pleuritic chest pain, cough, and hemoptysis; tachypnea, crackles, tachycardia, and S_4 gallop are the most common findings. Although these symptoms and signs are sensitive, they lack specificity. Arterial blood gases often are obtained, but the distributions of arterial Po_2 and the alveolar-arterial oxygen gradient are similar in patients with and without PE; approximately one of every four patients with PE has an arterial Po_2 ≥80 mm Hg (10.6 kPa).

Obtain a chest radiograph in all patients. Look for atelectasis, pleural effusion, focal oligemia (lack of vascularity), peripheral wedge-shaped density above the diaphragm, and an enlarged right descending pulmonary artery. An electrocardiogram often is abnormal, but positive findings lack sensitivity and specificity.

The simplified Wells criteria can be used to estimate the pretest probability of PE. Predictive factors are scored as follows: clinical signs/symptoms of DVT (3 points); no alternative diagnosis more

Table 1. Differential Diagnosis of Venous Thromboembolism

Disorder	Notes
Deep Venous Thrombosis	
Venous insufficiency (venous reflux)	Usually due to venous hypertension from such causes as venous reflux or obesity. Obtain ultrasound to diagnose venous reflux.
Muscle strain, tear, or trauma	Pain occurring with range of motion more characteristic of orthopedic problem due to trauma.
Ruptured Baker cyst	Pain localized to popliteal region of leg. Diagnosed with ultrasonography.
Cellulitis	Skin tenderness, erythema, and warmth. Normal ultrasound.
Lymphedema	Toe edema is more characteristic of lymphedema than of venous edema. Lymphedema can occur in one leg or both legs.
Pulmonary Embolism	
Acute coronary syndrome (see Chapter 3)	Chest pain associated with specific ECG and echocardiographic changes. Elevated cardiac enzymes can be seen in both acute coronary syndrome and large pulmonary emboli.
Pericarditis (see Chapter 1)	Substernal pain that is sharp, dull, or pressure-like, often relieved with sitting forward; usually pleuritic. ECG usually shows ST-segment elevation (usually diffuse) or PR-segment depression.
Aortic dissection (see Chapter 1)	Substernal chest pain with radiation to the back or mid-scapular region. Chest radiograph may show a widened mediastinal silhouette, a pleural effusion, or both.
Acute pulmonary edema (see Chapter 7)	Elevated venous pressure, S_3, bilateral crackles, and characteristic chest radiograph.
Pleurisy	Sharp, localized chest pain and fever. Pleural effusion may be present. Diagnosis of exclusion.
Pneumothorax	Sudden onset of chest pain and dyspnea. Chest radiograph establishes the diagnosis.
Asthma or chronic obstructive pulmonary disease exacerbation	Dyspnea and wheezing; positive response to bronchodilator (asthma). History of these disorders with a compatible course of illness is helpful.
Panic attack	Diagnosis of exclusion. Patient may have a history of somatization.

ECG = electrocardiogram, electrocardiographic.

Table 2. Laboratory and Other Studies for Suspected Deep Venous Thrombosis (DVT)

Test	Notes
D-dimer assay (ELISA)	Sensitivity for proximal DVT 98%, specificity 45%. Usually used in combination with ultrasonography or clinical scoring.
Duplex Doppler ultrasonography	Sensitivity for proximal DVT 96%, specificity 94%. Combines Doppler audio measurements of blood flow with visual ultrasonography.
Compression ultrasonography	Sensitivity for proximal DVT 94%, specificity 98%. The compressibility of the proximal veins is assessed with the ultrasound probe.
Venography	Sensitivity 100%, specificity 100%. Of limited value if there is poor contrast filling of the deep veins; historical "gold standard."

ELISA = enzyme-linked immunosorbent assay.

likely than PE (3 points); pulse rate >100/min (1.5 points); immobilization or surgery in the prior 4 weeks (1.5 points); previous history of DVT or PE (1.5 points); hemoptysis (1 point); cancer actively treated in the prior 6 months (1 point). Pretest probability categories are assigned as follows: low probability (<2 points); moderate probability (2-6 points); high probability (>6 points). The posttest probability of PE depends on pretest clinical probability and the results of diagnostic testing (Table 3).

In clinically stable patients (e.g., outpatients without hemodynamic compromise) with low probability of PE, a normal D-dimer value is correlated with an excellent outcome without further workup or treatment. However, in patients with a higher probability of PE or clinical instability, D-dimer results should not be used to confirm or exclude the diagnosis.

As an initial imaging test for PE, contrast-enhanced CT (also called CT angiography) or ventilation-perfusion (V/Q) scan is appropriate. Either test can reliably diagnose a large PE; however, only a totally normal V/Q scan excludes PE. CT scans that do not disclose intraluminal filling defects or V/Q scans with matched or small defects are nondiagnostic, and the decision about whether to pursue further workup should be based on a consideration of the pretest probability. If the patient's pretest probability is moderate or high, additional diagnostic tests are required, such as lower extremity ultrasonography or pulmonary angiography.

Because a V/Q scan detects alterations in pulmonary blood flow rather than providing a direct image of a clot (as does contrast-enhanced CT), there are many more indeterminate studies,

Table 3. Laboratory and Other Studies for Pulmonary Embolism (PE)

Test	Notes
Plain chest radiography	Sensitivity 84%, specificity 44%. Atelectasis and parenchymal abnormalities are most common (68%), followed by pleural effusion (48%), pleural-based opacity (35%), elevated diaphragm (24%), decreased pulmonary vascularity (21%), prominent central pulmonary artery (15%), cardiomegaly (12%), and pulmonary edema (4%).
Electrocardiography (12 lead)	Sensitivity 50%, specificity 88%. Most common abnormalities are ST-segment and T-wave changes (49%). P pulmonale, right axis deviation, right bundle branch block, and right ventricular hypertrophy occur less frequently. T-wave inversions in precordial leads may indicate more severe right ventricular dysfunction.
Arterial Po_2 and alveolar-arterial oxygen gradient	Sensitivity 81%, specificity 24%. Distributions of arterial Po_2 and alveolar-arterial oxygen gradient are similar in patients with and without PE.
D-dimer assay (ELISA)	Sensitivity 80%-100%, specificity 10%-64%. D-dimer levels <500 ng/mL (500 µL/L) have a high negative predictive value and are useful to exclude PE in patients with low pretest probability or a nondiagnostic lung scan. D-dimer measurement is less useful in patients with malignancy, recent surgery or trauma, and liver disease, because only a few have D-dimer levels <500 ng/mL (500 µL/L).
Ventilation-perfusion lung scan	Normal scan excludes PE. High-probability scan with high pretest clinical probability almost certainly confirms PE. Other scan results should be considered nondiagnostic and indicate need for further testing. PE is present in 87% of patients with a high-probability scan, 30% of patients with an intermediate-probability scan, and 14% of patients with a low-probability scan. Independent assessment of pretest probability is combined with lung scan results to improve diagnostic accuracy.
Pulmonary angiography	Indicated when noninvasive evaluation is nondiagnostic and clinical suspicion is high. Considered the gold standard.
Contrast-enhanced spiral CT of the chest	Sensitivity (53%-100%) and specificity (81%-100%) of CT are higher for main, lobar, and segmental vessel emboli. An advantage of CT is the diagnosis of other pulmonary parenchymal, pleural, or cardiovascular processes causing or contributing to symptoms.
Echocardiography	Echocardiography is most useful in the evaluation of acute cardiopulmonary syndromes to help diagnose or exclude pericardial tamponade, aortic dissection, myocardial ischemia or infarction, valvular dysfunction, and myocardial rupture.

ELISA = enzyme-linked immunosorbent assay.

because many cardiopulmonary diseases affect pulmonary blood flow. However, V/Q scans have several favorable characteristics. There is no radiocontrast agent load; therefore, renal failure and low perfusion states are not a contraindication. Also, V/Q scans are less affected by obesity than contrast-enhanced CT. Contrast-enhanced CT has excellent specificity and ability to provide alternative diagnoses but may not visualize small subsegmental pulmonary emboli.

Therapy

Deep Venous Thrombosis

Therapy for DVT requires an immediate-acting anticoagulant, usually unfractionated heparin, low-molecular-weight heparin (LMWH), or fondaparinux. All of these drugs, including unfractionated heparin, are effective and safe for VTE treatment when given subcutaneously in a weight-adjusted dose without adjustment by laboratory monitoring. LMWH and fondaparinux are metabolized in the kidney. If these drugs are used in patients with renal impairment, therapy must be monitored and the dosage adjusted by measuring plasma anti-Xa levels, thereby increasing the cost of therapy. Direct thrombin inhibitors, such as lepirudin and argatroban, have been used to treat DVT and PE, but because of their uncertain safety and efficacy, they are generally used only in patients with heparin-induced thrombocytopenia and thrombosis or with other contraindications to the use of unfractionated heparin and LMWH. Intravenous or catheter-directed thrombolysis with tissue plasminogen activator (thrombolytic therapy) may reduce the risk of postphlebitic syndrome in selected patients with iliofemoral DVT.

Warfarin is initiated simultaneously with heparin, and both therapies are overlapped for a minimum of 4 to 5 days and until the INR has reached the therapeutic range (2.0 to 3.0) for two measurements taken 24 hours apart. The duration of therapy is determined on the basis of whether DVT is associated with reversible or irreversible inciting factors or is idiopathic (Table 4). DVT associated with transient reversible factors is associated with a low risk for recurrence after 3 to 6 months of anticoagulant therapy. DVT that is idiopathic or associated with certain congenital thrombophilic conditions has a rate of recurrence as high as 8% to 10% per year after 6 to 12 months of therapy; therefore, longer-term therapy is recommended for these patients, and in some situations, lifelong therapy is appropriate. Results of D-dimer assay performed after 6 months of anticoagulation therapy have been shown to be predictive of thrombotic recurrence. An elevated high-sensitivity D-dimer assay result predicts an increased risk for recurrence by at least fourfold compared with a normal result. Thus, a positive assay provides further impetus to continue long-term anticoagulation, whereas a normal assay might lead to cessation of therapy. The assay must be done 3 to 4 weeks after warfarin therapy is stopped.

In patients with VTE and active cancer, several studies have shown the potential benefit of LMWH over warfarin in preventing recurrence without a significant difference in major bleeding or death between these two groups.

DVT damages the venous valves in the lower limbs, resulting in chronic venous insufficiency that manifests as lower extremity edema and discoloration and, in many cases, chronic venous stasis ulcers. All patients with DVT should wear graduated compression stockings to reduce the risk of postphlebitic syndrome,

Table 4. Duration of Treatment of Patients with VTE[a]

Type of VTE	Duration of Therapy
Associated with a transient reversible risk factor	3-6 mo of anticoagulation with warfarin
Associated with major continuing risk factor	≥6-12 mo of anticoagulation with warfarin, with consideration of long-term, indefinite anticoagulation
Associated with major thrombophilic defect (APS, AT or PC deficiency)	Same as above
Recurrent	Same as above
Idiopathic	Same as above
Associated with cancer	3-6 mo of anticoagulation with LMWH followed by warfarin if anticoagulation still required

APS = antiphospholipid syndrome; AT = antithrombin; LMWH = low-molecular-weight heparin; PC = protein C; VTE = venous thromboembolism.

[a] Patients must be assessed regularly for indefinite or long-term anticoagulation, and the duration is determined by assessing the risk of bleeding while receiving warfarin versus the risk for recurrent VTE after cessation of warfarin.

which develops within 2 years in about 50% of patients after a first episode of proximal DVT.

Pulmonary Embolism

If the hemodynamic and gas exchange effects of PE are not severe, PE can be treated with the same regimens used for DVT. Unfractionated heparin, LMWH, and fondaparinux are all safe and effective.

Hemodynamic instability from PE is a result of the acutely elevated pulmonary arterial resistance, which may lead to right ventricular strain, ischemia, and catastrophic cardiac dysfunction. The high mortality rate in these patients justifies a more intensive approach. Thrombolytic therapy may be effective in patients with circulatory shock due to PE and in patients with acute embolism and pulmonary hypertension or right ventricular dysfunction but without arterial hypotension or shock. Rapid clot lysis may lead to hemodynamic improvement and resolution of right ventricular dysfunction. The most important complication of thrombolytic therapy is bleeding.

Surgical embolectomy for massive PE is indicated if the patient is unstable or if drug therapy has been unsuccessful. Surgical embolectomy requires the immediate availability of cardiopulmonary bypass; the operative mortality ranges from 10% to 75%.

Inferior vena cava filters prevent PE in patients with DVT within the first 2 weeks of filter placement. Indications include failure of medical therapy (evidence of PE despite adequate anticoagula-

tion) and contraindications to anticoagulant therapy due to unacceptably high bleeding risk. After 1 year, patients may have a higher incidence of postphlebitic syndrome and increased risk of recurrent lower extremity thromboses.

Follow-Up

Once the level of anticoagulation with warfarin is stable, monitor INR every 4 weeks for the duration of warfarin therapy. Patients with unresolved risk factors for VTE and who are therefore at high risk for recurrence may require prolonged (possibly lifelong) anticoagulation. Persistent risk factors may reflect such chronic conditions as immobility, heart failure, persistent venous obstruction, or even an unrecognized hypercoagulable state.

Book Enhancement

Go to www.acponline.org/essentials/pulmonary-section.html. In *MKSAP for Students 5*, assess your knowledge with items 32-35 in the **Pulmonary Medicine** section.

Bibliography

Agnelli G, Becattini C. Acute pulmonary embolism. N Engl J Med. 2010; 363:266-274. [PMID: 20592294]

Bounameaux H, Perrier A, Righini M. Diagnosis of venous thromboembolism: an update. Vasc Med. 2010;15:399-406. [PMID: 20926499]

Chapter 88

Approach to Joint Pain

Thomas M. DeFer, MD

Joint pain can be characterized in several overlapping ways that are helpful in formulating a differential diagnosis, including the specific joints involved, the number and symmetry of involved joints, whether the source of pain is articular or periarticular, the time course and pattern of joint involvement, and whether the process is inflammatory or noninflammatory. The presence or absence of extra-articular manifestations also can provide important diagnostic clues to joint pain.

In some clinical situations, the cause of joint pain can be determined quickly, but in other cases the patient will need to be seen multiple times before the diagnosis is apparent. This is particularly true in the early stages of systemic conditions that may initially present solely as joint pain. Nonspecific rheumatologic tests (e.g., rheumatoid factor, antinuclear antibodies, erythrocyte sedimentation rate) should be ordered only to confirm a diagnosis suggested by the history and physical examination. Specific serologic studies associated with particular rheumatologic conditions in which joint pain may be a major manifestation are presented in Table 1. These tests also have limited diagnostic utility in the setting of low pretest probability. Likewise, plain radiographs are indicated only when there is a likelihood that the results will change management. In patients with joint effusion, joint fluid analysis can establish the diagnosis of infection or narrow the differential diagnosis. Table 2 categorizes joint fluid findings.

Location and Pattern

The particular joint or joints involved may suggest certain diagnoses, such as the first metatarsophalangeal joint, gout; the knee, osteoarthritis; and the metacarpophalangeal joints, rheumatoid arthritis. The spondyloarthropathies characteristically involve the axial skeleton (i.e., spine and sacroiliac, sternoclavicular, and manubriosternal joints) and large appendicular joints. Ankylosing spondylitis is the most common example of a spondyloarthropathy; others include reactive arthritis, psoriatic arthritis, and enteropathic arthritis (associated with inflammatory bowel disease). Joint pain can affect a single joint (monoarticular), two to four joints (oligoarticular), or multiple joints (polyarticular). Common monoarthropathies include gout, calcium pyrophosphate dihydrate crystal deposition disease (pseudogout), septic arthritis, and avascular necrosis. The spondyloarthropathies are characteristically oligoarticular. Rheumatoid arthritis, systemic lupus erythematosus (SLE), and osteoarthritis usually are polyarticular. Acute gout occasionally can present in a polyarticular manner, which may

Table 1. Disease Associations of Certain Serologic Studies in Patients with Joint Pain

Test	Association
ANA, centromere pattern	CREST syndrome
ANA, nucleolar pattern	Sjögren syndrome
ANA, peripheral pattern	Systemic lupus erythematosus
ANA, speckled and diffuse patterns	Nonspecific
Anti-CCP antibody	Rheumatoid arthritis
Anti-dsDNA antibody	Systemic lupus erythematosus
Antihistone antibody	Drug-induced lupus erythematosus
Anti-Jo-1 antibody	Polymyositis/dermatomyositis
Anti-La (SSB) antibody	Sjögren syndrome
Anti-U1-RNP antibody	Mixed connective tissue disease
Anti-Ro (SSA) antibody	Sjögren syndrome
Anti-Scl-70 (anti-topoisomerase I) antibody	Systemic sclerosis (scleroderma)
Anti-Sm antibody	Systemic lupus erythematosus
Anti-ssDNA antibody	Nonspecific
Rheumatoid factor	Rheumatoid arthritis

ANA = antinuclear antibody; CCP = cyclic citrullinated peptide; CREST = calcinosis, Raynaud phenomenon, esophageal dysmotility, sclerodactyly, telangiectasia; dsDNA = double-stranded DNA; RNP = ribonucleoprotein; ssDNA = single-stranded DNA.

Table 2. Joint Fluid Categories

Characteristic	Normal	Group I[a] (Noninflammatory)	Group II[b] (Inflammatory)	Group III[c] (Septic)
Volume (knee)	<3.5 mL	>3.5 mL	>3.5 mL	>3.5 mL
Viscosity	Very high	High	Low	Variable
Color	Clear	Straw	Straw to opalescent	Variable with organism
Clarity	Transparent	Transparent	Translucent, opaque at times	Opaque
Leukocyte count (cells/μL and cells × 10^6/L)	200	200-2000	2000-100,000	>50,000 (usually >100,000)
Neutrophils (%)	<25	<25	>50	>75
Culture	Negative	Negative	Negative	Usually positive

[a] Examples include osteoarthritis, avascular necrosis, hemochromatosis, and sickle cell disease.
[b] Examples include crystal-induced arthritis, rheumatoid arthritis, spondyloarthropathy, and systemic lupus erythematosus.
[c] Infectious arthritis (e.g., staphylococcal infection, gonococcal infection, tuberculosis).

Table 3. Patterns of Joint Involvement in the Differential Diagnosis of Inflammatory Arthritis

Differential Diagnosis	Pattern of Joint Involvement							
	Sym-metric	Asym-metric	Spinal	Mono-articular	Oligo-articular	Poly-articular	Migratory	Common Locations and Presentations
Bacterial (non-GC) infection	−	++++	++	++++	+++	+	−	Knee, hip, shoulder, wrist
Crystal-induced arthritis								
Gout	+	++++	+	+++	+++	+	+	First MTP joint, top of foot, heel, ankle, knee
Pseudogout[a]	++	+++	−	+++	++	++		Knee, wrist, shoulder, ankle, elbow
Rheumatoid arthritis	++++	−	+++	−	+	++++		Wrist, MCP joints, PIP joints, MTP joints, ankle, knee, elbow, shoulder, cervical spine
Psoriatic arthritis	++	+++	+	++	+++	++		Knee, DIP joints, spondylitis, sacroiliitis, dactylitis, enthesitis
IBD	++	+++	+	++	+++	++		Spondylitis, sacroiliitis, knee, MCP joints
Disseminated GC infection		++++			++++		++++	Knee, wrist, ankle, tenosynovitis
Lyme disease		++++			++++		++++	Knee, shoulder, ankle, elbow, wrist, temporomandibular joint
Acute rheumatic fever		++++			++	+++	++++	Knee, ankle, elbow, wrist

DIP = distal interphalangeal; GC = gonococcal; IBD = inflammatory bowel disease; MCP = metacarpophalangeal; MTP = metatarsophalangeal; PIP = proximal interphalangeal.
[a] Calcium pyrophosphate dihydrate crystal deposition disease.

cause diagnostic confusion. Determine symmetry if more than one joint is involved; joint involvement in rheumatoid arthritis, SLE, and osteoarthritis typically is symmetric. Table 3 presents a differential diagnosis of inflammatory arthritides based on the pattern and location of joint involvement.

Articular and Nonarticular Disorders

Differentiate articular from nonarticular sources of joint pain. Articular disorders are characterized by internal/deep joint pain that is exacerbated by active and passive motion and by reduced range of motion; joint pain may be accompanied by joint effusion, synovial thickening, joint deformity or instability, crepitations, clicking, popping, or locking. Periarticular disorders are associat-ed with greater joint pain with active rather than passive motion; in addition, range of motion often is preserved, and tenderness and signs of inflammation are removed from the actual joint. Common periarticular disorders include bursitis, tendinitis, polymyalgia rheumatica, fibromyalgia, and enthesopathies (inflammation of tendinous or ligamentous attachments to bone). Enthesopathies are characteristic of the spondyloarthropathies; the most common are Achilles tendonitis and plantar fasciitis. Dactylitis ("sausage digits") is another classic feature of the spondyloarthropathies, particularly psoriatic arthritis and reactive arthritis; dactylitis is caused by synovitis and enthesitis of the fingers and toes (Plate 63). Pain also may be referred or radiate to the joints from nonarticular sources (e.g., shoulder pain associat-ed with cervical radiculopathy) or other local pathology.

Time Course and Development

Determine the time course and pattern of development of the joint pain. Some arthropathies present in an acute manner (e.g., infection, gout, pseudogout); all patients with acute monoarticular arthritis require arthrocentesis and joint fluid analysis to establish the diagnosis. Other arthropathies have subacute or chronic presentations, such as osteoarthritis. Occasionally, some chronic arthropathies, such a rheumatoid arthritis, may have an abrupt onset.

Ongoing development of joint pain follows one of three major patterns: additive, migratory, or intermittent. With an additive pattern, new joints become involved while the previous sites remain affected (e.g., osteoarthritis, rheumatoid arthritis). A migratory pattern describes a sequential arthritis, in which a newly inflamed joint appears simultaneously with or immediately after a prior joint's improvement (e.g., gonococcal arthritis). With an intermittent pattern, affected joints improve completely, and then at a later time the same or different joints become affected in a similar manner (e.g., gout, pseudogout, SLE).

Inflammatory and Noninflammatory Pain

Joint pain is divided into inflammatory and noninflammatory categories (Table 4). Inflammatory joint pain is characterized by the presences of synovitis (soft-tissue swelling, tenderness, warmth, and effusion) and defines true arthritis. Inflammatory arthritides include septic arthritis, gout, pseudogout, rheumatoid arthritis, SLE, and the spondyloarthropathies. Inflammatory conditions are notable for more severe and prolonged (often ≥1 hour) morning stiffness and gelling (stiffness after a period of inactivity) that improve with activity. Inflammatory signs also are present in some periarticular conditions (e.g., bursitis, tenosynovitis, enthesopathies) but are less pronounced. Noninflammatory conditions are associated with less morning stiffness, typically <30 to 60 minutes. Osteoarthritis is by far the most common noninflammatory joint disorder.

Inflammatory arthropathies can be accompanied by systemic symptoms, including malaise, fatigue, weight loss, and fever. Laboratory manifestations indicative of inflammation also are seen (e.g., elevated erythrocyte sedimentation rate and/or C-reactive protein, anemia).

Extra-articular Manifestations

Focal signs of inflammation or organ dysfunction beyond the joints have important diagnostic value. Concominant findings involving the skin, eyes, mucous membranes, nervous system (central or peripheral), kidneys, gastrointestinal system, or heart all are suggestive of systemic inflammatory disease. For example, in addition to rheumatoid nodules, the major extra-articular manifestations of rheumatoid arthritis are pulmonary (pleuritis, interstitial lung disease, pulmonary nodules), cardiac (pericarditis, carditis), and ocular (scleritis, episcleritis). SLE can have renal, hematologic, neurologic, and serosal manifestations. Psoriatic arthritis occurs in 5% to 8% of patients with psoriasis. Reactive arthritis appears 1 to 4 weeks after a genitourinary or gastrointestinal infection (i.e., urethritis, cervicitis, or diarrhea). Spondyloarthropathy can be associated with ulcerative colitis and Crohn disease.

Book Enhancement

Go to www.acponline.org/essentials/rheumatology-section.html. In *MKSAP for Students 5*, assess your knowledge with items 1-3 in the **Rheumatology** section.

Bibliography

Mies Richie A, Francis ML. Diagnostic approach to polyarticular joint pain [published errata appear in Am Fam Physician. 2006;73:776 and Am Fam Physician. 2006;73:1153]. Am Fam Physician 2003;68:1151-60. [PMID: 14524403]

Table 4. Features of Inflammatory Versus Noninflammatory Arthritis

Feature	Type of Arthritis	
	Inflammatory	Noninflammatory
Physical examination findings	Joint inflammation (warmth, erythema, soft-tissue swelling, effusion)	No signs of inflammation; bony proliferation in osteoarthritis
Morning stiffness	>1 h (generally)	<1 h
Systemic symptoms	Low-grade fever, fatigue, rash	None
Synovial fluid findings	Leukocyte count >2000/μL [2000 × 10^6/L], predominantly neutrophils	Leukocyte count <2000/μL [2000 × 10^6/L], <50% neutrophils
Other laboratory studies	ESR and/or CRP often (but not always) elevated, anemia of inflammation, positive rheumatoid factor or anti-CCP antibody	Normal findings
Radiographs	Erosions, periostitis, joint-space narrowing	Joint-space narrowing, osteophytes, subchondral sclerosis

CCP = cyclic citrullinated peptide; CRP = C-reactive protein; ESR = erythrocyte sedimentation rate.

Chapter 89

Approach to Knee and Shoulder Pain

Joseph Rencic, MD

Knee Pain

Osteoarthritis is by far the most common cause of chronic knee pain in older persons. Acute knee pain may be due to inflammation (e.g., crystal-induced arthritis, rheumatoid arthritis), trauma, overuse syndromes, or infection. The knee is the most commonly infected joint, and septic arthritis must be considered in all patients with unilateral knee pain.

Evaluation

Determine location, duration, and precipitating and relieving factors. Ask about a locking (meniscus tear) or "popping" sensation (ligament rupture). Consider the direction of force on the knee in traumatic knee pain to predict the most likely structural injury. Joint effusion occurring <2 hours after trauma suggests anterior cruciate ligament rupture or tibial fracture.

Inspect the knee for structural changes or swelling both in the standing and supine positions, then palpate for warmth, tenderness, and effusion. Palpate the medial and lateral joint line for medial and lateral collateral ligament injury. Also palpate the anserine bursa and popliteal fossa if symptoms are present in these areas. Small effusions may be noted by "milking" joint fluid into the suprapatellar pouch and then pushing medially on the lateral knee just inferior to the patella with the knee extended. A fluid wave or bulge will be apparent in the medial compartment. Observe gait and assess range of motion, normally 160 degrees of flexion to full extension. Check for stability of major ligaments by performing stress maneuvers. Ask the patient to squat and walk in the squatting position; if this can be performed, even if painful, the integrity and stability of the joint are intact. Arthrocentesis should be performed when diagnostic uncertainty exists or when symptomatic relief will result (Table 1).

Knee Pain Syndromes

The most common cause of knee pain in patients aged <45 years, especially in women, is patellofemoral syndrome. The pain is peripatellar and exacerbated by overuse (e.g., running), descending stairs, or prolonged sitting. Diagnosis is confirmed by firmly compressing the patella against the femur and moving it up and down along the groove of the femur, reproducing pain or crepitation. The condition is self-limited; minimizing high-impact activity and use of NSAIDs improve symptoms.

Prepatellar bursitis is associated with anterior knee pain and swelling anterior to the patella; it often is caused by trauma or repetitive kneeling. Range of motion is not limited. Infectious prepatellar bursitis can be subtle; if warmth and erythema are present, aspirate to rule out infection. Located medially, about 6 cm below the joint line, the anserine bursa also can cause pain, which is worse with activity and at night. In general, treatment of bursitis includes avoidance of the inciting activity, ice, NSAIDs, and local corticosteroid injection for persistent symptoms.

Iliotibial band syndrome is a common cause of knife-like lateral knee pain that occurs with vigorous flexion-extension activities of the knee (e.g., running). Treat with rest and stretching exercises.

Trauma may result in fractures or ligament tears, which produce a noticeable "popping" sensation in 50% of patients. Typically, a large effusion collects rapidly after trauma. Obtain radiographs only in patients who fulfill ≥1 of the Ottawa knee rules (Table 2).

Anterior cruciate ligament tears occur with sudden twisting and hyperextension injuries. Collateral ligament tears occur with medial or lateral force without twisting. Posterior cruciate ligament tears occur with trauma to a flexed knee (e.g., dashboard injury). Check for stability of major ligaments by placing the knee in 160 degrees of extension and performing medial and lateral stress maneuvers; normal knees will have minimal give. Flex the knee 20 degrees. Grasp the patient's thigh above the patella with one hand, and with the opposite hand placed behind the patient's knee exert forward pressure to the back of the knee in an attempt to move the tibia forward (Lachman test). A full tear of the anterior cruciate ligament is associated with joint laxity (compared with the other knee) without a firm end point (positive likelihood ratio = 25; negative likelihood ratio = 0.1). With the knee in 90 degrees of flexion and the patient's foot resting on the examination table, check for

Table 1. Arthrocentesis Indications

Unexplained monoarthritis

Suspected joint infection

Unexplained joint effusion

Suspected crystal-induced arthritis

Hemarthrosis

Symptomatic relief from large painful effusion

Table 2. Ottawa Knee Rules

Obtain a knee radiograph following trauma for:

1. Patient aged >55 y

2. Isolated tenderness of the patella

3. Tenderness at the head of the fibula

4. Inability to flex knee to 90 degrees

5. Inability to bear weight immediately after injury or in the emergency department

posterior cruciate rupture by applying posterior force to the leg. Posterior movement of the leg with respect to the thigh, joint laxity, and lack of a firm end point support a diagnosis of posterior cruciate ligament rupture.

Meniscus tears present as pain, locking, and clicking. Tenderness usually localizes to the joint line on the affected side, with pain elicited with tibial rotation as the leg is extended. No physical examination maneuver reliably rules in or rules out the diagnosis.

Referred hip pain due to L_5-S_1 radiculopathy can cause knee pain. In this case, the knee examination will be normal, but findings consistent with radiculopathy (e.g. weakness, sensory abnormalities, and/or diminished deep tendon reflexes) may be present. In chronic pain syndromes, radiographs are unlikely to alter management. The decision to order an MRI usually should be made by a specialist.

Shoulder Pain

Shoulder pain occurs in up to 35% of the general population. It often evolves into a chronic, disabling problem (Table 3). The most common cause is irritation of the subacromial bursa or rotator cuff tendons from mechanical impingement between the humeral head and the coracoacromial arch, which includes the acromion, coracoacromial ligament, and the coracoid process (Figure 1). Chronic overhead activity may contribute to narrowing of this space, which can lead to recurrent microtrauma and chronic local inflammation of rotator cuff tendons.

Evaluation

Determine whether the pain is acute or chronic, and investigate possible mechanisms of injury (e.g., trauma, occupational or recreational activities). Ask for precipitating and relieving factors. Stiffness or loss of motion suggests glenohumeral arthritis or adhesive capsulitis, whereas referred pain is not exacerbated by shoulder movement.

Inspect the shoulder; asymmetry indicates a possible dislocation. Palpate the major anatomic landmarks, including the subacromial space below the tip of the acromion process, the acromioclavicular joint, the biceps tendon groove, the cervical spine, and the scapula. Ask the patient to raise both arms straight above the head (testing flexion and abduction), put both hands on the back of the head (testing external rotation), and put both hands behind the back (testing extension and internal rotation). The ability to perform all these maneuvers, even if painful, indicates normal joint anatomy and muscle strength. If the patient cannot perform these maneuvers actively, check passive range of motion; inability to perform passive maneuvers suggests an articular (glenohumeral or capsular) rather than a periarticular cause. Perform a neurologic examination to rule out radiculopathy as a cause of referred pain.

Shoulder Pain Syndromes

Patients with rotator cuff tendonitis and subacromial bursitis typically have gradually worsening pain that limits motion, is worse at night, and may extend down the arm but rarely extends below the elbow.

On examination, use one hand to passively raise the arm in forward flexion while depressing the scapula with the other hand. This action pushes the greater tuberosity into the anterior acromion process and will elicit pain when impingement is present (impingement sign). The circumduction-adduction shoulder maneuver (Clancy test) is helpful for diagnosing acromioclavicular disease and rotator cuff pathology (positive likelihood ratio = 19, negative likelihood ratio = 0.05). The patient stands with the head turned to the contralateral (uninvolved) shoulder. The affected shoulder is circumducted and adducted across the body to shoulder level, with the elbow extended and the thumb pointing toward the floor. Exert a uniform downward force on the patient's distal forearm/wrist while the patient resists the movement. Anterolateral shoulder pain and/or weakness constitutes a positive test. Pain without weakness is consistent with tendonitis; pain with weakness is consistent with tendon tear. Check internal rotation by having the patient move the thumb up the spine as far as possible, looking for pain or restricted movement.

Severe pain and frank weakness (inability to maintain the arm at 90 degrees of abduction) suggest complete rupture of the rotator cuff tendons. MRI is the most sensitive and specific imaging modality for complete or partial rotator cuff tears, although ultrasonography is quite good and more cost-effective.

Table 3. Common Causes of Shoulder Pain

Disorder	Notes
Rotator cuff tendonitis	Lateral shoulder pain aggravated by reaching, raising the arm overhead, or lying on the side. Subacromial pain to palpation and with passive/resisted abduction.
Rotator cuff tear	Shoulder weakness, loss of function, tendonitis symptoms, and nocturnal pain. Similar to tendonitis examination, plus weakness with abduction and external rotation. Positive drop arm test; in this test, the patient lowers the arms from a fully abducted position; inability to lower the affected arm smoothly is highly specific (but not sensitive) for rotator cuff tear.
Bicipital tendonitis/rupture	Anterior shoulder pain with lifting, overhead reaching, and flexion; reduced pain after rupture. Bicipital groove tenderness and pain with resisted elbow flexion. "Popeye" lump in antecubital fossa following rupture.
Adhesive capsulitis	Progressive decrease in range of motion, more from stiffness than from pain. Loss of external rotation and abduction (unable to scratch lower back or fully lift arm straight overhead).
Acromioclavicular syndromes	Anterior shoulder pain and deformity, usually from trauma or overuse. Localized joint tenderness and deformity (osteophytes, separation); pain with adduction.
Glenohumeral arthritis	Gradual onset of anterior pain and stiffness. Anterior joint-line tenderness, decreased range of motion, and crepitation.

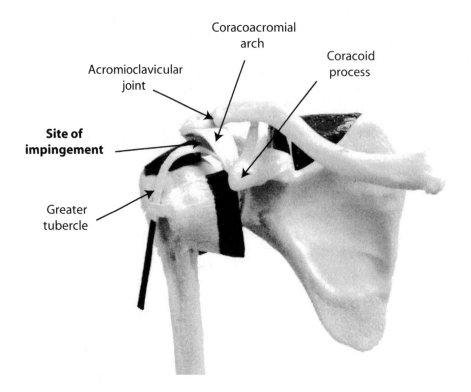

Figure 1. Shoulder anatomy as it relates to impingement syndrome.

A 2-week trial of an NSAID and rest is reasonable initial therapy for tendinitis or bursitis. If no improvement occurs within 4 to 6 weeks, physical therapy, subacromial corticosteroid injection, or (rarely) surgery may be helpful. Because it is unlikely to change management, imaging plays a limited role in most cases of chronic shoulder pain. If there is no response to conservative therapy in 6 weeks, consultation with a rheumatologist or an orthopedist is the appropriate next step.

Other causes of shoulder pain include glenohumeral instability, inflammatory arthropathies (e.g., rheumatoid arthritis), septic arthritis, acromioclavicular degeneration, and myofascial pain (e.g., trapezius strain). Shoulder pain in the setting of a normal shoulder examination suggests referred pain from a nerve injury, such as a spinal nerve root compression syndrome (e.g., cervical spondylosis, herniated disc) or brachial plexus pathology (e.g., viral infection, superior sulcus tumor). A careful neurologic examination may demonstrate weakness, decreased sensation, or altered deep tendon reflexes, which support the diagnosis of cervical radiculopathy. Osteoarthritis of the glenohumeral joint is relatively uncommon. These other causes of shoulder pain usually require management by an orthopedist or a rheumatologist, who will treat the pain based on the specific pathology.

Book Enhancement

Go to www.acponline.org/essentials/rheumatology-section.html. In *MKSAP for Students 5*, assess your knowledge with items 4-8 in the **Rheumatology** section.

Bibliography

Matsen FA 3rd. Clinical practice. Rotator-cuff failure. N Engl J Med. 2008; 358:2138-2147. [PMID: 18480206]

Schraeder TL, Terek RM, Smith CC. Clinical evaluation of the knee. N Engl J Med. 2010;363:e5. [PMID: 20660399]

Chapter 90

Septic Arthritis

J. Michael Finley, DO

Septic (infectious) arthritis is a medical emergency. Failure to promptly diagnose a joint infection can lead to joint destruction, chronic disability, or death.

Approximately 80% of joint infections are monoarticular; any joint can be affected. Acute monoarthritis, particularly of a large joint such as the hip, knee, ankle, or wrist, should prompt consideration of septic arthritis. Septic arthritis is more likely to have a polyarticular presentation in patients with preexisting rheumatoid arthritis than in other patients.

Many pathogens can cause septic arthritis, including fungi and mycobacteria, but bacterial infections are the most significant, and nongonococcal infections are the most serious. Bacterial joint infection typically is acquired hematogenously. The synovium lacks a basement membrane, and bloodborne bacteria can easily access the joint space, where they deposit on the synovial membrane and incite a swift inflammatory response. Septic arthritis may be a presenting feature of bacterial endocarditis. Joint infection also may result from direct inoculation of bacteria into the joint space following surgery, trauma, or arthrocentesis or from contiguous infection from soft tissue or bone. Within days, cytokines and proteases can cause cartilage degradation and bone loss. Delay in diagnosis or misdiagnosis of septic arthritis as rheumatoid arthritis or an acute gout flare not only postpones appropriate treatment but also may result in poor functional outcomes and even death.

Prevention

Preexisting arthritis, particularly rheumatoid arthritis, and prosthetic joint replacement predispose to septic arthritis. Treatment of rheumatoid arthritis with corticosteroids also increases a patient's vulnerability to infection. Other risk factors for septic arthritis are age >80 years, injection drug use, indwelling catheters, alcoholism, diabetes mellitus, and an immunocompromised state (e.g., HIV infection). Skin and wound infections are frequent sources of bacteria that seed diseased or prosthetic joints, resulting in septic arthritis. Treat all skin and wound infections promptly and vigorously in patients predisposed to septic arthritis, particularly patients with inflammatory arthropathies and on treatment with immunotherapy or biologic agents. There is no evidence to support the use of antibiotic prophylaxis to prevent septic arthritis in patients with prosthetic joints undergoing procedures.

Diagnosis

Acute monoarthritis should prompt a thorough history and physical examination and arthrocentesis for synovial fluid analysis.

Consider septic arthritis when a patient with rheumatoid arthritis has a monoarticular flare and in patients with acute gouty arthritis; crystal-induced arthritis and septic arthritis may coexist. Large joints most often are affected, with the knee involved in about 50% of cases; however, any joint can be involved. Septic arthritis may affect the axial skeleton, including the sternoclavicular and sacroiliac joints and symphysis pubis. Clues such as fever, joint pain, joint swelling, and recent trauma can be helpful but may be absent, particularly in elderly patients with multiple comorbidities and in immunosuppressed patients. Examine all joints for redness, warmth, swelling, and limitation of movement. Distinguish joint involvement from other causes of pain around a joint (e.g., bursitis, tendonitis) and from referred pain. Septic arthritis usually results from bacteremia; look carefully for potential sources, such as wound, skin, urinary tract, and intra-abdominal infections and pneumonia. Table 1 summarizes the differential diagnosis of septic arthritis.

The definitive diagnostic test in all cases of suspected septic arthritis is identification of bacteria in the synovial fluid. Therefore, it is necessary to obtain a joint fluid specimen for culture, Gram stain, polarized microscopy for crystals, and leukocyte count and differential (Table 2). In most patients, the synovial fluid leukocyte count is approximately 50,000/µL (50 x 10^9/L) or higher, with 90% neutrophils. A synovial fluid leukocyte count near 100,000/µL (100 x 10^9/L) with 90% neutrophils is specific for acute bacterial infection. However, patients who are immunosuppressed, have infection caused by *Mycobacterium* or *Neisseria* species, or have a prosthetic joint infection may have a lower synovial fluid leukocyte count. A count between 10,000/µL and 30,000/µL (10 and 30 x 10^9/L) with 50% neutrophils suggests mycobacterial or fungal arthritis. Confirm the diagnosis of nongonococcal septic arthritis by isolation of microorganisms from the synovial fluid; *Staphylococcus aureus* and *Streptococcus pneumoniae* are the most common causative organisms. Culture the blood and any extra-articular sites of possible infection to establish a microbiologic diagnosis. Synovial biopsy occasionally is indicated for patients with an indolent infection who have persistently negative cultures and a poor response to empiric therapy.

Plain radiographs of the infected joint are indicated to identify joint damage and possible concomitant osteomyelitis. CT or MRI may be more sensitive than radiography for diagnosing early osteomyelitis and are particularly useful in the evaluation of the hip, sternoclavicular, and sacroiliac joints. CT helps to guide aspiration of the hip; MRI helps to reveal adjacent soft-tissue edema and periarticular abscesses and to facilitate adequate debridement and drainage.

Table 1. Differential Diagnosis of Septic Arthritis

Disorder	Notes
Crystal-induced synovitis (see Chapter 91)	In gout, the first metatarsophalangeal joint most often is affected, and monosodium urate crystals are present in the synovial fluid. In CPPD deposition disease (pseudogout), the knee or wrist is the most common site of acute synovitis, and CPPD crystals are present in the synovial fluid. Consider the possibility that crystal-induced arthritis and septic arthritis may coexist.
Rheumatoid arthritis (see Chapter 93)	Rheumatoid arthritis usually is a symmetric polyarthritis affecting large and small joints; it rarely presents as monoarthritis. Rheumatoid factor is positive in 80% of cases. Flares may be monoarticular and present as pseudoseptic arthritis. Synovial fluid analysis including Gram stain and culture usually will distinguish a flare from septic arthritis.
Systemic lupus erythematosus (see Chapter 95)	Acute arthritis, especially monoarthritis, in an immunosuppressed patient with systemic lupus erythematosus requires a diligent workup to rule out septic arthritis. Search for opportunistic infections in addition to the common pathogens.
Reactive arthritis	Reactive arthritis can be precipitated by gastroenteritis or a genitourinary infection. Patients may present with urethritis, conjunctivitis, and arthritis; heel pain with enthesitis; keratoderma blennorrhagicum on the palms or soles; or circinate balanitis on the penis. Upon initial presentation, initiating antibiotic therapy is reasonable until culture results are known and the diagnosis of reactive arthritis can be substantiated.
Sickle cell disease (see Chapter 44)	Acute joint pain is seen with a painful crisis. Arthralgia is common, but frank arthritis can be encountered. In the event of an acute inflammatory arthritis, septic arthritis, bone infarction, and osteomyelitis must be considered. In addition to arthrocentesis, joint and bone imaging may be helpful in establishing a diagnosis.
Hemarthrosis	Blood in a joint may lead to an intense inflammatory reaction that mimics septic arthritis. The source of the blood may be from trauma, overanticoagulation, hemophilia, or another bleeding disorder (e.g., thrombocytopenia, severe liver disease, acquired clotting factor deficiency).
Other cause of infectious arthritis	Although subacute or chronic in many cases, infectious arthritis can be caused by fungi, viruses, parasites, tuberculosis, and Lyme disease.

CPPD = calcium pyrophosphate dihydrate.

Table 2. Laboratory and Other Studies for Septic Arthritis

Test	Notes
Complete blood count	The lack of leukocytosis does not rule out septic arthritis.
Synovial fluid leukocyte count	Synovial fluid leukocyte counts vary in septic arthritis. Most fall into the moderately (10,000-50,000/μL [10-50 × 10^9/L]) to highly (50,000 to >100,000/μL [50 to >100 × 10^9/L]) inflammatory range.
Synovial fluid Gram stain	The rate of finding gram-positive cocci varies from 50% to 75%; these organisms are more easily seen than gram-negative organisms. The rate of finding gram-negative bacilli is only 50%. From 70% to 90% of synovial fluid specimens show positive culture results in cases of septic arthritis not due to *Neisseria gonorrhoeae*; <50% of synovial fluid specimens are positive for *N. gonorrhoeae* arthritis. In the remaining cases, the diagnosis is established by culturing *N. gonorrhoeae* at an extra-articular site (e.g., blood, skin pustule, urethra, cervix, rectum, throat).
Synovial fluid culture	Gram-positive organisms cause 75%-80% of cases of septic arthritis. *Staphylococcus aureus* accounts for 50% of all cases; streptococci, 25%; gram-negative organisms, 20%; and other organisms (e.g., *Staphylococcus epidermidis*, *Haemophilus influenzae*), 5%.
Blood culture	Culture blood and extra-articular sites of possible infection to establish a microbiologic diagnosis.
Radiography and MRI	Changes seen on joint radiographs and bone damage due to infection are relatively late findings. In acute septic arthritis, soft-tissue fullness and joint effusions often are the only initial findings on radiographs. MRI of the affected joint is especially useful in detecting avascular necrosis, soft-tissue masses, and collections of fluid not appreciated by other imaging modalities.

Migratory arthralgia or arthritis settling in one inflamed joint and the presence of tenosynovitis (wrist or ankle) and/or typical dermatitis (Plate 48) in a sexually active young adult raises the suspicion of disseminated gonococcal infection. Confirm the diagnosis by isolation of the microorganism from the synovial fluid, blood, urethra, cervix, rectum, or throat or from a skin pustule. Patients suspected of having disseminated gonococcal infection should be tested for other sexually transmitted diseases.

Maintain a high index of suspicion for prosthetic joint infection, because common symptoms and signs of infection, other than pain, may be absent. Most patients with septic arthritis will be febrile; however, chills and spiking fevers are uncommon. Elderly patients frequently do not develop a fever. Failure to diagnose infection may lead to excess morbidity, prosthesis removal, and death. *Staphylococcus epidermidis* is much more common in prosthetic joint infections than in native joint infections.

Therapy

Hospitalize patients with suspected septic arthritis to confirm the diagnosis, initiate prompt intravenous antibiotic therapy, and closely monitor response to treatment. Management is directed toward drainage of the purulent joint fluid, preservation of joint integrity and function, and initiation of antibiotic therapy.

Use repeated needle aspiration to drain purulent joint fluid as completely as possible; arthroscopic drainage may be necessary when needle aspirates fail. Surgery may be indicated for suspected infection in patients who report pain in a previously painless and functioning joint prosthesis.

Because of increasing prevalence of community-associated methicillin-resistant *Staphylococcus aureus* infections, many experts recommend initiating vancomycin and ceftazidime or a quinolone antibiotic if the Gram stain is positive for gram-positive cocci or if the Gram stain is negative and the risk for *Neisseria gonorrhoeae* infection is low. If the Gram stain shows gram-negative cocci or the risk for *N. gonorrhoeae* infection is high, ceftriaxone is an appropriate first choice; also treat empirically with azithromycin for concurrent *Chlamydia* infection. Ceftazidime is recommended for infection with gram-negative bacilli. If *Pseudomonas* infection is possible (e.g., injection drug use), gentamicin is added to ceftazidime. As culture results become available, the antibiotic choice can be narrowed. Table 3 summarizes an empiric treatment approach for septic arthritis.

Duration of treatment is based on the initial response to antibiotic treatment, the specific microorganism, and patient characteristics. Shorten the duration of antibiotic administration to 2 weeks or less when the microorganism is exquisitely sensitive to the drug used (e.g., *N. gonorrhoeae*) and the patient responds promptly. Administer antibiotics for 4 weeks or longer for virulent microorganisms (e.g., *S. aureus*) or difficult-to-treat pathogens (e.g., *Pseudomonas aeruginosa*). Consider chronic suppressive antibiotic treatment of an infected prosthesis without removal only under certain circumstances, such as if the prosthesis is not loose or the patient is a poor surgical candidate.

Follow-Up

Perform serial synovial fluid examinations to help monitor the response to therapy. Serial synovial fluid specimens usually show a decrease in total leukocyte count, conversion to a negative culture result, and a decrease in the amount of fluid reaccumulation—findings that parallel other clinical signs of response. Pain with range of motion should decrease, and function of the joint should improve or be regained.

Book Enhancement

Go to www.acponline.org/essentials/rheumatology-section.html. In *MKSAP for Students 5*, assess your knowledge with items 9-11 in the **Rheumatology** section.

Bibliography

Mathews CJ, Weston VC, Jones A, Field M, Coakley G. Bacterial septic arthritis in adults. Lancet. 2010;375:846-855. [PMID: 20206778]

Table 3. Empiric and Definitive Antibiotic Therapy for Septic Arthritis in a Native Joint

Gram Stain Results	Likely or Identified Pathogen	First-Line Therapy	Second-Line Therapy
Gram-positive cocci	*Staphylococcus aureus*, other staphylococcal species	Oxacillin/nafcillin or cefazolin	Cefazolin or nafcillin
	Possible MRSA	Vancomycin or linezolid	Teicoplanin
Gram-negative cocci	*Neisseria gonorrhoeae*	Ceftriaxone (add azithromycin for *Chlamydia* infection)	Fluoroquinolone
Gram-negative bacilli	Enteric gram-negative bacilli	Ceftriaxone or cefotaxime	Fluoroquinolone
	Pseudomonas aeruginosa	Ceftazidime (plus gentamicin, if proven)	Carbapenem, cefepime, piperacillin-tazobactam, or fluoroquinolone
Gram stain unavailable	At risk for *N. gonorrhoeae*	Ceftriaxone or cefotaxime plus azithromycin	Fluoroquinolone
	No risk for *N. gonorrhoeae*; *S. aureus* or gram-negative bacilli likely	Nafcillin plus ceftazidime	Nafcillin plus fluoroquinolone

MRSA = methicillin-resistant *Staphylococcus aureus*.

Chapter 91

Crystal-Induced Arthritis

Katherine Nickerson, MD

The two most common forms of crystal-induced arthritis are gout and calcium pyrophosphate dihydrate (CPPD) deposition disease. Gout (monosodium urate deposition disease) refers to the group of clinical disorders associated with hyperuricemia (Table 1). The solubility of urate at physiologic pH is approximately 6.7 mg/dL (0.4 mmol/L). If the serum uric acid concentration increases above this level, urate deposits may develop in synovial tissue, bursae, tendon sheaths, kidney interstitium, and the urinary collection system. These deposits develop over time but may be reabsorbed if the serum uric acid level decreases below 6.7 mg/dL (0.4 mmol/L). Gout attacks occur when urate crystals are released from preexisting tissue deposits and are almost always associated with chronically elevated levels of serum uric acid. Gout includes a range of clinical disorders from acute, exquisitely painful, monoarticular arthritis to chronic, crippling, destructive polyarthritis. The risk of developing gout is directly related to the level and duration of elevated serum uric acid. Uric acid levels increase with increasing age, weight, and serum creatinine concentration. These increases may be accelerated by secondary factors, such as chronic kidney disease, alcohol consumption, diuretics, and low doses of aspirin, all of which inhibit uric acid excretion by the kidneys. Hyperuricemia more often is related to underexcretion (90%) than to overproduction (10%) of uric acid. Polymorphisms of several different genes related to renal handling of uric acid play an important role in underexcretion. Acute attacks often are triggered by events that precipitously raise or lower serum uric acid level, such as dehydration, postoperative fluid shifts, or initiation of uric acid–lowering agents. Gouty arthritis progresses through three distinct stages: asymptomatic hyperuricemia, which may last several decades; acute intermittent gout; and chronic tophaceous gout (Plate 64), which usually develops only after years of acute inter-

mittent gout. Estrogen promotes uric acid excretion, so that women usually do not develop gout until the postmenopausal period, whereas men often develop gout in the fourth or fifth decade. During intercritical periods (asymptomatic periods between gout attacks), crystals may still be detected in the synovial fluid. Therefore, the presence of crystals in synovial fluid is not always sufficient to provoke an attack.

CPPD deposition disease is caused by crystallization of calcium pyrophosphate dihydrate in articular tissues. The cause of this crystallization is unknown but clearly is related to aging; a few cases are associated with metabolic abnormalities. Many patients with CPPD deposition disease are asymptomatic. Symptom presentation varies and may include pseudogout, pseudo-osteoarthritis, and pseudo–rheumatoid arthritis. CPPD deposition disease is commonly known as pseudogout because acute mono- or pauci-articular inflammatory joint attacks of this condition mimic acute attacks of gout. Pseudogout attacks may be precipitated by surgery or illness. Pseudo-osteoarthritis, which is a more common presentation than pseudogout, mimics osteoarthritis but involves the wrist, metacarpophalangeal, shoulder, ankle, hip, and knee joints. Pseudo–rheumatoid arthritis is a rare presentation of CPPD deposition disease that manifests as a symmetric polyarticular disease accompanied by morning stiffness, fatigue, and joint swelling.

Prevention

There are no primary prevention measures for gout or CPPD deposition disease. However, administration of uric acid–lowering drugs to patients receiving chemotherapy for hematologic malignancies is recommended to prevent tumor lysis syndrome (acute hyperuricemia, hyperphosphatemia, hypocalcemia, hyperkalemia,

Table 1. Disorders Associated with Hyperuricemia

Disorder	Clinical Presentation	Cause
Gouty arthritis	Inflammatory erosive arthritis	Inflammatory response to monosodium urate crystals deposited into synovial tissue, bursae, and tendon sheaths due to chronic uric acid supersaturation of serum. Urate deposits cause joint and tissue destruction over time.
Tophi	Painless, persistent, generally noninflammatory nodules that develop in tissues and tendons, that are palpable on physical examination but also may occur as nodular lesions within joints or tissues	Tophi develop concomitantly with progressive gouty arthritis. Although typically noninflammatory, acute inflammatory response and local damage can occur at these sites, analogous to the acute gouty flares in the joints.
Nephrolithiasis	Formation of uric acid and calcium oxalate kidney stones	Increased uric acid levels in the urinary collecting system serve as a nidus for both uric acid and calcium oxalate stone formation.
Nephropathy	Loss of kidney function secondary to severe, typically acute increases in serum uric acid levels, such as occur in patients with tumor lysis syndrome	Deposition of monosodium urate crystals in the kidney interstitium.

and acute kidney injury). Effective secondary prevention of gout requires decreasing serum uric acid levels. However, it is not clear that all patients need such intervention.

Screening

Do not screen for asymptomatic hyperuricemia. Potential reactions to uric acid–lowering drugs may outweigh treatment benefits, and hypersensitivity reactions to allopurinol can be fatal.

Diagnosis

Perform arthrocentesis in patients presenting with acute monoarticular arthritis to diagnose infection or crystal-induced arthritis, being aware that the two conditions can coexist in rare cases (Table 2). A definitive diagnosis of gout is made by demonstrating negatively birefringent monosodium urate crystals within synovial fluid leukocytes or in a suspected tophus. Arthrocentesis of an affected joint during the intercritical period also may establish the diagnosis of gout. If joint fluid cannot be obtained, clinical criteria can be used. Rapid symptom onset, intense joint inflammation, complete resolution between attacks, involvement of the first metatarsophalangeal joint (podagra), and radiographs demonstrating subcortical erosions are distinguishing features of gout.

The diagnosis of CPPD deposition disease is made by finding positively birefringent rhomboid intracellular crystals in the synovial fluid. Radiographs can reveal chondrocalcinosis (linear calcifications along the articular cartilage and fibrocartilage; Figure 1), degenerative changes, and osteophytes. Screen patients aged <50 years with CPPD deposition disease for associated metabolic conditions (e.g., hemochromatosis, hyperparathyroidism, hypothyroidism, gout, hypomagnesemia, hypophosphatasia, familial hypocalciuric hypercalcemia, acromegaly, ochronosis).

Therapy

Advise patients with gout to avoid alcohol, which increases uric acid production and may impair uric acid excretion. Foods high in purine (e.g., organ meats, red meat, scallops, anchovies, sardines) also should be avoided. However, dietary interventions rarely are adequate to reverse hyperuricemia and prevent attacks of gout.

Effective treatment of acute attacks of gout involves high-dose therapy with nonselective or cyclooxygenase-2-selective NSAIDs, corticosteroids, or colchicine. The choice of agent for acute gout depends on patient characteristics and on the presence or absence of concomitant disease (Table 3). NSAIDs are effective but must be avoided in older patients; patients with chronic kidney disease, heart failure, or peptic ulcer disease; and patients on concurrent anticoagulation or other drugs that may interact with NSAIDs.

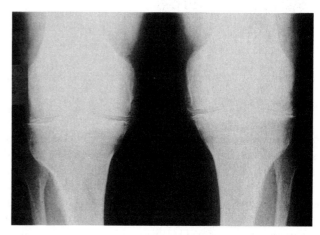

Figure 1. Linear calcification of the menisci and articular cartilage characteristic of calcium pyrophosphate dihydrate deposition disease.

Table 2. Differential Diagnosis of Gout

Disorder	Notes
Calcium pyrophosphate dihydrate (CPPD) deposition disease	May be asymptomatic or have a varied presentation resembling rheumatoid arthritis, osteoarthritis, or gout-like inflammation. Cartilage calcification, especially in fibrocartilage of knee meniscus, symphysis pubis, glenoid and acetabular labra, and triangular cartilage of wrist, are pathognomonic. Osteoarthritis in unusual places (wrist, elbow, metacarpophalangeal joints, shoulder) without a history of trauma suggests CPPD deposition. Defined by finding CPPD crystals in synovial fluid and by chondrocalcinosis on radiographs.
Osteoarthritis (see Chapter 92)	Characterized by bony enlargement with no acute signs of inflammation. Patients may have acute exacerbation of joint symptoms, especially after use. Radiographs may show focal joint-space narrowing, bony repair with osteophytes, and subchondral sclerosis.
Psoriatic arthritis	Characterized by joint distribution and appearance similar to that of reactive arthritis. Predilection for distal interphalangeal joints, often with concomitant nail changes. Elevated serum uric acid levels are proportional to skin involvement.
Reactive arthritis	Presents as inflammatory oligoarthritis, most often involving weight-bearing joints; may include tendon insertion inflammation. Extra-articular manifestations include conjunctivitis, urethritis, stomatitis, and psoriaform skin changes. Infection with *Salmonella, Shigella, Yersinia, Campylobacter,* or *Chlamydia* species within 3 wk prior to onset of initial attack.
Rheumatoid arthritis (see Chapter 93)	Symmetric polyarthritis most often involving small joints of the hands and feet. About 30% of patients have subcutaneous rheumatoid nodules. Radiographic changes include soft-tissue swelling, diffuse joint-space narrowing, marginal erosions of small joints, and absence of osteophytes. Acute rheumatoid arthritis sometimes mimics gout. The greater the number of joints involved, the more likely that rheumatoid arthritis is the diagnosis.
Septic arthritis (see Chapter 90)	Characterized by fever, arthritis, and exquisite joint tenderness. Up to half of patients have concomitant rheumatoid arthritis. The source of infection (skin, lungs) often is evident. Usually occurs in previously abnormal joints. Gout and septic arthritis may coexist.

Table 3. Drug Treatment of Gout

Agent	Notes
Acute Gout	
NSAIDs	Block formation of inflammatory prostaglandins and have analgesic effects. Effective within 12-24 h of onset. The NSAID used is less important than the rapidity with which the NSAID is started. Any NSAID *except* aspirin is appropriate. Start at high dose and taper rapidly over several days.
Colchicine (oral)	Colchicine decreases L-selectin expression by neutrophils, making them less able to adhere to vascular endothelium and egress into tissues. Nausea, vomiting, and diarrhea are dose-related. Bone marrow suppression can be life-threatening if maximum doses are exceeded. Myopathy and neuropathy can occur at any dose. Modify dose according to kidney function. Colchicine is not removed by dialysis and, thus, should be avoided in patients on dialysis.
Corticosteroids (oral)	Suppress inflammation by several mechanisms. Useful when NSAIDs are contraindicated (chronic kidney disease). Contraindicated in active peptic ulcer disease. May interfere with control of diabetes.
Corticosteroids (intra-articular)	Especially useful if only one joint is inflamed and patient has contraindications to other agents. Rule out infectious cause before administering injection.
Chronic Gout	
Allopurinol	Xanthine oxidase inhibitor; inhibits uric acid synthesis. Dose is increased over 2-3 wk to minimize acute gout attacks that may occur with abrupt fluctuations in serum uric acid levels. Initial dose is modified according to creatinine clearance. Target serum uric acid levels ≤6.0 mg/dL (0.35 mmol/L).
Febuxostat	Xanthine oxidase inhibitor useful in patients allergic to allopurinol. Does not appear to cause hypersensitivity reactions, but cardiovascular events are more common. Much more expensive than allopurinol.
Probenecid, sulfinpyrazone	Uricosuric agents effective in long-term treatment of chronic gout if sodium urate levels are maintained at ≤6.0 mg/dL (0.35 mmol/L). Not effective in chronic kidney disease.

In these situations, intra-articular or systemic corticosteroids are used. High-dose oral colchicine has a variable response rate and almost always is associated with severe diarrhea; therefore, oral administration should rarely be used and is contraindicated in the presence of kidney or liver disease. Intravenous colchicine has an unacceptable rate of serious adverse reactions and, therefore, has been removed from the U.S. market. In patients for whom NSAIDs and colchicine are contraindicated, oral corticosteroids may be the safest, most effective option.

Patients with recurrent episodes of gout who are at risk for joint damage are candidates for uric acid–lowering therapy. Chronic tophaceous gout is the only form of destructive arthritis that is preventable. Management or prevention of recurrent gout and chronic tophaceous gout requires drug therapy to achieve and maintain serum uric acid levels between 5 and 6 mg/dL (0.3 and 0.4 mmol/L). The xanthine oxidase inhibitor allopurinol is effective, but therapy must be lifelong and is associated with a 1% to 2% incidence of allergic reactions, which can be severe and life-threatening. Febuxostat is a newer, more expensive agent that can be used in patients with allopurinol allergy. Initiate therapy with a uric acid–lowering agent after resolution of an acute attack, sometimes with concomitant low-dose colchicine, which is then continued for approximately 6 months to prevent acute attacks.

Uricosuric agents (e.g., probenecid, sulfinpyrazone) occasionally are used but are less effective at lowering serum uric acid level, are not effective in patients with an estimated glomerular filtration rate of <40 mL/min/1.73 m^2, and should be used only in patients who excrete <600 mg (35.4 mmol) of uric acid daily.

Treatment of CPPD deposition disease is symptomatic. There is no agent that successfully reverses formation or deposition of CPPD crystals. Joint fluid aspiration, NSAIDs, and intra-articular corticosteroids are useful in managing an acute attack. Colchicine may be used, as it is in gout, as prophylaxis following an acute attack.

Book Enhancement

Go to www.acponline.org/essentials/rheumatology-section.html. In *MKSAP for Students 5*, assess your knowledge with items 12-14 in the **Rheumatology** section.

Bibliography

Wilson JF. In the clinic. Gout [published erratum appears in Ann Intern Med. 2010;152:479-480]. Ann Intern Med. 2010;152:ITC2-1-ITC2-16. [PMID: 20124228]

Chapter 92

Osteoarthritis

Amanda Cooper, MD

Osteoarthritis is characterized by breakdown of articular cartilage, subchondral bone alterations, meniscus degeneration, and bone repair (osteophytes) with minimal synovial inflammatory response. Loss of articular cartilage causes pain and loss of joint mobility. Osteoarthritis can involve any joint but most often affects the weight-bearing joints (knee, hip, spine) as well as the distal and proximal interphalangeal and first carpometacarpal joints of the hand. Osteoarthritis increases markedly with age and causes a significant burden of lost time at work and early retirement. After age 50 years, men are more likely to be affected by hip osteoarthritis, whereas women are more likely to develop hand, knee, and foot osteoarthritis. There is a familial tendency, indicating at least a partial genetic effect.

Prevention

Obesity and repetitive joint strain may be modified to decrease the risk of developing osteoarthritis. Counsel patients with a BMI >25 to lose weight. For each additional pound of body weight, the force across the knee increases by 0.9 to 1.4 kg (2 to 3 lb), thus increasing the risk of cartilage damage. Avoiding repetitive knee bending and heavy lifting helps reduce excessive loading of the knee and may reduce osteoarthritis. Advise athletes to follow graduated training schedules to build muscle strength, which helps improve joint stability and avoid intrinsic damage.

Diagnosis

In clinical practice, the diagnosis of osteoarthritis should be based primarily on history and physical examination findings. Laboratory tests are not helpful for diagnosis.

Osteoarthritis pain is a poorly localized, deep, aching sensation. Pain initially occurs with joint use; as the disease progresses, pain occurs at rest. Morning stiffness lasts <30 minutes. Joint examination findings may include tenderness, swelling, crepitation, bony enlargement or deformity, restricted motion, pain with passive movement, and instability. Bony enlargement of the distal interphalangeal joints (Heberden nodes) and proximal interphalangeal joints (Bouchard nodes) are particularly characteristic of osteoarthritis (Plate 65). Osteoarthritis of the first carpometacarpal joint is very common. It causes pain at the base of the thumb and bony enlargement, producing a squared appearance to the base of the hand. Crepitation and pain may be elicited with passive circular motion of the carpometacarpal joint ("grind test"). According to the American College of Rheumatology, the following clinical criteria should be applied when diagnosing osteoarthritis of the knee:

age >50 years, morning stiffness <30 minutes, crepitation, bony tenderness, bony enlargement, and no palpable warmth. The combination of knee pain plus at least 3 of these criteria is associated with a sensitivity of 95% and specificity of 69% for diagnosis of knee osteoarthritis.

Radiographs are most helpful in diagnosing osteoarthritis in the hip but only help to confirm osteoarthritis in the knee and have lower sensitivity and specificity than physical examination for osteoarthritis of the hand. Due to the low sensitivity, the absence of radiographic findings does not rule out symptomatic disease in any joint. Osteophytes, subchondral sclerosis, and joint-space narrowing seen on radiographs are indicative of osteoarthritis (Figure 1). If these findings are seen in the knee, specificity for diagnosis increases from 69% to 86%.

Joint aspiration should be considered if an effusion is present and the diagnosis is in question or a concomitant infection is suspected. Synovial fluid typically is clear, with a leukocyte count <2000 /μL (2000×10^6/L) (Table 1). Symptoms of inflammatory arthritis, such as symmetric peripheral polyarthropathy, soft-tissue swelling, morning stiffness >1 hour, or significant spine and sacroiliac joint involvement should be evaluated for other causes of arthritis. Secondary causes of osteoarthritis must be considered in patients who present with osteoarthritis in an unusual joint, at a young age, or with other symptoms (Table 2).

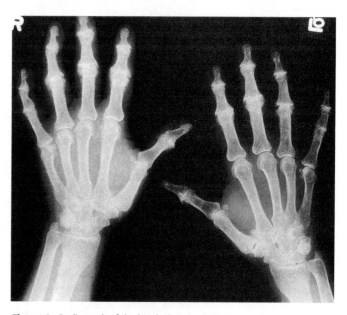

Figure 1. Radiograph of the hands showing joint-space narrowing, subchondral sclerosis, and osteophyte formation indicative of osteoarthritis.

Table 1. Differential Diagnosis of Osteoarthritis

Disorder	Notes
CPPD deposition disease (see Chapter 91)	Chondrocalcinosis of the knee, triangular fibrocartilage of the wrist, and symphysis pubis; attacks of pseudogout; and osteoarthritis in the second and third MCP joints. CPPD crystals may be identified in synovial fluid.
Rheumatoid arthritis (see Chapter 93)	Soft tissue (synovial) swelling rather than bony enlargement of the PIP and MCP joints (rarely involves the DIP joints), inflammatory signs (fatigue, prolonged morning stiffness), rheumatoid nodules, and inflammatory synovial fluid. Marginal erosions and juxta-articular osteopenia seen on radiographs.
Psoriatic arthritis	Synovial and entheseal swelling; may involve the DIP joints; dactylitis (sausage digits) present. Erosions and periostitis seen on radiographs.
Trochanteric bursitis	Pain and tenderness over the greater trochanter; pain may radiate down the lateral aspect of the thigh. Hip range of motion is normal.
Anserine bursitis (see Chapter 89)	Pain and tenderness over the anteromedial aspect of the lower leg below the joint line of the knee. May be a confounding cause of knee pain in patients with knee osteoarthritis.
Osteonecrosis	Joint pain out of proportion to radiographic changes. Risk factors include corticosteroids, alcohol abuse, systemic lupus erythematosus, and hemoglobinopathies. Usually involves the hip or knee. Diagnosis confirmed by MRI.
Gout (see Chapter 91)	History of acute attacks of monoarthritis with joint erythema. Bony enlargement of joints and tophi may be present on examination. Radiographs show large erosions with overhanging edges. Uric acid crystals may be identified in synovial fluid. Chronic tophaceous gout may involve the DIP and PIP joints and first MTP joint, causing deformities and bony enlargement akin to osteoarthritis.

CPPD = calcium pyrophosphate dihydrate; DIP = distal interphalangeal; MCP = metacarpophalangeal; MTP = metatarsophalangeal; PIP = proximal interphalangeal.

Table 2. Secondary Causes of Osteoarthritis

Cause	Notes
Trauma	Injury may predispose a joint to development of osteoarthritis. This is especially true for intra-articular fractures but also is true for fractures at distant sites that result in altered joint loading, such as fracture of the femoral shaft (hip), scaphoid (wrist), tibia (ankle), or humerus (shoulder).
Hemochromatosis	Hemochromatosis occurs due to iron overload and predominantly affects men aged 40-60 y. Osteoarthritis in the second and third MCP joints and radiographs showing hook-like osteophytes are characteristic. Early findings include arthralgia and elevated aminotransferase levels. Late findings may include hepatomegaly, bronze skin coloration, pituitary insufficiency, and diabetes. Serum transferrin saturation >60% in men or >50% in women suggests the diagnosis.
Wilson disease	Some patients with Wilson disease develop an arthropathy and, occasionally, chondrocalcinosis, most commonly in the knee. Laboratory findings include elevated aminotransferase levels. Diagnosis is suggested by a low serum ceruloplasmin level, high serum copper level, and Kayser-Fleischer rings on slit-lamp examination.
Ochronosis	In ochronosis, deficiency of homogentisic acid oxidase causes excretion of excess homogentisic acid in the urine and deposition of dark pigment in connective tissues. When the urine stands or is alkalinized, it turns dark (alkaptonuria). Associated arthropathy involves large joints and spares hands and feet; patients may present with early-onset lumbar spondylosis and calcification and ossification of the lumbar disks.
Acromegaly	In addition to increased size of the hands, feet, nose, and jaw, disease of the knee, hip, shoulder, and elbow joints occurs in 60% of patients with acromegaly; spine disease also is common. Radiographs may show widened joint space followed later by typical features of osteoarthritis.
Hyperparathyroidism	Most patients are asymptomatic but musculoskeletal symptoms may include proximal weakness, bone pain, nontraumatic fractures
Neuropathic joints	Most commonly associated conditions are syringomyelia, diabetes, and neurosyphilis. Patients may present with massive joint swelling. Pain is less severe than would be expected from the appearance of the joint. Radiographs show large unusually shaped osteophytes, transverse fractures, osteolysis, and large loose bodies. Synovial fluid is noninflammatory or bloody.
Ehlers-Danlos syndrome	Several subtypes exist but all have in common hyperelastic skin and joint hypermobility. Other features (depending on the subtype) include keratoconus, scoliosis, and sudden death secondary to rupture of large blood vessels.

MCP = metacarpophalangeal.

Therapy

In overweight patients with hip or knee osteoarthritis, weight loss combined with exercise has been shown to be superior to either intervention alone. Strengthening muscles around the involved joint is of significant importance in reducing pain. A low-impact exercise program is recommended, which can both increase muscle strength and promote weight loss. Specifically, quadriceps-strengthening exercises are prescribed for knee osteoarthritis, because they can reduce pain and improve physical function. Patients with medial knee compartment osteoarthritis may benefit from heel inserts (5-10 degrees of lift), which help relieve the pressure on the medial compartment. Use of a cane in the hand contralateral to the painful joint may help by unloading forces on the knee or hip. Knee taping or bracing improves knee alignment, thus improving pain. Referral to physical or occupational therapy for active and passive range of motion exercise instruction or joint protection education may be helpful.

Consider pharmacologic agents when conservative measures fail to relieve pain and improve function. Recommend acetaminophen as initial drug therapy for osteoarthritis in doses ≤4000 mg/day. Acetaminophen is an effective, safe, and relatively inexpensive treatment. Patients with inadequate response can be started on NSAIDs, preferably at the lowest effective dose to limit side effects (e.g., gastritis, renal insufficiency). Cylcooxygenase-2-selective NSAIDs are not more effective than nonselective NSAIDs, but they are less likely to cause gastrointestinal ulcers, significantly more expensive, and associated with an increased risk for adverse cardiovascular events. Concomitant use of a proton pump inhibitor with an NSAID should be considered in patients with risk factors for gastrointestinal bleeding (e.g., age >65 years, history of peptic ulcer disease or gastrointestinal bleeding, anticoagulant use).

Glucosamine sulfate is the building block of proteoglycans, the ground substance of articular cartilage. However, two recent meta-analyses show that oral glucosamine is similar to placebo in improving symptoms of osteoathritis. Substance P has been implicated in the pathogenesis of osteoarthritis pain. Topical capsaicin depletes substance P and may be used in addition to or as an alternative to oral medications. For full efficacy, capsaicin should be applied three times daily for 3 weeks. Opiate analgesics or tramadol may play an additional role in the treatment of patients whose pain is not well-controlled by NSAIDs or who have a contraindication to NSAIDs. Tramadol is a centrally acting synthetic opioid agonist that has comparable efficacy to NSAIDS in treating hip and knee pain due to osteoarthritis. Significant abuse has not been identified with tramadol, although nausea, constipation, and drowsiness may limit its use.

Pain unresponsive to systemic medications may respond to local therapy. Intra-articular corticosteroid injections are particularly effective in relieving pain from an acute exacerbation of osteoarthritis. Whenever joint fluid is aspirated, a sample should also be sent for analysis to rule out infection or crystal-induced arthritis. Never administer intra-articular corticosteroids when infection is suspected. The benefit from intra-articular corticosteroids for knee osteoarthritis varies, but statistically significant pain relief has been documented only up to 1 week after injection. In patients with osteoarthritis of the hip, intra-articular corticosteroid therapy has been shown to effectively relieve pain for up to 3 months. The efficacy of this therapy in treating osteoarthritis of joints other than the knee and hip remains uncertain. Do not inject corticosteroids more frequently than every 4 months due to the risk of tendon rupture. Studies generally have shown that intra-articular hyaluronan injection has comparable efficacy to NSAID therapy in patients with osteoarthritis of the knee. Patients may not experience relief until several weeks after undergoing injection, but the effects of this therapy can last for 6 months or longer.

Consider total joint arthroplasty for patients who do not adequately respond to nonsurgical methods. Replacement of the damaged joint restores normal biomechanics and often results in dramatic improvements in quality of life. Arthroscopic lavage with or without debridement is not beneficial. Joint fusion is an option that may successfully alleviate osteoarthritis pain; it is typically reserved for joints not critical for mobility (e.g., spine, small joints of the hand and foot). Although meniscus tears are almost universally present in knee osteoarthritis, they are not necessarily a cause of increased symptoms, and surgery is not recommended unless a patient experiences significant knee locking or loss of knee extension.

Book Enhancement

Go to www.acponline.org/essentials/rheumatology-section.html. In *MKSAP for Students 5*, assess your knowledge with items 15-18 in the **Rheumatology** section.

Bibliography

Hunter DJ. In the clinic. Osteoarthritis. Ann Intern Med. 2007;147:ITC8-1-ITC8-16. [PMID: 17679702]

Chapter 93

Rheumatoid Arthritis

Kyla Lokitz, MD
Seth Mark Berney, MD

Rheumatoid arthritis is a chronic, systemic inflammatory disease primarily involving the joints. Rheumatoid arthritis affects 1% to 1.5% of the worldwide population. The incidence increases during adulthood and peaks between the ages of 40 and 60 years. The ratio of female to male patients ranges from approximately 2:1 to 4:1. The hallmark features of rheumatoid arthritis are symmetric polyarthritis (synovitis) affecting the fingers, hands, wrists, and feet and the formation of autoantibodies. In addition, patients may experience constitutional symptoms (weight loss, low-grade fever, malaise, fatigue) and develop rheumatoid nodules and other extra-articular manifestations. If untreated, chronic rheumatoid arthritis results in joint deformity, significant decline in functional status, and premature death.

Although the precise cause of rheumatoid arthritis is unknown, several factors have been associated with development of the disease, including genetic susceptibility, infections (e.g., atypical bacteria, Epstein-Barr virus, human parvovirus B19, or retroviruses), hormones, trauma, cigarette smoking, and autoantibodies. Mediators of inflammation, including cytokines, growth factors, chemokines, adhesion molecules, and matrix metalloproteinases, play a pivotal role in the pathogenesis of rheumatoid arthritis by attracting and activating immune cells, promoting angiogenesis, and contributing to activation and proliferation of synoviocytes to form pannus. A pannus behaves similar to a locally invasive tumor, invading and eroding articular cartilage, subchondral bone, tendons, and ligaments. Edema of the synovium and periarticular structures contributes to joint stiffness in rheumatoid arthritis by interfering with normal joint biomechanics.

Screening

No adequate screening test for rheumatoid arthritis currently exists. However, in a patient with joint swelling typical of rheumatoid arthritis, testing for the presence of rheumatoid factor (RF) and anti–cyclic citrullinated peptide (anti-CCP) antibody is helpful in the diagnosis. RF, an antibody directed against the Fc fragment of IgG, is present in serum in more than 75% of patients with rheumatoid arthritis. However, RF also is found in patients with other conditions (e.g., infections, malignancies, other autoimmune diseases) as well as 10% of the normal population. Anti-CCP antibody is thought to be highly specific for rheumatoid arthritis. The presence of both RF and anti-CCP antibody is considered highly specific for rheumatoid arthritis.

Diagnosis

Previously, rheumatoid arthritis was diagnosed by the presence of 4 of the following 7 features: morning stiffness, arthritis in three or more joint areas, involvement of the joints of the hand, symmetric arthritis, rheumatoid nodules, RF-positive serum, and radiographic changes. However, the American College of Rheumatology in collaboration with the European League Against Rheumatism recently developed a score-based classification scheme for rheumatoid arthritis (Table 1) in an effort to detect early disease and initiate early therapy. The classification scheme takes into consideration the number and size of joints involved, presence of anti-CCP antibody, and erythrocyte sedimentation rate (ESR) and C-reactive protein (CRP) measurements. Because patients may not understand the distinction between their joints "feeling swollen" and the presence of synovitis, the synovitis must be observed by a physician.

The initial presentation of rheumatoid arthritis may be insidious or acute. Patients usually experience morning stiffness lasting >1 hour, joint pain and swelling, and difficulty performing activities of daily living. Symmetric and additive joint involvement is typical. Rheumatoid arthritis most commonly involves the metacarpophalangeal, proximal interphalangeal (Plate 66), wrist, elbow, knee, and metatarsophalangeal joints and the cervical spine while sparing the distal interphalangeal joints and the lumbosacral spine. The presence of C_1-C_2 subluxation can cause spinal instability and cord impingement and is a general anesthesia risk.

Laboratory studies in patients with active rheumatoid arthritis often reveal normocytic anemia, thrombocytosis, and elevated ESR and CRP levels typically paralleling the joint inflammation. The earliest radiographic abnormalities include soft-tissue swelling, uniform joint-space narrowing, and juxta-articular demineralization in the wrists or feet. Marginal erosions, found at the attachment of the synovium to the bone, may be observed initially at the head of the fifth metatarsal bone or ulnar styloid. Plain radiographs may not reveal articular erosions for months or longer. MRI and ultrasonography are more sensitive imaging modalities for early erosive disease compared with radiography. However, these studies currently are not widely used because of cost and lack of high-quality performance and interpretation.

Extra-articular features of rheumatoid arthritis include rheumatoid nodules and pulmonary, cardiovascular, ocular, hematologic, and neurologic manifestations. Rheumatoid nodules, associated with more severe disease, occur in 30% of patients and are commonly located on the extensor surfaces of the forearms. Rheumatoid nodules may be clinically indistinguishable from tophi and are best identified by aspiration and analysis of the aspirate with a polarizing microscope; monosodium urate crystals indicate tophi, whereas cholesterol crystals indicate rheumatoid nodules. Pulmonary manifestations occur in 20% to 25% of patients and include pleuritis, pleural effusions, interstitial fibrosis, nodular lung disease, bronchiolitis, and arteritis with pulmonary hypertension. The most

Table 1. The 2010 ACR/EULAR Classification Criteria for Rheumatoid Arthritis

Target population consists of patients who:

1. have at least 1 joint with definite clinical synovitis (swelling) *and*

2. the synovitis is not better explained by another disease

Classification Criteria	Score
Add score of categories A-D; a score of ≥ 6/10 is needed for classification of a patient as having definite rheumatoid arthritis	
A. Joint involvement (swollen or tender)	
1 large joint[a]	0
2-10 small joints[b]	1
1-3 small joints (with or without involvement of large joints)	2
4-10 small joints (with or without involvement of large joints)	3
>10 joints (at least 1 small joint)	5
B. Serology (at least 1 test result needed for classification)	
Negative RF and anti-CCP antibody	0
Low-positive RF or low-positive anti-CCP antibody	2
High-positive RF or high positive anti-CCP antibody	3
C. Acute-phase reactants (at least 1 test result needed for classification)	
Normal CRP and normal ESR	0
Abnormal CRP or abnormal ESR	1
D. Duration of symptoms[c]	
<6 wk	0
≥6 wk	1

ACR/EULAR = American College of Rheumatology/European League Against Rheumatism; CCP = cyclic citrullinated peptide; CRP = C-reactive protein; ESR = erythrocyte sedimentation rate; RF = rheumatoid factor.
[a] Large joints refers to shoulders, elbows, hips, knees, and ankles.
[b] Small joints refers to metacarpophalangeal joints, proximal interphalangeal joints, second through fifth metatarsophalangeal joints, thumb interphalangeal joints, and wrists.
[c] Duration of symptoms refers to patient self-report of the duration of signs and symptoms of synovitis of joints that are clinically involved at time of assessment.
Adapted from Aletaha D, Neogi T, Silman AJ, et al. 2010 Rheumatoid arthritis classification criteria: an American College of Rheumatology/European League Against Rheumatism collaborative initiative. Arthritis Rheum. 2010;62:2569-2581. [PMID: 20872595]

common ocular manifestation is keratoconjunctivitis sicca, which affects approximately 30% of patients with rheumatoid arthritis. Accelerated atherosclerotic disease and pericarditis are potential cardiac manifestations. Felty syndrome (rheumatoid arthritis, neutropenia, and splenomegaly) occurs in approximately 1% of patients. Extra-articular manifestations of rheumatoid arthritis are associated with increased mortality.

The differential diagnosis of rheumatoid arthritis includes the spondyloarthropathies (e.g., ankylosing spondylitis, reactive arthritis, psoriatic arthritis), viral infections (e.g., Epstein-Barr virus, human parvovirus B19, HIV, hepatitis C virus), bacterial infections (e.g., endocarditis, gonococcal infection, Lyme disease), metabolic disorders (e.g., gout, calcium pyrophosphate dihydrate deposition disease, hemochromatosis), connective tissue diseases (e.g., systemic lupus erythematosus, systemic sclerosis [scleroderma], dermatomyositis/polymyositis), sarcoidosis, amyloidosis, and malignancy. Osteoarthritis may present as joint swelling but generally is characterized by bony joint enlargement (Table 2).

Therapy

The goal of treatment is to suppress inflammation and preserve joint structure and function. Nonpharmacologic modalities such as heat and joint range-of-motion exercises can help to alleviate the joint stiffness that limits many patients with rheumatoid arthritis. Referral to other providers, including physical therapists, occupational therapists, and psychologists, also may help many patients with early rheumatoid arthritis. Counseling regarding joint protection techniques, use of assistive devices, and therapeutic exercises is essential.

In early rheumatoid arthritis, NSAIDs and systemic low-dose corticosteroids can help control symptoms but do not adequately prevent disease progression. Intra-articular corticosteroids are useful to control localized disease that is unresponsive to systemic therapy. Early, aggressive use of disease modifying anti-rheumatic drugs (DMARDs) and biologic response modifiers, alone or in combination, is most effective in achieving the treatment goal (Table 3). The initial choice of DMARD should be based on the severity of inflammation. DMARDs include methotrexate, sulfasalazine, leflunomide, hydroxychloroquine, gold, and, occasionally, minocycline. Monotherapy with hydroxychloroquine or sulfasalazine or combination therapy with these agents is indicated to treat early, mild, and nonerosive disease. Use of methotrexate or leflunomide may benefit patients with early mild to moderate rheumatoid arthritis but is most clearly indicated in patients with rapid disease progression or functional limitations. Combination

Table 2. Differential Diagnosis of Rheumatoid Arthritis

Disease	Notes
Ankylosing spondylitis (see Chapter 94)	Inflammatory disorder of the axial skeleton; may have peripheral involvement; apical pulmonary fibrosis; back pain. Differs from rheumatoid arthritis because ankylosing spondilitis uncommonly has peripheral involvement and usually involves the lumbar spine.
CPPD deposition disease (see Chapter 91)	Deposition of CPPD crystals in and around joints, most commonly the wrist, MCP joints, shoulder, and knee. May be monoarticular or acute oligoarticular, with hot and red joints; may be chronic polyarticular in 5% of cases. CPPD deposition disease can have a pseudo–rheumatoid arthritis pattern. Polarized microscopy reveals weakly positive birefringent crystals in synovial fluid. Radiographs show chondrocalcinosis.
Gout (see Chapter 91)	Deposition of monosodium urate crystals in and around joints. Initial attack is monoarticular, most commonly in the first MTP joint. Chronic form may have symmetric involvement of small joints of the hands and feet, with tophi. Gout can have a pseudo–rheumatoid arthritis pattern. Polarized microscopy reveals strongly negative birefringent crystals in synovial fluid or tophi. Gout is highly uncommon in premenopausal women with normal kidney function.
Infective endocarditis (see Chapter 58)	Characterized by involvement of large proximal joints, fever with leukocytosis, and heart murmur. Obtain blood cultures in all patients with fever and polyarthritis. RF is a common finding in patients with endocarditis.
Lyme disease	Multisystem inflammatory disease caused by *Borrelia burgdorferi*. Early disease: erythema migrans rash and cardiac abnormalities. Late disease: intermittent monoarthritis or oligoarthritis that may become chronic. Rash and tick exposure or travel to an endemic area are important for the diagnosis. Obtain ELISA test; confirm a positive result with Western blot.
Osteoarthritis (see Chapter 92)	Degeneration of articular cartilage, most often affecting the DIP, PIP, first CMC, first MTP, hip, and knee joints and the cervical and lumbar spine. Pain occurs with use; minimal soft-tissue swelling and morning stiffness. Radiographs show osteophytes with joint-space narrowing. Laboratory studies are normal.
Psoriatic arthritis	Multiple presentations: monoarthritis, oligoarthritis (asymmetric), polyarthritis (symmetric), arthritis mutilans, and axial disease. Common involvement of DIP joints, with fusiform swelling of digits and skin and nail changes consistent with psoriasis. Psoriatic arthritis can have a pseudo–rheumatoid arthritis pattern but tends to be RF-negative.
Peripheral arthritis associated with IBD	Up to 20% of cases of IBD involve arthritis. The arthritis usually is nondestructive, involves the lower extremities, and reflects active bowel disease. May be indistinguishable from ankylosing spondilitis.
Reactive arthritis (Reiter syndrome)	Can be precipitated by infection (usually gastroenteritis or genitourinary infection) with one of several bacterial organisms. Patients may present with urethritis, conjunctivitis, and arthritis; heel pain with enthesitis; keratoderma blennorrhagicum on the palms or soles; or circinate balanitis on the penis. Differs from rheumatoid arthritis in that it is oligoarticular and asymmetric.
Septic arthritis (see Chapter 90)	Usually monoarticular but may be oligoarticular; may be migratory; more often affects large joints. Patients present with hot, red, and swollen joints with limited range of motion. Joint fluid analysis is essential. Septic arthritis may develop in joints affected by rheumatoid arthritis.
Systemic lupus erythematosus (see Chapter 95)	Clinically indistinguishable from the arthritis of rheumatoid arthritis; however, the arthritis in systemic lupus erythematosus is non-nodular and nonerosive.
Viral arthritis	Possible causes include Epstein-Barr virus, adenovirus, human parvovirus B19, rubella, HIV, HBV, and HBC. Patients may have morning stiffness, with symmetric involvement of the hands and wrists; they also may be RF-positive (a pseudo–rheumatoid arthritis pattern). Most cases (except those caused by human parvovirus B19) resolve in 4-6 wk.

CMC = carpometacarpal; CPPD = calcium pyrophosphate dihydrate; DIP = distal interphalangeal; ELISA = enzyme-linked immunosorbent assay; HBV = hepatitis B virus; HCV = hepatitis C virus; IBD = inflammatory bowel disease; MCP = metacarpophalangeal; MTP = metatarsophalangeal; PIP = proximal interphalangeal; RF = rheumatoid factor.

therapy generally is more effective than monotherapy and may include use of two or three DMARDs. Regular use of alcohol and presence of hepatitis B or C are contraindications to the use of methotrexate or leflunomide.

When adequate disease control is not achieved with oral DMARDs or if erosive disease is present, biologic therapy should be initiated. Currently available biologic response modifiers include tumor necrosis factor α (TNF-α) inhibitors (adalimumab, etanercept, certolizumab pegol, golimumab, infliximab), an interleukin-1 receptor antagonist (anakinra), a T-cell costimulatory blocker (abatacept), a B-cell depleting agent (rituximab), and an interleukin-6 receptor antagonist (tocilizumab). Biologic therapy usually begins with a TNF-α inhibitor, which generally is added to baseline methotrexate therapy, because the rate of radiographic progression has been shown to decrease with combination

therapy. Use of the biologic response modifiers requires initial screening for tuberculosis and hepatitis B and monitoring for invasive fungal infection. Most of the life-threatening conditions are treated with DMARDS, high-dose corticosteroids, and/or immunosuppressants (azathioprine, cyclosporine, cyclophosphamide). Surgical therapy may be indicated for patients with destructive rheumatoid arthritis that cannot be managed pharmacologically. End-stage disease of the hip or knee often is treated with total joint arthroplasty.

Follow-up

The strategy recommended by the American College of Rheumatology for monitoring methotrexate or leflunomide toxicity is to screen patients for hepatitis A, B, and C and to

Table 3. Drug Treatment of Rheumatoid Arthritis

Drug	Mechanism	Indication	Notes
Anti-inflammatory agents			
NSAIDs	Inhibit cyclooxygenase	Mild disease without erosions; as an adjunctive analgesic in more serious disease	NSAIDs do not prevent disease progression. Use with caution in patients with chronic kidney disease or ulcer disease.
Corticosteroids	Suppress inflammation at multiple points along the inflammatory cascade	Low-dose or intra-articular injections when NSAIDs do not control symptoms and when DMARDs have not yet produced an effect	High-dose corticosteroids are useful in treating serious extra-articular manifestations (e.g., vasculitis).
DMARDs			
Methotrexate	Folic acid antimetabolite	DMARD that is most likely to provide durable long-term response; often the initial choice	Takes 1-2 mo to see benefit; frequently used in combination. Use with caution in patients who are pregnant or who have underlying liver or lung disease, immunosuppression, or infection. Folic acid supplementation prevents toxicity without interfering with efficacy.
Hydroxychloroquine	Antimalarial agent with lysosomotropic action that affects immune regulation and inflammation	Early, mild, and nonerosive disease; in combination with methotrexate or when methotrexate is contraindicated	Takes 2-6 mo to see benefit; frequently used in combination regimens. Use with caution in patients who are pregnant or who have antimalarial allergy, G6PD deficiency, or retinal abnormality. Perform ophthalmologic examination every 12 mo.
Sulfasalazine	Unknown	Early, mild, and nonerosive disease; in combination with methotrexate or when methotrexate is contraindicated	Takes 1-2 mo to see benefit. Use with caution in patients with sulfonamide or aspirin allergy, G6PD deficiency, kidney or liver disease, blood disease, or asthma.
Leflunomide	Pyrimidine synthesis inhibitor	In combination with methotrexate or when methotrexate is contraindicated for progressive disease	Use with caution in patients who are pregnant (known teratogen) or who have liver disease.
Biologic agents			
TNF inhibitors (adalimumab, etanercept, certolizumab pegol, golimumab, infliximab)	Immunomodulation	Uncontrolled disease despite use of DMARDs	Tuberculin skin test is required before starting therapy.
Interleukin-1 receptor antagonist (anakinra)	Immunomodulation	Uncontrolled disease despite use of DMARDs	Tuberculin skin test is required before starting therapy.
T-cell costimulatory blocker (abatacept)	Immunomodulation (down-regulation of T cells)	Uncontrolled disease despite use of DMARDs	Tuberculin skin test is required before starting therapy.
B-cell depleting agent (rituximab)	Monoclonal antibody against CD20	Uncontrolled disease despite use of DMARDs	Tuberculin skin test is required before starting therapy.

DMARD = disease-modifying anti-rheumatic drug; G6PD = glucose-6-phosphate dehydrogenase.

measure serum aspartate or alanine aminotransferase, albumin, and creatinine levels and complete blood count every 4 to 8 weeks. Coronary artery disease is the leading cause of death in patients with rheumatoid arthritis. Aggressive treatment of the underlying inflammatory process in rheumatoid arthritis has been shown to decrease the development of atherosclerotic disease and the associated morbidity and mortality. Management of traditional cardiovascular risk factors (smoking, hyperlipidemia, diabetes, hypertension, obesity) also is recommended.

Book Enhancement

Go to www.acponline.org/essentials/rheumatology-section.html. In *MKSAP for Students 5*, assess your knowledge with items 19-22 in the **Rheumatology** section.

Acknowledgment

We would like to thank Dr. Kathryn A. Naus, who contributed to an earlier version of this chapter.

Bibliography

Aletaha D, Neogi T, Silman AJ, et al. 2010 Rheumatoid arthritis classification criteria: an American College of Rheumatology/European League Against Rheumatism collaborative initiative. Arthritis Rheum. 2010;62:2569-2581. [PMID: 20872595]

Huizinga TW, Pincus T. In the clinic. Rheumatoid arthritis. Ann Intern Med. 2010;153:ITC1-1-ITC1-15; quiz ITC1-16. [PMID: 20621898]

Chapter 94

Spondyloarthropathies

J. Michael Finley, DO

The spondyloarthropathies are a heterogeneous group of related disorders that include ankylosing spondylitis, reactive arthritis (formerly known as Reiter syndrome), psoriatic arthritis, and enteropathic arthritis. *Undifferentiated spondyloarthropathy* refers to the clinical features of a spondyloarthropathy in patients who do not meet the criteria for an individual disease process. Manifestations vary widely among these conditions, but common features include a genetic predisposition, the potential for an infectious trigger, the presence of enthesitis (inflammation at the attachment site of tendon to bone), and extra-articular involvement. The results of serologic studies, including rheumatoid factor assays, are characteristically negative in affected patients.

Various cytokines mediate the local inflammatory and destructive processes affecting the synovium, entheses, and bone. The significant efficacy of tumor necrosis factor α (TNF-α) inhibitors in the treatment of the spondyloarthropathies suggests that TNF-α is a key mediator in this inflammatory process. T-cell activation is characteristic of the pathogenesis of the spondyloarthropathies, particularly psoriatic arthritis.

The class I histocompatibility antigen HLA-B27 is the strongest genetic risk factor for the spondyloarthropathies. HLA-B27 is a strong risk factor for ankylosing spondylitis and reactive arthritis but is not as strongly associated with enteropathic arthritis and psoriatic arthritis. Less than 5% of HLA-B27–positive persons actually develop ankylosing spondylitis. Testing for HLA-B27 positivity generally is not helpful diagnostically, because most HLA-B27–positive persons do not develop disease. In addition, not all patients with ankylosing spondylitis have this allele.

Infectious triggers have been suspected in all of the spondyloarthropathies. These triggers include the potential immunostimulatory properties of gastrointestinal flora in enteropathic arthritis and the bacteria harbored in psoriatic skin plaques. Nongonococcal genitourinary tract infections (primarily caused by *Chlamydia*) and infectious diarrhea (caused by *Shigella*, *Salmonella*, *Yersinia*, and *Campylobacter*) can be associated with reactive arthritis. Antibiotic treatment does not alter the course of arthritis in patients with nongonococcal disease. Patients with HIV infection have an increased incidence of reactive arthritis, psoriasis, and psoriatic arthritis. Testing for HIV infection is indicated for patients newly diagnosed with severe psoriatic or reactive arthritis.

Diagnosis

The cardinal feature of spondyloarthropathy is enthesitis, with subsequent reactive new bone and spur (osteophyte) formation. Spinal manifestations include sacroiliitis and spondylitis, which typically cause insidious-onset pain in the gluteal region. In affected patients, pain often persists for >3 months and may progress over time to involve the rest of the spine. Unlike mechanical back pain, pain and stiffness associated with the spondyloarthropathies are characteristically worse in the morning or after sedentary periods and are alleviated with exercise.

In patients with spondyloarthropathy, progressive limitation in spinal mobility may occur over years and ultimately result in spinal fusion, often in a forward-flexed position, with decreased chest expansion. Prior to fusion, sacroiliac joints may be tender to palpation. Patients also may have a loss of cervical spinal mobility. Inflammation of the ligamentous attachments erodes the corners of the vertebral bodies, which produces a squared-off appearance. Ossification of spinal ligaments leads to the development of a rigid "bamboo spine," named because the vertebrae resemble bamboo on radiography. MRI is the most sensitive method for detecting early inflammatory changes in the sacroiliac joints and spine.

Enthesitis and bone spurs can occur at any site of tendon attachment. Commonly seen in the plantar fascia and Achilles tendon, involvement at these sites often causes episodes of inflammation and heel pain. However, most cases of isolated plantar fasciitis are not related to spondyloarthropathy. Enthesitis contributes to dactylitis, which can cause the characteristic sausage-shaped digits associated with psoriatic and reactive arthritis (Plate 67).

The pattern and degree of peripheral joint involvement among the spondyloarthropathies vary widely, as summarized in Table 1. The most common pattern is an asymmetric oligoarthritis that predominantly involves the large joints of the lower extremities. However, psoriatic arthritis may potentially manifest as a predominantly peripheral arthritis that involves the small joints.

Extra-articular manifestations of the spondyloarthropathies include inflammatory disease involving the skin, eyes, lungs, gastrointestinal and genitourinary tracts, and vascular system. The most noticeable skin manifestation is psoriasis, but other mucocutaneous manifestations can include oral ulcers, keratoderma blennorrhagicum (pustular psoriasis on the soles and palms), and circinate balanitis (plaques or ulcers involving the glans and shaft of the penis), all of which are most typical in reactive arthritis. Erythema nodosum (Plate 2) and pyoderma gangrenosum (Plate 3) are typical in enteropathic arthritis. Inflammatory eye disease (conjunctivitis, uveitis, keratitis) can be recurrent and is the most common extra-articular manifestation of the spondyloarthropathies.

Genitourinary manifestations of the spondyloarthropathies include noninfectious urethritis, prostatitis, cervicitis, and salpingitis. Inflammatory bowel disease (IBD) is a form of gastrointestinal involvement. Pulmonary fibrosis, when present, characteristically

Table 1. Pattern of Peripheral Synovitis in the Spondyloarthropathies

Condition	Pattern of Involvement
Ankylosing spondylitis/reactive arthritis	Asymmetric oligoarthritis primarily involving the large joints of the lower extremities
Enteropathic arthritis	Asymmetric oligoarthritis primarily involving the large joints of the lower extremities; peripheral joint flares parallel the course of the bowel disease
Psoriatic arthritis	Oligoarticular disease: asymmetric pattern, primarily involving the large joints of the lower extremities
	Polyarticular disease: symmetric pattern resembling rheumatoid arthritis, involving both the large and small joints
	Distal interphalangeal joint disease: arthritis associated with characteristic psoriatic nail changes
	Arthritis mutilans: severely destructive arthritis involving the hands, with shortening of the digits

involves the lung apices. Aortitis with aortic root dilatation, conduction abnormalities, and myocardial dysfunction may occur. Both pulmonary and cardiac complications are rare and more characteristic of ankylosing spondylitis than of other types of seronegative spondyloarthropathy.

Ankylosing Spondylitis

Ankylosing spondylitis is the prototypical spondyloarthropathy. The prevalence of this condition in the United States is less than 1%. Males are affected more often than females; however, the disease tends to be milder in females and may go undiagnosed.

The onset of ankylosing spondylitis is marked by persistent low back pain and occurs in the teenage years or twenties. Although occasionally limited to the pelvis and sacroiliac joints, inflammatory spinal disease in ankylosing spondylitis typically progresses cephalad, resulting in a characteristic stooped posture and loss of spinal mobility seen in late disease. Fractures, including those caused by minor trauma to the rigid spine, and spinal cord and nerve root impingement (e.g., cauda equina syndrome) may complicate spinal involvement. Arthritis of the hips is common in this disease and further worsens function. Relatively common extra-articular manifestations of ankylosing spondylitis include uveitis, aortic regurgitation, chest wall restriction, and apical pulmonary fibrosis.

Early diagnosis has become particularly important with the availability of newer therapeutic agents that can alter the debilitating course of this disease. Early in the disease course, plain radiographs of the pelvis and spine often are normal. Symptomatic patients with suspected ankylosing spondylitis should undergo MRI of the sacroiliac joints to detect early inflammatory and erosive changes.

Reactive Arthritis

Reactive arthritis is an inflammatory arthritis occurring within 2 months of an episode of bacterial gastroenteritis or nongonococcal urethritis or cervicitis. Diagnosis is more difficult when there is no history of a preceding infection, as occurs in asymptomatic sexually transmitted diseases.

Reactive arthritis typically has an acute onset and presents as an asymmetric oligoarthritis predominantly of the lower extremities, inflammatory back pain, or a combination of these symptoms. Symptoms of enthesitis (heel pain, dactylitis) may be present. Extra-articular manifestations, particularly ocular (conjunctivitis, anterior uveitis), genitourinary (urethritis, cervicitis), and mucocutaneous (oral ulcers, keratoderma blennorrhagicum, circinate balanitis), are common and may precede the development of the arthritis. Only one third of affected patients have the classic triad of arthritis, urethritis/cervicitis, and conjunctivitis associated with reactive arthritis.

Acute episodes of reactive arthritis typically resolve within 4 to 6 months. In some patients, these episodes recur or evolve into a chronic destructive arthritis or progressive spinal disease. As many as 50% of affected patients have recurrent or progressive disease.

Enteropathic Arthritis

Up to 20% of patients with IBD (Crohn disease, ulcerative colitis) develop inflammatory arthritis. IBD-associated peripheral arthritis may manifest as either a polyarticular arthritis resembling rheumatoid arthritis or an asymmetric oligoarthritis predominantly of the lower extremities, resembling reactive arthritis. The peripheral arthritis may precede the development of gastrointestinal symptoms. The course of arthritis often fluctuates with the activity of the underlying bowel inflammation.

Approximately 10% to 20% of patients with IBD have spinal involvement ranging from asymptomatic sacroiliac disease seen on radiographs to a clinical presentation identical to that of ankylosing spondylitis, with progressive spinal fusion. Unlike the peripheral arthritis, the progression of spinal involvement in enteropathic arthritis is independent of the course of the bowel disease.

Additional extra-articular manifestations of enteropathic arthritis include inflammatory eye disease and erythema nodosum, which occur in up to 20% of patients with this condition. The course of the extra-articular manifestations typically parallels peripheral joint and bowel inflammation.

Psoriatic Arthritis

Psoriasis affects approximately 1% to 2% of the general population, and 20% to 40% of affected patients develop arthritis. The highest incidence of arthritis occurs in patients with extensive skin involvement. However, arthritis can develop even in patients with minimal skin disease, such as psoriasis that is limited to the nails. In psoriatic arthritis, psoriasis typically predates arthritis, whereas arthritis develops before skin disease in 15% of patients.

Psoriatic arthritis should be considered in patients with dactylitis, marked distal interphalangeal (DIP) joint involvement, asymmetric joint involvement, symptoms of enthesitis, or joint ankylosis. In these patients, a thorough skin examination should be performed to verify the diagnosis, looking for nail changes or undetected small patches of psoriasis in areas such as the scalp, periumbilical region, and intertriginous skin folds.

Psoriatic arthritis often presents as a symmetric polyarticular arthritis resembling rheumatoid arthritis in distribution, with the exception that psoriatic arthritis also is associated with involvement of the DIP joints. In some patients, the arthritis is limited almost exclusively to the DIP joints, often with associated psoriatic nail changes, such as pitting and onycholysis (Plate 63).

Therapy

Many of the treatments used in rheumatoid arthritis also suppress inflammation in the joints and extra-articular structures and provide long-term prevention of joint damage and functional loss in spondyloarthropathy. Current treatment of the spondyloarthropathies emphasizes aggressive use of immunosuppressive, disease-modifying agents such as methotrexate or sulfasalazine and, more recently, use of TNF-α inhibitors. NSAIDs are used as adjunctive therapy for joint inflammation and pain; they do not alter the disease course or prevent progression. NSAIDs also may exacerbate IBD and should be used with caution in patients with enteropathic arthritis.

Ankylosing Spondylitis

TNF-α inhibitors are first-line therapy for ankylosing spondylitis. TNF-α inhibitors significantly suppress inflammation in the axial skeleton, improve back pain, and potentially halt progressive ankylosis and subsequent loss of mobility and function. TNF-α inhibitors also are effective for peripheral arthritis and extra-articular disease. Traditional immunosuppressants (e.g., methotrexate, sulfasalazine) benefit patients with peripheral joint and extra-articular disease but are not effective for spinal involvement.

Reactive Arthritis

Antibiotics are indicated primarily for acute infection and generally are of little benefit for reactive joint disease. NSAIDs are first-line therapy for symptom management in reactive arthritis. Disease-modifying agents such as sulfasalazine or methotrexate may be beneficial in recurrent or chronic inflammatory disease. TNF-α inhibitors should be considered if other interventions are ineffective or if patients have significant axial skeletal involvement or severe disease.

Enteropathic Arthritis

The immunosuppressive therapies that benefit IBD also have efficacy in the treatment of the associated peripheral joint and extra-articular manifestations of enteropathic arthritis. These therapies include corticosteroids, sulfasalazine, azathioprine, methotrexate, and TNF-α inhibitors. In patients with axial skeletal disease, TNF-α inhibitors should be considered as first-line therapy.

Psoriatic Arthritis

The therapeutic options in psoriatic arthritis are similar to those in rheumatoid arthritis. Generally, immunosuppressive agents that have efficacy in psoriatic skin disease also benefit patients with joint disease. Methotrexate is beneficial for both skin and joint disease and has dominated therapy for many years. TNF-α inhibitors increasingly have been shown to be effective in psoriatic arthritis and are the preferred intervention for patients with predominant axial skeletal disease.

Book Enhancement

Go to www.acponline.org/essentials/rheumatology-section.html. In *MKSAP for Students 5*, assess your knowledge with items 23-26 in the **Rheumatology** section.

Bibliography

Khan MA. Update on spondyloarthropathies. Ann Intern Med. 2002; 136:896-907. [PMID: 12069564]

Chapter 95

Systemic Lupus Erythematosus

Saba Khan, MD
Seth Mark Berney, MD

Systemic lupus erythematosus (SLE) is an autoimmune disease characterized by immune complex deposition, autoantibody formation, and organ inflammation. Patients with SLE have abnormalities in immune tolerance to self-antigens and in the ability to clear cellular debris containing these antigens. In patients with SLE, autoantibodies can take the form of immune complexes that deposit in tissues or bond to target cells. Autoantibodies can cause damage by fixing complement on the surface of a cell (causing cell lysis), by binding to Fc receptors on circulating cells (leading to cell clearance in the liver or spleen), or by binding to Fc receptors on macrophages (initiating cell-mediated inflammation). SLE is most common in women of childbearing age; women are nine times more likely than men to be affected by SLE. People of certain races (e.g., black, Asian, Hispanic) also are more commonly affected by SLE. The clinical course of SLE is variable and may be characterized by alternating periods of remission and relapse (with either acute or chronic onset).

Although the cause of SLE is unknown, the disease appears to be multifactorial. A genetic association exists, with 25% to 50% concordance in monozygotic twins but only 5% concordance in dizygotic twins and nontwin siblings. Environmental influences (e.g., ultraviolet [UV] light), infections, and hormonal factors likely contribute to SLE development or disease flares. Additionally, many drugs can trigger an SLE-like illness or autoantibody formation. However, drug-induced lupus erythematosus tends to be milder than SLE and is temporally related to the causative drug. The most common agents associated with drug-induced lupus are procainamide, hydralazine, isoniazid, and quinidine.

SLE commonly involves the blood components, skin, kidneys, lungs, joints, serosal tissues, and central and peripheral nervous systems. The most characteristic laboratory abnormality is the presence of antinuclear antibody (ANA) in serum.

Screening

Screening for SLE in asymptomatic patients or in patients with atypical symptoms is not indicated. ANA is found in 95% to 99% of patients with SLE but lacks specificity. ANA also is found in patients with viral and bacterial infections, other autoimmune diseases, malignancies, and cirrhosis and in up to 10% of the normal population.

Diagnosis

The diagnosis of SLE depends on obtaining an appropriate history and physical examination and supportive laboratory data. A patient is classified as having SLE if 4 of the 11 American College of Rheumatology criteria for SLE diagnosis are confirmed by a physician. Patients may present with an explosive onset of multiple findings or have a more subtle presentation over a long period of time. To establish the diagnosis of SLE, patients need not manifest all the diagnostic criteria simultaneously; the criteria can be fulfilled over time. The differential diagnosis of SLE is broad and is summarized in Table 1.

Diagnostic Criteria

The mnemonic SOAP BRAIN MD is useful for recalling the diagnostic criteria for SLE.

- Serositis includes pleuritis, pericarditis, and peritonitis. Patients may report pleuritic chest pain or positional pain consistent with pericarditis, and they must have radiographic, electrocardiographic, or echocardiographic findings consistent with serositis.
- Oral ulcers are painless and usually seen on the hard palate or nasal mucosa.
- Arthritis is clinically indistinguishable from rheumatoid arthritis but does not cause nodules or erosions. Some patients may develop ulnar deviation, flexion, and hyperextension. These deformities (called *Jaccoud arthropathy*) generally are reducible and secondary to involvement of the para-articular tissues, such as the joint capsule, ligaments, and tendons.
- Photosensitive rash is any rash caused or worsened by UV light exposure. Patients will develop this rash in tanning beds and in direct sunlight. Because clouds do not block UV radiation, photosensitive rashes can appear or worsen on cloudy days.
- Blood dyscrasias associated with SLE include leukopenia, lymphopenia, thrombocytopenia, and Coombs-positive (autoimmune) hemolytic anemia with reticulocytosis. The presence of any of these findings on two separate occasions fulfills this criterion. The cytopenias are believed to be secondary to peripheral destruction of circulating cells, not bone marrow suppression.
- Renal disease is very common in SLE. A patient satisfies this criterion by having a 24-hour urine protein excretion >500 mg, by urinalysis showing >10 erythrocytes per high-power field or erythrocyte or leukocyte casts in a sterile urine sample (proven by culture), or by kidney biopsy. There are six subtypes of lupus nephritis, and treatment varies with the subtype. Patients with class I or class II lupus nephritis have no evidence of altered kidney function and may have a normal biopsy (by light microscopy), minimal mesangial deposits (by immunofluorescence or electron microscopy), or mesangio-

Table 1. Differential Diagnosis of Systemic Lupus Erythematosus (SLE)

Disorder	Notes
Fibromyalgia, chronic fatigue syndrome	About 30% of patients with SLE may have fibromyalgia; most patients with SLE have chronic fatigue syndrome. Fibromyalgia diagnosis requires characteristic tender points, with chronic pain above and below the waist.
Rheumatoid arthritis (see Chapter 93)	Rheumatoid arthritis causes symmetric polyarthritis, similar to SLE, but deforming arthritis and erosions are more common. Patients with SLE may be seropositive for rheumatoid factor.
Drug-induced lupus	Certain drugs (minocycline, hydralazine, procainamide, isoniazid) may cause a syndrome of fever, serositis, and arthritis.
Hepatitis B or C (essential mixed cryoglobulinemia)	Essential mixed cryoglobulinemia can cause palpable purpura, nephritis, and neuropathy. Although 30% of patients with SLE have mildly elevated transaminase levels, these findings should lead to a search for hepatitis B or C.
Wegener granulomatosus (see Chapter 97)	Sinus disease, lung nodules, and kidney disease. Patients usually are seropositive for ANCA.
Polyarteritis nodosa (see Chapter 97)	Vasculitis, kidney disease, and mononeuritis multiplex. Biopsy shows medium-vessel vasculitis.
Erythema infectiosum (fifth disease)	Can cause a symmetric polyarthritis, usually self-limited. May be associated with fifth disease outbreak in the local school system.
Serum sickness	May mimic SLE, with fever, rash, and complement consumption.
Thrombotic thrombocytopenic purpura (see Chapter 45)	May mimic SLE, with fever, CNS changes, thrombocytopenia, and kidney failure. Finding schistocytes on peripheral smear is a major clue.
Malignancy	May be associated with positive ANA, anemia, high ESR, polyarthritis, pleural effusions, fever, and other symptoms.
HIV/AIDS (see Chapter 54)	Can lead to production of antiphospholipid antibodies, a positive Coombs test, and thrombocytopenia. Some patients with SLE will have false-positive results for HIV infection on ELISA; confirmation on Western blot is essential.

ANA = antinuclear antibody; ANCA = antinuclear cytoplasmic antibody; CNS = central nervous system; ELISA = enzyme-linked immunosorbent assay; ESR = erythrocyte sedimentation rate.

proliferative glomerulonephritis. Class III, class IV, and class V lupus nephritis are associated with deteriorating kidney function and focal (III) or diffuse (IV) proliferative nephritis or membranous (V) nephritis. Class VI disease (advanced sclerosing lupus nephritis) is associated with irreversible kidney damage.

- ANA titer ≥1:80 is compatible with SLE. Immunofluorescence pattern is no longer used in the diagnosis of SLE, because specific antibodies correlate with the patterns, allowing more precise identification.
- Immunologic findings include anti–double-stranded DNA (anti-dsDNA) and anti-Smith (anti-Sm) antibodies, which are very specific but insensitive for the diagnosis of SLE. Other immunologic findings are antiphospholipid antibody (which may be detected by a positive test for lupus anticoagulant), a false-positive rapid plasma reagin or VDRL test, or anticardiolipin antibody. The presence of any one of these findings fulfills the immunologic criterion.
- Neurologic syndromes that fulfill the diagnostic criteria are limited to seizure and psychosis. However, SLE is associated with various neurologic and psychiatric manifestations, including cerebritis, cranial and peripheral neuropathies, transverse myelitis, mood disorders (e.g., depression), and acute confusional state.
- Malar rash (butterfly rash) is a photosensitive maculopapular or erythematous rash that usually involves the cheeks and the bridge of the nose but spares the nasolabial folds (Plate 33).
- Discoid lesions occur as slowly progressive, scaly, infiltrative papules and plaques or atrophic red plaques on sun-exposed skin surfaces. Other lesions may be hypertrophic or verrucous

and may leave scars after healing (Plate 34). Many patients have discoid lesions without systemic manifestations (termed *discoid lupus*) and negative or low ANA titers. These patients have an increased risk of developing SLE, which usually is heralded by the presence of a positive ANA (titer ≥1:80).

In addition, nonspecific constitutional features of SLE—some of which dominate the clinical picture—include fatigue, fever, and weight loss. SLE also is associated with Raynaud phenomenon, which is characterized by the fingers or toes becoming white then blue when cold and then red when warmed (Plate 68), and by keratoconjunctivitis sicca (or sicca) symptoms seen in Sjögren syndrome, which causes dry mucous membranes (mouth, nose, eyes, vagina).

Physical Examination and Laboratory Studies

A patient suspected of having SLE requires a thorough physical examination to identify specific organ involvement, with emphasis on the diagnostic criteria. Nonspecific findings (e.g., fever, tachycardia, lymphadenopathy) are common but must not automatically be attributed to SLE. The most common cause of fever in SLE is infection, which may result from chronic immunosuppression caused by the disease or medications used to treat the disease. Closely inspect nasal and oral mucous membranes for painless ulcers. Dentures should be removed to inspect the hard palate. Discoid rashes commonly occur on the external ear, forearm, and scalp; scalp lesions may cause alopecia. Funduscopic examination may reveal grayish white fluffy exudates (cytoid bodies or cotton-wool spots) indicating focal retinal infarctions. Pleuritis or pericarditis may be detected by auscultating a friction rub or by identifying signs of a pleural effusion. Hepatosplenomegaly may be seen in SLE. Intestinal perforation (resulting from corticosteroids, vasculitis, or infection) must also be considered as a cause of abdominal pain. On musculoskeletal examination, patients may have joint tenderness or synovitis. Neurologic deficits, seizures, or confusion may indicate central nervous system infection, ischemia, or brain or spinal cord inflammation (cerebritis or transverse myelitis) or the more subtle neuropsychiatric manifestations of SLE. Sensory or motor symptoms may be due to peripheral neuropathy, muscle inflammation, or ischemia caused by vasculitis.

In active SLE, the circulating immune complexes activate complement, causing their consumption and resulting in a decrease of C3, C4, and total hemolytic complement (CH50 or CH100). Serial C3 and C4 or CH50, or CH100 measurements may help determine whether SLE is becoming more active or is responding to therapy. In addition, the level of anti-dsDNA antibody may reflect disease activity, with higher levels corresponding to more active disease.

Therapy

Patient education is fundamental to the management of SLE and is directed toward understanding the disease and its treatment. Patients should try to avoid stress and UV radiation (e.g., sun exposure) and strive to maintain good nutrition. To minimize the risk of SLE exacerbation by solar radiation, patients should use sunscreen with an SPF of 15 or higher and wear a hat and protective clothing to cover as much skin as possible. Patients with SLE are at increased risk for premature atherosclerosis and corticosteroid-induced osteoporosis. To help reduce these risks, patients should eat a balanced diet low in saturated fats, exercise regularly, take calcium and vitamin D supplements, and avoid cigarettes. It was previously thought that oral contraceptives or pregnancy always caused SLE flares. However, recent data have contradicted this belief, and oral contraceptives and pregnancy now are considered acceptable for most patients.

Drug therapy for SLE depends on the manifestations in a particular patient. Arthralgia, arthritis, myalgia, fever, and mild serositis may improve with NSAIDs or hydroxychloroquine. Hydroxychloroquine may be continued indefinitely to prevent disease reactivation, even if the disease has been quiescent for many years, and is associated with decreased mortality. Methotrexate or, occasionally, low-dose corticosteroids may be necessary if a patient fails to respond to initial therapies or the initial manifestations are more severe.

Photosensitive rashes can be treated conservatively with a sunscreen that blocks UVA and UVB radiation, hydroxychloroquine, and topical corticosteroids. Intralesional corticosteroids may be helpful to treat discoid lupus erythematosus until hydroxychloroquine therapy becomes effective.

High-dose corticosteroids or pulse doses (high doses over a short period of time) of methylprednisone and other immunosuppressive agents (e.g., cyclophosphamide, mycophenolate mofetil, azathioprine) are used for the more severe manifestations of SLE, including nephritis, cerebritis, vasculitis, and life-threatening hematologic abnormalities.

Prior to or at the time of initiation of systemic corticosteroids or immunosuppressants, a tuberculin skin test or a *Mycobacterium tuberculosis* interferon-γ release assay must be performed to establish whether the patient is at risk for reactivation of latent tuberculosis. Because patients with SLE may have functional asplenia, vaccination against pneumococcal illness, *Haemophilus influenza* infection, influenza, and, possibly, meningococcal infection is indicated.

Follow-Up

Recent data indicate 80% to 90% survival rates for patients with SLE 10 years after diagnosis; 3 decades ago, the mortality rate was 50% 2 years after diagnosis. Early deaths are seen in patients with active disease and in patients who require high doses of corticosteroids and intense immunosuppression, whereas later deaths often are due to cardiovascular disease. Although SLE is not curable, extended periods of remission with no clinical activity frequently occur.

Patients need regular follow-up to detect disease flares. A complete blood count, serum creatinine level, C3 and C4 measurement, and urinalysis with culture and sensitivity should be performed at routine follow-up visits to screen for anemia, leukopenia, thrombocytopenia, and evidence of nephritis. Lifestyle modifications and pharmacologic therapies to reduce cardiovascular risk factors must be instituted, because cardiovascular disease is a major cause of death in patients with SLE.

Book Enhancement

Go to www.acponline.org/essentials/rheumatology-section.html. In *MKSAP for Students 5*, assess your knowledge with items 27-30 in the **Rheumatology** section.

Acknowledgment

We would like to thank Dr. Nicole Cotter, who contributed to an earlier version of this chapter.

Bibliography

Crow MK. Developments in the clinical understanding of lupus. Arthritis Res Ther. 2009;11:245. [PMID: 19849817]

Chapter 96

Other Rheumatologic Conditions

Kevin M. McKown, MD

Polymyositis and Dermatomyositis

Polymyositis and dermatomyositis are autoimmune inflammatory disorders that affect muscle and other tissues and typically present as subacute-onset, symmetric proximal weakness. Polymyositis and dermatomyositis are associated with significant morbidity and mortality and always need to be considered in a patient with proximal weakness. Other causes of proximal weakness also must be considered, especially medications (Table 1).

The cause of polymyositis and dermatomyositis is unknown, but the disorders are thought to be triggered by environmental factors (e.g., viral infection) in genetically susceptible individuals. Dermatomyositis (less frequently polymyositis) also may occur as a paraneoplastic phenomenon. There is evidence that at least some myositis-specific autoantibodies may play a role in disease pathogenesis. Involved muscles demonstrate muscle fiber necrosis, regeneration, and inflammatory infiltrates; however, histopathologic differences between polymyositis and dermatomyositis are thought to reflect differences in the pathophysiology of these disorders. The lymphocytic infiltration in polymyositis is predominantly composed of CD8 T cells within muscle fascicles. In dermatomyositis, inflammation occurs predominantly around the muscle fascicles and in the interfascicular and perivascular areas. In dermatomyositis, the terminal C5b-9 membrane attack complex can be found in vessel walls, and muscle damage may be due to infarction of small blood vessels supplying the muscle.

Diagnosis

Proximal weakness is suggested by difficulty rising from a chair, walking, and raising the arms or head. Pharyngeal and respiratory involvement is associated with higher mortality and is suggested by difficulty swallowing, nasal regurgitation, and dyspnea. Signs and symptoms suggesting peripheral nerve, spinal cord, or brain disorders rather than muscle disease include dysesthesia, numbness, tremor, stiffness, focal or asymmetric neurologic findings, or distal weakness.

Look for weakness raising the arms against resistance or rising from a chair, along with relative sparing of distal strength (e.g., grip strength). Oculomotor muscles are spared, sensation and reflexes are normal, and significant muscle tenderness is unusual, as is muscle atrophy. Look for scaly, purplish papules and plaques located on the extensor surfaces of the metacarpophalangeal and interphalangeal joints (Plate 69, Gottron papules) and an edematous, heliotrope (dusky purple) discoloration of the upper eyelids and periorbital tissues; both of these rashes are diagnostic for dermatomyositis (Plate 70). Patients also may have an erythematous rash in a V-shaped area over the lower neck and upper chest (V-sign) or over the upper back, back of the next, and shoulders (shawl sign). A pertinent hand finding is rough, cracked, dirty-appearing skin on the lateral surfaces and tips of the fingers (mechanic's hands).

Serum creatine kinase (CK), aldolase, and aspartate aminotransferase usually are elevated to at least twice the normal levels.

Table 1. Differential Diagnosis of Polymyositis and Dermatomyositis

Disorder	Notes
Hypothyroidism (see Chapter 12)	Can cause weakness, stiffness, and elevated CK level. Screen with serum TSH measurement.
Diabetes mellitus (see Chapter 9)	Can cause fatigue and generalized muscle weakness. Diabetes causes neuropathies and plexopathies.
Drug- and alcohol-induced muscle disease	Can cause weakness, pain, and elevated CK level. Consider statins, fibric acid derivatives, and organophosphate poisoning.
Inclusion body myositis	Causes asymmetric proximal and distal weakness; more common than polymyositis in older people; does not respond well to corticosteroids and immunosuppressants. Biopsy is essential to make the diagnosis.
Infections	Viruses often cause pain and may cause frank myositis. HIV can cause myositis. Consider bacterial infection, trichinosis, and other parasitic infections.
SLE, systemic sclerosis, Sjögren syndrome, amyloidosis, vasculitis, rheumatoid arthritis	May mimic myositis, have an element of myositis, or coexist independently of polymyositis.
Critical illness neuromyopathy	Profound generalized weakness following prolonged therapeutic paralysis in an intensive care unit; caused by a combination of muscle and nerve dysfunction.
Rhabdomyolysis	Acute muscle necrosis with myoglobinuria leading to acute kidney injury; caused by drugs, alcohol, trauma, seizures, and muscle disease. CK level usually is >10,000 U/L.

CK = creatine kinase; SLE = systemic lupus erythematosus; TSH = thyroid-stimulating hormone.

Table 2. Laboratory and Other Studies for Polymyositis and Dermatomyositis

Test	Notes
Creatine kinase (CK)	Elevated CK level is one of the diagnostic criteria; levels are 10 to 50 times normal. Myocardial muscle isoforms may be elevated. Exclude hypothyroidism, alcohol, medications, exercise, cardiac disorders, and muscular dystrophy as alternative causes for an elevated CK level.
Aldolase, aspartate aminotransferase (AST), alanine aminotransferase (ALT), lactate dehydrogenase (LDH)	AST, ALT, and LDH may be elevated in muscle disease but proportionately less than CK. Elevated AST, ALT, and LDH levels may mistakenly suggest liver dysfunction.
Electromyography	One of the diagnostic criteria. It supports the diagnosis of a muscle disorder or, alternatively, a neuropathic or spinal cord disorder.
Anti-Jo-1 antibody	Anti-Jo-1 antibody is present in 20%-25% of adult patients and is associated with higher likelihood of interstitial lung disease and higher mortality rates. The "antisynthetase syndrome" consists of acute onset of dermatomyositis or polymyositis with fever, rash, Raynaud phenomenon, arthritis, and interstitial lung disease.
Anti-Mi-2 antibody	Anti-Mi-2 antibody is present in 5%-10% of patients and is associated with good response to therapy. Seen in dermatomyositis in association with V-sign and shawl sign.
Antinuclear antibody (ANA) and rheumatoid factor (RF)	ANA and RF are positive in a fraction of patients with polymyositis but have no predictive value.
Muscle MRI	MRI helps to localize inflammation and to indicate a biopsy site and may be corroborative when the diagnosis cannot be confirmed by other criteria. Conversely, a negative MRI of a weak muscle makes polymyositis unlikely.
Muscle biopsy	A positive muscle biopsy is the definitive criterion for inflammation.
Chest radiography	Interstitial lung disease may be present before, at, or long after the onset of muscle disease and can follow a variable course.
Pulmonary function studies	In polymyositis and dermatomyositis, respiratory dysfunction can be caused by respiratory muscle weakness or, more often, by interstitial lung disease.

Other causes of elevated CK levels need to be considered, including drugs (e.g., statins) and hypothyroidism. Obtain a muscle biopsy in all patients with unexplained proximal muscle weakness and an elevated CK level.

Biopsy is the most definitive test to classify a myopathy as polymyositis, muscular dystrophy, inclusion body myositis, or another less common disease. Inflammatory infiltrates of lymphocytes invading nonnecrotic muscle cells (or interstitial and perivascular areas) will be seen in about 80% of cases of polymyositis or dermatomyositis. A clinically weak muscle that has not been damaged by electromyography should be chosen for biopsy. MRI is sometimes used to select the biopsy site, as muscle involvement can be patchy. Sometimes MRI or electromyographic studies are done to provide further evidence of a myopathy, especially if a biopsy cannot be obtained or the results are nondiagnostic. Electromyographic and nerve conduction velocity studies can suggest a myopathic process and can help identify neuropathic conditions. Myositis-specific autoantibodies may help predict manifestations (e.g., interstitial lung disease) as well as responsiveness to therapy and mortality (Table 2).

Interstitial lung disease, cardiomyopathy, arthritis, and photosensitive rashes are associated with polymyositis and dermatomyositis. Malignancies are increased in adults with dermatomyositis and in adults aged >45 years with polymyositis. The most commonly associated malignancies are adenocarcinomas of the cervix, lung, ovary, pancreas, bladder, and stomach. Patients from Southeast Asia also have an increased risk of nasopharyngeal carcinoma; the increased risk of malignancy extends from 2 years before to 2 years after the onset of myopathy. Many experts recommend upper and lower endoscopy and chest, abdominal, and pelvic imaging studies in these high-risk patients. For other patients, obtain age- and gender-appropriate cancer screening tests.

Therapy

Therapy consists of prednisone and immunosuppressive agents. Prednisone typically is started at doses of 1 mg/kg/day and is tapered as the patient responds. Methotrexate or azathioprine is used with prednisone to improve the response rate and to act as a corticosteroid-sparing agent.

Follow-Up

Monitor serum CK level and muscle strength to assess response to treatment. Monitor treatment-induced toxicities with serial complete blood counts and aminotransferase and blood glucose measurements. Corticosteroid-induced myopathy can occur during treatment and should be suspected when a patient on a moderate to high corticosteroid dose develops worsening proximal muscle weakness in the presence of a normal or minimally elevated CK level. Patients on high-dose or long-term corticosteroids need to be observed for infection and treated with a bisphosphonate, calcium, and vitamin D. Patients also need to be monitored for the development of cardiac or pulmonary manifestations, malignancy, and other autoimmune disease.

Systemic Sclerosis

Systemic sclerosis is a disease of unknown cause. The hallmarks of this condition are microangiopathy and fibrosis of the skin and visceral organs. Common pathophysiologic findings include endothelial cell dysfunction, abnormal fibroblast function, and autoantibody production. Systemic sclerosis most commonly affects women and has a peak initial presentation in the third to fourth decade of life.

Classification

Systemic sclerosis is classified according to the extent and pattern of skin involvement. Limited cutaneous systemic sclerosis (lcSSc) is characterized by skin thickening distal to the elbows or knees but can also involve the face and neck. A subset of this condition is the CREST syndrome (calcinosis, Raynaud phenomenon, esophageal dysmotility, sclerodactyly, and telangiectasia). Diffuse cutaneous systemic sclerosis (dcSSc) is characterized by skin thickening proximal to the elbows and/or knees. Pulmonary arterial hypertension is the major cause of disease-related mortality associated with lcSSc. Interstitial lung disease and kidney disease are the major causes of disease-related mortality associated with dcSSc.

Diagnosis

The diagnosis of systemic sclerosis is established in patients with sclerodermatous skin changes (tightness, thickening, and non-pitting induration) and sclerodactyly (sclerodermatous skin changes limited to the fingers and toes). In the absence of these findings, the diagnosis of systemic sclerosis may be established in patients with two of the following features: sclerodactyly, digital pitting (soft-tissue defects and scarring in the pulp space of the distal phalanges), or basilar fibrosis visible on chest radiography (Table 3).

Antinuclear antibody (ANA) is present in >95% of patients with systemic sclerosis; a centromere pattern is associated with lcSSc and with a lower incidence of interstitial lung disease. The presence of anti-topoisomerase I (anti-Scl-70) antibody is associated with dcSSc and with an increased risk interstitial lung disease (Table 4).

Early physical findings include puffiness or swelling in the hands and fingers. Later findings include hypo- or hyperpigmentation, telangiectases, and subcutaneous calcinosis. Raynaud phenomenon due to arterial vasospasm is the initial clinical manifestation in 70% of patients and eventually occurs in >95%. Episodes of Raynaud phenomenon usually are triggered by cold exposure. Look for sequelae of Raynaud phenomenon, such as digital pitting, ulceration, and gangrene (Plate 71). Inflammatory arthritis and inflammatory myositis are uncommon.

At least 80% of patients have esophageal dysfunction. Smooth muscle dysfunction results in dysphagia, and decreased lower esophageal sphincter pressure causes gastroesophageal reflux disease (GERD). Mucosal telangiectases in the stomach may cause significant blood loss. Small- and large-bowel involvement may cause a functional ileus that manifests as symptoms of bowel obstruction. Bacterial overgrowth due to dysmotility may cause chronic diarrhea, alternating diarrhea and constipation, and/or malabsorption. Patients with lcSSc also may develop biliary cirrhosis.

Scleroderma renal crisis is a life-threatening condition characterized by the acute onset of hypertension, kidney failure, and microangiopathic hemolytic anemia. Scleroderma renal crisis usually is seen with dcSSC and may be precipitated by corticosteroid therapy. Cardiac disease in patients with systemic sclerosis may be clinically silent or manifest as cardiomyopathy, pericarditis, or arrhythmias.

Therapy

Treatment of systemic sclerosis is directed at disease manifestations. No therapy has been shown to modify the underlying disease process. There is no clearly effective treatment for skin thickening. Raynaud phenomenon is best treated by avoiding cold exposure. Pharmacologic therapy for Raynaud phenomenon starts with the use of vasodilators, such as dihydropyridine calcium channel blockers. Antiplatelet agents, such as aspirin and dipyridamole, also are used. The phosphodiesterase type 5 inhibitor sildenafil reduces the development of digital ulcers. In patients with severe, refractory Raynaud phenomenon, surgical revascularization, sympathetic nerve blockade or sympathectomy, prostacyclin analogues, or endothelin antagonists may be used.

Gastric acid suppression with proton pump inhibitors is indicated for nearly all patients with systemic sclerosis, as most will

Table 3. Differential Diagnosis of Systemic Sclerosis

Disorder	Notes
Primary Raynaud disease	Patients have cold-induced vasospasm without an associated underlying disease. ANA test is negative.
Systemic lupus erythematosus (see Chapter 95)	Among other disease characteristics, patients have fatigue, arthralgia, and a positive ANA test.
Inflammatory myopathy	Patients have proximal muscle weakness caused by muscle inflammation, elevated muscle enzymes (creatine kinase, aldolase), abnormal electromyography results, and a positive ANA test.
Eosinophilic fasciitis	Eosinophilic fasciitis causes woody induration of the skin with thickening of the fascia, often with associated peripheral eosinophilia; the hands and feet typically are spared. Internal organs are not affected, Raynaud phenomenon is absent, and ANA test is negative. Full-thickness skin-to-muscle biopsy is helpful in making the diagnosis.
Generalized morphea	Confluence of plaques of morphea (localized scleroderma), with sparing of the hands and feet. Internal organs are not affected, and Raynaud phenomenon is absent. ANA test may be positive.
Idiopathic pulmonary fibrosis (see Chapter 86)	Patients have restrictive lung disease with pathologic changes identical to those seen in systemic sclerosis. However, Raynaud phenomenon, gastrointestinal and musculoskeletal symptoms, and systemic sclerosis–specific autoantibodies are absent.
Nephrogenic systemic fibrosis	Brawny hyperpigmentation, papular lesions; occurs in patients with chronic kidney disease exposed to gadolinium-containing contrast agents used for MRI procedures.

Table 4. Laboratory and Other Studies for Systemic Sclerosis

Test	Notes
Antinuclear antibody (ANA)	ANA is present in >95% of patients with systemic sclerosis.
ANA, centromere pattern	Typically associated with lcSSc. Patients tend to have a reduced frequency of pulmonary, renal, and cardiac involvement.
Anti-Scl-70 (anti-topoisomerase I) antibody	Most commonly seen in patients with dcSSc. Associated with interstitial lung disease.
Blood urea nitrogen, serum creatinine	Used to monitor kidney function, particularly in patients with dcSSc. Patients with dcSSc are at risk for scleroderma renal crisis.
Complete blood count with peripheral smear	Scleroderma renal crisis (a microangiopathic process) is associated with anemia, schistocytes on peripheral blood smear, and thrombocytopenia.
Chest radiography	Chest radiographs may reveal basilar pulmonary fibrosis.
Pulmonary function tests	Reduced forced vital capacity occurs in interstitial lung disease. Reduced diffusion capacity occurs in both interstitial lung disease and pulmonary hypertension. An isolated reduction of diffusion capacity may be indicative of pulmonary hypertension.
Doppler echocardiography	A noninvasive method to evaluate for pulmonary hypertension.
Nailfold capillaroscopy	Wide-field magnification of the nailfold capillaries shows characteristic changes in patients with systemic sclerosis. This procedure should be performed by a specialist trained in its use.

dcSSc = diffuse cutaneous systemic sclerosis; lcSSc= limited cutaneous systemic sclerosis.

have symptomatic GERD. Extended courses of antibiotics are useful in patients with bowel overgrowth. Scleroderma renal crisis is a medical emergency, and patients should be admitted to the hospital immediately for aggressive blood pressure control with ACE inhibitors. These agents should be continued even in patients with significant renal insufficiency, because kidney function may improve even after months of dialysis.

Cyclophosphamide may improve pulmonary symptoms in patients with interstitial lung disease and has been shown to modestly improve lung function in this setting. Treatment for isolated pulmonary arterial hypertension is vasodilation (e.g., sildenafil, bosentan, epoprostenol) and, if needed, oxygen.

Follow-Up

Screen patients for end-organ involvement, including interstitial lung disease, pulmonary arterial hypertension, and chronic kidney failure. Judicious follow-up can aid in detecting internal organ involvement at an early stage.

Sjögren Syndrome

Sjögren syndrome is a chronic autoimmune inflammatory disorder associated with mononuclear cell infiltration of the exocrine glands, with resultant decreased lacrimal and salivary gland function. There is a 9:1 female predominance, and onset typically is in mid life. Although Sjögren syndrome may be a primary disorder, it commonly occurs secondary to another autoimmune disease. Secondary Sjögren syndrome can be seen in association with rheumatoid arthritis, systemic lupus erythematosus, systemic sclerosis, inflammatory myopathy, autoimmune liver disease, and autoimmune thyroid disease.

Diagnosis

The combination of the sicca complex (i.e., dry eyes [xerophthalmia] and dry mouth [xerostomia]), an abnormal Schirmer test (confirming dry eyes), and positive anti-Ro/SSA and anti-La/SSB antibodies has both a sensitivity and a specificity of 94% for the diagnosis of primary Sjögren syndrome. Clues to this condition include a patient report of a dry, gritty feeling in the eyes or use of eye drops multiple times daily. Patients with dry mouth typically awaken at night to drink water and often keep water at their bedside.

Look for red sclerae, a decreased salivary pool, periodontal disease, dental caries, and parotid gland enlargement. Other possible features include an inflammatory polyarthritis, cutaneous vasculitis, interstitial lung disease, interstitial nephritis with associated distal renal tubular acidosis, vasculitis associated with mononeuritis multiplex, and peripheral neuropathy. Pathologic diagnosis of Sjögren syndrome can be confirmed if biopsy specimens of a labial salivary gland reveal focal lymphocytic infiltration. Because Sjögren syndrome is associated with B-cell clonal expansion, affected patients have an increased risk for developing lymphoma (5% lifetime risk), which typically involves the salivary glands.

Therapy

Frequent use of lubricant eye drops (artificial tears) is the primary treatment for symptomatic dry eyes. Oral pilocarpine or cevimeline can be helpful for dry mouth symptoms. Aggressive dental prophylaxis can reduce the incidence of periodontal disease and dental caries. NSAIDs or hydroxychloroquine may be helpful for arthralgias. Systemic corticosteroid therapy or other immunosuppressants may be warranted in patients with severe extraglandular manifestations of Sjögren syndrome.

Follow-Up

Regularly scheduled follow-up visits are needed to monitor the lymphatic system and to consider biopsy of persistently enlarged parotid or submandibular glands, to look for malignant lymphoproliferation.

Fibromyalgia

Fibromyalgia is characterized by chronic, widespread musculoskeletal pain. Affected patients almost always have fatigue and nonrestorative sleep; they also have an increased prevalence of anxiety and major depression. Fibromyalgia affects women more frequently than men and typically has an onset between the ages of 20 and 50 years. The cause of fibromyalgia is unknown but may be related to central nervous system (CNS) mechanisms, such as dysregulation of neurotransmitter function and central pain sensitization.

Diagnosis

Patients with fibromyalgia demonstrate widespread tenderness, but the number of tender points may vary from day to day. The location of tender points is arbitrary, as patients typically are tender elsewhere, and expert opinion holds that the presence of specific tender points is not essential in the diagnosis of fibromyalgia. Table 5 summarizes a differential diagnosis of fibromyalgia. Fibromyalgia can occur in association with autoimmune disorders, such as rheumatoid arthritis, systemic lupus erythematosus, and Sjögren syndrome. Laboratory studies are useful only in excluding conditions that may mimic fibromyalgia and generally should include a complete blood count and measurement of serum thyroid-stimulating hormone level, erythrocyte sedimentation rate, and alanine and aspartate aminotransferase levels (chronic hepatitis). Routine testing for ANA or rheumatoid factor is not indicated and may be confusing, as these tests often are abnormal in normal individuals.

Therapy

Patient education and nonpharmacologic interventions form the cornerstone of therapy. Educating patients with fibromyalgia about the nature and course of the disease is imperative. Regular low-impact aerobic exercise, such as walking and water aerobics, has demonstrated effectiveness. Cognitive behavioral therapy has been shown to be beneficial. Tricyclic antidepressants are the most-studied pharmacologic agents in the treatment of fibromyalgia. Pregabalin, which disrupts neuronal signaling in the CNS, and the serotonin-norepinephrine reuptake inhibitors duloxetine and milnacipran are approved by the FDA for the treatment of fibromyalgia. All of these agents have been shown to decrease pain and, to various degrees, to improve fatigue, sleep, depression, and quality of life compared with placebo. NSAIDs may provide some patients additional pain relief when used in combination with these agents. Opioid analgesics and corticosteroids have no demonstrated efficacy in fibromyalgia.

Follow-Up

Follow-up is important to determine progress, reinforce positive health behavior, and appropriately diagnose a new disease or condition that might have developed since the last visit.

Book Enhancement

Go to www.acponline.org/essentials/rheumatology-section.html. In *MKSAP for Students 5*, assess your knowledge with items 31-34 in the **Rheumatology** section.

Bibliography

Arnold LM, Clauw DJ. Fibromyalgia syndrome: practical strategies for improving diagnosis and patient outcomes. Am J Med. 2010;123:S2. [PMID: 20569735]

Gabrielli A, Avvedimento EV, Krieg T. Scleroderma. N Engl J Med. 2009;360:1989-2003. [PMID: 19420368]

Mammen AL. Dermatomyositis and polymyositis: Clinical presentation, autoantibodies, and pathogenesis. Ann N Y Acad Sci. 2010;1184:134-153. [PMID: 20146695]

Papiris SA, Tsonis IA, Moutsopoulos HM. Sjögren's syndrome. Semin Respir Crit Care Med. 2007;28:459-471. [PMID: 17764063]

Table 5. Differential Diagnosis of Fibromyalgia

Disorder	Notes
Rheumatoid arthritis, osteoarthritis	Patients with arthritis have objective joint swelling. Look for findings related to the specific type of arthritis (e.g., positive rheumatoid factor and bony erosions in rheumatoid arthritis; characteristic crepitation and radiographic findings in osteoarthritis).
Polymyalgia rheumatica	Patients generally are older (>60 y) and have diffuse pain (mostly in hip and shoulder girdles), prominent stiffness, constitutional symptoms (fever, malaise, loss of appetite and weight), and elevated ESR (usually >50 mm/h).
Hypothyroidism (see Chapter 12)	Patients have fatigue, lethargy, muscle stiffness or cramping, constipation, dry skin, delayed relaxation phase of deep tendon reflexes, low T_4, and elevated TSH. Tender points are uncommon in hypothyroidism.
Myopathy	Patients have muscle weakness and fatigue, objective muscle weakness on examination, increased muscle enzymes, and typical muscle biopsy and electromyographic findings.
Ankylosing spondylitis (see Chapter 94)	Patients (most often males) have back pain, decreased mobility of the lumbar spine, characteristic radiographic findings of sacroiliitis, and elevated ESR.
Chronic fatigue syndrome	Patients have severe fatigue, postexertional malaise, musculoskeletal pain, impaired memory or concentration, sore throat, and tender cervical or axillary lymph nodes.

ESR = erythrocyte sedimentation rate; T_4 = thyroxine; TSH = thyroid-stimulating hormone.

Chapter 97

Vasculitis

Patrick C. Alguire, MD

Vasculitis is an inflammation of blood vessels that causes stenosis, obstruction, or attenuation with subsequent tissue ischemia, aneurysm, or hemorrhage. Vasculitis may be secondary to an underlying process or occur as a primary disease of unknown cause. Primary vasculitides may be categorized based on the size of the blood vessel that is predominantly involved (small, medium, or large), the pattern of organ involvement, and the histopathology. Systemic vasculitis often is a diagnosis of exclusion in patients with multisystem disease. Clinical clues often point to the diagnosis, especially if there are signs of skin, kidney, or large-vessel involvement. The diagnosis of vasculitis requires biopsy of an affected site or arteriography (if medium-sized or large vessels are involved).

A vasculitis of particular relevance to general internal medicine is giant cell arteritis (GCA). GCA is relatively common (prevalence of 1.5%) and found almost exclusively in the elderly. The disorder frequently is in the differential diagnosis of perplexing geriatric symptoms; it rarely occurs in those aged <50 years. GCA causes localized inflammation in the smaller branches of the external carotid artery but typically spares the intracranial vessels. Involvement of the ophthalmic artery can cause blindness. Subclinical involvement of the proximal and distal aorta also is common. The release of inflammatory cytokines contributes to the prominent constitutional symptoms of malaise, fever, and weight loss seen with GCA; the disorder often is associated with anemia of inflammation.

Polyarteritis nodosa, a necrotizing vasculitis of the medium-sized arteries, also is particularly relevant to internal medicine. Approximately 50% of cases are associated with hepatitis B virus infection and, less frequently, hepatitis C virus infection.

Diagnosis

Consider a diagnosis of vasculitis in patients with systemic symptoms and single- or multiple-organ dysfunction. Exclude infectious, hematologic, drug-related, and other organ-specific processes that can mimic vasculitis. Ask specifically about previous thrombotic events, cocaine abuse, endocarditis, hepatitis, and HIV infection. Look for recent invasive arterial procedures (e.g., cardiac catheterization), because cholesterol emboli can mimic vasculitis. Use of vasoconstrictive drugs (e.g., phenylpropanolamine, ephedra alkaloids) also can mimic vasculitis (Table 1).

On physical examination, look for the more common features of vasculitis: rashes (Plate 31), nail bed infarcts, or digital tuft ulcers; pulse asymmetry, bruits, or aortic regurgitation; muscle weakness or tenderness; nasal, oral, or genital ulcers; and sinusitis.

Obtain the following tests in all patients with suspected vasculitis: complete blood count, serum creatinine level, aminotransferase levels, and erythrocyte sedimentation rate (ESR) or C-reactive protein (CRP). Obtain a urinalysis and assess for erythrocytes, erythrocyte casts, and mixed cellular casts. Urinalysis is

Table 1. Differential Diagnosis of Vasculitis

Disorder	Notes
Infection (e.g., sepsis, endocarditis, hepatitis)	Heart murmur, rash, and/or musculoskeletal symptoms can occur in bacterial endocarditis or viral hepatitis. Obtain blood cultures, hepatitis B and C serologic studies, and an echocardiogram.
Drug toxicity/poisoning	Cocaine, amphetamines, ephedra alkaloids, and phenylpropanolamine may produce vasospasm, resulting in symptoms of ischemia. Perform a toxicology screen.
Coagulopathy	Occlusive diseases (disseminated intravascular coagulation, antiphospholipid syndrome, thrombotic thrombocytopenic purpura) can produce ischemic symptoms. Perform a coagulation panel, and test for hypercoagulability.
Malignancy	Paraneoplastic vasculitis is rare. Any organ system may be affected, but the skin and nervous system most commonly are involved. Vasculitic symptoms may precede, occur simultaneously with, or follow diagnosis of cancer. Lymphoma occasionally may involve the blood vessels and mimic vasculitis. Consider malignancy in patients with incomplete or no response to therapy for idiopathic vasculitis.
Atrial myxoma	Classic triad of symptoms: embolism, intracardiac obstruction leading to pulmonary congestion or heart failure, and constitutional symptoms (fatigue, weight loss, fever). Skin lesions can be identical to those seen in leukocytoclastic vasculitis. Atrial myxomas are rare, but they are the most common primary intracardiac tumor. Myxomas also can occur in other cardiac chambers.
Multiple cholesterol emboli	Typically seen in patients with severe atherosclerosis. Embolization may occur after abdominal trauma, aortic surgery, or angiography. May also occur after heparin, warfarin, or thrombolytic therapy. Patients may have livedo reticularis, petechiae, purpuric lesions, and localized skin necrosis.

essential, because glomerulonephritis is common in many systemic vasculitides and is clinically silent until uremia develops. In suspected Wegener granulomatosis, the presence of c-ANCA (cytoplasmic antineutrophil cytoplasmic antibody) with enzyme immunoassay specificity for proteinase 3 provides strong support for the diagnosis. In suspected microscopic polyangiitis and Churg-Strauss syndrome, the combination of p-ANCA (perinuclear antineutrophil cytoplasmic antibody) and antibodies to myeloperoxidase is strong circumstantial evidence. Ultimately, it is the clinical pattern of disease and confirmatory biopsy that make the diagnosis of vasculitis (Table 2).

Most patients with GCA present with headache that typically involves the temporal area. Approximately 33% of affected patients have symptoms of polymyalgia rheumatica (PMR) or visual abnormalities. Some of these patients may develop visual loss, which is a medical emergency that requires immediate parenteral corticosteroid therapy. PMR is characterized by aching and morning stiffness in the proximal muscles of the shoulder and hip girdle

and may develop in patients with GCA or as a primary condition. The presence of temporal artery beading, prominence, or enlargement is the most predictive physical finding (positive likelihood ratio >4) for GCA, whereas the presence of synovitis makes the diagnosis much less likely.

GCA is associated with a markedly elevated ESR; an ESR <50 mm/h makes the diagnosis very unlikely (negative likelihood ratio = 0.35). Other common laboratory abnormalities include elevated CRP level, anemia, and thrombocytosis. However, only a temporal artery biopsy specimen showing destruction of the internal elastic lamina, intimal thickening, and inflammatory infiltrates is diagnostic of this condition. Giant cells are present in the inflammatory infiltrate in only 50% of affected patients. Duplex ultrasonography of the temporal artery can reveal a characteristic halo sign in patients with GCA, and positron emission tomography scanning often shows uptake in the thoracic aorta.

Patients with polyarteritis nodosa typically present with fever, abdominal pain, arthralgia, and weight loss that develop over days

Table 2. Categorization and Treatment of Vasculitis

Disorder	Notes
Large-Vessel Vasculitis	
Giant cell (temporal) arteritis	Granulomatous arteritis of the aorta and its major branches; commonly affects the temporal artery. Cardinal symptoms are headache, scalp tenderness, jaw claudication, carotidynia, and fever. Ocular symptoms, including blindness, may occur in 5%-30% of cases. Usually occurs in patients aged >50 y. Treated initially with prednisone 40-60 mg/d.
Takayasu arteritis	Chronic granulomatous inflammatory disease primarily of the aorta and its main branches. Affects women during their reproductive years. Cardinal symptom is claudication associated with pulse deficits, bruits, or asymmetric blood pressures. Treated with prednisone 1 mg/kg; methotrexate is added in resistant cases. Percutaneous transluminal angioplasty is performed for fixed vascular lesions causing ischemia.
Medium-Vessel Vasculitis	
Polyarteritis nodosa	Nongranulomatous necrotizing vasculitis of medium-sized or small arteries, without glomerulonephritis. Key features are kidney disease, hypertension, gastrointestinal pain, peripheral neuropathy, and skin lesions. Vasculitis also can cause testicular pain, cardiac disease, and stroke. May be related to hepatitis B. Treated with corticosteroids and cyclophosphamide for life-threatening disease. If secondary to viral hepatitis, antiviral treatment is indicated.
Small-Vessel Vasculitis	
Wegener granulomatosis	Granulomatous necrotizing inflammation of small to medium-sized vessels. Predilection for the upper and lower respiratory tracts and kidneys. Associated with positive c-ANCA; the antibody-targeted antigen usually is proteinase 3. Treated with corticosteroids and cyclophosphamide. Relapse is common.
Churg-Strauss syndrome	Granulomatous inflammation of small to medium-sized vessels, with key features of asthma and eosinophilia. Pulmonary involvement with transient, patchy, alveolar infiltrates is common. Kidney disease occurs in about 50% of cases. Can be confused with Wegener granulomatosis, which usually lacks asthma. Prednisone 1 mg/kg/d is effective; cyclophosphamide is added for resistant or life-threatening disease.
Microscopic polyangiitis	Nongranulomatous necrotizing inflammation of small vessels, with or without medium-vessel involvement. Commonly affects the lungs and kidneys. Distinguished from polyarteritis nodosa by the presence of pulmonary capillaritis or glomerulonephritis. Can be confused with the pulmonary-renal presentation of Wegener granulomatosis but is distinguished by lack of otolaryngologic features. Initial treatment is combination cyclophosphamide and prednisone 1 mg/kg/d.
Henoch-Schönlein purpura	Vasculitis of small vessels that typically involves the skin, gut, and kidneys (nephritis). Fever and arthralgia/arthritis are common. Gut involvement is less common in adults than in children. Biopsy shows predominantly IgA immune-complex deposition. Often initiated by an upper respiratory infection. Corticosteroids have no proven benefit.
Essential cryoglobulinemic vasculitis	Small-vessel inflammation characterized by the presence of cryoglobulins. Commonly affects the skin and kidneys. Most often due to hepatitis C. Treat hepatitis C; avoid corticosteroids.
Leukocytoclastic vasculitis	Vasculitis of small vessels that most commonly affects the skin (Plate 31). Can result from many conditions, including autoimmune disease (systemic lupus erythematosus, rheumatoid arthritis), infection (especially viral hepatitis), malignancy, and medications. Treatment is based on cause.

c-ANCA = cytoplasmic antineutrophil cytoplasmic antibody.

to months. Two thirds of these patients have mononeuritis multiplex, and one third have hypertension, testicular pain, and skin findings (nodules, ulcers, purpura, livedo reticularis). The kidneys and heart also are commonly affected. Aneurysm formation is common, especially in the mesenteric vessels. Ischemia, not glomerulonephritis, causes kidney disease in patients with polyarteritis nodosa.

Patients with polyarteritis nodosa usually have anemia, leukocytosis, and an elevated ESR. ANCA assays almost always are negative. Diagnosis usually is established with a skin or sural nerve biopsy. A definitive diagnosis also can be made by radiographic imaging of the mesenteric or renal arteries showing aneurysms and stenoses.

Therapy

Drug therapy depends on the specific type of vasculitis and the degree of end-organ involvement. In patients with a strong suspicion for GCA, high-dose prednisone therapy (40 to 60 mg/day) is indicated before biopsy to decrease the risk for visual loss; if biopsy is performed within 4 weeks of initiating this therapy, biopsy results will not be affected. Once the symptoms of GCA have resolved and the ESR has normalized, the corticosteroid dosage can be tapered. In addition, aspirin may lower the risk for cerebral ischemia. GCA recurs in more than 50% of affected patients during the first year. When symptoms recur, the corticosteroid dosage should be increased. Neither methotrexate nor infliximab is an effective corticosteroid-sparing agent for GCA.

Patients with PMR respond rapidly and dramatically to low-dose prednisone (10 to 20 mg/day). Once symptoms have subsided, the prednisone dosage can be tapered; the average patient requires treatment for 1 year. Methotrexate, but not infliximab, is an effective corticosteroid-sparing agent for PMR.

High-dose prednisone therapy (60 to 80 mg/day) is indicated initially to treat polyarteritis nodosa. Patients with severe disease or disease that is not controlled by corticosteroids should also receive cyclophosphamide. Short-term high-dose prednisone therapy accompanied by an antiviral agent (e.g., lamivudine) is indicated in patients with concomitant hepatitis B.

Follow-Up

Arrange follow-up every 1 to 4 weeks for patients with vasculitis to evaluate disease activity and monitor for medication toxicity. Although laboratory studies are not definitive markers of disease activity, most diseases can be monitored with the ESR or CRP level and urinalysis.

Book Enhancement

Go to www.acponline.org/essentials/rheumatology-section.html. In *MKSAP for Students 5*, assess your knowledge with items 35-37 in the **Rheumatology** section.

Bibliography

Smetana GW, Shmerling RH. Does this patient have temporal arteritis? JAMA. 2002;287:92-101. [PMID: 11754714]

Index

M

Color Plates

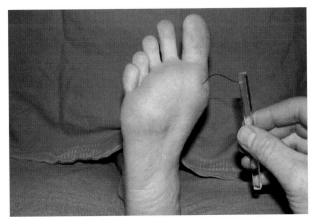

Plate 1   Testing for sensory neuropathy with a 5.07/10-g monofilament.

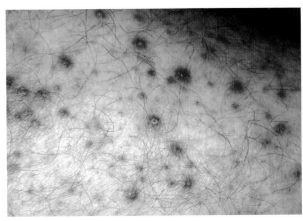

Plate 4   Cellulitis is a rapidly spreading subcutaneous-based infection characterized by a well-demarcated area of warmth, swelling, tenderness, and erythema.

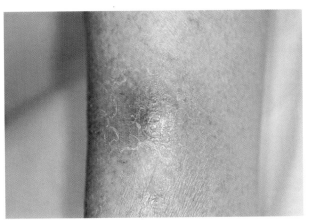

Plate 2   The typical clinical presentation of erythema nodosum is the sudden onset of one or more tender, erythematous nodules on the anterior legs.

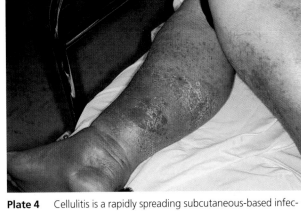

Plate 5   Folliculitis is characterized by pink papules and pustules centered on hair follicles.

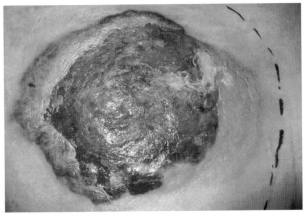

Plate 3   Pyoderma gangrenosum presents as a painful ulcer with a purulent base and undermined, ragged, violaceous borders.

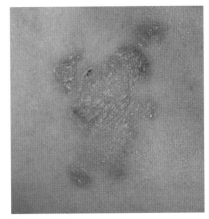

Plate 6   Impetigo is a superficial skin infection characterized by a yellowish, crusted surface. The infection may be caused by staphylococci or streptococci.

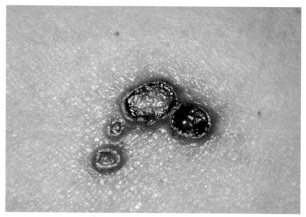

Plate 7 The classic lesions of ecthyma are superficial, saucer-shaped ulcers with overlying crusts.

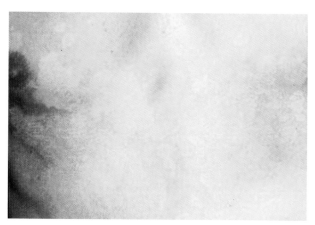

Plate 10 Tinea versicolor is characterized by slightly scaly hyper- or hypopigmented macules on the trunk and upper extremities.

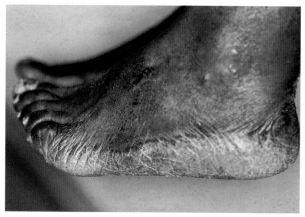

Plate 8 Tinea pedis is characterized by interdigital scaling and maceration or by blisters of the plantar arch, sides of the feet, and/or heel.

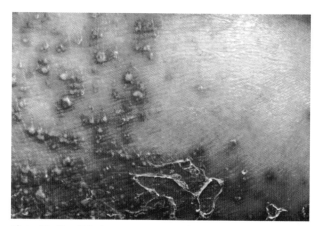

Plate 11 Candidiasis appears as an erythematous rash with scattered satellite papules and pustules.

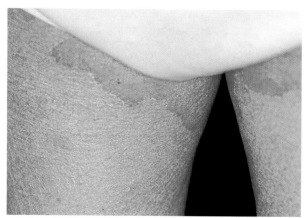

Plate 9 Tinea cruris characteristically presents as an annular lesion with a slight scale, an erythematous advancing edge, and central clearing.

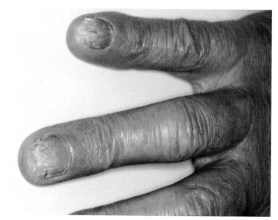

Plate 12 Onychomycosis usually is characterized by a thickened, yellow or white nail with scaling under the elevated distal free edge of the nail plate.

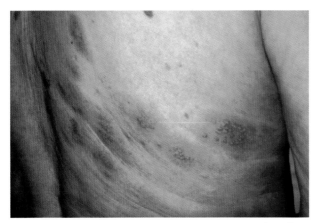

Plate 13 The classic herpes zoster morphology is grouped vesicles on an erythematous base.

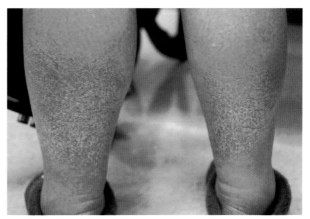

Plate 16 In acute venous stasis dermatitis, the skin is red, warm, and scaly.

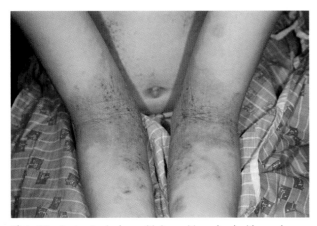

Plate 14 Acute atopic dermatitis is pruritic and red with poorly demarcated, eczematous, crusted, papulovesicular plaques and excoriations.

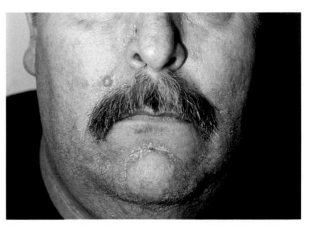

Plate 17 Seborrheic dermatitis is characterized by pink to red skin lesions with greasy scale, crusts, and, occasionally, small pustules.

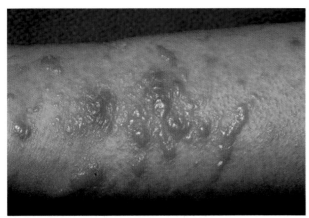

Plate 15 Allergic contact dermatitis usually is intensely pruritic. In acute reactions, the skin is red, edematous, weepy, and crusted, and there may be vesicles or bullae.

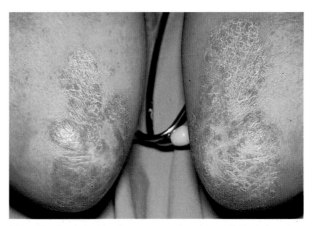

Plate 18 Psoriasis vulgaris appears as sharply marginated plaques with a thick, adherent, silvery scale.

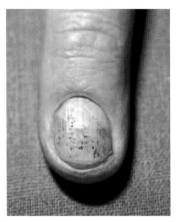

Plate 19   Nail pitting is a classic diagnostic finding associated with psoriasis.

Plate 22   Pityriasis rosea begins as a single thin, pink, oval, 2- to 4-cm plaque with a thin collarette of scale at the periphery; similar lesions subsequently develop.

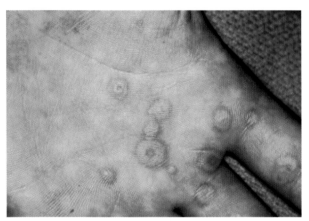

Plate 20   Erythema multiforme lesions range in size from several millimeters to several centimeters and consist of erythematous plaques with concentric rings.

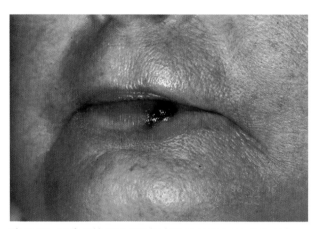

Plate 23   Orofacial herpes simplex lesions appear as a cluster of grouped, painful, pink papules that rapidly become vesicular and typically heal with crusting.

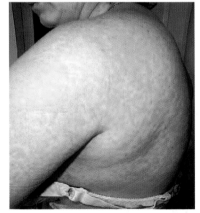

Plate 21   A morbilliform (measles-like) drug eruption consists of symmetrically arranged erythematous macules and papules, some discrete and others confluent.

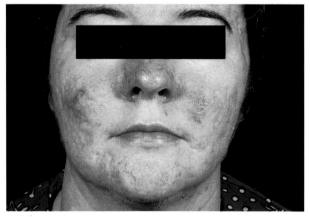

Plate 24   Rosacea is characterized by persistent central facial redness with telangiectasia, pink papules, pustules, and nodules.

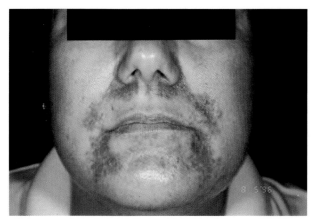

Plate 25 Perioral dermatitis is characterized by discrete papules and pustules on an erythematous base, centered around the mouth.

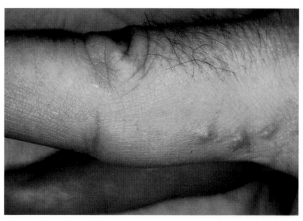

Plate 28 Scabies infestation causes intense pruritus and a papular or vesicular rash.

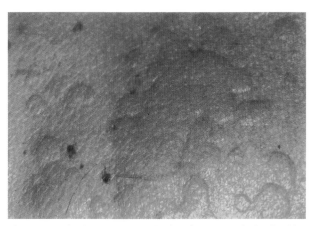

Plate 26 Urticaria presents as episodes of pruritic, red wheals with sharp borders; lesions can last from minutes to hours.

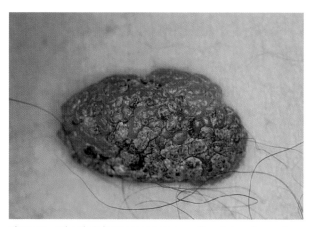

Plate 29 Seborrheic keratoses appear as yellow, tan, or brown to black, well-demarcated papules with a "stuck on" appearance.

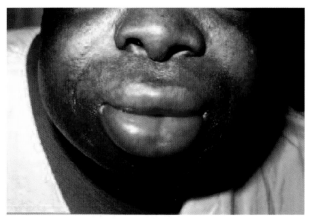

Plate 27 Angioedema, a severe, life-threatening form of urticaria, is characterized by localized edema of the skin or mucosa, usually involving the lips, face, hands, feet, penis, or scrotum.

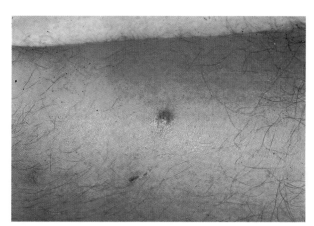

Plate 30 Dermatofibromas are benign skin lesions that appear as firm dermal nodules about the size of a pencil eraser.

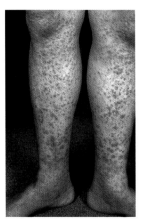

Plate 31 Leukocytoclastic vasculitis is characterized by palpable purpura.

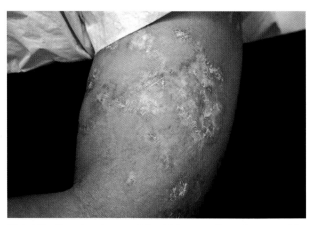

Plate 34 Chronic cutaneous (discoid) lupus erythematosus consists of slowly progressive, scaly infiltrative papules and plaques or atrophic red plaques on sun-exposed skin surfaces.

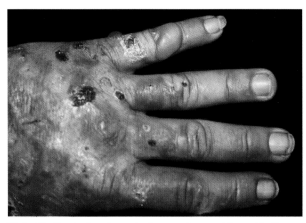

Plate 32 Porphyria cutanea tarda presents as vesicles and bullae on sun-exposed skin surfaces.

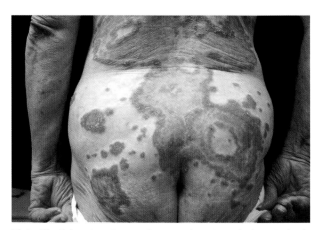

Plate 35 Subacute cutaneous lupus erythematosus is characterized by annular or papulosquamous (psoriasis-like) lesions on sun-exposed skin surfaces.

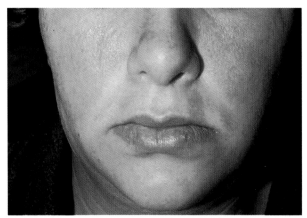

Plate 33 Acute cutaneous lupus erythematosus can present as the classic "butterfly rash," which is characterized by confluent malar erythema.

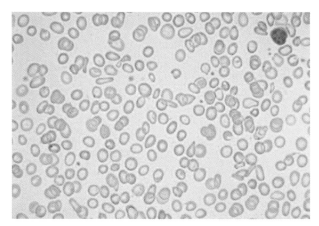

Plate 36 Erythrocyte hypochromia, anisocytosis, and "pencil cells" characteristic of iron deficiency anemia.

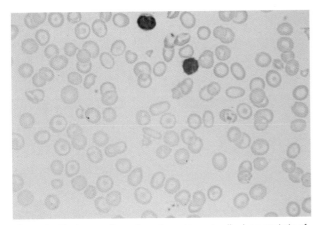

Plate 37 Erythrocyte hypochromia and target cells characteristic of thalassemia trait.

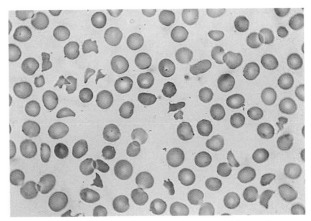

Plate 40 Marked anisocytosis and poikilocytosis with prominent schistocytes.

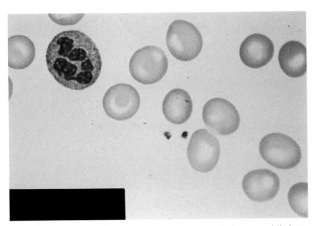

Plate 38 Macro-ovalocytes and a hypersegmented neutrophil characteristic of megaloblastic anemia.

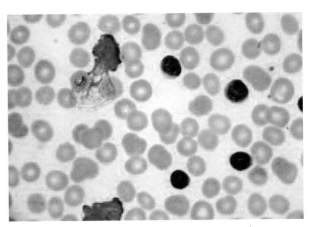

Plate 41 Increased number of mature lymphocytes and two "smudge" cells on peripheral smear (center and bottom) characteristic of chronic lymphocytic leukemia.

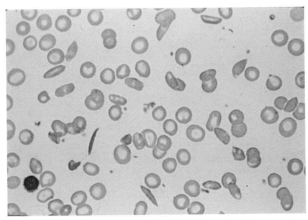

Plate 39 Erythrocyte anisocytosis and poikilocytosis with several sickle cells.

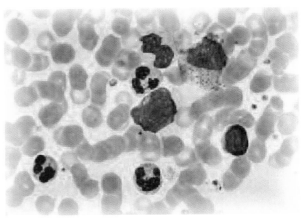

Plate 42 Increased number of granulocytic cells in all phases of development on the peripheral blood smear characteristic of chronic myeloid leukemia.

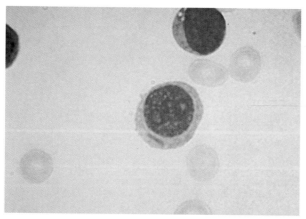

Plate 43 Peripheral blood smear showing an immature granulocyte with a rod-shaped inclusion body (Auer rod) characteristic of acute myeloid leukemia.

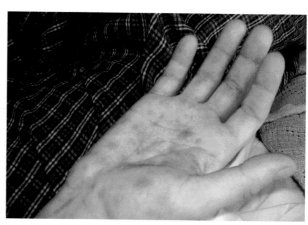

Plate 46 The skin findings of secondary syphilis consist of a generalized mucocutaneous rash (including palms and soles), generalized lymphadenopathy, and constitutional symptoms.

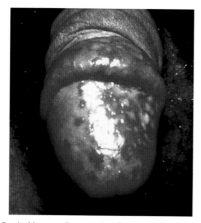

Plate 44 Genital herpes (herpes simplex virus infection) usually presents as a cluster of painful, pink papules that rapidly become vesicular.

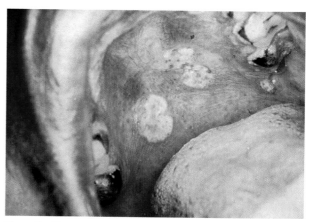

Plate 47 The mucous patches of secondary syphilis appear on mucous membranes and are highly infectious.

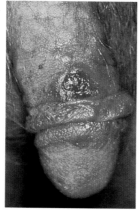

Plate 45 The primary ulcerative lesion (chancre) in syphilis has a clean appearance with heaped-up borders. The lesion usually is painless.

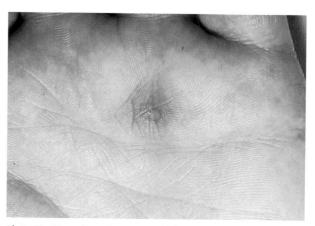

Plate 48 Disseminated gonococcal infection is associated with painless pustular or vesiculopustular skin lesions.

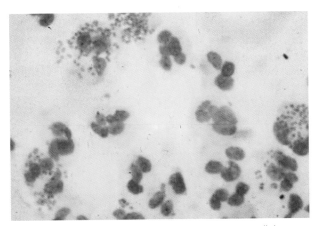

Plate 49 This image demonstrates gram-negative intracellular diplococci, an appearance characteristic of *Neisseria gonorrhoeae.*

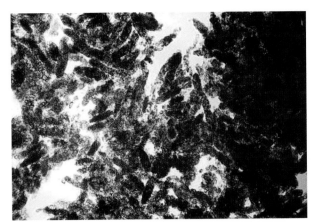

Plate 52 Muddy brown casts indicative of acute tubular necrosis.

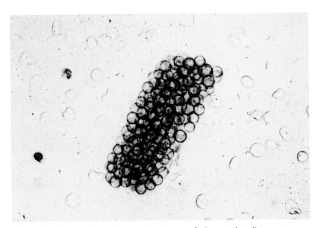

Plate 50 An erythrocyte cast indicative of glomerular disease.

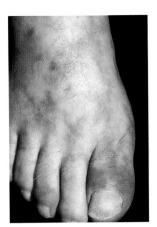

Plate 53 Livedo reticularis is a mottled discoloration of the skin that occurs in a netlike pattern and can be a manifestation of atheroemboli.

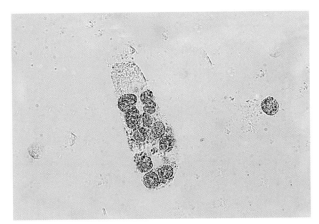

Plate 51 A leukocyte cast indicative of kidney interstitial disease.

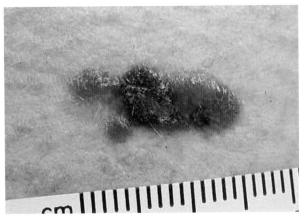

Plate 54 Malignant melanoma with characteristic asymmetric shape, irregular borders, and variegated coloration.

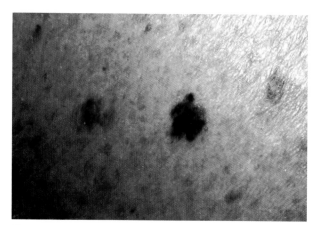

Plate 55 Superficial spreading melanomas typically are >6 mm, with irregular borders and pigmentation.

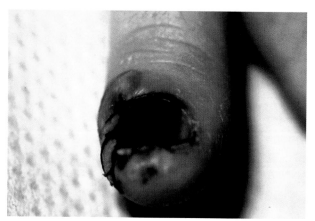

Plate 58 Acral lentiginous melanoma, with pigmentation involving the proximal nail fold and cuticle.

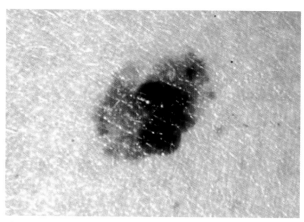

Plate 56 Nodular melanomas often present as uniformly dark blue or black "berry-like" lesions that most commonly originate from normal skin. They can also arise from a preexisting nevus, as did this melanoma. Nodular melanomas expand vertically rather than horizontally.

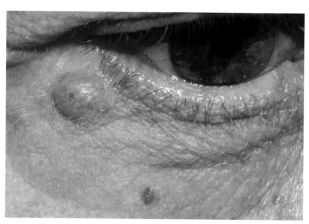

Plate 59 Basal cell carcinomas typically present as pearly papules with telangiectasias.

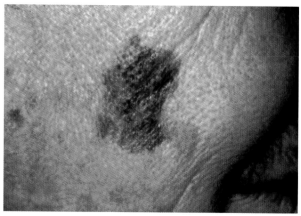

Plate 57 Lentigo maligna melanoma presents as a slowly enlarging, variegated, pigmented patch on sun-damaged skin.

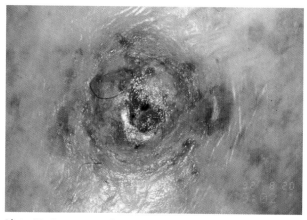

Plate 60 Squamous cell carcinomas present as hyperkeratotic scaly or crater-like lesions.

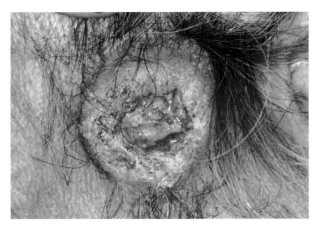

Plate 61 Fully developed keratoacanthoma, with a visible central keratotic plug.

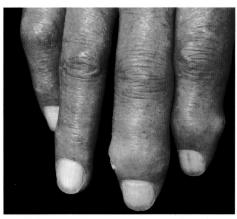

Plate 64 Milky white nodules characteristic of chronic tophaceous gout. Aspiration of the nodules will show sheets of monosodium urate crystals that are negatively birefringent and needle-shaped.

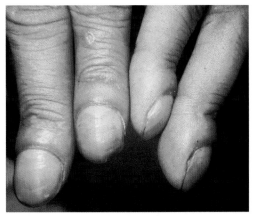

Plate 62 Example of clubbing, a painless enlargement of the connective tissues of the terminal digits. The angle of the nail to the digit is >190 degrees.

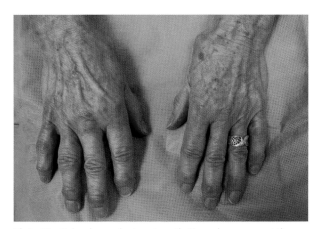

Plate 65 Heberden nodes in osteoarthritis are bony spurs at the dorsolateral and medial aspects of the distal interphalangeal joints.

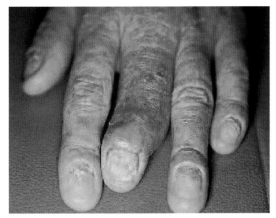

Plate 63 Small-joint polyarthritis with typical psoriatic skin lesions and nail pitting characteristic of psoriatic arthritis.

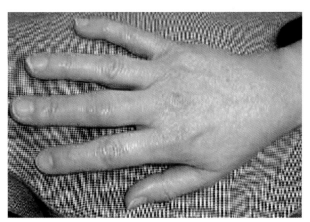

Plate 66 Typical fusiform swelling of the proximal interphalangeal joints with sparing of the distal interphalangeal joints characteristic of rheumatoid arthritis.

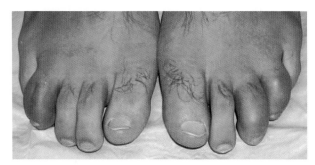

Plate 67 "Sausage digits" (dactylitis) in a patient with reactive arthritis.

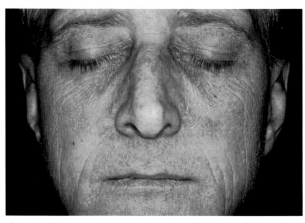

Plate 70 A dusky purple (heliotrope) rash on the eyelids characteristic of dermatomyositis.

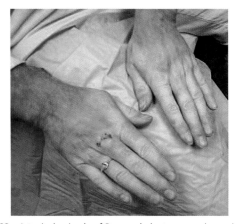

Plate 68 A typical episode of Raynaud phenomenon is precipitated by cold exposure, which is soon followed by distinctive color changes: white (ischemic phase), blue (cyanotic phase), and then red (with rewarming).

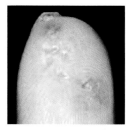

Plate 71 Digital pitting (soft-tissue defects and scarring in the pulp space of the distal phalanges) in a patient with systemic sclerosis.

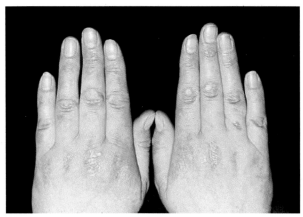

Plate 69 Discrete red plaques over the knuckles and fingers (Gottron papules) characteristic of dermatomyositis.